WO 200

KU-112-631

Vascular Access
Principles and Practice

FIFTH EDITION

Samuel Eric Wilson, MD
Professor of Surgery
Department of Surgery
University of California, Irvine
Irvine, California

Wolters Kluwer | Lippincott Williams & Wilkins
Health

Philadelphia · Baltimore · New York · London
Buenos Aires · Hong Kong · Sydney · Tokyo

Acquisitions Editor: Brian Brown
Product Manager: Ryan Shaw/Erika Kors
Senior Manufacturing Manager: Benjamin Rivera
Marketing Manager: Lisa Parry
Design Coordinator: Holly McLaughlin
Production Service: Spearhead Global, Inc.

Printed in China

Library of Congress Cataloging-in-Publication Data
Vascular access : principles and practice / [edited by] Samuel Eric Wilson. — 5th ed.
    p. ; cm.
  Includes bibliographical references and index.
  ISBN-13: 978-1-60547-203-4
  ISBN-10: 1-60547-203-4
  1. Blood-vessels--Cutdown. I. Wilson, Samuel E., 1941-
  [DNLM: 1. Vascular Surgical Procedures. WG 170 V32758 2010]
  RD598.5.V34 2010
  617.4'13—dc22
                        2009023983

Care has been taken to confirm the accuracy of the information presented and to describe generally accepted practices. However, the authors, editors, and publisher are not responsible for errors or omissions or for any consequences from application of the information in this book and make no warranty, expressed or implied, with respect to the currency, completeness, or accuracy of the contents of the publication. Application of the information in a particular situation remains the professional responsibility of the practitioner.

The authors, editors, and publisher have exerted every effort to ensure that drug selection and dosage set forth in this text are in accordance with current recommendations and practice at the time of publication. However, in view of ongoing research, changes in government regulations, and the constant flow of information relating to drug therapy and drug reactions, the reader is urged to check the package insert for each drug for any change in indications and dosage and for added warnings and precautions. This is particularly important when the recommended agent is a new or infrequently employed drug.

Some drugs and medical devices presented in the publication have Food and Drug Administration (FDA) clearance for limited use in restricted research settings. It is the responsibility of the health care provider to ascertain the FDA status of each drug or device planned for use in their clinical practice.

To purchase additional copies of this book, call our customer service department at (800) 638-3030 or fax orders to (301) 223-2320. International customers should call (301) 223-2300.

Visit Lippincott Williams & Wilkins on the Internet: at LWW.com. Lippincott Williams & Wilkins customer service representatives are available from 8:30 am to 6 pm, EST.

10 9 8 7 6 5 4 3 2 1

Contributors

Michael T. Alkire, MD

Associate Professor of Anesthesiology and Perioperative Care, University of California, Irvine, Irvine, California

Anesthesia for Vascular Access Surgery

Jeffrey L. Ballard, MD, FACS

Clinical Professor of Surgery, University of California, Irvine, Irvine, California; Staff Vascular Surgeon, St Joseph Hospital, Orange, California

Surgical Anatomy for Hemodialysis Access

Cyril H. Barton, MD

Associate Professor of Medicine, University of California, Irvine, Irvine, California

Epidemiology and Pathophysiology of Chronic Renal Failure and Guidelines for Initiation of Hemodialysis

Robert S. Bennion, MD

Professor of Surgery, University of California, Los Angeles (UCLA) School of Medicine; Attending Physician, UCLA Hospitals and Clinics, Los Angeles, California

Socioeconomic Implications of Vascular Access Surgery

Ankit Bharat, MD

Surgical Resident, Washington University School of Medicine; Surgical Resident, Barnes-Jewish Hospital, St Louis, Missouri

Assessment and Intervention for Arteriovenous Fistula Maturation

John A.C. Buckels, CBE, MD

Professor of Hepatobiliary and Transplant Surgery, College of Medicine, University of Birmingham; Consultant Surgeon, Liver Surgery, Queen Elizabeth Hospital, Birmingham, England, United Kingdom

Infection in Vascular Access Procedures

Nikunj K. Chokshi, MD

Surgical Resident, University of Southern California, Los Angeles, California

Access in the Neonatal and Pediatric Patient

Marianne E. Cinat, MD, FACS

Professor of Surgery, University of California, Irvine (UCI), Irvine, California; Director, UCI Regional Burn Center and Director, Surgical Critical Care Fellowship Program, Orange, California

Access in the Neonatal and Pediatric Patient

Patrick S. Collier

Research Associate, Department of Surgery, University of Miami, Miami, Florida

Reflections on Four Decades of Experience in Vascular Access Surgery

Richard Brad Cook, MD

Chief Resident, General Surgery, University of California, Los Angeles, Los Angeles, California

Vascular Access for Trauma, Emergency Surgery, and Critical Care

Peter W. Crooks, MD

Physician Director of Renal Program, Kaiser Permanente Southern California, Los Angeles, California

Organizing Hemodialysis Access: The Kaiser Permanente Southern California Experience

Louis F. D'Amelio, MD, FACS

Associate Clinical Professor of Surgery, New York College of Osteopathic Medicine, Old Westbury, New York; Director of Surgical Services, Capital Health, Trenton, New Jersey

Biologic Properties of Venous Access Devices

Matthew D. Danielson, MD

Chief Resident, Radiology, University of California, Davis, Sacramento, California

Central Venous Cannulation for Hemodialysis Access

Stephen F. Derose, MD, MS

Research Scientist, Research and Evaluation, Kaiser Permanente Southern California, Pasadena, California

Organizing Hemodialysis Access: The Kaiser Permanente Southern California Experience

Larry-Stuart Deutsch, MD, CM, FRCPC, FACR, FSIR

Professor of Vascular and Interventional Radiology, University of California, Davis (UCD); Clinical Operations Director of Interventional Radiology Service, UCD Medical Center, Sacramento, California

Central Venous Cannulation for Hemodialysis Access

Jean T. Diesto, RN, BSN

Director of Renal Program, Kaiser Permanente Southern California, Los Angeles, California

Organizing Hemodialysis Access: The Kaiser Permanente Southern California Experience

Michael Farooq, MD

Staff Vascular Surgeon, Vascular Surgery, Kaiser Permanente Orange County, Anaheim, California

Organizing Hemodialysis Access: The Kaiser Permanente Southern California Experience

Richard L. Feinberg, MD

Assistant Professor of Vascular Surgery, Johns Hopkins University School of Medicine, Baltimore, Maryland; Chief Resident, Vascular Surgery, Howard County General Hospital, Columbia, Maryland

Peritoneal Dialysis

Clarence E. Foster III, MD, FACS

Associate Clinical Professor of Surgery, University of California, Irvine (UCI), Irvine, California; Chief of Transplantation, UCI Medical Center, Orange, California

Basilic Vein Transposition: A Modern Autogenous Vascular Access for Hemodialysis

Julie A. Freischlag, MD

Chair, Department of Surgery, Johns Hopkins Medical Institutions; Surgeon-in-Chief, Department of Surgery, Johns Hopkins Hospital, Baltimore, Maryland

Peritoneal Dialysis

Joseph C. Fuller

Research Assistant, Department of Surgery, University of Miami, Miami, Florida

Reflections on Four Decades of Experience in Vascular Access Surgery

Dmitri V. Gelfand, MD

Clinical Instructor, Vascular Surgery, Stony Brook University; Clinical Instructor, Vascular Surgery, Stony Brook University Medical Center, Stony Brook, New York

Surveillance, Revision, and Outcome of Vascular Access Procedures for Hemodialysis

Sidney M. Glazer, MD

Clinical Associate Professor of Vascular Surgery, University of California, Irvine, Irvine, California; Vascular Surgeon, Kaiser Permanente Orange County, Anaheim, California

Organizing Hemodialysis Access: The Kaiser Permanente Southern California Experience

Marc H. Glickman

Assistant Professor of Vascular Surgery, Eastern Virginia Medical School; Director of Vascular Services, Sentara HealthCare, Norfolk, Virginia

Should the KDOQI Guidelines for First Time Dialysis Access Apply to All Patients?

H. Earl Gordon, MD†

Professor of Surgery, Emeritus, University of California, Los Angeles, School of Medicine; Consultant in General Surgery, VA Greater Los Angeles Healthcare Center, Los Angeles, California

Development of Vascular Access Surgery

Ian L. Gordon, PhD, MD

Associate Clinical Professor of Surgery, University of California, Irvine, College of Medicine, Irvine, California

Physiology of the Arteriovenous Fistula

Ralph S. Greco, MD

Professor of General Surgery, Stanford University, Stanford, California

Biologic Properties of Venous Access Devices

Sukgu Han, MD

Vascular Surgery Research Fellow, University of Southern California Keck School of Medicine, Los Angeles, California

Axillosubclavian Vein Thrombosis

Aladdin Hassanein, MD

Surgical Resident, University of California, San Diego, San Diego, California

Dialysis Access–Associated Ischemic Steal Syndrome; Infection in Vascular Access Procedures

Michael S. Hayashi, MD

Surgical Resident, University of California, Irvine, Irvine, California

Autogenous Vein for Fistulas and Interposition Grafts

Jonathan R. Hiatt, MD

Robert and Kelly Day Professor and Chief of General Surgery, Vice Chair for Education, David Geffen School of Medicine at University of California, Los Angeles, Los Angeles, California

Vascular Access for Trauma, Emergency Surgery, and Critical Care

Victoria E. Holmes, RN, MSN, CNN, CNS

Clinical Nurse Specialist, Nursing Service, Good Samaritan Hospital, Cincinnati, Ohio

Coordination and Patient Care in Vascular Access

Robert J. Hye, MD, FACS

Voluntary Clinical Professor of Surgery, University of California, San Diego; Chief of Vascular Surgery, Kaiser Foundation Hospital, San Diego, California

Complications of Percutaneous Vascular Access Procedures and Their Management

---

†Deceased.

Todd S. Ing, MD

Professor of Medicine, Emeritus, Loyola University of Chicago Stritch School of Medicine, Maywood, Illinois; Courtesy Staff Physician, Hines VA Hospital, Hines, Illinois

Cardiovascular Consequences of Rapid Hemodialysis

James G. Jakowatz, MD

Associate Professor of Surgery, University of California, Irvine, Irvine, California

Placement of Indwelling Venous Access Systems

Juan Carlos Jimenez, MD

Assistant Professor of Vascular Surgery, David Geffen School of Medicine at University of California, Los Angeles (UCLA); Attending Surgeon, Department of Vascular Surgery, Ronald Reagan–UCLA Medical Center, Los Angeles, California

Socioeconomic Implications of Vascular Access Surgery

Ashish Kalthia, MD

Assistant Clinical Professor of Medicine, University of California, Irvine (UCI), Irvine, California; Assistant Clinical Professor, Division of Nephrology and Hypertension, UCI Medical Center, Orange, California

Epidemiology and Pathophysiology of Chronic Renal Failure and Guidelines for Initiation of Hemodialysis

Khushboo Kaushal, BS

Student, University of California, San Diego School of Medicine, La Jolla, California; Research Associate, Department of Surgery, Long Beach VA Medical Center, Long Beach, California

Thrombophilia as a Cause of Recurrent Vascular Access Thrombosis in Hemodialysis Patients; Biologic Response to Prosthetic Dialysis Grafts; New Synthetic Grafts and Early Access

Thomas B. Kinney, MD, MSME

Professor of Clinical Radiology, University of California, San Diego; Interventional Radiologist, University of California, San Diego, Medical Center, San Diego, California

Complications of Percutaneous Vascular Access Procedures and Their Management

Ted R. Kohler, MD

Professor of Surgery, University of Washington; Chief of Vascular Surgery, VA Puget Sound Health Care System, Seattle, Washington

Strategies to Reduce Intimal Hyperplasia in Dialysis Access Grafts

Orly F. Kohn, MD, FACP

Associate Professor of Medicine, The University of Chicago; Medical Director, Home Dialysis Unit, The University of Chicago Medical Center, Chicago, Illinois

Cardiovascular Consequences of Rapid Hemodialysis

Eric D. Ladenheim, MD, MBA

Medical Director, Dialysis Access Research Center; Medical Director, Ladenheim Dialysis Access Center, Fresno, California

Ten Mistakes to Avoid in Dialysis Access Surgery

Sarah J. Madison, MD

Resident and Research Fellow, Department of Anesthesiology and Perioperative Care, University of California, Irvine, Irvine, California

Anesthesia for Vascular Access Surgery

Brian Mailey, MD

General Surgery Resident, University of California, Irvine, Irvine, California

New Synthetic Grafts and Early Access

Nam X. Nguyen, MD

Associate Clinical Professor of Surgery, University of Southern California Keck School of Medicine; Director of Minimally Invasive Surgery, Childrens Hospital Los Angeles, Los Angeles, California

Access in the Neonatal and Pediatric Patient

Peter D. Peng, MD

Chief Resident, Department of Surgery, Stanford University; Chief Resident, Department of Surgery, Stanford University Hospital, Stanford, California

Biologic Properties of Venous Access Devices

Merisa Piper

Research Associate, Department of Surgery, University of California, Irvine, Irvine, California

Basilic Vein Transposition: A Modern Autogenous Vascular Access for Hemodialysis

Subhash Popli, MD, FACP

Clinical Professor of Medicine, Loyola University School of Medicine, Maywood, Illinois; Director, Renal Dialysis Unit, Hines VA Hospital, Hines, Illinois

Cardiovascular Consequences of Rapid Hemodialysis

Andrew R. Ready, MD

Consultant Surgeon, Queen Elizabeth Hospital, Birmingham, England, United Kingdom

Infection in Vascular Access Procedures

Albert I Richardson II, MD

Vascular Surgeon, John D. Archbold Memorial Hospital, Thomasville, Georgia

Should the KDOQI Guidelines for First Time Dialysis Access Apply to All Patients?

Vincent L. Rowe, MD

Associate Professor of Surgery, University of Southern California (USC); Chief of Vascular Surgery and Endovascular Therapy, CardioVascular Thoracic Institute, USC Medical Center, Los Angeles, California

Axillosubclavian Vein Thrombosis

Larry A. Scher, MD

Professor of Clinical Surgery, Montefiore Medical Center;
Professor of Clinical Surgery, Vascular Surgery, Albert
Einstein College of Medicine, Bronx, New York

*Vascular Access Neuropathic Syndrome: Ischemic Monomelic
Neuropathy*

A. Frederick Schild, MD, FACS

Professor of Surgery, University of Miami Leonard M.
Miller School of Medicine; Vascular Surgeon, Jackson
Memorial Hospital, Miami, Florida

*Reflections on Four Decades of Experience in Vascular Access
Surgery*

Amit R. Shah, MD

Fellow, Division of Vascular Surgery, Montefiore Medical
Center, Bronx, New York

*Vascular Access Neuropathic Syndrome: Ischemic Monomelic
Neuropathy*

Surendra Shenoy, MD, PhD

Professor of Surgery, Washington University School of
Medicine; Professor of Surgery, Barnes-Jewish Hospital, St
Louis, Missouri

*Assessment and Intervention for Arteriovenous Fistula
Maturation; Ultrasound in Vascular Access*

Kimberly S. Stone, MD

Resident Physician, Department of General Surgery,
Stanford University, Stanford, California

Endovascular Management of Dialysis Graft Stenosis

Apostolos K. Tassiopoulos, MD, FACS

Associate Professor of Surgery, Stony Brook University;
Chief of Vascular Surgery, Stony Brook University Medical
Center, Stony Brook, New York

*Surveillance, Revision, and Outcome of Vascular Access
Procedures for Hemodialysis*

Gail T. Tominaga, MD

Critical Care Surgeon, Department of Trauma Services,
Scripps Memorial Hospital, La Jolla, California

Placement of Indwelling Venous Access Systems

Nosratola D. Vaziri, MD, MACP

Professor of Medicine, Physiology, and Biophysics and
Chief of Nephrology and Hypertension, University of
California, Irvine (UCI), Irvine, California; Chief of
Nephrology and Hypertension, UCI Medical Center,
Orange, California

*Epidemiology and Pathophysiology of Chronic Renal Failure
and Guidelines for Initiation of Hemodialysis;
Cardiovascular Consequences of Rapid Hemodialysis*

Fred A. Weaver, MD, MMM

Professor of Surgery and Chief of Vascular Surgery and
Endovascular Therapy, University of Southern California
(USC) Keck School of Medicine; Chief of Vascular
Surgery and Endovascular Therapy, CardioVascular
Thoracic Institute, USC University Hospital, Los Angeles,
California

Axillosubclavian Vein Thrombosis

Jason Wellen, MD

Assistant Professor of Transplant Surgery, Washington
University in St Louis; Assistant Professor of Transplant
Surgery, Barnes-Jewish Hospital, St Louis, Missouri

Ultrasound in Vascular Access

Geoffrey H. White, MB, BS, FRACS

Associate Professor of Surgery, University of Sydney; Head
of Vascular Surgery, Royal Prince Alfred Hospital, Sydney,
New South Wales, Australia

*Patient Assessment and Planning for Vascular Access
Surgery; Autogenous Vein for Fistulas and Interposition
Grafts; Central Venous Cannulation for Hemodialysis Access*

Rodney A. White, MD

Professor of Surgery, David Geffen School of Medicine at
University of California, Los Angeles (UCLA), Los
Angeles, California; Chief of Vascular Surgery, Harbor-
UCLA Medical Center, Torrance, California

Biologic Response to Prosthetic Dialysis Grafts

Russell A. Williams, MD, FACS

Professor of Surgery, University of California, Irvine
(UCI), Irvine, California; Attending Surgeon at UCI
Medical Center, Orange, California, and at Long Beach VA
Medical Center, Long Beach, California

Endovascular Management of Dialysis Graft Stenosis

Samuel Eric Wilson, MD

Professor of Surgery, University of California, Irvine
(UCI), Irvine, California; UCI Medical Center, Orange,
California; Chief of Surgical Service, Long Beach VA
Medical Center, Long Beach, California

*Development of Vascular Access Surgery; Patient Assessment
and Planning for Vascular Access Surgery; Thrombophilia as
a Cause of Recurrent Vascular Access Thrombosis in
Hemodialysis Patients; Autologous Arteriovenous Fistulas:
Direct Radiocephalic Anastomosis for Hemodialysis Access;
Interposition Arteriovenous Grafts (Bridge Fistulas) for
Hemodialysis; New Synthetic Grafts and Early Access;
Surveillance, Revision, and Outcome of Vascular Access
Procedures for Hemodialysis; Complications of Vascular
Access: Thrombosis, Venous Hypertension, Congestive Heart
Failure, Neuropathy, and Aneurysm; Dialysis
Access–Associated Ischemic Steal Syndrome; Infection in
Vascular Access Procedures*

James E. Wiseman, MD
Resident, General Surgery, Department of Surgery, University of California, Irvine, Irvine, California
Placement of Indwelling Venous Access Systems

Karen Woo, MD
Vascular Surgery Fellow, Scripps Clinic–University of California, San Diego, La Jolla, California
Complications of Percutaneous Vascular Access Procedures and Their Management

Preface

I had not planned on a fifth edition of *Vascular Access: Principles and Practice*, but in the seven years since the last edition so much has changed that an updating and rewriting seemed imperative. Indeed, from the first edition, 30 years ago, the field of vascular access has changed entirely. No longer strictly a surgical endeavor, interventional radiologists, nephrologists, and critical care specialists all play an important role. Edward Passaro Jr, my mentor, understood how the field would evolve and enlarge. In the preface to the first edition he wrote that vascular access was then everyone's skill—"physicians at the periphery of problems, working at the periphery of the vascular system"—but predicted this era would soon pass. He was right again.

Two early editions described the new operations of arteriovenous fistula and prosthetic graft implantation, and later editions considered the sequence of vascular access procedures, assessment of outcome, and the growing role of interventional radiology. Now, in this latest edition, we continue to emphasize fundamental knowledge of vascular anatomy and the hemodynamic changes attendant to construction of the arteriovenous fistula. The text provides detailed information on the specialized technical skills necessary for successful vascular access operations. The contributors evaluate the importance of surveillance, the role of interventional percutaneous transluminal angioplasty and stenting, and provide information on efforts to combat intimal hyperplasia and thrombophilia. Much of the text has been rewritten, with new authors discussing axillosubclavian vein thrombosis, neuropathic syndrome, ultrasound imaging, and myointimal hyperplasia. The impact of "ex cathedra" guidelines on fistula construction and the still-high frequency of central venous catheterization are critically analyzed.

I am indebted to the authors for their generous and timely contributions. Some have endured through five editions of the text. My colleagues at the University of California, Irvine, who have written almost half of the chapters, have been most gracious and considerate in recording their expertise. More so than in previous editions, I have called on contributions of specialists across the country, all members of the Vascular Access Society of the Americas (VASA).

The editorial team at Lippincott, Williams and Wilkins has been very patient and most helpful. Khushboo Kaushal, a student at the University of California, San Diego School of Medicine, has been an invaluable manager of correspondence, reference accuracy, and editing.

Surgeons continue to approach me at scientific meetings to comment on how useful and practical they have found *Vascular Access*. No one can expect a better reward. If we can improve the surgical care of the almost half a million patients requiring vascular access, and especially those on maintenance hemodialysis, our authors' efforts will have been very worthwhile.

Samuel Eric Wilson, MD

Contents

GENERAL PRINCIPLES OF VASCULAR ACCESS

CHAPTER 1

Development of Vascular Access Surgery

H. Earl Gordon* and Samuel Eric Wilson

The remarkable achievements in access to venous and arterial circulation have been directly responsible for prolonging or saving the lives of countless patients. The emergence of the need for repeated and long-term access as required for chronic hemodialysis and total parenteral nutrition (TPN) served as an impetus for a myriad of technical advances and clinical applications.

In the broadest of terms, *vascular access* must include blood transfusions and intravenous therapy. Although these procedures are taken for granted by laypersons and clinicians alike, their origin represents the first step in the evolution of long-term access to the circulatory system.

Intravenous injection of drugs into animals antedated the first transfusion by at least a decade. Richard Lower, in his *Tractatus de Corde,*[1] (see the frontispiece) commented in 1669, "For many years at Oxford I saw others at work, and myself, for the sake of experiment, inject[ing] into the veins of living animals various opiate and emaetic solutions, and many medicinal fluids of that sort."

Although Sir Christopher Wren was best known for his architectural feats (Fig. 1-1), he invented an instrument for intravenous therapy in 1657 that was used to inject drugs into the veins of dogs. The instrument consisted of a cannula made from a quill with a pointed tip, which permitted penetration of the skin and underlying vein. In 1663, Robert Boyle (Fig. 1-2) described and published Wren's experiments. Boyle was the first person to extend intravenous infusions from animals to humans, using prison inmates in London as subjects.[2]

Considering the aura of fascination that always accompanied the heart and circulatory system, it is not surprising that attempts at transfusions would soon follow. In May 1665, Lower[1] reported a successful direct transfusion between two dogs. By using a series of quills, he transferred blood from the carotid artery of one dog into the jugular vein of a second dog that had previously been phlebotomized. At the conclusion of the experiment, the recipient dog "promptly jumped down from the table, and apparently oblivious of its hurts, soon began to fondle its master . . . ."

In Paris on June 15, 1667, Jean Denys, professor of philosophy and mathematics at the University of Montpellier, performed the first successful transfusion into humans.[3] Animal blood was used in this experiment. During November of that same year, Lower performed the first successful human transfusion in England. Arthur Coga,

variously described as a "harmless lunatic" and an "eccentric scholar," was the subject, and Lower administered 9 or 10 ounces of blood from the artery of a sheep. Although the patient survived without any apparent physical harm, Lower's comment reflected disappointment by the absence of expected benefits: "In order to make further experiments on him with some profit also to himself, I decided to repeat the treatment several times in an effort to improve his mental condition, he, on the other hand, consulted his instinct rather than the interest of his health, and completely eluded our expectations."

These efforts were soon doomed to failure. One of the patients transfused by Denys developed all of the signs that we recognize today as those of a transfusion reaction. After the death of another patient, an investigation terminated in a verdict against Denys. The infusion of animal blood into humans was rapidly abandoned, and no significant work in this area was reported for the next 150 years.

James Blundell performed the first transfusion of human blood on December 22, 1818.[3] Using a syringe, he injected 12 to 14 ounces of blood from several donors into his patients. Because blood typing was unknown at that time, it is not surprising that Blundell's experiments met with uncertain success. Although Karl Landsteiner discovered the ABO blood groups in 1901, it was another decade before his discovery led to practical application. Additional milestones were achieved in 1914, when Richard Lewisohn of New York and other investigators introduced the use of sodium citrate as an anticoagulant, and in 1937, when Landsteiner and Wiener discovered the Rh factor. Charles Drew (1904–1950) carried on research in blood preservation and was a major force in the organization of blood banks.

One of the first published papers on hemodialysis was by Abel, Rowntree, and Turner, who coined the term *artificial kidney* in 1913.[4] They circulated the blood of a dog through multiple celloidin tubes that allowed the toxins to pass out into the surrounding liquid while keeping the blood substances inside. Later, Necheles conceived the prototype of all machines by using membranes between screens or mats.[1]

Fortunately, Dr. Willem J. Kolff of the Netherlands had access to both heparin and a high-quality cellophane and is credited with developing the first practical model for humans in 1943.[5] Initially, he used only venipuncture needles for outflow and inflow to the artificial kidney. He later used a glass cannula inserted into the radial artery through a small incision above the wrist. In the absence of a pump, the return of the blood to the patient was accomplished via gravity, using a buret that could be raised to the ceiling with

---

*Deceased

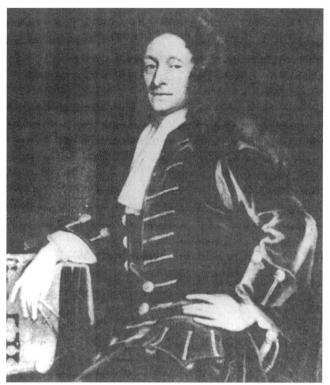

Figure 1-1.
Sir Christopher Wren (1632-1723), one of the most famous English architects, who designed St. Paul's Cathedral and more than 50 other London churches after the great fire, also invented a cannula for vascular access. (Courtesy of National Library of Medicine, Bethesda, MD.)

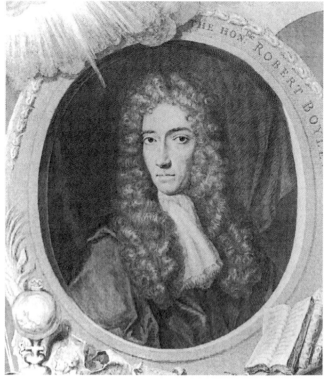

Figure 1-2.
Robert Boyle (1627-1691), an Irish physicist, studied the compression and expansion of gases to formulate Boyle's law and extended intravenous infusions from animals to humans. (Courtesy of National Library of Medicine, Bethesda, MD.)

a pulley. During a visit to Boston in 1947, he presented a copy of the blueprints of his machine to Dr. Carl Walter, who then built the Peter Bent Brigham version of the rotating kidney. Dr. Kolff left the Netherlands for the United States in 1950 to accept an appointment at the Cleveland Clinic to continue his investigations. Kolff's revised model, built in his basement in 1955, included seven beer cans, a fruit juice can, and window screening to keep the cellophane in place.[6] Obvious refinements were made for commercial production, which was under way by the next year (Fig. 1-3).

Early enthusiasm for the unit was dampened, however, by the technical problems associated with intermittent hemodialysis. The necessity for cutdowns on the artery and vein for each dialysis and the necessity for ligation of these vessels at the termination of each procedure essentially limited hemodialysis to short-term therapy for acute renal failure. Even with the introduction of plastic cannulas (eg, the Scribner shunt), the average life of the arterial and venous lines was 7 to 10 days.

Chronic access to the circulation finally became a reality in 1960 through the combined talents of an internist, a surgeon, and an engineer. Scribner, Dillard, and Quinton[7] introduced the Teflon-Silastic arteriovenous shunt (Fig. 1-4), which brought new hope to the patient with end-stage renal disease. Their first six consecutive patients were successfully cannulated without any clotting in the external

bypass that connected the artery with the vein. In the seventh patient, however, repeated attempts ended in failure (D. Dillard, personal communication, 1979). One can only speculate how the course of events might have been altered if the latter patient had been their initial subject.

For the next 6 years, this ingenious device was universally adopted, and regular dialysis became a standard method of treatment. Because of interference of the external appliance with normal activity and because of the risks of infection, thrombosis, and other complications, the search continued for improved techniques.

Many of these disadvantages were overcome through introduction of the subcutaneous arteriovenous fistula by Brescia, Cimino, Appel, and Hurwich in 1966.[8] They surgically created a fistula between the radial artery above the wrist and the largest available vein in close proximity. This procedure enabled them to achieve blood flow rates of 250 to 300 mL/min. Their innovative approach remains the initial procedure of choice in patients who are candidates for long-term hemodialysis and who have suitable vessels. Unfortunately, many of these individuals have thrombosed arteries and veins as a result of repeated venipuncture and arterial puncture in the distal forearm. Consequently, a number of techniques have evolved in bridging the gap between artery and vein at more proximal levels in the arm, using transposition procedures and synthetic grafts.

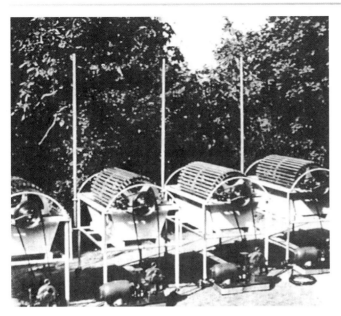

Figure 1-3.
Four rotating drum kidneys made during German occupation of the Netherlands. After the war in 1946, one was sent to London, one to New York, and one to Montreal. (Courtesy of Milton Owens, MD, San Pedro, CA, who was given this photograph by Willem J. Kolff, MD, PhD, designer of the first practical dialysis machine.)

An innovation essential to the development of cardiac catheterization was carried out by Werner Forssman, a young intern in a German hospital in 1929. While standing behind a fluoroscopic machine and looking into a mirror, he threaded a thin catheter inserted into his own arm vein and into his heart. After intracardiac catheterization led to critically important physiologic studies, Forssman was named as a corecipient of a Nobel prize in 1976.[4]

In the 1940s, cardiac surgery was limited to the readily accessible great vessels in the region of the heart. General hypothermia with inflow occlusion was developed in the early 1950s. This allowed the closure of simple congenital cardiac defects under direct vision within a 6-minute time interval.[9]

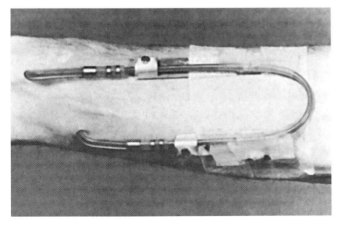

Figure 1-4.
Early external arteriovenous shunt, using metal plates on rings to secure tubing.

Still to be conquered was the necessity to provide cerebral oxygenation to the brain during cardiac surgery. Dr. John Gibbon and his coworkers finally achieved this in 1953 after 21 years of experimentation in the development of a heart-lung machine. This enabled Gibbon to successfully close a septal defect within the heart under direct vision.[9] Cardiopulmonary bypass has been responsible for the phenomenal success of cardiac surgery and cardiac transplantation.

During the 1950s, attention was focused on the nutrition of the surgical patient in preparation for surgery and during the postoperative period. Inasmuch as hypertonic additives to TPN solutions led to sclerosing of peripheral veins, it served as an impetus to search for other modalities of therapy. Dudrick was one of the pioneers in this field. In 1968, he and his colleagues[10] were the first to administer hypertonic TPN solutions via catheter introduced into the subclavian vein through a percutaneous infraclavicular route. His approach was patterned after that of Aubaniac, a French military surgeon who in 1952 described his 10-year experience with the use of subclavian vein catheters for the rapid infusion of resuscitation fluids in military casualties.[11]

The increasing demand for long-term use of TPN as an artificial gut led Broviac, Cole, and Scribner[12] to develop an indwelling right atrial catheter in 1973. This silicone rubber catheter was tunneled subcutaneously from the lower chest wall and into the central venous system through the cephalic or internal jugular vein. In 1979, Hickman and colleagues[6] reported their modification of the Broviac catheter by increasing the diameter to facilitate the needs of patients undergoing bone marrow transplantation. The larger bore allowed for the infusion of blood products, plasmapheresis, and hyperalimentation. It continues to be widely used for access into the central venous system for chemotherapeutic agents, antibiotics, and other drugs, as well as for nutritional support.

Technologic advances in improved catheters focused interest on improving drug delivery systems. The external arterial catheters and those used for venous access all had the potential for infection and sepsis through the skin exit site. In addition, they limited patient activity and required frequent dressing changes. It is not surprising that totally implantable delivery systems would be forthcoming. Most of the studies on the first implantable pumps were directed to arterial perfusion using the Infusaid system.[13,14]

Because of the limited success with hepatic artery infusions in controlling metastatic disease to the liver, increased attention was directed to implantable devices for venous access. Bothe and colleagues[15] reported their experience in 1984 with the use of the "Port-a-Cath" in 74 patients for long-term chemotherapy. This unit consisted of a small stainless steel reservoir inserted into the subcutaneous space of the chest wall with a Silastic catheter introduced into the central venous system in a manner similar to that used with Broviac-Hickman catheters. The implantable devices in use today are primarily for venous access to provide long-term administration of chemotherapeutic agents, antibiotics, nutrition, and other therapeutic agents.

In the future, the volume of patients requiring long-term circulatory access will undoubtedly escalate. With our aging population, the demand for chronic hemodialysis will continue to increase at a time when organ donations have reached a plateau. It has been reported that vascular access thrombosis accounts for at least several billion in annual expenses and 25% of hospitalizations for chronic hemodialysis patients.[16] Consequently, it is imperative that every dialysis center establish a quality assurance program to ensure that they are operating at a cost-effective level while maintaining a high quality of life for their patients. The use of such methods as blood flow measurements,[16] endovascular techniques,[17] and angioplasty may help to achieve these objectives. Meanwhile, the search will continue for further technologic refinements and new clinical applications.

REFERENCES

1. Lower R. Tractatus de Corde, 1669. In: Gunther RT. *Early Science in Oxford*. Vol 9. Franklin KJ, trans-ed. London: Oxford Press; 1932.
2. Wheatley HB. *The Diary of Samuel Pepys*. Vol 2. New York: Random House; 1966.
3. Erskine AG, Wladyslaw WS. *The Principles and Practice of Blood Grouping*. 2nd ed. St. Louis: Mosby; 1978.
4. Lyons AS, Petrucelli RJ. *Medicine: An Illustrated History*. New York: Harry N. Adams; 1987.
5. Graham WB. Historical aspects of hemodialysis. *Transplant Proc*. 1977;9:xlix.
6. Hickman RO, Buckner CD, Clift RA, Sanders JE, Stewart P, Thomas ED. A modified right atrial catheter for access to the venous system in marrow transplant recipients. *Surg Gynecol Obstet*. 1979;148:871-875.
7. Quinton WE, Dillard D, Scribner BH. Cannulation of blood vessels for prolonged hemodialysis. *Trans Am Soc Artif Intern Organs*. 1960;6:104-113.
8. Brescia MJ, Cimino JE, Appel K, Hurwich BJ. Chronic hemodialysis using venipuncture and a surgically created arteriovenous fistula. *N Engl J Med*. 1966;275:1089-1092.
9. Fedak PW. Open hearts. The origins of direct-vision intracardiac surgery. *Tex Heart Inst J*. 1998;25:100-111.
10. Dudrick SJ, Wilmore DW, Vars HM, Rhoads JE. Long-term total parenteral nutrition with growth development and positive nitrogen balance. *Surgery*. 1968;64:134-142.
11. Aubaniac R: L'infection intraveineuse sousclaviculaire: avantages et technique. *Presse Ivied*. 1952;60:1456.
12. Broviac JW, Cole JJ, Scribner BH. A silicone rubber atrial catheter for prolonged parenteral alimentation. *Surg Gynecol Obstet*. 1973;136:602-606.
13. Blackshear PJ, Dorman FD, Blackshear PL Jr, Varco RL, Buchwald H. The design and initial testing of an implantable infusion pump. *Surg Gynecol Obstet*. 1972;134:51-56.
14. Niederhuber JE, Ensminger W, Gyves JW, Liepman M, Doan K, Cozzi E. Totally implanted venous and arterial access system to replace external catheters in cancer treatment. *Surgery*. 1982;92:706-712.
15. Bothe A Jr, Piccione W, Ambrosino JJ, Benotti PN, Lokich JJ. Implantable central venous access system. *Am J Surg*. 1984;147:565-569.
16. Neyra NR, Ikizler TA, May RE, et al. Change in access blood flow over time predicts vascular access thrombosis. *Kidney Int*. 1988;54:1714-1719.
17. Holzenbein TJ, Miller A, Gottlieb MN, Gupta SK. The role of routine angioscopy in vascular access surgery. *J Endovasc Surg*. 1995;2:10-25.

CHAPTER 2

Patient Assessment and Planning for Vascular Access Surgery

Geoffrey H. White and Samuel Eric Wilson

One of the primary determinants of successful vascular access surgery is the preoperative planning process, which must be based on a thorough assessment of the patient and on knowledgeable selection of the appropriate access technique. Because the age, prevalence, and long-term survival of patients who receive dialysis for end-stage renal failure are all increasing, the requirement for multiple access procedures over many years is common.[1,2] It is thus advantageous to not only consider the first procedure but to also have in mind a long-term plan that includes stepwise, multiple access procedures.

Sound planning helps to avoid complications and the necessity for multiple procedures or revisions. Nothing is more frustrating and discouraging to the dialysis patient, nephrologist, and surgeon than multiple revisions early in the course of chronic renal disease. Early failures of the access site can be minimized by careful preoperative choice of the inflow and outflow vessels. Patients should not be submitted to an exploration of various vessels in an attempt to decide on a procedure at the time of the surgery. Preoperative ultrasound examination is invaluable in the identification of suitable vasculature and patency of the central veins. In addition, patient comfort during hemodialysis can be greatly improved by correct positioning of the access site in the extremity.

This chapter is intended to describe a strategy for planning these procedures on the basis of a systematic assessment of the patient and a policy of preservation of the appropriate vessels in patients who may later require dialysis. The details of individual techniques are covered in other chapters.

General Principles of Access Surgery

Several guiding principles should be followed.

- It is preferable to use the arm vessels for access rather than the leg vessels, and when possible the nondominant arm should be used. Infection and arterial occlusion are less common in the upper extremities.
- In general, access sites should be placed as distally as practical in the limb so proximal sites will be available for subsequent procedures.
- Although not always possible, inadequate or atherosclerotic arteries should be avoided, and a suitable length of

patent runoff vein is required to accommodate multiple cannulation sites.

- The chosen site should allow for ease of access for cannulation and should be positioned so patient comfort is ensured during hemodialysis.
- Before secondary constructions are performed, the patient should be re-evaluated for the feasibility of arteriovenous (AV) fistula construction.
- The complications of percutaneous central venous dialysis catheter insertion may be life threatening.
- Technical precision and gentle tissue handling are mandatory; the use of optical magnification, fine monofilament suture materials, atraumatic clamps, and microvascular instruments is recommended.[3]
- An arteriovenous anastomosis is unlikely to provide satisfactory flow for hemodialysis if the vein is less than 3 mm in diameter.
- A temporary access procedure, such as placement of a double-lumen venous catheter (usually in the internal jugular, subclavian, or femoral veins) or peritoneal catheter, may be required during the time that an AV fistula is maturing before use. The interval should be kept as brief as possible to prevent central venous stenosis.
- Anticoagulation may not be necessary during routine access operations, except for graft thrombectomy and revision procedures or for patients who do not have the usual platelet dysfunction of chronic renal failure.
- Infection is a major cause of morbidity and the second leading cause of death in patients undergoing hemodialysis.[4,5] Prophylactic antibiotics are used perioperatively for all operations that involve insertion of prosthetic material. Although controversial, the incidence of infection at the operative access site may be decreased by temporary decolonization with short-term perioperative antimicrobials and mupirocin ointment directed at nasal carriage of methicillin-resistant *Staphylococcus aureus*.[6]

Preservation of Access Vessels

The autogenous AV fistula constructed at the wrist or forearm is the procedure of first choice.[2] Most second-choice procedures also make use of the forearm, with the principal access vessels being the radial and brachial arteries, cephalic vein, and veins of the cubital fossa (basilic, antecubital, and cephalic). Once the diagnosis is known, these primary access vessels are preserved through the avoidance of venipuncture, intravenous cannulation, or invasive monitoring lines in all patients with acute or progressive renal disease.[7] The patient and all involved hospital personnel must be instructed in the need to preserve the selected vessels from the time of the earliest indication of renal failure. In particular, the placement of intravenous lines into the cephalic vein must be avoided, because thrombosis or sclerosis prevents its use for an AV fistula. When the patient is hospitalized, these policies may be emphasized by marking the arm vessels with an indelible pen or by posting a sign over the patient's bed. Educate the patient as to the importance of preserving the veins of at least one arm. Adequate hydration, weight control, hypertension treatment, avoidance of smoking, and control of local dermatitis or cellulitis are all measures that may help increase the likelihood of performing and maintaining a radiocephalic autogenous AV fistula.[7,8]

The importance of planning is illustrated by the reported experience of Hinsdale, Lipkowitz, and Hoover,[9] who could only attempt Brescia-Cimino fistulas in 25% of their patients, in part because of iatrogenic destruction of suitable peripheral veins by personnel in a teaching hospital environment. This percentage was subsequently improved to 50% after the introduction of strict protocols in the selection of patients for autogenous construction. In contrast, reviews of the collected European vascular access experience have shown high rates of autogenous fistula construction (85% to 95%), which are attributed to patient selection and careful planning.[10] In the Japanese hemodialysis network, the majority of patients have dialysis via an autogenous AV fistula. The Dialysis Outcome Quality Initiative guidelines of the National Kidney Foundation also emphasize the autogenous fistula as the first choice.[8]

Planning Strategy: Choice of Procedure

A rational sequence of procedure choices, based on our practice, is listed in Table 2-1. The radial artery-to-cephalic vein fistula at the wrist, as originally described by Brescia and associates in 1966,[11] remains firmly established as the procedure of choice, although the fistula may also be placed more distally in the anatomic snuff box at the base of the thumb.[12] This procedure is often possible in the mid-forearm when the distal cephalic vein is too small. Approximately half of patients referred for primary access procedures should be suitable for direct fistula at the wrist or mid-forearm, especially if measures for the preservation of vessels, as discussed, have been followed. The radiocephalic autogenous fistula lasts longer than other access sites, is convenient for the patient, and has the lowest rate of complications. However, poor patient selection or errors in technique may result in early thrombosis, so patients with narrow or diseased vessels as determined by physical examination or ultrasound should not be selected for this technique. The brachiocephalic autogenous fistula in the cubital fossa is also a first-choice procedure but is more likely to cause a late "steal" phenomenon.

We consider a second-choice procedure to be an AV graft bridge fistula using prosthetic polytetrafluoroethylene

Table 2-1

Procedure Choices in Vascular Access Surgery

First Choice

Radiocephalic direct autogenous arteriovenous (AV) fistula
Brescia-Cimino at the wrist or forearm AV fistula
Brachiocephalic AV fistula, cubital fossa

Second Choice

Upper arm transposed AV fistula
Brachial to basilic (basilic vein transposed after anastomosis to brachial artery)
Forearm arteriovenous graft (bridge) fistula (6-mm-diameter polytetrafluoroethylene [PTFE]) (Note: When this construction is under consideration, re-evaluate patient for possibility of autologous brachial artery to cubital vein AV fistula)
Straight
Radial artery to largest superficial vein of cubital fossa
Loop
Brachial artery to largest superficial vein of cubital fossa
Brachioaxillary AV graft

Third Choice

Femorosaphenous AV graft, loop in upper thigh
Femorofemoral AV graft, loop in upper thigh

Others

Axilloaxillary AV graft
Iliac-femoral AV graft or iliac-iliac AV graft

(PTFE) material in the upper arm. As shown in Table 2-1, forearm bridge grafts (eg, a straight graft from the radial artery at the wrist to one of the major cubital fossa veins, a looped graft from the brachial artery curving onto the dorsum of the forearm and returning to nearby antecubital veins), are possible. One should carefully reassess patients in whom this construction is being considered for the possibility of a direct, autogenous AV fistula in the forearm. If the patient has no visible or palpable veins in the forearm or elbow region, an alternative outflow vein is often available adjacent to the brachial artery. Usually two or more brachial venae comitantes are found here, medial and lateral to the brachial artery, and in most cases, one of these veins is of sufficient diameter to allow for good long-term graft patency.[13] Other second-choice procedures favored in some dialysis units are the alternative techniques of direct AV fistula that are discussed in detail elsewhere in this text, especially the upper arm basilic vein-to-brachial artery transposed fistula.[14] This method allows the avoidance of a prosthetic graft. Dagher[14] reported 70% patency rate at 8 years for this upper arm AV fistula. The brachioaxillary bridge graft is the most reliable second-choice prosthetic procedure.[15] At least three sites for revision are accessible along the proximal axillary vein.

We reserve grafts that involve the larger vessels of the thoracic outlet and leg as third choices, although in selected patients, the use of these vessels at an early stage may be

Table 2-2

Ischemic Steal Resulting from Arteriovenous Access Procedures

Category	No. of Procedures	Incidence of Symptomatic Steal
Procedure		
Brescia-Cimino fistula	83	0
Forearm access graft	57	3 (5.2%)
Upper arm access graft	20	2 (10%)
Others	6	0
TOTAL		5
Inflow Artery		
Radial	125	1 (0.8%)
Brachial	35	4 (11.4%)
Axillary or femoral	6	0
TOTAL		5
Related Factors		
Diabetes mellitus	35	4 (11.4%)
No diabetes	131	1 (0.7%)

This table shows the relative incidence and distribution of five cases of ischemic steal occurring in 166 procedures during a 2-year period.

indicated because of the large diameter, high flow rates, and consequent low early thrombosis rate.[9] Balancing these factors is a higher rate of surgical complications due to the proximity of important structures in the axilla or groin, higher rates of infection, and an increased incidence of significant steal (Table 2-2). Moreover, incontinence is a relative contraindication to constructions in the upper thigh. For these reasons, we prefer to reserve such techniques for the patient with inadequate vessels elsewhere or for the patient who has previously had multiple procedures. It is wise to avoid vessels that cannot be ligated if subsequent problems arise; for example, anastomosis to the superficial femoral artery is preferred to that of the common femoral for grafts in the thigh.

When the above measures have been exhausted, alternative sites as detailed elsewhere in this text are considered, or peritoneal dialysis may be instituted.

Planning the Graft Site and Course

The site and course of a dialysis graft must be planned so it will be easily accessible for cannulation, comfortable for the patient while on dialysis, and free of compression by adjacent structures or joint movements, and not in proximity to major structures that may be subsequently damaged by attempts to place needles. Occasionally, the cosmetic appearance of the graft must also be considered in the decision of an appropriate site.

A graft in the forearm should be positioned toward the lateral aspect so that dialysis may be carried out with the arm in a comfortable neutral position. The subcutaneous tunnel is formed in the shape of a gentle loop, avoiding excess angulation at the anastomosis. The straight forearm graft is curved dorsally from the line of the vessels, and a loop graft is angulated laterally so that its apex also lies dorsally. If these grafts are positioned on the medial, volar aspect, the arm must be held in a less-comfortable, extended, and supinated position during dialysis.[16] In the upper arm, anterolateral positioning allows easier cannulation than does a medial, inner arm position and avoids both compression of the graft against the chest wall and accidental needling of the radial nerve.[16] It is helpful to mark the proposed graft position on the skin before surgery.

Planning Fistula Maturation

Ideally, when a fistula or graft has been fashioned, a period of maturation is necessary to allow for dilatation and thickening of the vein wall or for incorporation of the prosthetic graft material into the surrounding subcutaneous tissues closing the graft tunnel. In the best situation, in which a patient with progressive renal failure is being followed in a nephrology clinic, an access should be established several months before the need for hemodialysis (ie, when the serum creatinine reaches 4%).[17] Without maturation of the AV fistula, early puncture renders the patient susceptible to episodes of hemorrhage, subcutaneous hematoma, pseudoaneurysm formation, and early thrombosis.[18] If a prosthetic graft is not allowed to incorporate into its surrounding tissue, puncture may produce leakage into the graft tunnel, with subsequent hematoma formation.[19] For these reasons, if the patient's condition permits, we sometimes delay use for 2 weeks for a PTFE graft and for up to 6–8 weeks for a Brescia-Cimino fistula. A temporary dialysis technique must be used during this time unless the patient has not yet reached the point of requiring dialysis. Large-bore, double-lumen, cuffed venous cannulas serve the purpose, but prolonged use causes central vein occlusion.[20] A polyethylene terephthalate (Dacron) cuffed type of catheter is useful if more than 4 to 6 weeks is required for graft or fistula maturation. Peritoneal dialysis is another alternative.

Modifications in stretch PTFE manufacturing aimed at allowing cannulation within the first 24 hours have not been completely successful in clinical trials owing to increased thrombosis and technical difficulty in thrombectomy, which requires an incision in the graft wall. Concerned that the placement of central venous dialysis catheters carries a considerable risk of serious complications such as pneumothorax and arterial puncture or laceration with subsequent hemorrhage into the mediastinum pleural space, some surgeons recommend early puncture (within 24 hours) of PTFE grafts. Clinical reports, including one comparative trial, indicate that the incidence of graft thrombosis and subcutaneous hematoma and infection with early puncture, given the use of careful technique, is not significantly increased compared with waiting for access site maturation.[21] In any event, should such complications occur, they are minor compared with the complications of percutaneous dialysis catheter placement. Accordingly, in our practice, we recommend early puncture of new dialysis grafts with the provision that it be undertaken by experienced dialysis personnel. Newer grafts composed of PTFE and a self-sealing membrane show promise of routine, "safe," early puncture in clinical trials.

Patient Assessment for Primary Access Procedure

The initial priority when assessing a patient who has been referred for a first hemodialysis access procedure is to determine whether this patient will be suitable for a Brescia-Cimino or forearm autogenous AV fistula. Recent recommendations by a committee of the Society for Vascular Surgery are shown in Table 2-3.[22] The patency and size of the radial artery and cephalic vein within the forearm are checked, and the veins of the cubital fossa should also be accurately assessed so that an alternative procedure plan can be formulated. The adequacy of collateral supply via the ulnar and interosseous arteries and palmar arches is assessed clinically by Allen's test and may be confirmed by noninvasive vascular laboratory techniques if there is doubt.[23] Atherosclerosis or diabetes mellitus will occasionally render the radial artery unsuitable for a fistula. Documentation of collateral circulation is important, because digital gangrene has occurred after radial artery cannulation.[24] The cephalic vein should be widely patent to above the elbow, without evidence of previous venipuncture or intravenous infusion and with a diameter of at least 3 mm. Inadequate assessment of the patency and size of this vein is a common error. Duplex scanning can be used routinely to map veins of the forearm and serves as a useful guide to a successful construction. Obesity may result in the veins being deeply embedded and difficult to cannulate.[2] Other factors involved in the assessment for radial cephalic fistula include an inspection of the condition of the skin in the area and the exclusion of previous deep vein obstruction

(especially if the patient has had a subclavian catheter).[25] A duplex scan of the axillosubclavian veins should be obtained in patients who have risk factors for thrombosis of these vessels, such as prolonged central venous catheterization (>3 weeks).

Assessment of the Failing Access Graft

Decreasing function of a graft will often be heralded by a rise in venous outflow resistance or high intragraft pressures during dialysis. Usually, this is caused by progressive stenosis of the venous anastomosis, which may also be suspected if a pulse becomes stronger and easily palpable near the venous end. (In a well-functioning graft, the pulse should decrease in force just beyond the arterial anastomosis.[2]) On-table angiography is most helpful in confirming and localizing the stenosis so that corrective surgery or percutaneous intervention can be planned. A simple method for the correction of graft venous anastomic narrowing is an outflow patch angioplasty. Percutaneous angioplasty and stenting are also employed for this purpose, although long-term success (patency) may be less than with operative revision.

Patient Assessment for Secondary Access Procedures

Secondary procedures are required when there are failures of primary access sites or the patient has advanced peripheral vascular disease or inadequate veins. To assess the patient who has had previous access procedures, notes must be made of the position of previous incisions, the site and type of graft materials, and evidence of complications such as aneurysmal dilation, embolism or steal, vein thrombus or stenosis, and infection.

It is critical to determine whether thrombectomy or revision will allow salvage in patients with thrombosis or poor flow within the prior access vessels. A new AV access site is also planned, in the event of immediate failure of the thrombectomy or revision. If the patient has previously had an AV fistula, it may be possible to fashion a new direct AV fistula at a more proximal level. Even if a prosthetic graft was used for the previous procedure, nearby veins may have become well developed because of the associated high flow, to the extent that the patient may now be suitable for a direct AV fistula technique. Rescue of a failing fistula has the major advantage of not interrupting regular hemodialysis or requiring a temporary percutaneous catheter.

When a direct autogenous fistula occludes after some years of use, salvage attempts are often unproductive, and we usually prefer a new site.

Special Problems

The Patient With Peripheral Vascular Disease

Patients with atherosclerosis or diabetic calcification of vessels present special problems for several reasons: (1) the distal vessels are likely to be occluded or severely stenotic, rendering them unusable, and (2) use of the larger proximal

Table 2–3
Clinical Recommendation of the Society for Vascular Surgery[22]
Timing of referral to surgeon and timing of placement of permanent vascular access
Advanced chronic renal disease, creatinine >4 mg/dl (late stage 4, glomerular filtration rate <20 to 25 mL/min) Upper extremity autogenous arteriovenous (AV) access preferred Prosthetic access should be delayed until just before the need for dialysis
Placement of autogenous AV fistula accesses
As far distally in the upper extremity as possible to preserve proximal sites for future accesses Nondominant arm given preference over the dominant arm only when access opportunities are equal in both extremities
Forearm autogenous AV access as the first choice for primary access for hemodialysis
Autogenous radial-cephalic direct wrist access (Brescia-Cimino-Appel) or autogenous posterior radial branch-cephalic direct wrist access (snuffbox) is preferred

vessels (brachial or axillary) is associated with a higher incidence of vascular steal.[26]

In addition to the decreased number of vessels available for access, the systemic nature of the disease makes occlusion of any access site more common, and long-term patency rates are poor. Steal in these patients tends to be severely symptomatic and may precipitate digital gangrene because of poor small vessels and inadequate collateralization. Diabetic patients are especially prone to experience steal.[27] Similarly, an episode of arterial thrombosis or embolization that has only a minor clinical effect in the normal limb may precipitate severe distal ischemia in the presence of arterial disease. An analysis of the incidence of ischemic and steal complications in a teaching hospital setting over a 2-year period is presented in Table 2-2.

When the radial artery is occluded or stenotic, use of the larger vessels in the thigh or brachium may be necessary. Use of the basilic vein transposition fistula technique in the upper arm is often possible, and the alternative of long-term peritoneal dialysis should also be considered. A detailed discussion of the indications for continuous ambulatory peritoneal dialysis is presented in Chapter 28. Patients with hypotension may also require peritoneal dialysis because of frequent thrombosis of vascular access.[18]

There is no accurate method of predicting steal, although the application of clinical and/or noninvasive vascular laboratory testing of collateral supply via the palmar arterial arches is recommended for this patient group. Angiography may help in devising an access plan in the particularly challenging patient with advanced peripheral occlusive disease.

The Patient Who Has Undergone Multiple Previous Access Procedures

Patients who have had most of their access vessel sites previously used present major problems to both the nephrologist and the vascular surgeon. The position of all previous access grafts should be carefully examined, because the inflow and outflow vessels may still be patent. In this case, reuse of the same vessels is often possible with a new graft positioned adjacent to the old graft. Occasionally, when only prosthetic grafts have previously been used, it may still be possible to fashion an autogenous AV fistula using one of the recommended alternative techniques. Otherwise, the use of proximal vessels or those within the thigh is recommended. We avoid attaching grafts to the subclavian or iliac arteries, because infection can be catastrophic, but recognize that in rare patients this may be the only site for maintaining life.

The Patient With Recurrent Thrombosis of Fistula or Graft

Patients who have access grafts for reasons other than chronic renal failure (eg, plasmapheresis or chemotherapy) are particularly liable to experience repeated episodes of thrombosis, as are patients with systemic lupus erythematosus, collagen diseases, or hypercoagulable blood states.[28] There remains a small group of chronic renal failure patients for whom access sites repeatedly thrombose for unknown reasons. It has been postulated that a consumptive deficiency of antithrombin III associated with repeated heparinization for hemodialysis may occur.[29] Fortunately, erythropoietin has not been found to be thrombogenic to vascular grafts.[30]

Prophylactic use of daily low-dose aspirin or aspirin and dipyridamole combinations has been recommended, because these drugs reduce aggregation and adherence of platelets to vascular endothelium and graft surfaces[31] and were shown to decrease the incidence of thrombotic episodes in external hemodialysis shunts.[32] We have successfully prolonged access patency with the use of warfarin in some patients. In the patient who has repeated thrombotic episodes within a prosthetic graft—without technical etiology, often caused by hypotensive episodes—renewed attempts to use autogenous construction and peritoneal dialysis should be considered or, as a last resort, a permanent percutaneous catheter can be placed.

REFERENCES

1. Gotch FA, Uehlinger DE. Mortality rates in U.S. dialysis patients. *Dial Transplant.* 1991;20:255-257.
2. Scribner BH. Circulatory access: still a major concern. *Proc Eur Dial Transplant Assoc Eur Ren Assoc.* 1982;19:95-98.
3. Harder F, Landmann J. Trends in access surgery for hemodialysis. *Surg Annu.* 1984;16:135-149.
4. Churchill DN, Taylor DW, Cook RJ, et al. Canadian Hemodialysis Morbidity Study. *Am J Kidney Dis.* 1992;19:214-234.
5. Lowrie EG, Lazarus JM, Mocelin AJ, et al. Survival of patients undergoing chronic hemodialysis and renal transplantation. *N Engl J Med.* 1973;288:863-867.
6. Brunner FP, Brynger H, Chantler C, et al. Combined report on regular dialysis and transplantation in Europe, IX, 1978. *Proc Eur Dial Transplant Assoc Eur Ren Assoc.* 1979;16:2-73.
7. Kinnaert P, Vereerstraeten P, Toussaint C, Van Geertruyden J. Nine years' experience with internal arteriovenous fistulas for haemodialysis: a study of some factors influencing the results. *Br J Surg.* 1977;64:242-246.
8. Vascular Access Work Group: NKF-DOQI clinical practice guidelines for vascular access. *Am J Kidney Dis.* 1997;30(suppl 3):S150-S191.
9. Hinsdale JG, Lipkowitz GS, Hoover EL. Vascular access for hemodialysis in the elderly: results and perspectives in a geriatric population. *Dial Transplant.* 1985;14:560-565.
10. White GH. Use of the brachial venae comitantes for hemodialysis access procedures. Unpublished data, 1995.
11. Brescia MJ, Cimino JE, Appel K, Hurwich BJ. Chronic hemodialysis using venipuncture and a surgically created arteriovenous fistula. *N Engl J Med.* 1960;275:1089-1092.
12. Mehigan JT, McAlexander RA. Snuffbox arteriovenous fistula for hemodialysis. *Am J Surg.* 1982;143:252-253.
13. Weitzig GA, Gough IR, Furnival CM. One hundred cases of arteriovenous fistula for haemodialysis access: the effect of cigarette smoking on patency. *Aust N Z J Surg.* 1985;55:551-554.
14. Dagher FJ. The upper arm AV hemoaccess: long-term follow-up. *J Cardiovasc Surg (Torino).*1986;27:447-449.
15. Bittner HB, Weaver JP. The brachioaxillary interposition graft as a successful tertiary vascular access procedure for hemodialysis. *Am J Surg.* 1994;167:615-617.
16. Gifford RM. Improved positioning of the upper arm graft fistula for hemodialysis. *Am J Surg.* 1986;151:407-408.
17. Friedman EA, Butt KM, Pascua LJ, Hardy MA, Lawton RL, Uldall PR. Panel conference: vascular access update. *Trans Am Soc Artif Intern Organs.* 1979;25:526-531.
18. Giacchino JL, Geis WP, Buckingham JM, Vertuno LL, Bansal VK. Vascular access: long-term results, new techniques, *Arch Surg.* 1979;114:403-409.
19. Tellis VA, Kohlberg WI, Bhat DJ, Driscoll B, Veith FJ. Expanded polytetrafluoroethylene graft fistula for chronic hemodialysis. *Ann Surg.* 1980;180:101-105.

20. Uldall PR, Dyck RF, Woods F. A subclavian cannula for temporary vascular access for hemodialysis or plasmapheresis. *Dial Transplant.* 1979;8:963-968.
21. Taucher LA. Immediate, safe hemodialysis into arteriovenous fistulas created with a new tunneler. *Am J Surg.* 1985;150:212-216.
22. Sidawy AN, Spergel LM, Besarab A, et al. The Society for Vascular Surgery: Clinical practice guidelines for the surgical placement and maintenance of arteriovenous hemodialysis access. *J Vasc Surg.* 2008; 48(suppl 5): 2S-25S.
23. Duncan H, Ferguson L, Faris I. Incidence of the radial steal syndrome in patients with Brescia fistula for hemodialysis: its clinical significance. *J Vasc Surg.* 1986;4:144-147.
24. Sprung J, et al. A rare complication of radial artery cannulation: gangrene in the distribution of radial artery supply. *Res Staff Physician.* 1993;39:31–33.
25. Purcell RR, Pena FG. Venous hypertension associated with asymptomatic bilateral axillary vein thrombosis and graft arteriovenous fistula. *Vasc Endovascular Surg.* 1985;19:270-273.
26. Matolo N, Kastagir B, Stevens LE, Chrysanthakopoulos S, Weaver DH, Klinkman H. Neurovascular complications of brachial arteriovenous fistula. *Am J Surg.* 1971;121:716-719.
27. Connolly JE, Brownell DA, Levine EF, McCart PM. Complications of renal dialysis access procedures. *Arch Surg.* 1984;119:1325-1328.
28. Humphries AL, Nesbit RR Jr, Caruana RJ, Hutchins RS, Heimburger RA, Wray CH. Thirty-six recommendations for vascular access operations: lessons learned from our first thousand operations. *Am J Surg.* 1981;47:145-151.
29. Brandt P, Jespersen J, Sorensen LH. Antithrombin III and platelets in haemodialysis patients. *Nephron.* 1981;28:1-3.
30. Standage BA, Schuman ES, Ackerman D, Gross GF, Ragsdale JW. Does the use of erythropoietin in hemodialysis patients increase dialysis graft thrombosis rates? *Am J Surg.* 1993;165:650-654.
31. Oblath RW, Buckley FO Jr, Green RM, Schwartz SI, DeWeese JA. Prevention of platelet aggregation and adherence to prosthetic vascular grafts by aspirin and dipyridamole. *Surgery.* 1978;84:37-44.
32. Harter HR, Burch JW, Majerus PW, et al. Prevention of thrombosis in patients on hemodialysis by low-dose aspirin. *N Engl J Med.* 1979; 301:577-579.

CHAPTER 3

Anesthesia for Vascular Access Surgery

Sarah J. Madison and Michael T. Alkire

Vascular access is required in patients undergoing hemodialysis or chronic infusion for chemotherapeutic agents, antimicrobials, and total parenteral nutrition. Candidates for vascular access surgery usually present significant anesthesia risks. In managing any seriously ill patient, meticulous preoperative preparation plays an important role, and teamwork between the surgeon and the anesthesiologist greatly improves the outcome. Every effort should be made to restore patients to optimal physiologic condition before subjecting them to the stress of surgery and the risks of anesthesia. Because an overwhelming majority of those presenting for vascular access procedures are chronic renal failure (CRF) patients, this chapter focuses on the anesthetic concerns in this patient group.

CRF

The end result of chronic renal disease is complete renal failure that requires dialysis or renal transplantation. The majority of surgical procedures for patients on dialysis are performed to establish vascular access for dialysis. Rational anesthetic management in these patients requires a thorough understanding of the functional changes characteristic of CRF, as listed in Table 3-1. A discussion of the implications of each dysfunction follows.

Table 3-1
Characteristic Changes of Chronic Renal Failure

Chronic anemia
Coagulopathies (platelet dysfunction)
Increased susceptibility to infection
Cardiovascular abnormalities (pericardial effusion, tamponade)
Hypertension
Unpredictable intravascular fluid volume
Electrolyte disturbances (hyperkalemia, hypermagnesemia, hypocalcemia)
Metabolic acidosis
Nervous system abnormalities (autonomic dysfunction, encephalopathy)
Gastrointestinal abnormalities (delayed emptying time, increased acid production)

Chronic Anemia

Hemoglobin values of less than 8 g/dL (hematocrit <24%) are commonly encountered in the functionally anephric patient. The primary causes of the normochromic, normocytic anemia of end-stage renal failure are decreased renal production of erythropoietin and a decrease in erythrocyte survival time of up to 50%. Other contributing factors include increased bleeding tendency (gastrointestinal and genitourinary), bone marrow toxicity from uremia, iron deficiency, and deficiencies of folate and vitamin B_{12} that develop from the combination of poor dietary intake and removal of these vitamins through dialysis.[1,2]

Anemia can lead to tissue hypoxia secondary to a reduction in blood oxygen-carrying capacity. Because the anemia develops slowly, compensatory mechanisms (increased cardiac output, decreased venous saturation, and decreased blood viscosity) can be used to maintain tissue oxygen delivery.[3] In addition, at the tissue level, oxygen dissociation from the blood is enhanced by a rightward shift in the oxyhemoglobin dissociation curve that is caused by the combined effects of metabolic acidosis and increased concentrations of 2,3-diphosphoglycerate. Renal failure patients often live in a perpetual state of abnormally high cardiac output, which reduces their available cardiac reserves for dealing with the stresses of anesthesia and surgery.

Hemoglobin levels of 6 to 8 g/dL are generally well tolerated by these patients because of the slow onset of anemia, and routine preoperative transfusion of blood is not recommended. However, if indicated (eg, owing to acutely decreasing hematocrit value or symptomatic patients), there is no need to withhold red blood cell transfusions. This population has a high incidence of concomitant coronary artery disease, and any signs of cardiac ischemia (eg, angina) coupled with anemia are strong indications for transfusion. It is possible that multiple transfusions sensitize a patient to histocompatibility antigens, which worsens the outcome for future transplants.[4] When transfusions are required, administer leukocyte-poor, packed red blood cells during dialysis. Transfusion during dialysis allows for the removal of excess potassium and fluid.

Exogenous administration of human recombinant erythropoietin can correct the anemia of CRF, improving the patient's ability to function and decreasing the need for blood transfusions.[5] Patients for whom anemia is corrected with this treatment usually have their cardiac function normalize. However, patients treated with erythropoietin may have increased problems with hypertension and thrombosis of arteriovenous (AV) fistulas. Risk of cardiovascular events in patients with chronic kidney disease does not change with correction of anemia.[6] In fact, a "black box" warning was issued by the U.S. Food and Drug Administration (FDA) in 2007 on erythropoietic agents, citing increased risk of thrombotic events and death. Recent guidelines dictate judicious use of erythropoietic agents for correction of hemoglobin levels in the 10- to 12-g/dL range.[7]

Coagulopathies

Suspect bleeding tendencies in all patients with CRF. Although platelet count and thrombopoietic (coagulation factor) activity are normal or only mildly decreased, platelet dysfunction occurs.[8] This dysfunction appears to be responsible for most of the coagulation abnormalities of CRF. Bleeding time prolongation and abnormal thromboelastograph (TEG) are usually the only tests that correlate with the risk of clinical bleeding in CRF patients. The cause of platelet dysfunction may be related to increased plasma levels of guanidinosuccinic acid, which causes a decline in platelet factor 3 availability. Lack of factor 3 inhibits secondary platelet aggregation. Dialysis partially corrects platelet dysfunction, and dialysis within 24 hours before surgery remains the standard preoperative hemostatic therapy in patients with CRF.[9] In addition to platelet dysfunction, the vitamin K–dependent factors (II, VII, IX, and X) and factor V tend to be low. Coexisting liver disease and heparinization from dialysis may also contribute to clotting abnormalities. Hemostatic therapy options in patients with CRF include platelet transfusion, fresh-frozen plasma, cryoprecipitate,[10] conjugated estrogen,[11] and 1-deamino-8-D-arginine vasopressin (DDAVP).[12] DDAVP decreases bleeding time by elevating circulating levels of factor VIII–von Willebrand complex.

Increased Susceptibility to Infection

CRF patients have increased susceptibility to infectious agents. In fact, sepsis is the most common cause of death in these patients. Although the basis of their susceptibility is unclear, multiple factors have been implicated in dialysis patients, including protein calorie malnutrition, cutaneous anergy, and functional abnormalities of neutrophils, monocytes, and macrophages.[13,14] CRF patients also have a high incidence of viral hepatitis (types B and C), often followed by residual hepatic dysfunction.[15]

Cardiovascular Abnormalities

Patients with CRF who have been on long-term hemodialysis develop atherosclerosis at an accelerated rate. The high incidence of ischemic heart disease may be the consequence of the nearly uniform presence of multiple cardiac risk factors, including diabetes and peripheral vascular disease. Goldman and colleagues[16] demonstrated that a serum creatinine level greater than 3 mg/dL was an independent cardiac risk factor for patients undergoing noncardiac surgery. A revision of the initial "Goldman criteria" retained serum creatinine greater than 2 mg/dL as a predictor of risk, but not an independent correlate of major cardiovascular

complications.[17] Congestive heart failure, pulmonary edema, pericarditis, and pericardial effusion are often seen in patients with CRF. The incidence of uremic pericarditis with or without cardiac tamponade has decreased with the availability of dialysis.

Hypertension

Hypertension is almost always present in patients with CRF. Intravascular volume expansion and activation of the renin-angiotensin-aldosterone system are the most probable explanations, although others have been proposed more recently.[18,19] Hemodialysis, fluid restriction, and dietary sodium reduction may control hypertension in many of these patients. However, in a few patients, hypertension is secondary to increased renin levels, and potent antihypertensive agents may be needed to control the blood pressure. The increased anesthetic risks associated with uncontrolled hypertension are well documented.

Unpredictable Intravascular Fluid Volume

Dialysis-dependent patients are at risk for both volume overload and hypovolemia. However, as with any other surgical patient, intravascular volume must be adequately maintained throughout the perioperative period. Intravascular volume status can be estimated by correlating body weight changes with changes in arterial blood pressure and heart rate before and after dialysis. Regardless of blood volume status, these patients often respond to induction of anesthesia as if they were hypovolemic. Intraoperative fluid losses should usually be replaced with potassium-free solutions.

Electrolyte Disturbances

Hyperkalemia is the most serious electrolyte abnormality in patients with CRF. Elective surgery should be postponed if the serum potassium concentration exceeds 5.5 mEq/L.[20] If surgery cannot be delayed, treat hyperkalemia with glucose-insulin infusion, hyperventilation, sodium bicarbonate, and calcium chloride. All patients on hemodialysis should receive dialysis therapy within 12 to 24 hours before surgery. The use of succinylcholine should probably be avoided when the potassium concentration exceeds 5.5 mEq/L. Rocuronium is a suitable alternative for rapid-sequence induction, but it may have prolonged effects in patients with renal failure.[21] This restriction may place the anesthesiologist in a difficult situation because these patients often have gastroparesis and other conditions that place them at high risk for aspiration during anesthesia induction. Other electrolyte abnormalities are also common, including hypermagnesemia, hyperphosphatemia, and hypocalcemia. The latter can predispose these patients to hypotension during general anesthesia.

Metabolic Acidosis

In patients with CRF, a metabolic acidosis with increased anion gap develops secondary to accumulation of fixed acids (sulfates and phosphates) that are produced through normal metabolic processes. Chronic metabolic acidosis stimulates compensatory hyperventilation, and acidosis may alter the efficacy of local anesthetics used during surgery. Dialysis is generally effective in correcting acidosis. For patients who require emergency surgery in the presence of severe metabolic acidosis (pH < 7.15), it is generally recommended that the pH be increased to greater than 7.25 and the bicarbonate level be increased to greater than 18 mEq/L through administration of sodium bicarbonate. Exercise caution during bicarbonate administration because of its potentially serious side effects, which may include volume overload, precipitation of tetany in patients with preexisting hypocalcemia, and acute hypokalemia.

Nervous System Abnormalities

Autonomic nervous system dysfunction commonly accompanies CRF (particularly in diabetics) and may contribute to attenuated compensatory responses to intravascular volume changes. Furthermore, autonomic nervous system dysfunction independently increases anesthetic risk, and adverse events have been reported after induction of regional anesthetics.[22] In patients with severe CRF, uremic encephalopathy may occur. Manifestations vary from subtle personality changes to lethargy, seizures, and coma.[23] Dialysis may be effective in improving both uremic encephalopathy and autonomic neuropathy.

Gastrointestinal Abnormalities

Patients with CRF often have delayed gastric-emptying time; increased gastric juice volume and acid production; and increased incidence of nausea, vomiting, and peptic ulceration. Pulmonary aspiration of stomach contents is a potentially fatal complication, so aspiration precautions must be taken during general anesthesia induction and emergence. This usually implies a rapid-sequence induction of anesthesia, to minimize the time during which the unconscious patient has an unprotected airway.

Pharmacology

Many drugs used in the perioperative period depend on renal excretion for elimination. In the presence of CRF, standard dosages may have an exaggerated or prolonged effect. The systemic effects of azotemia can stimulate the pharmacologic actions of many of these agents. Some drugs, such as metacurine and gallamine, are exclusively dependent on renal excretion and thus are contraindicated in these patients.

The administration of succinylcholine, a depolarizing neuromuscular blocking agent, increases serum potassium concentration by 0.5 mEq/L or more in patients with or without renal failure. Succinylcholine should probably be avoided in anephric patients when serum potassium is greater than 5.5 mEq/L.[24] Pretreatment with a small dose of a nondepolarizing muscle relaxant does not reliably attenuate the succinylcholine-induced release of potassium. Dialysis treatment may lower the levels of plasma cholinesterase, the enzyme responsible for metabolizing succinylcholine, producing a slightly prolonged response to succinylcholine. Despite these hazards, succinylcholine

remains the most rapid onset muscle relaxant for obtaining intubation conditions in the shortest possible time.

Rocuronium is a rapidly acting, nondepolarizing muscle relaxant that may be used for rapid-sequence induction. Its effects last much longer than those of succinylcholine, especially in patients with renal failure, which may be disadvantageous for operations lasting less than 1 hour.[21] Atracurium is eliminated by ester hydrolysis and Hofmann degradation (a nonenzymatic degradation independent of renal function) and, therefore, is a neuromuscular blocking agent useful in patients with renal failure. The duration of action of atracurium is not prolonged in renal failure. cis-Atracurium is an isomer of atracurium with similar pharmacokinetics, but it has twice the potency of the former drug and, hence, a lower incidence of side effects, which are primarily caused by histamine release.

Volatile anesthetic agents are good choices in patients with CRF because of their lack of dependence on the kidneys for elimination and their ability to control blood pressure, facilitate neuromuscular blockade, and withstand modest effects on renal blood flow. Classically, it has been thought that with some volatile anesthetics, biotransformation by oxidative dehalogenation to inorganic fluoride may result in nephrotoxicity. Fluoride-induced nephrotoxicity depends on the extent of anesthetic metabolism and the duration of exposure. This toxicity is characterized by an inability to concentrate urine, which may result in polyuria, hypernatremia, and elevated serum osmolality. Owing to its fluoride nephrotoxicity, methoxyflurane (Penthrane) is no longer used in the United States. Methoxyflurane can produce toxic fluoride levels in only 2.5 to 3 (MAC)-hours. The biotransformation of enflurane may also lead to release of free fluoride; however, the usual levels of fluoride required to produce nephrotoxicity (50 μmol/L) are rarely exceeded in clinical conditions. Sevoflurane can be metabolized to produce the nephrotoxic "compound A," and there is conflicting evidence as to whether this is ever clinically significant.[25] Biotransformation of halothane, isoflurane, and desflurane to inorganic fluoride is insufficient to produce even a theoretical risk of fluoride-induced nephrotoxicity. More recent work, however, suggests that fluoride may not be the culprit it was once thought to be.

Most narcotic agents used today are inactivated by the liver through conjugation or metabolic breakdown. Significant accumulation of active metabolites generally does not occur, with the exception of morphine and meperidine.[26,27] The accumulation of morphine and meperidine metabolites (normorphine and normeperidine) has been associated with prolonged respiratory depression and excessive sedation. Normeperidine has also been associated with seizures in animal models.

Preoperative Evaluation

A comprehensive preoperative history and physical examination are essential. In addition, preoperative dialysis is commonly required to normalize volume status and electrolyte levels. Give special attention to preoperative volume status. A review of the patient's predialysis and postdialysis weights may be helpful. Assessment of cardiac risk for patients undergoing major or minor noncardiac surgery

Table 3-2

Major Cardiac Complications Among Patients With Individual Risk Factors

Risk Factor	Risk Percent
High-risk surgery	3-4
Ischemic heart disease	4-5
History of congestive heart failure	5-7
History of cerebrovascular disease	6-7
Insulin therapy for diabetes	5-6
Preoperative serum creatinine >2.0 mg/dL	5-9

From Lee TH, Marcantonio ER, Mangione CM, et al. Derivation and prospective validation of a simple index for prediction of cardiac risk of major noncardiac surgery. *Circulation*. 1999;100:1043-1049.

may be guided by the American Heart Association Cardiac Risk Index (Table 3-2). Presence of two or more of these factors is associated with higher complication rates in the perioperative period.[17] Most recently, the guidelines for definitive preemptive cardiac evaluation and treatment have been greatly revised (Table 3-3). Evaluation guidelines now suggest further workup is generally reserved for the sickest patients.

Laboratory evaluation of the patient with CRF should include a complete blood count to determine baseline hemoglobin level and platelet count. Generally, reserve preoperative red blood cell transfusions for severely anemic patients (hemoglobin < 6–7 g/dL), those with symptoms of tissue hypoxia (eg, angina), or those in whom significant blood loss is anticipated. If regional anesthesia is being considered, obtain bleeding time and coagulation studies. Remember that a TEG or bleeding time may be the only abnormal coagulation test. Evaluate serum electrolytes, especially potassium, after dialysis. Evaluate blood urea nitrogen and creatinine measurements after dialysis for adequacy of dialysis. Carefully examine an electrocardiogram for evidence of ischemic heart disease, hypertensive cardiovascular disease, pericardial effusion, and electrolyte abnormalities. Obtain a chest radiograph when indicated by the patient's medical condition or other risk factors (eg, smoking).

Anesthetic premedication agents are usually limited to alert patients who are relatively stable. Benzodiazepines, barbiturates, and narcotics may cause excessive sedation in patients with CRF because of relative hypoproteinemia, which may result in decreased protein binding and impaired renal elimination of active metabolites. Continue the patient's usual medications through the perioperative period, with the possible exception of certain antidepressant drugs such as monoamine oxidase inhibitors and tricyclic antidepressants.

Monitoring

Base intraoperative monitoring for patients with CRF on the same physiologic considerations applied to all patients. Invasive hemodynamic monitoring may be indicated by

Table 3-3

American Heart Guidelines 2007: Active Cardiac Conditions for Which the Patient Should Undergo Evaluation and Treatment

Condition	Examples
Unstable coronary syndromes	Unstable or severe angina (CCS class III or IV) Recent myocardial infarction
Decompensated HF (NYHA functional class IV; worsening or new-onset HF)	
Significant arrhythmias	High-grade atrioventricular block Mobitz II atrioventricular block Third-degree atrioventricular heart block Symptomatic ventricular arrhythmias Supraventricular arrhythmias (including atrial fibrillation) with uncontrolled ventricular rate (HR > 100 beats/min at rest) Symptomatic bradycardia Newly recognized ventricular tachycardia
Severe valvular disease	Severe aortic stenosis (mean pressure gradient >40 mm Hg, aortic valve area <1.0 cm², or symptomatic) Symptomatic mitral stenosis (progressive dyspnea on exertion, exertional presyncope, or HF)

Canadian Cardiovascular Society HF, heart failure; HR, heart rate; NYHA, New York Heart Association. From Fleisher LA, Beckman JA, Brown KA, et al. ACC/AHA 2007 guidelines on perioperative cardiovascular evaluation and care for noncardiac surgery: a report of the American College of Cardiology/American Heart Association Task Force on Practice Guidelines. *Circulation*. 2007;116:e418-e499.

the presence of concomitant diseases (especially cardiac), anticipated volume shifts, and overall clinical impression. Standards for intraoperative monitoring during general anesthesia, as established by the American Society of Anesthesiologists (ASA), include the electrocardiogram, blood pressure, body temperature, respiratory rate, oxygen saturation, end-tidal carbon dioxide, stethoscope, and inspired oxygen concentration. Noninvasive blood pressure should not be measured in a limb with a functioning vascular shunt.

Anesthesia Management

All appropriate forms of anesthesia, including general, regional, and local infiltration anesthesia, may be used safely in patients who require vascular access.[28] Procedures to establish vascular access are usually well tolerated in most patients. Regardless of the anesthetic method used, surgical deaths are rare. Because of the increased risk of pulmonary aspiration and the high incidence of concomitant coronary artery disease in many of these patients, regional or local anesthesia is often advantageous. Furthermore, a prospective observational study by Glover and coworkers[29] showed that brachial plexus block may improve patency and graft survival.

General Anesthesia

All patients with CRF who are scheduled for general anesthesia should be considered to have a full stomach and should undergo rapid-sequence induction with cricoid pressure (the Sellick maneuver). The induction of anesthesia can be accomplished safely with propofol, etomidate, barbiturates, narcotics, or midazolam plus succinylcholine (see previously mentioned precautions). Patients with CRF tend to respond to the induction of anesthesia as if they were hypovolemic, regardless of their actual blood volume status. Patients who are hypovolemic or those on antihypertensive medications that attenuate sympathetic nervous system responses may have exaggerated reductions in blood pressure. Institution of positive-pressure ventilation and abrupt changes in body position may contribute to decreased blood pressure. Also, these patients often have autonomic dysfunction that may impede their ability to compensate for anesthetic-induced vasodilation.

Brachial Plexus Blockade[30,31]

Brachial plexus blocks are the most commonly used anesthetic technique for patients undergoing vascular access procedures. Brachial plexus blocks may offer greater intraoperative hemodynamic stability than general anesthesia. Because of their effects, these blocks are associated with higher blood flows in newly created AV fistulas than are general or local techniques.[32] It has been suggested that the duration of brachial plexus anesthesia is shortened in patients with CRF; however, controlled studies have not confirmed this. Difficulty in placing brachial plexus blocks using nerve stimulation techniques alone may arise in patients with severe neuropathy. Ultrasound-only techniques have been used with success in such cases.[33]

The four commonly used techniques for blocking the brachial plexus are the axillary, supraclavicular, infraclavicular, and interscalene blocks. The latter three approaches can be used for any operation at the shoulder level and distal. The axillary approach is used primarily for surgery distal to the elbow, because it covers the more caudad nerves of the brachial plexus. The supraclavicular and infraclavicular approaches give a more homogeneous coverage, and the interscalene approach results in blockade of the cephalad portions of the brachial plexus as well as the caudad portions of the cervical plexus.[34]

Axillary Brachial Plexus Block

The axillary approach is the simplest and most commonly performed block of the brachial plexus. Although the axillary block has the best success rate in the distribution of the ulnar nerve (C7-T1), with anesthesia also in the median and the radial distributions, axillary techniques often fail to block the musculocutaneous (C5) and intercostobrachial (T1-T4) nerves. Supplemental block of the musculocutaneous nerve is necessary for complete anesthesia of the forearm and wrist. It is most useful for surgeries of the forearm and hand. The axillary brachial plexus block may be performed using paresthesia, nerve stimulation, ultrasound, or a combined technique, but success rates appear to be higher when ultrasound is used.[35] First identify the pulse of the axillary artery just anterior to the posterior axillary fold next to the coracobrachialis muscle and trace it proximally into the apex of the axilla.

If ultrasound is used, place a linear probe perpendicular to the axillary fold to identify in short axis the axillary artery, vein, and brachial plexus. Anatomic landmarks in this view include the humerus deep and lateral to the neurovascular bundle (NVB), biceps muscle superficial and lateral to the NVB, and coracobrachialis muscle lateral to the NVB. Identify the axillary artery and vein using Doppler if necessary, and visualize the nerves within the sheath with median nerve anterior and lateral to the artery, ulnar nerve posterior and medial to the artery, and radial nerve posterior and lateral to the artery. The musculocutaneous nerve is located just lateral and anterior to the NVB in the fascial plane between the biceps and the coracobrachialis muscles.

For nerve stimulation and combined out-of-plane ultrasound techniques, place a short (5-cm) 22-gauge stimulating needle just overlying the axillary pulse at an angle 45 degrees cephalad and advanced 1 to 2 cm. End-points for stimulation include a twitch of the hand in median, radial, or ulnar distribution at 0.2 to 0.4 mA. Multiple-injection techniques may speed onset and improve block quality.[36,37] Acceptance of stimulation greater than 0.6 mA is associated with a lower success rate.[38] Alternatively, a paresthesia may be elicited in the same distribution without stimulation. Use a transarterial technique if arterial blood is aspirated during needle placement; this technique was shown to be both effective and safe in a review by Hudson and associates.[39]

The musculocutaneous nerve can be blocked by a separate needle insertion above the artery toward the coracobrachialis muscle just deep to the insertion of the pectoralis major muscle. Elicit biceps muscle twitch at 0.2 to 0.4 mA and inject 5 mL of local anesthetic.

For a pure ultrasound in-plane technique, needle placement is more anterior with the needle advancing posteriorly, parallel to the ultrasound probe. Inject local anesthetic within the NVB under direct visualization, usually with three injections next to each of the three target nerves.[40] Musculocutaneous nerve can also be identified and blocked under ultrasound guidance.[41,42] If a stimulating needle is used, D_5W can be used for fluid dissection during ultrasound guidance.[43]

Regardless of technique, inject a large volume of local anesthetic (35–40 mL) with aspiration every 5 mL to avoid inadvertent intravascular injection, a potentially catastrophic event.[44-47] Block onset is usually around 15 to 25 minutes, with loss of coordination of the arm as the first sign of a potentially successful block. The axilla is a highly vascularized area with potential for local anesthetic toxicity by intravascular injection and channeling of local anesthetic into small veins traumatized by needle insertion. The use of bupivicaine is thus not recommended. For any brachial plexus block, pain on injection or needle placement, high injection pressure, and stimulation currents below 0.2 mA are indicative of possible intraneural needle placement, which could potentially lead to peripheral nerve injury. After arterial puncture, pressure should be held for at least 5 minutes. Frequent and careful aspiration during performance of the block, as well as gentle injection of local anesthetic, is recommended to avoid complications.

Supraclavicular Brachial Plexus Block

The supraclavicular brachial plexus block, placed at the level of trunks and divisions of the brachial plexus, offers high success rates for hand surgery. Previously noted complications using traditional techniques are significantly reduced with the use of ultrasound.[48,49] The quality and speed of onset of the block are probably superior with an ultrasound technique as well. In a retrospective review of ultrasound-guided supraclavicular blocks with and without nerve stimulation, Beach and colleagues[50] observed that nerve stimulation does not improve block success and may be an unnecessary extra step.

Position the patient supine with the head turned away from the side to be blocked. The clavicular head of the sternocleidomastoid muscle and the pulse of the subclavian artery are useful surface landmarks because the brachial plexus lies posterolateral to these structures. A small, high-frequency probe that is either curved or linear is often used. Local structures include the first rib located just inferior to the brachial plexus, the apex of the lung medial to the first rib, and the subclavian artery, which courses medial to the plexus and passes laterally over the first rib. Place the probe just above the clavicle over the area of the subclavian artery, which may be confirmed by Doppler. A cluster of hypoechoic trunks can be visualized superolateral to the artery. Medial and deep to the artery is the first rib, which is hyperechoic and linear in appearance. The pleura is just deep to the first rib and appears as a hyperechoic line.

Needle placement for an in-plane technique (recommended) is just lateral to the probe immediately above the clavicle, in a lateral-to-medial direction (a medial-to-lateral approach has been described). The needle may be angled slightly cephalad to avoid the apex of the lung. If a stimulating needle is used for confirmation, acceptable twitches may include pectoralis, deltoid, biceps, triceps, forearm, and hand at 0.4 mA or less. Injection around the lower trunks may yield better anesthesia of the hand. Injection of D_5W may be useful to visualize the spreading of injectate around the plexus without compromising nerve stimulation.

Limitations of this block include the higher risk of subclavian artery puncture and pneumothorax (≤1% of cases). Additional complications with this block include unintended paralysis of the phrenic and the recurrent laryngeal nerves, owing to their proximity.[51,52] In addition, the proximity of the stellate ganglion to the site of injection can sometimes result in Horner's syndrome.

Infraclavicular Brachial Plexus Block

The infraclavicular approach to the brachial plexus has gained popularity in recent years over other approaches, especially with the advent of ultrasound.[53-57] It provides adequate coverage for procedures involving the hand, wrist, forearm, elbow, and distal arm, including areas supplied by the ulnar and often musculocutaneous and intercostobrachial nerves.[58] It is not associated with the pulmonary complications often seen with the interscalene approach.[59,60] The cords of the brachial plexus lie beneath the pectoralis muscles surrounding the subclavian artery, inferior to the clavicle and coracoid process.

Position the patient supine with the head turned away from the side to be blocked, with the arm on the side to be blocked either abducted with the elbow flexed or resting at the patient's side.[61] The clavicle, coracoid process, and sternal notch should be palpated easily. Ultrasound probe placement is below the clavicle in the parasagittal plane, lateral to mid-clavicle and medial to the coracoid process.[61] The subclavian artery and vein should be identified as anechoic structures, confirmed with Doppler. The lateral cord lies cephalad and superficial to the artery, the medial cord caudad to the artery, and the posterior cord posterior and slightly cephalad. The pleura may be visible as a hyperechoic line just posterior to the NVB. For an in-plane ultrasound technique, needle placement is just cephalad to the ultrasound probe at an angle of 45 to 60 degrees to the skin. To avoid complications, visualization of the entire shaft of the needle is recommended during the entire block procedure. Deposition of local anesthetic may be divided between the three cords, with visualization of local anesthetic spread around the hyperechoic structures, although a single-injection technique about the posterior cord may be adequate.[62-64] If a combined technique is used, D_5W may be used for visualization of injectate before deposition of local anesthetic.

For a nerve stimulation or combined out-of-plane ultrasound technique, place a 10-cm 22-gauge stimulating needle 2 cm inferior to the midpoint of the clavicle and advance it laterally at a 45-degree angle. Insertion points above the coracoid process have also been described.[58] Advance the needle slowly until the brachial plexus is encountered, indicated by distal twitches.[65] Injection of a large volume of local anesthetic (35–40 mL) should yield an adequate block within 5 to 15 minutes.

Complications with infraclavicular block are rare, especially with the use of ultrasound. Vascular puncture and pneumothorax are of primary concern to most practitioners, and performance of brachial plexus block at any level carries the risk of local anesthetic toxicity with or without intravascular injection, damage to local structures, and nerve injury.

Interscalene Brachial Plexus Block

The interscalene brachial plexus block creates anesthesia of the shoulder, arm, and elbow (local supplementation may be required for shoulder surgeries). It fails to fully block the ulnar nerve 10% to 20% of the time, which makes it suboptimal for surgeries distal to the elbow. The brachial plexus lies between the anterior and the middle scalene muscles in the interscalene groove, with the internal jugular vein and common carotid artery located anteromedially. The phrenic nerve generally runs alongside the anterior scalene muscle anteriorly.

Generally, perform the block with the patient positioned supine, with the head of the bed elevated slightly and the patient's head turned away from the side to be blocked. First identify the sternal notch, clavicle, sternal head of the sternocleidomastoid muscle, and the mastoid process. If ultrasound is used, place a linear probe transversely over the interscalene groove at the level of C6. Identifiable structures at this level include the common carotid artery and internal jugular vein in short axis, which may be confirmed with Doppler, appearing as anechoic structures deep to the sternocleidomastoid muscle. The anterior scalene muscle lies just posterior to the sternocleidomastoid muscle, with the middle and posterior scalene muscles immediately posterolateral to it. The roots of the brachial plexus may be identified posterolateral to the vessels between the anterior and the middle scalene muscles, appearing as small, round, hypoechoic structures.[66]

If an in-plane ultrasound technique is used, needle placement is just lateral to the probe, angled medially so as to be aligned with the ultrasound beam. The needle should be visualized passing through the middle scalene muscle and into the plexus sheath. If nerve stimulation is used, a D_5W solution may be injected to confirm appropriate spread of injectate around the plexus before injection of local anesthetic.

For an out-of-plane ultrasound technique, needle placement is overlying the brachial plexus at the level of C6. Angle the needle in a slightly caudad direction, parallel to the ultrasound beam. For a nerve stimulation technique, place the nondominant hand firmly between the anterior and the middle scalene muscles (scalene muscles are more easily identified by asking the patient to sniff). Needle insertion is between the anterior and the middle scalene muscles at the level of the cricoid cartilage (C6) with the needle directed at an angle perpendicular to the skin surface. A twitch should be elicited at a depth of 1 to 2 cm. Acceptable end-points for stimulation include twitches of the pectoralis, deltoid, triceps, biceps, forearm, or hand at 0.2 to 0.4 mA.[67-69] Inject a large volume (35–40 mL) of local anesthetic with aspiration every 5 mL to avoid inadvertent intravascular injection. Block onset is usually around 15 to 25 minutes, with loss of coordination of the arm as the first sign of a potentially successful block.

Complications with this block are rare,[70] but two that are unique to this approach are the intra-arterial injection of local anesthetic agent into the vertebral artery and the injection of local anesthetic agent into the epidural, subarachnoid, or subdural spaces, or even into the spinal cord, which may result in total spinal anesthesia especially with injection at stimulation less than 0.2 mA.[71-73] Pain on injection or needle placement, high injection pressure, and stimulation currents below 0.2 mA are indicative of possible intraneural needle placement. It is recommended that a shorter needle be used for safety in block performance.[73] Frequent and careful aspiration during performance of the block, as well as gentle injection of local anesthetic, is recommended to avoid complications. Undesirable side effects of interscalene brachial plexus block include Horner's syndrome, hoarse voice, nasal congestion, and phrenic nerve paralysis. Forced expiratory volume in 1 second (FEV1) and forced vital capacity (FVC) may be reduced by as much as 30%, which may make interscalene block less suitable for patients with reduced pulmonary reserve.[74]

Lower Extremity Blockade

Some vascular access procedures are performed on the lower extremities. Available regional anesthetic techniques include spinal, epidural, caudal, and lumbar plexus anesthesia and peripheral nerve block. Care must be taken with the neuraxial regional techniques (spinal and epidural) because the resultant loss of vascular tone may cause hypotension. Other potential side effects include high block, accidental intravascular injection of anesthetic agent or epinephrine, and toxicity from anesthetic overdose. Contraindications to regional anesthesia include lack of patient consent or cooperation, hypovolemia, coagulopathy, infection at the skin entry site, sepsis or bacteremia, elevated intracranial pressure, and allergy to local anesthetics.

Monitored Anesthesia Care

Monitored anesthesia care (also called MAC), formerly called "local-standby," refers to the administration of intravenous sedatives, analgesic agents, and amnesic agents as supplements to a primarily local anesthetic technique. Patients scheduled for local or regional anesthesia require the same preoperative evaluation as patients scheduled for general anesthesia because any regional or monitored anesthesia care procedure might become a general anesthesia procedure. Patients undergoing surgery with local or regional anesthesia are usually more comfortable with the use of additional medications. The proper administration of monitored anesthesia care is a skill that avoids depression of protective airway reflexes while maintaining the patient's comfort and ability to respond. During monitored anesthesia care, the anesthesiologist monitors the level of patient awareness by speaking to the patient frequently. The anesthesiologist's role includes being reassuring and alerting the patient of upcoming surgical events. The ASA standards for basic intraoperative monitoring apply to sedation techniques that are a part of monitored anesthesia care. Specific and diligent monitoring by the anesthesiologist is necessary because of the synergistic interactions between sedative and analgesic drugs with respect to respiratory

Table 3-4

Local Anesthetic Agents: Dosages for Infiltration Anesthesia

Drug	Usual Concentration (%)	Plain Solution		Epinephrine-Containing Solution	
		Maximum Dose (mg)	Duration (min)	Maximum Dose (mg)	Duration (min)
Esters					
Procaine	1.0	1000	30-60		
Chloroprocaine	1.0-2.0	800	30-45	1000	30-90
Amides					
Lidocaine	0.5-2.0	300	30-120	500	120-360
Mepivacaine	0.5-1.0	300	45-90	500	120-360
Prilocaine	0.5-1.0	500	30-90	600	120-360
Bupivacaine	0.25-0.5	175	120-240	225	180-420
Ropivacaine	0.2-1.0	300	360-600	Not used	
Etidocaine	0.5-1.0	300	120-180	400	180-420

A 0.5% solution contains 5 mg/mL, a 1.0% solution contains 10 mg/mL, and a 2.0% solution contains 20 mg/mL.

and cardiovascular depression. These cases can be very challenging for the anesthesia care provider.

Local Anesthetic Agents

The choice of local anesthetic agent must take into consideration the duration of surgery, regional technique used, surgical requirements, and potential for local or systemic toxicity. Local anesthetic agents, which block impulse conduction by reversible inhibition of sodium ion influx, can be separated chemically into two groups: amino ester and amino amide agents (Table 3-4). Ester local anesthetics are hydrolyzed by esterase in the liver and by cholinesterase in the plasma. The liver exclusively metabolizes amide local anesthetics. The use of propofol for sedation after brachial plexus blockade may prolong the effects of amide local anesthetics by competitive inhibition of the cytochrome P-450 (CYP-450) system.[75]

Epinephrine (or, less commonly, phenylephrine) can be added to local anesthetics to prolong the duration of action, decrease systemic toxicity, increase the intensity of the block, and decrease surgical bleeding.[76] Do not use epinephrine in peripheral nerve blocks in areas with poor collateral blood flow (eg, fingers, toes, nose, genitals), particularly in patients with peripheral vascular disease. Clonidine is an alternative adjuvant for prolonging duration of blockade and has been used safely in patients with renal failure.[77] Alkalinization of local anesthetics with bicarbonate has been shown to result in a more rapid onset and a more profound degree of conduction blockade.[78] The addition of sodium bicarbonate to local anesthetics raises the pH and increases the concentration of nonionized free base, increasing the rate of diffusion and speed of neural blockade onset.[79]

True allergic reactions to local anesthetics are rare. Allergic reactions are primarily due to methylparaben (preservative) or to ester local anesthetics, which produce the metabolite para-aminobenzoic acid (PABA). Amide local anesthetics have essentially no allergic potential, with ropi-

vacaine as a possible exception. An easy way to differentiate the local anesthetics is to note that all amides have the letter i in the first part of the word before the "-caine."

Accidental intravascular injection of a local anesthetic agent can result in systemic toxicity that involves the central nervous system (producing light-headedness, dizziness, tinnitus, metallic taste, visual disturbances, perioral numbness, seizures, and unconsciousness)[80] and the cardiovascular system (producing myocardial depression, decreased cardiac output, dysrhythmias, loss of vasomotor tone, decreased conduction, and cardiac arrest).[47,81] Ropivacaine is less likely to cause central nervous system and cardiovascular toxicity than bupivacaine, although toxicity has been reported at doses as low as 6.25 mg/kg for brachial plexus blockade.[82] The formation of methemoglobin is a side effect associated with prilocaine and benzocaine. Rescue from local anesthetic overdose can be facilitated by the infusion of 20% intralipid.[83,84]

Topical Anesthesia

Topical anesthesia can be used as a supplement to the administration of local infiltration anesthesia. Methods for the topical application of local anesthetic agents include ointment-based and iontophoresis techniques. The ointment-based techniques include EMLA cream, patch-based techniques, and gel-based techniques. EMLA cream is a eutectic mixture of local anesthetic (EMLA) following "agents" that contains equal amounts of lidocaine (2.5%) and prilocaine (2.5%).[85] It has been formulated to penetrate intact skin and provide anesthesia to a depth sufficient for the performance of needle puncture and superficial skin procedures. It is gaining popularity as a method for allowing painless venipuncture and is only limited by a few side effects related to local circulation, primarily pallor, erythema, or edema. To be fully effective, EMLA requires 30 to 60 minutes of elapsed time after application.

Concluding Remarks

Patients who require vascular access surgery usually have additional risk factors that make the selection and administration of anesthesia particularly important. Most of these patients are in CRF, which by itself creates a number of important anesthetic considerations. Furthermore, renal failure patients often have serious coexisting diseases including diabetes, hypertension, coronary artery disease, and peripheral vascular disease. All of these increase anesthesia risk and influence the selection of techniques and monitoring. Vascular access surgical procedures, which often seem minor in themselves, require a skilled anesthesiologist and a close working relationship between the anesthesiologist and the surgeon.

This updated and expanded chapter was revised from a version written by Mark R. Ezekiel, MD, Michael T. Alkire, MD, and Steven J. Barker, PhD, MD.

REFERENCES

1. Bansal VK, Popli S, Pickering J, Ing TS, Vertuno LL, Hano JE. Protein-calorie malnutrition and cutaneous anergy in hemodialysis maintained patients. *Am J Clin Nutr.* 1980;33:1608-1611.
2. Young GA, Swanepoel CR, Croft MR, Hobson SM, Parsons FM. Anthropometry and plasma valine, amino acids, and proteins in the nutritional assessment of hemodialysis patients. *Kidney Int.* 1982;21: 492-499.
3. Capelli JP, Kasparian H. Cardiac work demands and left ventricular function in end-stage renal disease. *Ann Intern Med.* 1977;86:261-267.
4. Poli F, Scalamogna M, Cardillo M, Porta E, Sirchia G. An algorithm for cadaver kidney allocation based on a multivariate analysis of factors impacting on cadaver kidney graft survival and function. *Transpl Int.* 2000;13(suppl 1):S259-S262.
5. Eschbach JW, Egrie JC, Downing MR, Downing MR, Browne JK, Adamson JW. Correction of the anemia of end-stage renal disease with recombinant human erythropoietin. Results of a combined phase I and II clinical trial. *N Engl J Med.* 1987;316:73-78.
6. Drueke TB. Normalization of hemoglobin level in patients with chronic kidney disease and anemia. *N Engl J Med.* 2006;355:2071-2084.
7. Moist LM, Foley RN, Barrett BJ, et al. Clinical practice guidelines for evidence-based use of erythropoietic-stimulating agents. *Kidney Int Suppl.* 2008;110:S12-S18.
8. Gafter U, Bessler H, Malachi T, Zevin D, Djaldetti M, Levi J. Platelet count and thrombopoietic activity in patients with chronic renal failure. *Nephron.* 1987;45:207-210.
9. Di Minno G, Martinez J, McKean ML, et al. Platelet dysfunction in uremia. Multifaceted defect partially corrected by dialysis. *Am J Med.* 1985;79:552-559.
10. Janson PA, Jubelirer SJ, Weinstein MJ, Deykin D. Treatment of the bleeding tendency in uremia with cryoprecipitate. *N Engl J Med.* 1980;303:1318-1322.
11. Livio M, Mannucci PM, Viganò G, et al. Conjugated estrogens for the management of bleeding associated with renal failure. *N Engl J Med.* 1986;315:731-735.
12. Kentro TB, Lottenberg R, Kitchens CS. Clinical efficacy of desmopressin acetate for hemostatic control in patients with primary platelet disorders undergoing surgery. *Am J Hematol.* 1987;24:215-219.
13. Lewis SL, Van Epps DE. Neutrophil and monocyte alterations in chronic dialysis patients. *Am J Kidney Dis.* 1987;9:381-395.
14. Ruiz P, Gomez F, Schreiber AD. Impaired function of macrophage Fc gamma receptors in end-stage renal disease. *N Engl J Med.* 1990;322: 717-722.
15. Shusterman N, Singer I. Infectious hepatitis in dialysis patients. *Am J Kidney Dis.* 1987;9:447-455.
16. Goldman L, Caldera DL, Nussbaum SR, et al. Multifactorial index of cardiac risk in noncardiac surgical procedures. *N Engl J Med.* 1977;297:845-850.
17. Lee TH, Marcantonio ER, Mangione CM, et al. Derivation and prospective validation of a simple index for prediction of cardiac risk of major noncardiac surgery. *Circulation.* 1999;100:1043-1049.
18. Hoy WE, Hughson MD, Bertram JF, Douglas-Denton R, Amann K. Nephron number, hypertension, renal disease, and renal failure. *J Am Soc Nephrol.* 2005;16:2557-2564.
19. Ketteler M, Gross M-L, Ritz E. Hypertension and cardiovascular diseases in progressive renal failure. Calcification and cardiovascular problems in renal failure. *Kidney Int.* 2005;s120.
20. Weir PH, Chung FF. Anaesthesia for patients with chronic renal disease. *Can Anaesth Soc J.* 1984;31:468-481.
21. Robertson EN, Driessen JJ, Booij LHDJ. Pharmacokinetics and pharmacodynamics of rocuronium in patients with and without renal failure. *Eur J Anaesthesiol.* 2005;22:4-10.
22. Lucas LF, Tsueda K. Cardiovascular depression after brachial plexus block in two diabetic patients with renal failure. *Anesthesiology.* 1990;73:1032-1035.
23. Brouns R, De Deyn PP. Neurological complications in renal failure: a review. *Clin Neurol Neurosurg.* 2004;107:1-16.
24. Thapa S, Brull SJ. Succinylcholine-induced hyperkalemia in patients with renal failure: an old question revisited. *Anesth Analg.* 2000;91: 237-241.
25. Ebert TD, Frink EJ, Kharasch ED. Absence of biochemical evidence for renal and hepatic dysfunction after 8 hours of 1.25 minimum alveolar concentration sevoflurane anesthesia in volunteers. *Anesthesiology.* 1998;88:601-610.
26. Chauvin M, Sandouk P, Scherrmann JM, Farinotti R, Strumza P, Duvaldestin P. Morphine pharmacokinetics in renal failure. *Anesthesiology.* 1987;66:327-331.
27. Szeto HH, Inturrisi CE, Houde R, Saal S, Cheigh J, Reindenberg MM. Accumulation of normeperidine, an active metabolite of meperidine, in patients with renal failure of cancer. *Ann Intern Med.* 1977;86: 738-741.
28. Solomonson MD, Johnson ME, Ilstrup D. Risk factors in patients having surgery to create an arteriovenous fistula. *Anesth Analg.* 1994;79: 694-700.
29. Glover GW, Bowie R, Stoves J, et al. Brachial plexus block for formation of arteriovenous fistula is associated with improved patency. *Anaesthesia.* 2007;62:425-425.
30. Tsui BC-H. *Atlas of Ultrasound and Nerve Stimulation-Guided Regional Anesthesia.* New York: Springer; 2007.
31. Hadzic A, Vloka J. *Peripheral Nerve Blocks: Principles and Practice.* New York: McGraw-Hill/Professional; 2004.
32. Mouquet C, Bitker MO, Bailliart O, et al.: Anesthesia for creation of a forearm fistula in patients with end-stage renal failure. *Anesthesiology.* 1989;70:909-914.
33. Sheppard DG, Iyer RB, Fenstermacher MJ. Brachial plexus: Demonstration at US. *Radiology.* 1998;208:402-406.
34. Lanz E, Theiss D, Jankovic D. The extent of blockade following various techniques of brachial plexus block. *Anesth Analg.* 1983;62:55-58.
35. Chan VWS, Perlas A, McCartney CJL, Brall R, Xu D, Abbas S. Ultrasound guidance improves success rate of axillary brachial plexus block. *Can J Anaesth.* 2007;54:176-182.
36. Partridge BL, Katz J, Benirschke K. Functional anatomy of the brachial plexus sheath: implications for anesthesia. *Anesthesiology.* 1987;66: 743-747.
37. Koscielniak-Nielsen ZJ, Nielsen PR, Mortensen CR. A comparison of coracoid and axillary approaches to the brachial plexus. *Acta Anaesthesiol Scand.* 2000;44:274-279.
38. Carles M, Pulcini A, Macchi P, et al. An evaluation of the brachial plexus block at the humeralcanal using a neurostimulator (1417 patients): the efficacy, safety, and predictive criteria of failure. *Anesth Analg.* 2001;92:194-198.
39. Hudson SJ, Emamdee RI, Htut Y, Pal SK. The transarterial brachial plexus block for hand and forearm surgery: a review of 1062 cases. *Eur J Anaesthesiol.* 2007;24:470-472.
40. Casati A, Danelli G, Baciarello M, et al. A prospective, randomized comparison between ultrasound and nerve stimulation guidance for multiple injection axillary brachial plexus block. *Anesthesiology.* 2007; 106:992-996.
41. Schafhalter-Zoppoth I, Gray AT. The musculocutaneous nerve: ultrasound appearance for peripheral nerve block. *Reg Anesth Pain Med.* 2005;30:385-390.
42. Spence BC, Sites BD, Beach ML. Ultrasound-guided musculocutaneous nerve block: a description of a novel technique. *Reg Anesth Pain Med.* 2005;30:198-201.
43. Tsui BCH, Kropelin B. Regional Anesthesia Case Reports: The electrophysiological effect of dextrose 5% in water on single-shot peripheral nerve stimulation. *Anesth Analg.* 2005;100:1837.

44. Khan H, Atanassoff PG. Accidental intravascular injection of levo-bupivacaine and lidocaine during the transarterial approach to the axillary brachial plexus. *Can J Anaesth.* 2003;50:95.

45. Gould DB, Aldrete JA. Bupivacaine cardiotoxicity in a patient with renal failure. *Acta Anaesthesiol Scand.* 1983;27:18-21.

46. Albright GA. Cardiac arrest following regional anesthesia with etidocaine or bupivacaine. *Anesthesiology.* 1979;51:285-287.

47. Moller RA, Covino BG. Cardiac electrophysiologic effects of lidocaine and bupivacaine. *Anesth Analg.* 1988;67:107-114.

48. Kapral S, Krafft P, Eibenberger K, Fitzgerald R, Gosch M, Weinstabl C. Ultrasound-guided supraclavicular approach for regional anesthesia of the brachial plexus. *Anesth Analg.* 1994;78:507-513.

49. Kobayashi I, Takahashi H, Hatakeyama Y, et al. Ultrasound-guided supraclavicular approach to brachial plexus. *Anesthesiology.* 1994;81: A906.

50. Beach ML, Sites BD, Gallagher JD. Use of a nerve stimulator does not improve the efficacy of ultrasound-guided supraclavicular nerve blocks. *J Clin Anesth.* 2006;18:580-584.

51. Bigeleisen PE. Anatomical variations of the phrenic nerve and its clinical implication for supraclavicular block. *Br J Anaesth.* 2003;91: 916-917.

52. Mak PHK, Irwin MG, Ooi CGC, Chow BF. Incidence of diaphragmatic paralysis following supraclavicular brachial plexus block and its effect on pulmonary function. *Anaesthesia.* 2001;56:352-356.

53. Deleuze A, Gentili ME, Marret E, Lamonerie L, Bonnet F. A comparison of a single-stimulation lateral infraclavicular plexus block with a triple-stimulation axillary block. *Reg Anesth Pain Med.* 2003;28:89-94.

54. Heid FM, Jage J, Guth M, Bauwe N, Brambrink AM. Efficacy of vertical infraclavicular plexus block vs. modified axillary plexus block: a prospective, randomized, observer-blinded study. *Acta Anaesthesiol Scand.* 2005;49:677-682.

55. Koscielniak-Nielsen ZJ, Rasmussen H, Hesselbjerg L, et al. Infraclavicular block causes less discomfort than axillary block in ambulatory patients. *Acta Anaesthesiol Scand.* 2005;49:1030-1034.

56. Niemi TT, Salmela L, Aromaa U, Pöyhiä R, Rosenberg PH. Single-injection brachial plexus anesthesia for arteriovenous fistula surgery of the forearm: a comparison of infraclavicular coracoid and axillary approach. *Reg Anesth Pain Med.* 2007;32:55-59.

57. Arcand G, Williams SR, Chouinard P, et al. Ultrasound-guided infraclavicular versus supraclavicular block. *Anesth Analg.* 2005;101:886-890.

58. Raj P. Infraclavicular approaches to brachial plexus anesthesia. *Tech Reg Anesth Pain Manag.* 1997;1:169-177.

59. Dullenkopf A, Blumenthal S, Theodorou P, Roos J, Perschak H, Borgeat A. Diaphragmatic excursion and respiratory function after the modified Raj technique of the infraclavicular plexus block. *Reg Anesth Pain Med.* 2004;29:110-114.

60. Rodriguez J, Barcena M, Rodriguez V, Aneiros F, Alvarez J. Infraclavicular brachial plexus block effects on respiratory function and extent of the block. *Reg Anesth Pain Med.* 1998;23:564-568.

61. Bigeleisen P, Wilson M. A comparison of two techniques for ultrasound guided infraclavicular block. *Br J Anaesth,* 2006;96:502-507.

62. Gaertner E, Estebe JP, Zamfir A, Cuby C, Macaire P. Infraclavicular plexus block: Multiple injection versus single injection. *Reg Anesth Pain Med,* 2002;27:590-594.

63. Desgagnes MC, Levesque S, Dion N, et al. Single versus triple injections ultrasound-guided infraclavicular block: a prospective randomized trial. American Society of Regional Anesthesia and Pain Medicine Spring Meeting, May 1-4, Cancun, Mexico.

64. Porter JM, McCartney CJL, Chan VWS. Needle placement and injection posterior to the axillary artery may predict successful infraclavicular brachial plexus block: a report of three cases. *Can J Anaesth.* 2005;52:69-73.

65. Borgeat A, Ekatodramis G, Dumont C. An evaluation of the infraclavicular block via a modified approach of the Raj technique. *Anesth Analg.* 2001;93:436-441.

66. Chan VW. Applying ultrasound imaging to interscalene brachial plexus block. *Reg Anesth Pain Med.* 2003;28:340-343.

67. Silverstein WB, Saiyed MU, Brown AR. Interscalene block with a nerve stimulator: a deltoid motor response is a satisfactory endpoint for successful block. *Reg Anesth Pain Med.* 2000;25:356-359.

68. Coleman MM, Peng P. Pectoralis major in interscalene brachial plexus blockade. *Reg Anesth Pain Med.* 1999;24:190-191.

69. Tonidandel WL, Mayfield JB. Successful interscalene block with a nerve stimulator may also result after a pectoralis major motor response. *Reg Anesth Pain Med.* 2002;27:491-493.

70. Borgeat A, Ekatodramis G, Kalberer F, Benz C. Acute and nonacute complications associated with interscalene block and shoulder surgery: a prospective study. *Anesthesiology.* 2001;95:875-880.

71. Passannante AN. Spinal anesthesia and permanent neurologic deficit after interscalene block. *Anesth Analg.* 1996;82:873-874.

72. Dutton RP, Eckhardt WF 3rd, Sunder N. Total spinal anesthesia after interscalene blockade of the brachial plexus. *Anesthesiology.* 1994;80:939-941.

73. Benumof JL. Permanent loss of cervical spinal cord function associated with interscalene block performed under general anesthesia. *Anesthesiology.* 2000;93:1541-1544.

74. Gottardis M, Luger T, Florl C, et al. Spirometry, blood gas analysis and ultrasonography of the diaphragm after Winnie's interscalene brachial plexus block. *Eur J Anaesthesiol.* 1993;10:367-369.

75. Osaka Y, Inomata S, Tanaka E, et al. Effect of propofol on ropivacaine metabolism in human liver microsomes. *J Anesth.* 2006;20:60-63.

76. Scott DB, Jebson PJ, Braid DP, Ortengren B, Frisch P. Factors affecting plasma levels of lignocaine and prilocaine. *Br J Anaesth.* 1972;44: 1040-1049.

77. Adnan T, Elif AA, Ayse K, Gülnaz A. Clonidine as an adjuvant for lidocaine in axillary brachial plexus block in patients with chronic renal failure. *Acta Anaesthesiol Scand.* 2005;49:563-568.

78. Bokesch PM, Raymond SA, Strichartz GR. Dependence of lidocaine potency on pH and PCO_2. *Anesth Analg.* 1987;66:9-17.

79. DiFazio CA, Carron H, Grosslight KR, Moscicki JC, Bolding WR, Johns RA. Comparison of pH-adjusted lidocaine solutions for epidural anesthesia. *Anesth Analg.* 1986;65:760-764

80. Scott DB. Toxic effects of local anaesthetic agents on the central nervous system. *Br J Anaesth.* 1986;58:732-735.

81. Lynch C 3rd. Depression of myocardial contractility in vitro by bupivacaine, etidocaine, and lidocaine. *Anesth Analg.* 1986;65:551-559.

82. Kimura Y, Kamada Y, Kimura A, Orimo K. Ropivacaine-induced toxicity with overdose suspected after axillary brachial plexus block. *J Anesth.* 2007;21:413-416.

83. Litz RJ, Popp M, Stehr SN, Koch Tl. Successful resuscitation of a patient with ropivacaine-induced asystole after axillary plexus block using lipid infusion. *Anaesthesia.* 2006;61:800-801.

84. Turner-Lawrence DE, Kerns W. Intravenous fat emulsion: a potential novel antidote. *J Med Toxicol.* 2008;4:109-114.

85. Lund PC, Cwik JC. Propitocaine (Citanest) and methemoglobinemia. *Anesthesiology.* 1965;26:569-571.

CHAPTER 4

Surgical Anatomy for Hemodialysis Access

Jeffrey L. Ballard

Precise knowledge of surgical anatomy is crucial for decision making in hemodialysis access. Accurate incision placement and atraumatic dissection help to protect adjacent arterial or neural structures and to ensure long-term patency of the outflow vein and the inflow artery chosen for the dialysis access site. In addition, preoperative extremity vein mapping is essential for selection of good-caliber vein outflow sites and a complete noninvasive arterial study will ensure normal extremity perfusion, thereby greatly reducing the risk of ischemic steal syndrome.

This chapter reviews the anatomy of pertinent arteries and veins in the upper and lower extremities that are likely be used for temporary or permanent hemodialysis access. Various arteriovenous (AV) fistulas and synthetic graft configurations are detailed in brief.

Central Venous Anatomy for Hemodialysis Access

Vascular access for temporary or emergent hemodialysis is usually initiated with central venous cannulation while plans are made for a more permanent access site. Placement of central venous catheters requires accurate knowledge

of adjacent neurovascular structures; otherwise, serious vascular injury may result in patient morbidity as well as the inability to utilize the precious access site. The internal or external jugular vein, subclavian vein, and femoral vein are frequently used for temporary hemodialysis access. As a last resort, the large central neck veins can be used for permanent hemodialysis access with one of many different types of dual-lumen catheters (see Chapter 16).

The internal jugular vein (IJV) is the optimal central vein to use for venous access.[1] Cannulation of this vein using ultrasound guidance is straightforward and the right IJV in particular facilitates a straight route to the superior vena cava (SVC). Thrombosis of this vein, which is a well-recognized complication of chronic central venous access, does not preclude the use of upper extremity veins for hemodialysis access, as is the case when there is subclavian vein thrombosis. For this reason, long-term cannulation of the subclavian vein should be reserved for situations in which all other ipsilateral upper extremity vein outflow sites have been exhausted. Similarly, the femoral vein should be considered a secondary site for permanent hemodialysis access because of associated wound and/or catheter infection problems.[2] Knowledge of vascular anatomy at the thoracic outlet (Fig. 4-1) and femoral trian-

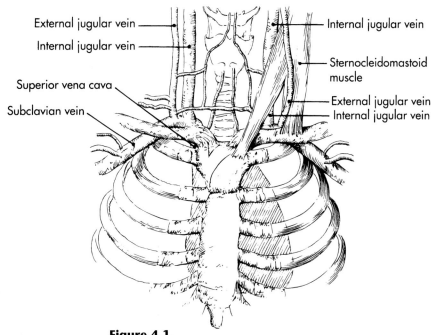

Figure 4-1.
Central venous anatomy at the thoracic outlet.

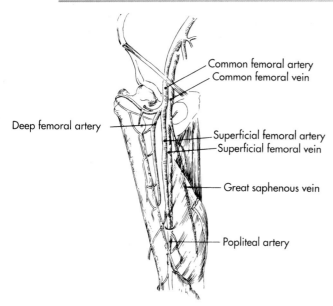

Figure 4-2.
Vascular anatomy at the femoral triangle.

gle (Fig. 4-2) is critical for appropriate placement of central venous hemodialysis catheters.

Jugular Venous Cannulation

The external jugular vein (EJV) can be located in the upper lateral aspect of the neck underlying the platysma muscle. Cannulation of this peripheral vein affords access to the central venous system because the EJV courses along the surface of the sternocleidomastoid (SCM) muscle and flows with the IJV into the subclavian vein at the base of the neck. The EJV may be cannulated directly at any point along its course. This vein is normally used for temporary hemodialysis access because it is a small-caliber conduit; however, some authors have reported excellent mid- to long-term success utilizing the EJV when the right IJV was not a usable access site.[3]

Either IJV is a suitable site for temporary or permanent central venous hemodialysis access. Ultrasound guidance facilitates vein cannulation and significantly decreases the risk of arterial injury and pneumothorax. In fact, both failure and complication rates are reported to be significantly lower when the physician guiding the sonographic probe is well versed using the method.[4] At the base of the neck, the IJVs are lateral and anterior to the common carotid arteries (see Fig. 4-1). The right IJV is preferred because its course to the SVC is short and relatively straight. In addition, the right IJV at the base of the neck is safer for cannulation than the left IJV because it is farther away from the common carotid artery.

Percutaneous access to the IJV can be obtained at the apex of the angle made by the sternal and clavicular heads of the SCM muscle. Direct the needle toward the ipsilateral nipple, lateral to the common carotid artery, and advanced at a 45-degree angle to the body surface. After entering the vein, a guidewire is passed through the needle into the SVC. For temporary access, the hemodialysis catheter can be advanced directly over the guidewire after incision of the skin puncture site and careful passage of a dilator to enlarge the subcutaneous tissue and vein puncture site. For permanent access, first tunnel the hemodialysis catheter from its exit site on the anterolateral chest wall to the skin puncture site. Then advance a dilator surrounded by a peel-away introducer sheath over the guidewire into the vein. Removal of the dilator/guidewire leaves the open introducer through which the catheter is passed to the level of the right atrium. Confirm catheter placement with fluoroscopy before securing the catheter at the skin exit site. An upright chest radiograph to rule out pneumothorax completes the procedure.

Alternative approaches to the IJV for percutaneous access are twofold. The vein can be cannulated from the posterior border of the SCM muscle at the level of the thyroid cartilage or at the anterior border of the SCM muscle with the neck in an extended but neutral position. For this latter approach, the common carotid artery must be palpated and kept medial to the needle insertion site; otherwise, the carotid artery can be inadvertently cannulated.

A horizontal incision made just above the clavicle between the sternal and the clavicular heads of the SCM muscle is used for direct IJV cutdown. Once the platysma layer is divided, the dense fascia of the carotid sheath can be located deep between the heads of the SCM muscle. Carefully divide the fascia longitudinally to expose the IJV. The vagus nerve normally lies posteromedial to the IJV, but its course can vary. The nerve should be observed and protected during the dissection to free the jugular vein from surrounding tissue. After securing proximal and distal control of the IJV, place a 5-0 Prolene suture widely in a pursestring manner, with room left for passage of the large-caliber, dual-lumen catheter. Create a small venotomy in the middle of the pursestring, and place the hemodialysis catheter into the IJV under direct vision after it has been tunneled from its exit site on the anterolateral chest wall. Check catheter location with fluoroscopy. The tip of the catheter should reside within the SVC and just above the right atrium.

Femoral Vein Cannulation

At the level of the femoral triangle (see Fig. 4-2), the femoral vein lies medial to the femoral artery. After shaving and preparing the groin with an antiseptic solution, cannulate the vein at a 45-degree angle to the body surface using ultrasound guidance.[2] Decrease the angle of the needle to advance a guidewire into the femoral vein. Then advance the hemodialysis catheter over the guidewire to avoid inadvertent vein puncture or laceration above the inguinal ligament.

Discussion

The Seldinger technique can be performed safely in the majority of patients for central vein cannulation.[1-4] The choice of any of these central venous cannulation methods depends on operator experience, venous anatomy, patient body habitus, and other medical problems (eg, coagulopathy). Temporary catheters placed using ultrasound guidance is optimal because this method greatly reduces the complication rate associated with the percutaneous procedure. Chronic indwelling central venous catheters that require tunneling from the skin exit site to the target central vein are best placed under fluoroscopic guidance in either the operating room or the angiographic suite. Similar success and complication rates are reported with either approach, and percutaneous methods are used in the overwhelming majority of cases as opposed to open IJV cutdown.

Many reports document the safety of percutaneous long-term central venous access; however, this procedure is not trouble-free.[1-4] Debate continues regarding the technique for central venous catheterization that is associated with the lowest complication rate and the highest success rate. Pittiruti and colleagues[1] reviewed a 7-year experience with 5479 central venous percutaneous punctures for the insertion of short-term ($N = 2109$), medium, and long-term ($N = 2627$) catheters, as well as double-lumen, large-bore catheters for hemodialysis ($N = 743$). They analyzed the incidence of the most frequent insertion-related complications by comparing different percutaneous approaches to the jugular vein, subclavian vein, EJV, and femoral vein. The "low-lateral" approach to the IJV as described in their report had the lowest incidence of inadvertent arterial puncture (1.2%) and malposition (0.8%), no instances of pneumothorax, and a low rate of required repeated attempts (3.3%) to successfully cannulate the vein.

In a large series reporting major complications of hemodialysis access surgery, Ballard and coworkers[5] noted that five patients required major vascular repair or emergent thoracotomy for complications of percutaneous central venous hemodialysis catheter placement. The large dilators and introducer sheaths required for permanent percutaneous access are quite stiff and unyielding. Either device can easily puncture through the IJV or SVC, leading to a variety of potential problems. Although infrequently used today, IJV cutdown does afford direct visual access to the central venous system and obviates the need for dilators and introducer sheaths.

Complications associated with central venous cannulation include venous laceration, pneumothorax, hemothorax, air embolism, catheter embolus or malposition, cardiac tamponade, venous thrombosis, and catheter sepsis.[5] Accidental cannulation of an adjacent major artery can lead to arterial dissection, laceration, or thrombosis with possible limb ischemia. For instance, this author has had to remove a central venous access catheter from the aortic arch that passed through the left subclavian vein and into the arch between the innominate and the left common carotid arteries. Permanent nerve injury may result from direct needle or catheter trauma or compression from an adjacent hematoma. Regardless of the access site, complications related to the central venous catheters can be minimized with attention to detail and a clear understanding of applied vascular anatomy.

Surgical Anatomy of Hemodialysis Access at the Wrist

Two anatomic sites are useful for the creation of permanent AV hemodialysis access at the wrist level. When the thumb is abducted and extended, the tendons of the extensor

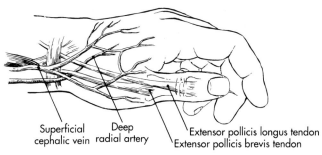

Figure 4-3.
Vascular anatomy at the anatomic snuffbox.

pollicis longus muscle and the extensor pollicis brevis muscle form the anatomic snuffbox. The radial artery can be palpated at the base of the first metacarpal bone. A short incision centered over the radial artery reveals the subcutaneous cephalic vein. The radial artery lies adjacent to the cephalic vein and continues onto the dorsum of the hand as the deep radial artery. At this level, the vein-to-artery anastomosis can be accomplished side-to-side, end-to-end, or end-to-side, depending on the arterial/venous anatomy and surgeon preference. Figure 4-3 shows the essential anatomy of this autogenous AV fistula.

The more common exposure for a primary radial artery–to–cephalic vein arteriovenous (RACV) fistula, also known as a *Brescia-Cimino fistula,* is proximal and medial to the anatomic snuffbox on the anterolateral wrist (Fig. 4-4). An incision made between the palpable radial artery and the cephalic vein affords access to both vessels. In the soft tissue between the vessels lies the superficial branch of the radial nerve, which supplies the skin of the dorsum of the thumb and the radial two and one-half digits. It is wise to protect this nerve during vessel exposure because inadvertent injury may lead to the loss of skin innervation over the dorsal thumb or chronic ill-defined pain in the same nerve distribution, which can be particularly annoying for the patient.

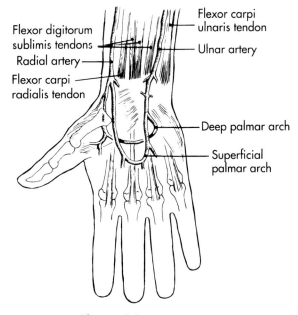

Figure 4-4.
Arterial anatomy at the wrist.

Incision of the deep forearm fascia lateral to the tendon of flexor carpi radialis muscle exposes the radial artery. Careful dissection of the artery is necessary because there are numerous small branches at this level that can be inadvertently injured and obscure the dissection field. Using the adjacent cephalic vein, a side-to-side, end-to-end, or end-to-side vein-to-artery fistula can be constructed. A palpable thrill over the anastomosis and within the cephalic vein in the more proximal forearm is a good indication that the fistula is functioning well and will mature in a timely fashion. A mature Brescia-Cimino fistula can be cannulated for hemodialysis anywhere along the course of the dilated cephalic vein, usually within 6 weeks of construction.

Discussion

A well-functioning autogenous RACV fistula at the wrist level is the ideal angioaccess. Pooled data confirm the superiority of autologous RACV fistulas compared with synthetic grafts.[6] A well-functioning primary fistula created at the wrist will ultimately have better long-term patency than a bridge graft, although RACV fistulas have a significantly higher early thrombosis rate.[7-9] Expanded polytetrafluoroethylene (PTFE) bridge grafts have better early patency rates because 12% to 24% of RACV fistulas never mature, for a variety of arterial and/or venous problems.[5,7-9] A useful alternative wrist fistula can be created at the anatomic snuffbox.[10] If the cephalic vein is sclerosed at this level, one of the rich collateral dorsal hand veins can provide adequate outflow. The limiting factor for the success of this type of primary fistula is the size of the distal veins of the hand. Despite early failure rates as high as 14%, long-term patency in a large patient series of snuffbox fistulas was 83% at 1 year and 46% at 6.5 years.[11]

Surgical Anatomy of Hemodialysis Access in the Forearm

In order to choose the best site for construction of a permanent hemodialysis access site in the forearm, accurate preoperative information regarding extremity arterial hemodynamics and vein caliber is of primary importance (Fig. 4-5; see also Fig. 4-4).[12-14] The venous circulation of the forearm involves two major veins. The cephalic vein begins approximately near the anatomic snuffbox on the posterolateral aspect of the wrist. It gradually swings

around the forearm as it ascends to become the lateral vein of the forearm. At the apex of the antecubital fossa, the median cubital vein courses variably and medially from the cephalic vein to meet the basilic vein. The cephalic vein continues up the anterolateral aspect of the arm and courses through the deltopectoral groove before emptying into the axillary vein.

The basilic vein begins on the posterior aspect of the forearm, courses upward to then swing around the proximal forearm. It then ascends onto the medial aspect of the distal arm before piercing the deep fascia. At the lower border of the teres major muscle, the basilic vein joins the brachial veins in the arm to form the axillary vein lateral to the pectoralis minor muscle. Another potentially useful outflow conduit is the median antebrachial vein, which drains the palmar surface of the hand. This vein ascends on the ulnar side of the forearm and terminates in the basilic vein near the elbow or in the median cubital vein at the apex of the antecubital fossa.

The radial artery is chosen as the primary arterial source for an arteriovenous fistula in the forearm because it is subcutaneous and nondominant compared with the ulnar artery. Use of this artery is less likely to cause arterial steal syndrome of the hand. The radial artery arises at the bifurcation of the brachial artery just below the flexion crease at the elbow. It is overlapped by the brachioradialis muscle in the upper portion of the forearm; however, in the distal half of its course, it is immediately beneath the deep fascia and is easily palpable. The ulnar artery follows a deep course in the forearm and is not easily accessible for surgical exposure.

Carefully protect the superficial radial nerve during exposure of the distal radial artery. This nerve passes anterior to the pronator teres muscle and lateral to the radial artery under the cover of the brachioradialis muscle in the upper and middle forearm. It then diverges away from the artery approximately 7 cm proximal to the wrist, where it passes beneath the tendon of the brachioradialis muscle and pierces the deep fascia to enter the posterior compartment of the forearm, where the superficial radial nerve divides into two branches. The smaller lateral branch supplies the skin of the radial side and the base of the thumb. The larger medial branch communicates with the dorsal branch of the lateral antebrachial cutaneous nerve on the back of the hand to innervate skin and fascia over the lateral side of the dorsum of the hand, dorsum of the thumb, and proximal lateral two and one-half fingers.

Discussion

The radial artery is immediately beneath the deep fascia in the distal half of the forearm and can be used as an arterial origin for an autogenous AV fistula, particularly if it is heavily diseased at the wrist. Silva and associates[13] described a number of forearm vein transpositions that can be used to create autogenous AV fistulas. These modifications of the previously described single-incision RACV fistula maximize the use of patent forearm veins that are not immediately adjacent to the radial artery. Cumulative primary patency for these alternate AV fistula configurations was reported to be 84% at 1 year and 69% at 2 years.[13]

The distal radial artery or hood of a failed Brescia-Cimino fistula can be used as the arterial origin of a straight

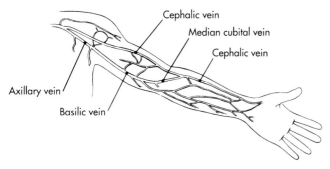

Figure 4-5.
Venous anatomy of the upper extremity.

radial artery–to–antecubital vein PTFE bridge graft. The latter is preferred because there is an excellent size match between the old anastomotic hood and a PTFE graft. However, the straight radial artery–to–antecubital vein PTFE graft configuration is controversial. Pontari and McMillen[15] noted that this straight bridge graft preserved ulnar collateral flow to the hand as well as the brachial artery for later access use, and in their 10-graft series, patency was 90% at 6 months. Six of 10 grafts remained patent after 12 to 24 months of follow-up, without the need for graft thrombectomy (3 patients died during follow-up).[15] However, in a much larger study, Schmidt and Field[16] demonstrated that a forearm loop PTFE bridge graft was superior to a straight graft. Despite similar primary and secondary patency rates, the straight grafts required more revisions and thrombectomies to maintain patency.[16]

Surgical Anatomy of Hemodialysis Access at the Antecubital Fossa

The antecubital fossa (Figs. 4-6 and 4-7) is roughly triangular in shape, with the base of the triangle formed by an imaginary line drawn between the humeral condyles. The pronator teres muscle forms the medial converging border, and the brachioradialis muscle forms the lateral border. The brachioradialis muscle overlaps the pronator teres muscle at the apex of the triangular fossa. The floor of the fossa is formed by the brachialis muscle and is covered by the deep fascia of the forearm.

Several important superficial veins course through the antecubital fossa. The median cubital vein is a continuation of the cephalic vein of the forearm. It courses from the apex of the triangle in a medial course to join the basilic vein in the distal arm. The forearm cephalic vein travels laterally through the antecubital fossa and ascends through the anterolateral aspect of the arm (see Fig. 4-6 for a diagram of these vessels). The communicating vein, which acts as a connector between the deep and the superficial veins of the proximal forearm, can be utilized for venous outflow in constructing a primary AV fistula. This vein, also known as the *perforating antecubital vein*, is demonstrated in the diagram.[17]

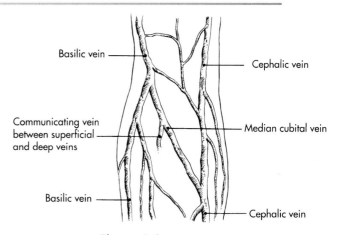

Figure 4-6.
Antecubital venous anatomy.

The lacertus fibrosus lies deep to the superficial veins described earlier. This structure represents the flat tendinous insertion of the biceps muscle that fuses with the fascia of the forearm. Exposure of the terminal brachial artery requires division of the lacertus fibrosus. This maneuver facilitates exposure of the brachial artery as it courses from its medial location to terminate at the apex of the antecubital fossa by dividing into the radial artery and the larger ulnar artery. The median nerve lies medial to the brachial artery as it travels into the forearm. No other important anatomic structures reside in the immediate vicinity of the brachial artery and the median nerve in the antecubital fossa.

Discussion

The antecubital fossa is a frequently used site for hemodialysis access because many patients with end-stage renal disease also have advanced peripheral vascular disease, diabetes mellitus, or both, and a more distal forearm or wrist fistula is often precluded owing to poor-caliber veins or heavily diseased arteries. Ballard and coworkers[5] and others[18,19] have reported high early failure rates with

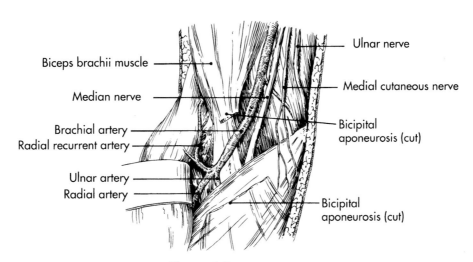

Figure 4-7.
Antecubital arterial anatomy.

Brescia-Cimino fistulas in this difficult-to-manage diabetic population. Because of this failure rate, subsequent hemodialysis access sites are often created at the antecubital fossa. The most common configuration is a primary brachial artery–to–cephalic vein AV fistula. An alternate plan if other forearm vein transpositions are also precluded would be to create a straight or loop forearm PTFE bridge graft as the next step after a failed RACV fistula. This maneuver facilitates dilation and arterialization of the superficial veins in the arm that can be used later for creation of a primary AV fistula. Primary AV fistulas created at the antecubital fossa are usually well functioning but are also associated with a high rate of hand ischemia due to the steal phenomenon. The steal syndrome is particularly likely if forearm and hand arteries are heavily diseased.[5]

Primary antecubital AV fistulas can be constructed in a variety of ways. Well-described configurations include a side-to-side anastomosis between the median cubital vein and the brachial artery, an end-to-side anastomosis between the cephalic vein and the brachial artery, and an end-to-side anastomosis between the communicating antecubital vein and the brachial or proximal radial artery.[17,20,21] These primary fistulas have excellent long-term patency; however, as mentioned previously, they are associated with an increased risk of hand ischemia. This is particularly true in elderly women who have diabetes.[5,18,19] Pseudoaneurysm formation from repeated cannulation of the fistula within a small area has also been reported.[17,20] This complication most likely occurs when the cephalic vein outflow is compromised thereby limiting cannulation sites or if the basilic vein lies in its anatomic position instead of being transposed to a more superficial site.

Brachiocephalic jump graft fistulas have also been used with success when the cephalic vein is too far away from the brachial artery.[22] A short segment of harvested vein or PTFE graft effectively bridges the gap between the two vessels. Cumulative primary patency rates at 1, 3, 5, and 7 years were reported to be 85%, 67%, 48%, and 34%, respectively.[22] Numerous authors have also confirmed the durability of longer forearm loop PTFE grafts that bridge the brachial artery to the cephalic vein or the brachial artery to the basilic vein.[23] A useful alternative to the abandonment of failed PTFE loop grafts that have venous outflow obstruction at the antecubital fossa has been described by Schulak and colleagues.[24] The technique entails construction of a new venous bypass extension to the basilic vein in the arm using the previous arterial inflow limb. The proximal portion of the transected inflow limb is then transposed to the transected old outflow limb. This essentially reverses blood flow direction in the PTFE graft and effectively bypasses the venous outflow obstruction at the antecubital fossa.

Surgical Anatomy of Hemodialysis Access in the Upper Arm

The brachial artery begins at the lower border of the teres major muscle and terminates approximately 2.5 cm below the transverse skin crease of the elbow (Fig. 4-8; see also Fig. 4-7). The two terminal branches are the radial and ulnar arteries; the latter is the larger branch. The

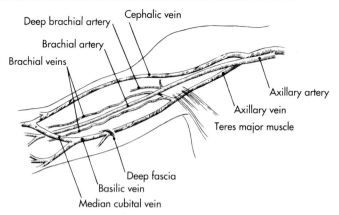

Figure 4-8.
Vascular anatomy of the arm.

pulsations of the brachial artery can be felt along the bicipital groove until this vessel disappears beneath the lacertus fibrosus. The subcutaneous location of this artery facilitates its surgical exposure. There are three major branches of this artery in the arm. The first is the profunda brachial artery, which rises as high as the teres major muscle. One would not ordinarily expect to see this large branch during the usual dissection because of its proximal location. The superior ulnar collateral artery arises in the middle aspect of the arm and accompanies the ulnar nerve. Here, it enters the posterior compartment and disappears from sight. The inferior ulnar collateral artery arises approximately 5 cm above the termination of the brachial artery. It passes inward behind the ulnar artery and out of the dissection field.

There are three major veins associated with the brachial artery (see Figs. 4-5 and 4-8). The medial and lateral brachial veins course with the artery and have numerous venous tributaries. The basilic vein ascends the arm in the groove on the medial side of the distal artery. In the distal arm, the vein pierces the deep fascia to become more closely related to the brachial artery. The basilic vein joins with the brachial veins to form the axillary vein at a variable level in the axilla.

Several important relationships should be kept in mind when exposing the brachial artery. The coracobrachialis muscle overlaps the brachial artery proximally, and the artery lies on the brachialis muscle and the insertion of the coracobrachialis muscle. The middle third of the artery is overlapped by the medial border of the biceps muscle. In the distal arm, the brachial artery courses in front of the humerus and is overlapped by the biceps tendon. Both the medial cutaneous nerve and the ulnar nerve lie to the medial side of the brachial artery and separate the artery from the basilic vein. The radial nerve lies posterior to the brachial artery. The median nerve courses closely to the artery throughout its course in the arm, and it crosses from lateral to medial in the middle aspect of the arm to reach the posterior compartment. The median nerve lies medial to the brachial artery in the distal arm. The medial cutaneous nerve of the forearm lies medial to the artery and should be protected because injury can cause annoying paresthesias or chronic discomfort.

Discussion

Sites on the upper arm should be reserved for patients for whom wrist, forearm, or antecubital fossa AV fistulas or other distal graft configurations have failed. In general, primary AV fistulas are created between the brachial artery and the cephalic or basilic vein.[25] Alternatively, brachial artery–to–basilic vein or brachial artery–to–cephalic vein bridge grafts can be created in straight or looped configurations.[26] The basilic vein can also be transposed above the deep fascia of the arm and anastomosed to the brachial artery to serve as a durable autogenous conduit for hemodialysis access.[27-31] Brachial artery–to–jugular vein PTFE bridge grafts have been described as a possible access site solution for patients who have axillary vein stenosis or occlusion.[32]

Similar to primary AV fistulas created in the antecubital fossa, upper arm AV fistulas have a relatively high rate of associated hand ischemia. Occasionally, fistula ligation is required to treat ischemic steal syndrome of the hand. However, the construction of a proximal bridge fistula based on inflow from axillary branch arteries may serve to limit upper extremity ischemia while maintaining a site for hemodialysis.[33] Hemodialysis access-induced ischemia of the hand can also be successfully treated with the distal revascularization interval ligation (DRIL) procedure.[34,35] This technique begins with arterial ligation just distal to the fistula origin. Distal revascularization is then reestablished by arterial bypass using harvested saphenous vein from a point at least 8 to 10 cm proximal to the fistula origin to a point distal to the arterial ligature. This author usually transects the terminal brachial artery to perform an end-to-end distal anastomosis. One report demonstrated salvage of 13 of 14 extremities *and* the fistulas in a series of very difficult-to-manage diabetic patients.[34] The interested reader is referred to the articles cited for a more detailed description of the surgical technique.[34,35]

In our practice, we have noticed that hemodynamic steal syndrome complicating brachial artery based dialysis access occurs with increasing frequency when the preoperatively measured mean finger/brachial index (MFBI) is less than 0.85. We always perform preemptive DRIL when there is preexisting finger ulceration/gangrene and often when the preoperative ipsilateral MFBI is less than 0.85. Nevertheless, we inform all patients about the symptoms of hemodynamic steal syndrome and advise them to seek immediate medical care should these symptoms develop.

Surgical Anatomy of Hemodialysis Access in the Thigh

The neurovascular structures that enter the thigh are located in the femoral triangle (see Fig. 4-2). The base of the femoral triangle is the inguinal ligament. The medial border of the sartorius muscle forms the lateral boundary, and the medial boundary is the medial border of the adductor longus muscle. The apex of the triangle is where these two muscles intersect. The common femoral artery enters this triangle midway between the anterosuperior iliac spine and the pubic tubercle. The common femoral vein lies medial to the artery, and the femoral nerve courses lateral to the artery.

The common femoral artery divides into the superficial femoral artery and the deep femoral artery at varying distances from its origin. The former continues distally until it disappears beneath the sartorius muscle to enter Hunter's canal. The superficial femoral artery is not usually exposed distally because of its deep location. Once it has passed through the adductor hiatus above the knee, the proximal popliteal artery can be exposed through a medial thigh approach. This incision is made in the groove between the vastus medialis and the sartorius muscles. Dissection is directed deeper by retracting the above muscles. The artery can be felt in a plane just posterior to the femur and dissected free from surrounding tissue for a considerable length.

The greater saphenous, superficial, and deep femoral veins empty into the common femoral vein. The saphenous vein enters the thigh in the subcutaneous tissues by coursing over the posterior aspect of the medial condyle of the femur. It continues its subcutaneous course upward and medial to terminate at the anteromedial surface of the common femoral vein near the inguinal ligament. It accumulates numerous and variable small and medium-sized tributaries as it ascends in the thigh. In a deeper plane, the superficial femoral vein lies medial to the artery throughout its course in the thigh. A large tributary of the deep femoral vein, the lateral femoral circumflex vein, passes between the superficial and the deep femoral arteries just distal to their origins. The vein can be easily entered unless one is cautious during the isolation of the common femoral artery bifurcation. The adjacent lateral femoral circumflex artery can be large enough to be considered as an arterial origin site for creation of a primary AV fistula.

The femoral nerve at the groin is not easily injured during exposure of the femoral artery or vein if its lateral location is kept in mind and protected. Likewise, medial exposure of the proximal popliteal artery does not place the tibial or peroneal nerves at risk of injury, because they are lateral and posterior to the popliteal vein and therefore well out of harm's way.

Discussion

Although it is preferable to avoid cannulation of the femoral vein for hemodialysis access or creation of an AV fistula at this level, occasionally a patient with multiple failed upper extremity access sites will require hemodialysis access in the thigh. Primary AV fistulas based on the mobilized saphenous vein are well described for chronic hemodialysis access.[36,37] The greater saphenous vein can be anastomosed to the side of the popliteal artery in a straight configuration or to the side of the proximal superficial femoral artery in a loop configuration. In these cases, the vein must be transposed to a subcutaneous plane so it can be more easily cannulated for dialysis. The reader is referred to the articles cited for details of the surgical procedures.[37,38]

Expanded PTFE grafts tunneled in a loop configuration also work well as a bridge graft in the thigh. The superficial femoral vein or the saphenofemoral junction is preferred for venous outflow. If these previously mentioned vein outflow sites are utilized, a revision can be performed by extending the venous outflow to the common femoral vein, using either a vein segment or a PTFE interposition graft.

Alternatively, the greater saphenous vein can be used for outflow. However, this author has revised a number of thigh loop grafts that have failed because of sclerosis of the intervening greater saphenous vein between the outflow anastomosis and the common femoral vein.

Concluding Remarks

By no means have all the possible hemodialysis access sites or configurations been exhausted in this chapter. A patient with multiple failed AV fistulas or PTFE grafts with stenosis or occlusion of the more common artery inflow or vein outflow sites can pose a very real clinical problem. Finding a patent outflow vein in a relatively superficial location is the usual challenge. Thorough preoperative arterial and venous ultrasound imaging greatly improves selection of a satisfactory inflow/outflow conduit. In-depth knowledge of the surgical anatomy pertinent to hemodialysis access and meticulous surgical technique will create a situation that is gratifying for the surgeon, the nephrologist, and the patient with end-stage renal disease.

REFERENCES

1. Pittiruti M, Malerba M, Carriero C, Tazza L, Gui D. Which is the easiest and safest technique for central venous access? A retrospective survey of more than 5,400 cases. *J Vasc Access.* 2000;1:100-107.
2. Zollo A, Cavatorta F, Galli S. Ultrasound-guided cannulation of the femoral vein for acute hemodialysis access with silicone catheters. *J Vasc Access.* 2001;2:56-59.
3. Cho SK, Shin SW, Do YS, Park KB, Choo SW, Choo IW. Use of the right external jugular vein as the preferred access site when the right internal jugular vein is not usable. *J Vasc Interv Radiol.* 2006;17:823-829.
4. Mey U, Glasmacher A, Hahn C, et al. Evaluation of an ultrasound-guided technique for central venous access via the internal jugular vein in 493 patients. *Support Care Cancer.* 2003;11:148-155.
5. Ballard JL, Bunt TJ, Malone JM. Major complications of angioaccess surgery. *Am J Surg.* 1992;164:229-232.
6. Wilson SE. Complications of vascular access procedures: thrombosis, venous hypertension, arterial steal, and neuropathy. In Wilson SE (ed). *Vascular Access: Principles and Practice.* 3rd ed. St. Louis: Mosby–Year Book; 1995:212-224.
7. Kherlakian GM, Roedersheimer LR, Arbaugh JJ, Newmark KJ, King LR. Comparison of autogenous fistula versus expanded polytetrafluoroethylene graft fistula for angioaccess in hemodialysis. *Am J Surg.* 1986;152:238-243.
8. Coburn MC, Carney WI Jr. Comparison of basilic vein and polytetrafluoroethylene for brachial arteriovenous fistula. *J Vasc Surg.* 1994;20:896-902.
9. Kawecka A, Debska-Slizien A, Prajs J, et al. Remarks on surgical strategy in creating vascular access for hemodialysis: 18 years of one center's experience. *Ann Vasc Surg.* 2005;19:590-598.
10. Wolowczyk L, Williams AJ, Donovan KL, Gibbons CP. The snuffbox arteriovenous fistula for vascular access. *Eur J Vasc Endovasc Surg.* 2000;19:70-76.
11. Bonalumi U, Cavalleri D, Rovida S, Adami GF, Gianetti E, Griffanti-Bartoli F. Nine years' experience with end-to-end arteriovenous fistula at the "anatomical snuffbox" for maintenance hemodialysis. *Br J Surg.* 1982;69:486-488.
12. Miller PE, Tolwani A, Luscy CP. Predictors of adequacy of arteriovenous fistulas in hemodialysis patients. *Kidney Int.* 1999;56:275-280.
13. Silva MB Jr, Hobson RW 2nd, Pappas PJ, et al. A strategy for increasing use of autogenous hemodialysis access procedures: impact of preoperative noninvasive evaluation. *J Vasc Surg.* 1998;28:302-307.

14. Silva MB Jr, Hobson RW 2nd, Pappas PJ, et al: Vein transposition in the forearm for autogenous hemodialysis access. *J Vasc Surg.* 1997;26: 981-986.
15. Pontari MA, McMillen MA. The straight radial-antecubital PTFE angio-access graft in an era of high-flux dialysis. *Am J Surg.* 1991;161: 450-453.
16. Schmidt SP, Field FI. Forearm vascular access: loop versus straight polytetrafluoroethylene grafts. In Sommer BG, Henry ML (eds): *Vascular Access for Hemodialysis. Vol 2.* Chicago: Precept Press; 1991: 179-185.
17. Sparks SR, VanderLinden JL, Gnanadev DA, Smith JW, Bunt TJ. Superior patency of perforating antecubital vein in arteriovenous fistulae for hemodialysis. *Ann Vasc Surg.* 1997;11:165-167.
18. Aman LC, et al. Vascular-access survival in diabetic and non-diabetic hemodialysis patients. In Kootstra G, Jorning PJG (eds). *Access Surgery.* Ridgewood, NJ: Bogden and Sons; 1983.
19. Palder SB, Kirkman RL, Whittemore AD, Hakim RM, Lazarus JM, Tilney NL.: Vascular access for hemodialysis. Patency rates and results of revision. *Ann Surg.* 1985;202:235-239.
20. Nazzal MM. The brachiocephalic fistula: a successful secondary vascular access procedure. *Vasa.* 1990;19:326-329.
21. Fitzgerald JT, Schanzer A, Chin AI, McVicar JP, Perez RV, Troppmann C. Outcomes of upper arm arteriovenous fistulas for maintenance hemodialysis access. *Arch Surg.* 2004;139:201-208.
22. Polo JR, Vázquez R, Polo J, Sanabia J, Rueda JA, Lopez-Baena JA. Brachiocephalic jump graft fistula: an alternative for dialysis use of elbow crease veins. *Am J Kidney Dis.* 1999;33:904-909.
23. Wilson SE: Vascular interposition (bridge fistulas) for hemodialysis. In Wilson SE (ed). *Vascular Access: Principles and Practice.* 3rd ed. St. Louis: Mosby–Year Book; 1995:157-169.
24. Schulak JA, Lukens ML, Mayes JT. Salvage of thrombosed forearm polytetrafluoroethylene vascular access grafts by reversal of flow direction and venous bypass grafting. *Am J Surg.* 1991;161:485-487.
25. Livingston CK, Potts JR 3rd. Upper arm arteriovenous fistulas as a reliable access alternative for patients requiring chronic hemodialysis. *Am Surg.* 1999;65:1038-1042.
26. Hill SL, Seeger JM. The arm as an alternative site for vascular access for dialysis in patients with recurrent access failure. *South Med J.* 1985;78:37-40.
27. Hatjibaloglou A, Grekas D, Saratzis N, et al. Transposed basilic vein–brachial arteriovenous fistula: an alternative vascular access for hemodialysis. *Artif Organs.* 1992;16:623-625.
28. Rivers SP, Scher LA, Sheehan E, Lynn R, Veith FJ. Basilic vein transposition: an underused autologous alternative to prosthetic dialysis angioaccess. *J Vasc Surg.* 1993;18:391-396.
29. Butterworth PC, Doughman TM, Wheatley TJ, Nicholson ML. Arteriovenous fistula using transposed basilic vein. *Br J Surg.* 1998;85: 653-654.
30. Hakaim AG, Nalbandian M, Scott T. Superior maturation and patency of primary brachiocephalic and transposed basilic vein arteriovenous fistulae in patients with diabetes. *J Vasc Surg.* 1998;27: 154-157.
31. Humphries AL Jr, Colborn GL, Wynn JL. Elevated basilic vein arteriovenous fistula. *Am J Surg.* 1999;177:489-491.
32. Polo JR, Sanabia J, Garcia-Sabrido JL, Luño J, Menarguez C, Echenagusia A. Brachial-jugular polytetrafluoroethylene fistulas for hemodialysis. *Am J Kidney Dis.* 1990;16:465-468.
33. Jendrisak MD, Anderson CB. Vascular access in patients with arterial insufficiency: construction of proximal bridge fistulae based on inflow from axillary branch arteries. *Ann Surg.* 1990;212:187-193.
34. Schanzer H, Skladany M, Haimov M. Treatment of angioaccess-induced ischemia by revascularization. *J Vasc Surg.* 1992;16: 861-864.
35. Berman SS, Gentile AT, Glickman MH, et al. Distal revascularization-interval ligation for limb salvage and maintenance of dialysis access in ischemic steal syndrome. *J Vasc Surg.* 1997;26:393-402.
36. De Rosa P, Romano G, Buonanno GM, Di Salvo E. A simple vascular access for hemodialysis in "desperate" cases. *Hal J Surg Sci.* 1986;16: 209-210.
37. Mandel SR, McDougal EG. Popliteal artery to saphenous vein vascular access for hemodialysis. *Surg Gynecol Obstet.* 1985;160:358-359.

CHAPTER 5

Physiology of the Arteriovenous Fistula

Ian L. Gordon

Much of what we understand regarding the physiologic effects of arteriovenous (AV) fistulas was first placed into the modern context by Emil Holman, Halsted's last resident at Johns Hopkins, who eventually became chair of surgery at Stanford. In the early part of his career, he participated in the surgical ablation of large AV fistulas in several patients who were in extremis from high-output cardiac failure. He reported these operations in a vivid style that incorporated precise descriptions of the changes in blood flow and cardiovascular dynamics achieved with fistula closure. The patients' dramatic improvement sparked a lifelong interest in these lesions before their practical value for hemodialysis access was appreciated. Holman and his research associates at Stanford created fistulas of various sizes in dogs, concentrating on the iliac and femoral systems. By comparing fistulas of different dimensions and configurations in different limbs of the same animal and carefully applying simple methods of pressure measurement and angiography, he was able to deduce many of the factors that control blood flow after fistula formation. His findings have been largely confirmed by those studying the dynamics of hemodialysis access fistulas in the modern era. His elegant

and lucid descriptions of both the clinical and the laboratory aspects of AV fistula physiology are worth seeking out by any student of this topic.[1-6]

In this chapter, a direct connection via anastomosis between artery and vein is referred to as a *fistula, AV fistula,* or *AVF*. A communication between artery and vein resulting from a conduit anastomosed separately to each vessel is referred to as an *AV shunt,* or *bridge fistula*. In general, the effects of AV communications are discussed with the understanding that little difference exists between shunts and fistulas, although, where possible, known differences are described. The physiologic effects of AVFs can be separated into local hemodynamic effects, systemic cardiovascular effects, and secondary effects on tissue metabolism due to local or systemic changes. Because the caliber of the AV access blood vessels increases for several weeks after surgical construction,[7] we discuss both the immediate hemodynamic consequences of opening an AVF and the chronic effects evident once a fistula has matured. A fistula constructed via side-to-side anastomosis between artery and vein has four limbs through which blood flows (Fig. 5-1). An example of such a fistula would be a side-to-side

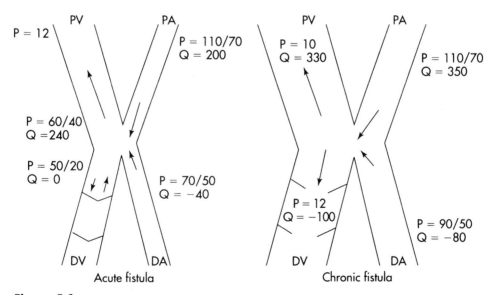

Figure 5-1.
Pressure and flow in idealized side-to-side acute and chronic arteriovenous fistulas. Compared with the acute fistula, the mature chronic fistula has higher distal artery (DA) pressures as a result of the development of arterial collaterals, and distal vein (DV) flow is retrograde as a result of valvular incompetence. *P,* Pressure in millimeters of mercury; *PA,* proximal artery; *PV,* proximal vein; *Q,* flow in milliliters per minute.

Brescia-Cimino fistula[8] employing the radial artery and the cephalic vein. Other variants are commonly constructed clinically to provide hemodialysis access—for example, the vein is divided and the proximal end is sewn to the side of the artery. Because local hemodynamic effects are critically influenced by anatomy, evaluation of clinical or experimental data requires consideration of the specific type of fistula constructed. In a four-limb fistula, the anatomic elements are the proximal artery (PA), distal artery (DA), proximal vein (PV), distal vein (DV), interconnecting fistula bridge in the case of shunts, arterial collateral vessels, venous collateral vessels, and the peripheral vascular bed (PVB), supplied by the DA. Each of these elements may have an influence on the blood flow patterns in an AVF.

Local Hemodynamic Effects Resulting from AVF Construction

The effect of creating a fistula on the PA is like making a hole in a dike. The minimal pressure gradient that normally exists between neighboring segments of an artery is changed at the fistula connection because of the large difference in pressure between arteries and veins. Flow in the PA increases dramatically in response to the sudden decrease in outflow pressure afforded by the fistula. Figure 5-1 depicts the typical patterns of flow and pressure present in both acute and chronic side-to-side fistulas.

The direction of flow in the PA remains antegrade, away from the heart, when an AVF is acutely opened, but increases dramatically. With forearm AVFs, brachial artery flows increase 5- to 10-fold compared with flows before opening the communication.[9] One factor affecting the magnitude of flow in the PA is the caliber of the fistula communication. In older experimental studies, the length (maximum diameter) of the fistula is generally substituted for cross-sectional area. As the dimensions of the fistula increase, flow in the PA increases until the anastomotic length approaches 75% or more of the PA diameter (Fig. 5-2). A recent study of canine femoral AVFs indicated, however, that as anastomotic length increased from 1.5 to 3 times greater than the PA diameter, total fistula flow increased from 5.6- to 8.4-fold greater than baseline.[10] The key concept is that increasing anastomotic length above a certain threshold leads to diminishing impact on PA and total fistula flow.

The situation in the DA is more complex. With small fistula communications, DA flow is maintained antegrade, away from the heart. With increasing fistula size, however, DA flow decreases until it reaches a standstill when the anastomotic length is about the same as the PA diameter. At this point, circus motion develops. Antegrade flow toward the PVB during systole is matched by retrograde flow during diastole through the fistula into the venous limbs. As the anastomotic length of the fistula communciation increases further, above the diameter of the artery, reversed flow in the DA increases until it exceeds antegrade DA flow.[3,11-13] With large fistulas, the absolute magnitude of acute retrograde DA flow is usually less than the antegrade flow that existed before opening the fistula. The relations between anastomotic size and DA flow have been characterized by flow measurements in both experimental animals

with peripheral fistulas and in patients with hemodialysis fistulas in the brachial, radial, and femoral systems.[12,14-17] Of note, clinical studies of radiocephalic fistulas indicate that retrograde DA flow is evident at the time of surgical construction in 75% to 80% of cases.[18] Normally reversed DA flow is about one quarter to one third of the magnitude of antegrade PA flow into the fistula. An example of reversal of flow in the distal artery caused by opening an AVF is illustrated in Figure 5-3.

With peripheral AVFs (eg, in the forearm), immediately after construction virtually all flow through the fistula is directly toward the heart via the PV—retrograde flow into the DV aimed distally is prevented or minimized by competent venous valves. With proximal AVFs involving central veins without valves, significant retrograde flow into the DV develops immediately after fistula opening. The acute influence of opening an AVF on local vessel pressures is also shown in Figure 5-1. Immediately after opening the fistula, there is a small decrement in PA pressure near the anastomosis and a larger decrease in neighboring DA pressure, which may fall to 50% of PA pressure.[13] The difference between systolic and diastolic pressure (pulse pressure) in the PA increases close to the fistula[19] because of the low resistance afforded by the fistula. Pressure in the midpoint of the fistula communication is intermediate between arterial and venous pressure. With bridge grafts, a gradient of pressure between the arterial and the venous anastomosis develops. With short shunts, and in true fistulas, the pressure waveform encountered just beyond the venous anastomosis usually shows significant arterial characteristics (Fig. 5-4). Immediately after AVF construction, the pressure in the PV is highest just at the anastomosis, but rapidly falls in the PV with movement toward the heart to basal values, reflecting the large capacitance of the venous circulation. With the high flows achieved in routine access surgery, the pressure gradient driving flow is usually sufficient to drive flow beyond Reynold's limit, and turbulence in the run-off vein or the bridging conduit is evidenced by a thrill or bruit. The absence of turbulence may indicate flow restriction from stenosis affecting the arterial inflow or venous run-off. In experimental animals, the flow through the PV may be so rapid that measurable pressure becomes less than zero from the Venturi effect.[6,13] In the distal vein, however, competent valves usually prevent flow retrograde—consequently, pressure in the DV is elevated in the vicinity of the fistula and shows arterial properties.

Several factors affect the magnitude of flow created by acutely opening an AVF. Proximity to the heart is important, because higher flows are found with fistulas between the aorta and the cava or other great vessels than with fistulas of comparable dimensions between more peripheral vessels.[3,8] Second, as indicated previously, the cross-sectional area or anastomotic length influences flow in a nonlinear manner (Fig. 5-5). Until the anastomotic diameter exceeds 20% of the PA diameter, fistula flow is relatively low. Between 20% to 75% of the PA diameter, total fistula flow rapidly rises. Above 75% of the PA diameter, further modest increases in total fistula flow are due to increasing retrograde DA flow into the fistula. More recent data from a canine femoral AV fistula model suggested, however, that as anastomotic length increases above 1.5 times the PA diameter, the increase in total fistula flow may be more a

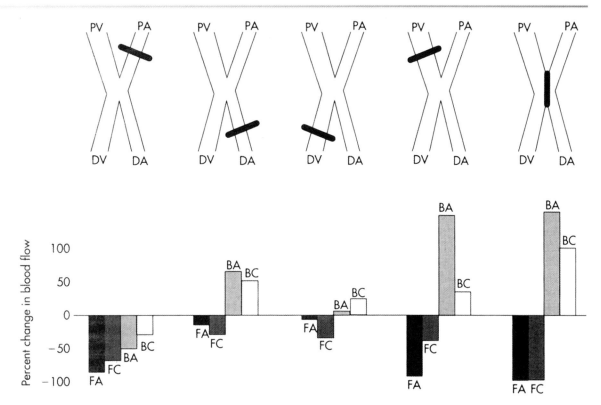

Figure 5-2.
Effect of occluding limbs of a side-to-side fistula. The effects of occluding individual limbs on total fistula flow and flow in the peripheral vascular bed are shown. The percent change in flow for each parameter is depicted for both acute and chronic fistulas. Proximal artery (PA) occlusion actually leads to decreased peripheral vascular bed flow by increasing reversal of flow through the distal artery (DA) and steal. The effect on the distal vascular bed is less pronounced in chronic fistulas because arterial collaterals are better able to maintain flow. DA occlusion enhances peripheral vascular bed flow and causes only a modest fall in total fistula flow. Distal vein (DV) occlusion causes minimal acute effects, only a moderate fall in total fistula flow, and a moderate increase in peripheral vascular bed flow in the mature fistula. Acute proximal vein (PV) occlusion causes near cessation of fistula flow, comparable with occlusion of the fistula opening, but has much less impact in the chronic fistula because of alternative venous return. Occluding the fistula communication *(right)* restores flows acutely to basal values, but has less effect on peripheral vascular bed flow in the chronic situation because of increased arterial collateral flow. *BA,* Acute peripheral vascular bed flow; *BC,* chronic peripheral vascular bed flow; *FA,* acute total fistula flow; *FC,* chronic total fistula flow.

consequence of increased PA flow, which continues to increase, with reversed DA flow reaching a maximum earlier in relation to anastomotic length.[10]

Smaller fistula openings tend to preserve antegrade flow away from the heart in the DA and flow toward the heart in the DV. Because such small fistulas have an increased risk for thrombosis or inadequate dialysis flow rates, the length of the anastomosis in access fistulas is generally at least the diameter of the donor artery, except when large arteries such as the axillary are employed and the anastomotic dimensions are deliberately constrained for fear of creating too high a flow and inducing high-output cardiac failure (see "Systemic Hemodynamic Effects **Resulting from AVF Construction**").

The relations summarized in Poiseuille's law govern the flow in fistulas. Relatively unappreciated clinically, arterial blood pressure is an independent variable influencing flow as venous pressure is relatively constant. All else being equal, access flow rates rise in hemodialysis patients in a linear fashion with increasing arterial pressure.[12,20] More appreciated clinically is the diameter of the veins and

arteries carrying the AV flow. Clinical data show that with small veins (≤3 mm in diameter), significantly lower flows are observed immediately after construction of radiocephalic AVFs. Similarly, when either the artery or the vein is less than 1.6 mm in diameter, significantly lower flow and increased risk for early access failure are found.[18] Another factor that influences flow is blood viscosity, primarily a consequence of hematocrit, which can be shown to influence measurable flows.[12]

Normal brachial artery flow in humans has a mean value of approximately 85 mL/min; opening an AVF multiplies brachial artery flow by a factor of 5 to 10.[9,21] Flow rates measured in the operating room may not accurately predict subsequent flows if the vessels are in spasm and do not reflect the increased flows that normally result from vessel dilatation as fistulas mature. Intraoperative flow measurements obtained immediately after AV access construction show mean flows to be about 300 mL/min for radiocephalic fistulas.[7,18,22] Flow is higher for shunts constructed based on the brachial or femoral arteries, and the mean value reported

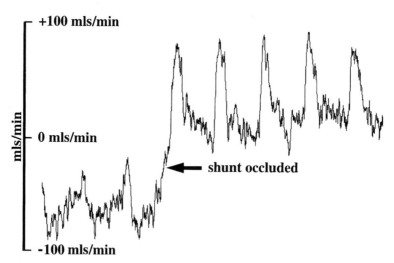

Figure 5-3.

Intraoperative flow measurements of the distal radial artery. The patient had a severe steal develop immediately after construction of a shunt between the radial artery and the antecubital vein. Pulse oximetry signals were absent in the affected hand unless the shunt was occluded by compression. Similarly, digital Doppler velocity waveforms were markedly blunted on the affected side. A 4-mm transit time ultrasound probe was placed on the radial artery just distal to the arterial anastomosis and flow was recorded with the shunt open and occluded *(arrow)*. Before occlusion, flow was directed in a retrograde fashion into the open shunt, with antegrade flow restored by shunt occlusion. Ligation of the distal radial artery led to satisfactory resolution of the patient's pain.

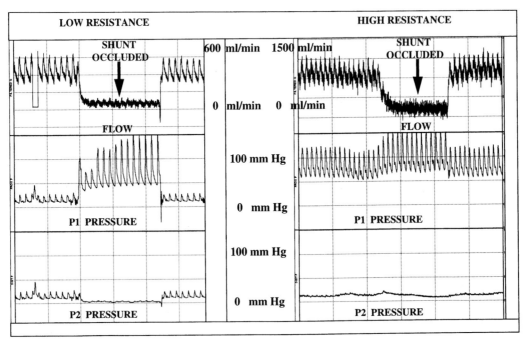

Figure 5-4.

Hemodynamic differences between low- and high-resistance AV shunts. Flow and pressure recordings, made with the technique shown in Figure 5-5, were obtained during revision of 6-mm polytetrafluoroethylene (PTFE) grafts. Note that in the low-resistance graft, temporary clamping causes a dramatic rise in P1 and a less dramatic but still marked fall in P2. In contrast, with high longitudinal resistance, clamping causes only a minor augmentation of P1 pressure and minimal effects on P2.

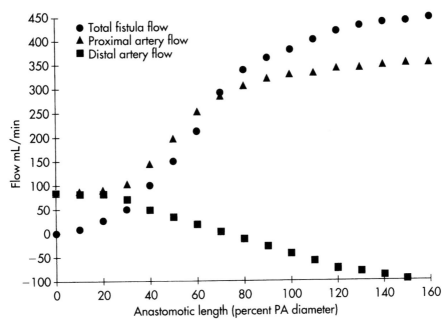

Figure 5-5.

Relation between anastomotic length and fistula flows. Depicted are the relations between the size of the fistula communication, total fistula flow, flow in the proximal artery, and flow in the distal artery. The anastomotic length as a percentage of proximal artery (PA) diameter is used to represent fistula size. Total fistula flow is the difference between PA and distal artery (DA) flows, so that when distal flow is reversed (ie, has a negative value), total flow is the sum of PA flow and the absolute magnitude of DA flow.

for early flow rates in these positions is 700 to 1000 mL/min.[22] Flows normally increase by 50% to 100% after access construction over a few weeks as vessels dilate.[23-27] Desirable flow rates for hemodialysis are 350 mL/min or higher; otherwise the efficiency of dialysis is reduced by recirculation within the fistula-dialysis machine circuit.[28] Patency of AVFs correlates with flow measurements taken intraoperatively as well as those taken after maturation but immediately before first cannulation.[29,30]

It should be appreciated that the resistance of both the distal PVB and the arterial collateral circulation contributes to the hemodynamic results of opening an acute fistula. Pressure in the DA falls to a minimum near the fistula communication and increases with increasing distance away from the fistula as a consequence of inflow from arterial collaterals. All else being equal, the lower the resistance to flow in the PVB, the more antegrade flow in the DA is promoted. High resistance in the PVB promotes retrograde flow in the DA toward the fistula. If resistance to flow in the arterial collaterals is low, more blood will flow into the DA, also promoting reversed flow. Conversely, poorly developed arterial collaterals, or high resistance in them, by deceasing peripheral perfusion, promotes antegrade flow in the DA, other factors being constant.

Reversed flow in the DA leads to diversion of flow from the distal vascular bed (eg, the hand in radiocephalic fistulas). This phenomenon underlies the rationale for ligating the DA or constructing end-artery–to–vein radiocephalic fistulas to prevent retrograde DA flow. Steal tends to develop in all side-artery–to–vein constructions with large communications, but local anatomy will influence the severity. When fistulas are based on the brachial artery, reversal of flow may be created in both the radial and the ulnar arteries, leading to a higher risk of severe steal than radial artery–based accesses, in which ulnar flow is maintained antegrade into the palmar arch, which in turn feeds retrograde radial flow.[31,32]

Studying the effect of temporary occlusion of the individual limbs of AVFs helps to better appreciate their hemodynamic properties. Figure 5-2 depicts how occlusion of each limb affects flow in the fistula and the distal vascular bed in both acute and chronic settings. In the acute AVF constructed peripherally, occlusion of the PV has essentially the same effect as occluding all four limbs, emphasizing the limited run-off through the DV when its valves are competent. For the same reason, with competent valves, occlusion of the DV has minimal impact in the acute AVF. Occlusion of the DA reduces acute fistula flow only modestly (20%-30%), because more flow into the fistula via the PA is one of the tendencies induced by DA occlusion, but flow in the PVB is enhanced by DA occlusion as steal is diminished. In contrast, occlusion of the PA with a patent DA leads to decreased flow in both the fistula and the PVB. The decrease in fistula flow caused by PA occlusion is less than that achieved with PV occlusion because the patent DA continues to supply flow. The decrease in PVB flow seen with PA occlusion is due more to enhanced steal from retrograde DA flow than to limitation of inflow into the PVB— combined occlusion of both PA and DA causes less decrease in PVB flow than PA occlusion alone.

Blood flow velocity profiles in and near AVFs have been studied with Doppler ultrasound. Before AVF construction, the velocity profiles of forearm arteries show the high-resistance characteristics of arteries supplying a muscular bed. Velocities are low during diastole, and reversal of flow during diastole is observed when the distal run-off resistance is high. The ratio of systolic-to-diastolic velocities is high. Exercise or skin warming may decrease resistance sufficiently to ablate reversal of flow during diastole. Opening an AVF changes the triphasic velocity waveform of the PA to a monophasic high-diastolic flow pattern typical of low resistance.[33] Normally, the mean brachial artery flow velocity is approximately 9 cm/sec. This velocity increases to about 90 cm/sec with an AVF.[21,34] Phasic velocities in the brachial artery proximal to the fistula range from 100 to 400 cm/sec in systole and 60 to 200 cm/sec in diastole. Velocity waveforms in the PV show an arterial pulsation pattern with mean velocities of 30 to 100 cm/sec, with minimal respiratory variation. Doppler ultrasound demonstration of triphasic waveforms in the artery feeding a fistula strongly suggests occlusion or stenosis in the fistula pathway creating high resistance to flow.[35]

Depending on the degree of reversed flow in the DA, its velocity profile may show continued antegrade flow, circus motion with approximately equal flows oriented in opposite directions in diastole and systole, or continuously reversed flow. When turbulent flow is found with ultrasound examinations, the evident pattern is a wide dispersion in the range of velocities present with increased maximal velocities characteristic of a jet. Flow proximal to valves in the DV may show a circus motion pattern characteristic of obstruction. Disturbed flow may persist for some distance away from the fistula opening into the PV before laminar flow is reestablished.[35] Vortices may fill the vein during systole and subside during diastole. The asymmetrical patterns of flow near the anastomosis lead to areas of high- and low wall shear stress (WSS) in the vein, which parallel the velocity vector profile.[36] Computational fluid dynamic models indicate flow through fistula anastomoses is asymmetrical, although the anastomotic geometry itself is symmetrical.[37] Computation fluid dynamics also indicate that in Cimino fistulas, WSS ranges from 20 and 36 dynes/cm^2, on the straight portion of the afferent radial artery, whereas on the inner surface of the bending zone, it is increased up to 350 dynes/cm^2. On the venous side, in the proximal vein, WSS oscillates between negative and positive values (from -12 dynes/cm^2 to 112 dynes/cm^2). Areas of the vessel wall with very high shear stress gradient were identified on the bending zone of the radial artery and on the venous side, just beyond the AV communication.[38]

Systolic pressures in the digits and thumb can be measured with inflatable cuffs and Doppler ultrasound. Normal digital pressures are generally 75% or more of brachial artery pressure (average, 86%).[39] Opening an AV fistula will cause a modest decrease in digital pressure from steal of flow via the DA. A fall in the ratio of digital-to-brachial pressure below 50% correlates with an increased risk of symptomatic steal, and a fall below 30% correlates with a high probability of ischemic necrosis. Digital pulse volume waveforms (pulse oscillometry) and Doppler velocity waveforms both show decreased magnitude when significant steal develops in hemodialysis fistulas.[40] Severe steal will lead to marked blunting or effacement of the digital waveforms.[41-43] A useful maneuver in evaluating steal with AV

shunts is to temporarily occlude the shunt conduit and compare digital artery pressures or Doppler velocity waveforms before and after. With fistulas, the comparable maneuver is to temporarily occlude the DA, because occlusion of the PA may actually enhance the steal. Another method for assessing the severity of steal is afforded by pulse oximetry. Normally, pulse oximeters placed on the fingers of a limb with an AVF yield measurements of arterial blood oxygen saturation (Sao$_2$) close to those measured contralaterally.[44] The difference in Sao$_2$ between hands can be 10% or more when severe steal is present and this difference is accentuated when hemodialysis circuit flow is induced.[45] Steal also induces a temperature gradient between the skin over a fistula and the hand, and coolness of the hand is another marker of steal (see "Chronic Consequences of AVF").

Systemic Hemodynamic Effects Resulting from AVF Construction

The immediate effect of opening a fistula is to divert blood flow away from the rest of the peripheral circulation and into a special low-resistance path directly connecting the left side to the right side of the heart. Cardiac output increases acutely via increased rate and stroke volume to provide this flow, but paradoxically, diversion of flow into this parasitic circulation depletes the volume in the rest of the vascular system. Arterial pressure falls, and heart rate increases; these changes are minimal with low-flow fistulas and increase with increasing fistula flow. Cardiac work ($\int PQ\delta t$) also increases.[46] Central venous pressures and pulmonary pressures tend to rise minimally in normal animals because of the large capacitance of the venous side of circulation, but pulmonary hypertension may develop in dialysis patients (see "Systemic Hemodynamic Effects of Chronic AVS").

Studies in experimental animals show that with modest fistula flows totaling 20% or less of baseline cardiac output, the net increase in cardiac output achieved by opening an AVF essentially equals fistula flow. As fistula flow increases above 20% of cardiac output, peripheral resistance rises to divert flow from the nonfistulous portion of the peripheral circulation into the fistula circuit. This rise is an acute effect, and peripheral resistance tends to return toward basal levels with chronic adaptation to the AVF. The net effect of this response is an acute steal of flow from other organ beds into the fistula circuit.[47-49]

With high-flow experimental AVFs, the heart contracts in size as if a state of relative hypovolemia has been induced. Cardiac output increases with increasing fistula diameter and proximity to the heart; increases of well over 100% are observed in experimental settings.[6,50,51] Relatively small fistulas (1 cm) between the aorta and the vena cava may induce shock and death in dogs.[46] AVFs of similar length in the extremities cause significantly lower increases in cardiac output and minimal and transient changes in blood pressure and pulse rate with opening. Temporary occlusion of an AVF or shunt (either acute or chronic) by compression may cause a decrease in pulse rate and a rise in blood pressure, the Nicoladoni-Branham sign, but this is not reliably present in fistulas with moderate flow rates. Interestingly, most of the cardiovascular changes induced by opening a fistula occur rapidly, within a few pulse beats, and do not require the participation of central reflexes. They are purely a consequence of the anatomic rearrangement of pressure and flow.[52]

In normal animals, experimental AVFs lead to salt and water retention to compensate for the hypovolemic state created by opening the fistula. This response is mediated in part through the renin-angiotensin-aldosterone axis[53-56] but does not entail changes in overall renal blood flow.[57] Both atrial and brain natriuretic peptide levels have been shown to increase in renal failure patients undergoing access surgery, with levels peaking around 10 days after surgery.[58] The increase in circulating volume is due to increased plasma volume, not red blood cell mass. Patients with renal failure cannot be relied on to compensate in the same manner, and thought must be given to expanding intravascular volume as an adjunct to operation, particularly if high-flow fistulas in the brachial or femoral systems are being constructed.

Large fistulas, such as aortocaval fistulas resulting from syphilitic aortitis, atherosclerotic abdominal aneurysm, or trauma during lumbar disk surgery,[59-61] have dramatic effects on the cardiovascular system. Patients suffering from these conditions have characteristic relative hypovolemia and a decreased cardiac silhouette on chest radiograph. The first symptom may be angina pectoris from increased myocardial work and decreased coronary perfusion related to the drop in diastolic pressure. The acute presentation of a large central AVF resembles shock as peripheral blood flow and intravascular volume are diverted to the fistula circuit, in contrast to the chronic large fistula in which the pattern is more like that of high-output cardiac failure.

Chronic Consequences of AVFs

Multiple morphologic changes develop in a typical side-to-side fistula with maturation. In small fistula, the anastomotic communication tends to become obstructed by the accumulation of platelets and fibrin. Subsequent myointimal proliferation leads to thrombosis and closure. In fistulas that remain patent, the PA, PV, and DV all tend to elongate and dilate to accommodate the increased blood flow. Dilatation of the DA is less pronounced, but it is enhanced if flow in the PA is limited by stenosis or occlusion. Arterial dilatation is accompanied by elongation, and tortuous aneurysmal degeneration may be the ultimate result. Histologically, the arterial changes are characterized by smooth muscle hypertrophy of the media, with aneurysm formation a result of smooth muscle atrophy in later stages. The PV undergoes arterialization with hypertrophy of subintimal smooth muscle and elastin and increased collagen and fibrous tissue content.[62] The DV undergoes similar changes when incompetent valves allow retrograde flow.

Holman attributed the dilatation of vessels in fistulas with maturation to distention from the blood volume shifted into the direct circuit connecting the left and the right sides of the heart.[3] The elongation observed has never been clearly explained and, possibly, is a consequence of a longitudinally oriented tension that develops secondary to the fistula pressure gradient or, alternately, is induced by the increase in vessel diameters.[63] Animal models suggest

that high WSS is responsible for development of elongation and tortuosity without causing medial thickening.[64] Part of the response of the arterial wall to increased blood flow appears to represent a homeostatic mechanism that conserves WSS. WSS is defined as $4\eta Q/\pi r^3$, where η is blood viscosity, Q is blood flow in milliliters per minute, and r is vessel radius. Studies in experimental animals show that after AVF construction, vessel radius increases over several weeks to a new equilibrium value that balances the increase in Q, so that WSS returns to its original level. Ultrasound studies measuring WSS in dialysis patients undergoing access construction indicate that radial artery dilatation restores peak WSS to basal levels, suggesting endothelial cell responses are sensitive to maximal shear stress rather than time-averaged shear stress.[65] Comparable studies in the brachial artery also show that dilatation after brachial-based fistula construction leads to conservation of peak WSS.[66] Dilatation appears to be dependent on endothelial cell elaboration of nitric oxide, because inhibition of nitric oxide synthesis in experimental animal models prevents both PA and PVn dilatation.[67,68] There also appears to be a necessary role for tissue matrix metalloproteinase activity for dilatation of the arterial wall, because nonspecific inhibition of these enzymes prevents dilatation in experimental animals with AVFs.[69] New synthesis of structural components in the arterial wall also is induced by increased flow, because the thickness of the donor artery wall remains either unchanged with progressive dilatation or actually increases.[67,70]

One of the most clinically important histologic changes that occur in AVFs is stenosis due to intimal hyperplasia or atherosclerotic degeneration. Although in most instances the tissue that develops at fistula communications is due to myointimal hyperplasia, histologic evaluation of tissue in several experimental and clinical observations confirm some similarities to atherosclerotic lesions.[71,72] Although high WSS has been associated with induction of intimal lesions in some settings,[73,74] a growing body of clinical and experimental evidence implicates low WSS as more important in the causation of anastomotic stenosis. Long-term exposure to low WSS induces medial smooth muscle proliferation and migration, with strong correlations observed between sites of low shear stress and sites of intimal thickening.[64,75,76]

The intuitive concept that repetitive exercise improves fistula flow is contradicted by understanding the effect of PVB resistance on fistula hemodynamics. As noted previously, retrograde flow through the DA falls with decreasing resistance through the distal vascular bed. Clinical measurements of fistula flow in hemodialysis patients during hand exercise (which decreases resistance in the hand) have confirmed that exercise does not increase fistula flow,[20,77,78] although it may possibly promote arterial collateral formation.

One of the striking differences between acute and chronic fistulas is the collateral arterial supply to the DA. In side-to-side AVFs, retrograde flow through the DA usually increases with time over several months. At the same time, PVB perfusion returns close to the level existing before shunt construction. Contrast angiography in experimental animals demonstrates prominent hypertrophy and hyperplasia of the collateral arterial circulation to the DA.

Ligation of the DA or end-artery–to–vein anastomosis prevents formation of increased arterial collaterals. With side-to-side AVFs, temporary occlusion of the PA decreases distal vascular bed perfusion less severely than in the acute setting because of the increased collateral supply (see Fig. 5-2).

As in the acute setting, retrograde flow through the DA in mature fistulas may comprise as much as one third of total flow. With time, flow increases in both PAs and DAs.[79] The incidence of steal is highest in side-to-side radial fistulas when the ulnar artery is obstructed. Of note, successful dialysis access without hand ischemia has been achieved using the stump of the radial artery after thrombosis of the proximal radial artery.[80] Because flow is generally higher in side-of-artery–to–vein fistulas than end-of-artery–to–vein configurations, and higher flows correlate with longer fistula patency, it appears that a good strategy when constructing AV access is to avoid ligation of the distal radial artery unless preoperative studies suggest compromise of the ulnar artery. An alternative approach is to measure digital pressures intraoperatively and ligate the DA only if they fall below a critical threshold after fistula opening.

In the rare case in which steal develops in the presence of a side-of-artery–to–vein fistulas, ligation of the fistula and restoration of distal flow is always the safest course.[81] When saving a fistula is paramount, ligation of the DA may improve distal perfusion sufficiently to allow preservation of both hand and fistula. When ulnar occlusion is present, ligating the radial artery just distal to the fistula communication with concomitant bypass to a distal segment of the radial artery has successfully preserved the hand and AV access.[82,83] Intraoperative monitoring of digital cuff pressures and Doppler waveforms while temporally occluding vessels is useful to help determine the exact modification of a fistula or shunt required to manage steal.[84]

Some advocate ligating the DV or end-of-vein–to–artery anastomosis during construction of access. DV ligation has little effect on flow in the acute setting and prevents the complication of hand edema.[9,85] Edema of the upper extremity after access construction generally is a consequence of obstruction in the lymphatic or venous drainage of the limb proximal to the fistula and is unlikely to result from the hemodynamic impact of AVF formation alone. In the mature fistula, repeated puncture may cause strictures and increased resistance in the PV, diverting flow into the retrograde vein and collaterals, which often are not accessible for hemodialysis. After DV ligation, flow rates via the accessible PV may be more satisfactory for dialysis. Similarly, branches of the PV that communicate with deeper veins may divert flow away from easily accessed superficial vein segments—in these cases, ligation of distal tributaries of the PV near the fistula can salvage a fistula with inadequate flow.[86]

Historically, the optimal strategy for control of an AVF was ligation of all four limbs. Current techniques allow more precise interventions, such as oversewing the arterotomy from inside the vein lumen, preserving distal arterial flow. In difficult situations, ligation of the inflow artery in conjunction with venous ligation may be the only choice available. Such a compromise approach should lead to a satisfactory outcome because adequate distal perfusion is normally preserved despite ligation of the PA as a consequence of the stimulation of arterial collaterals that accompanies chronic side-to-side fistulas. With modern fluoroscopically guided endovascular methods, fistulas can be ablated by deployment of stent grafts to line either the vein or the artery on one side of the fistula communication. Similarly, restriction of flow within fistulas and AV grafts to reverse steal can be precisely controlled by deployment of endoluminal stent grafts with circumferential ligatures to narrow the fistula conduit to the outer diameter of the stent graft.[87]

Blood flow can be modeled like electrical circuits[88] and because the effects of pulsatile blood flow on resistance are minimal (unpublished observations), they can be mostly ignored, such that direct current models are appropriate. Turbulence effects are hard to model, however, and probably do significantly influence AVF flow and pressure relations. Predictions of the models indicate that flows should be higher in side-to-side than in end-to-side or end-to-end fistulas. The effect of anastomotic diameter on flows in the chronic setting is theoretically similar to acute fistulas: 75% of the PA diameter remains a critical value. With shunts, both the diameter and the length of the bridge limb theoretically influence flow. Circuit models indicate that increased bridge lengths in shunts may limit flow and that the diameter of the conduit should be several times the PA diameter to achieve maximal flows. Although theoretically important, the diameter and length of the conduit bridge minimally affect flow in mature AV grafts compared with the effects of stenosis within the conduit or anastomoses or run-off vein caliber. Of note, flows measured in mature radial artery–to–antecubital vein shunts are fairly similar to those found in radiocephalic fistulas.[22,78,89-91] There is no clear evidence from either circuit models or clinical blood flow measurements of shunts and fistulas that significantly higher flows are routinely achieved in fistulas compared with shunts based on the same vessels. The implication is that the significantly better patency rates associated with fistulas[92] are probably more a consequence of stenosis arising within shunts or shunt anastomoses rather than differences in flow per se.

Studies of flow in hemodialysis AVFs indicate that flows tend to increase with time, but not invariably.[17,93] Increased flow is promoted by dilatation of the PA and the outflow veins, which expand to the degree allowed by their anatomic properties, limited by the caliber of the fistula communication and the pressure gradient. Collateral flow around the fistula also increases, with much of this being diverted retrograde via the DA into the fistula. Opposing the tendency for flow to increase is the propensity for stenosis to develop at the venous anastomosis and the neighboring PV. Contributing to the development of stenosis are access trauma, myointimal hyperplasia, and atherosclerotic degeneration with low WSS secondary to turbulence being important. Stenosis may occur at the arterial anastomosis in shunts, but is less common than venous stenosis as a cause of failure.[35,94]

The relation between flow rates and fistula patency is obscured by the factors that lead to stenosis in the fistula circuit. Within-graft and anastomotic stenoses develop unpredictably as a consequence of needle puncture for hemodialysis access, but conceivably, an AVF with a high initial flow could be at higher risk of subsequent failure from turbulence-induced myointimal hyperplasia than

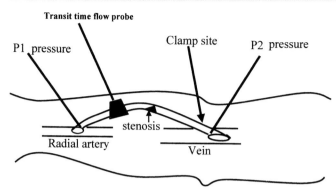

Figure 5-6.
Technique for measuring arteriovenous (AV) shunt resistance. Separate 22-gauge catheters are inserted into the graft near the arterial (P1) and venous (P2) anastomoses, and a transit time ultrasonic probe is placed on the graft to measure flow (Q). Mean P1, P2, and Q values are measured, and mean longitudinal resistance (R_L) calculated as {P1 – P2)/Q. Often, with newly implanted PTFE grafts, there is interference with the flow measurement from gas remaining in the conduit wall, so that the flow probe should be placed on the proximal vein. The technique works satisfactorily with previously implanted PTFE grafts undergoing revision as well as vein or collagen conduits. If the graft is occluded as part of the measurement, it is best to place the clamp close to the venous anastomosis to assess as much of the graft as possible.

would a fistula with less flow. Since the inception of AV access surgery for hemodialysis access, investigators have repeatedly demonstrated that patency rates correlate with measurable flow in the AV access. The consistent trend has been that accesses with low flows have significantly decreased subsequent patency.[18,22,24-27,86,92] Unfortunately, there is no agreed-upon standard method for measuring AV access flows, leading to a high degree of variability in measured flows for comparable access anatomy reported from different centers. Although a threshold value for access flow that should trigger prophylactic interventions has not reliably been established, it appears clear from the literature that low flow correlates with decreased patency, especially when serial measurements show falling flow rates.[92] Several new techniques for measuring flow are promising, including indicator dilution methods to monitor the washout of saline injected into the hemodialysis circuit with transit-time ultrasound, electrical resistance, or thermodilultion.[95-98]

We have become interested in the correlation between longitudinal resistance in AV shunts and subsequent patency. By placing small catheters into a PTFE graft near each anastomosis, the pressure at each end (arterial end = P1; venous end = P2) can be recorded, and bulk flow (Q) can be measured with perivascular transit-time probes (see Fig. 5-6). Longitudinal resistance (R_L) is calculated as the pressure gradient (P1 – P2) divided by Q. We have found that resistance varies (more than flow or pressure gradient) over a dynamic range of 200-fold in AV shunts, depending on the severity of focal stenoses within the conduit. The R_L measurement does not reflect the influence of anastomotic dimensions or the presence of stenosis in the outflow veins;

rather, it simply defines the resistance to flow between the two pressure catheters. We have reported how R_L strongly correlates with subsequent patency after thrombectomy and revision of clotted PTFE shunts.[99] As illustrated in Figures 5-4 and 5-6, clamping the conduit between the pressure catheters leads to different effects on the P1 and P2 pressure waveforms, depending on whether high or low resistance to flow is present. In the absence of stenosis, pressure at the arterial end (P1) dramatically rises with graft clamping, which ablates the effect of low resistance created by the venous anastomosis. When significant stenosis exists within the graft, clamping does not cause a marked increase in P1, which already is near inflow artery pressure. This effect can be detected clinically without formal pressure measurements by palpating near the arterial end of an AV shunt before and after occlusion near the venous end. The palpable pulse dramatically increases in a low-resistance conduit with occlusion. In contrast, there is only a minor increment in the force of the pulse palpated induced by occlusion when significant stenosis within the conduit causes high resistance to flow.

A comparable phenomenon is evident in the relation between longitudinal resistance and the P2 pressure. With low resistance, the P2 waveform shows marked arterial excursions because relatively high pressure is directed into the venous end. Clamping a low resistance graft near the arterial end leads to marked diminution in the P2 pressure waveform, which assumes pure venous morphology. In contrast, the P2 waveform in a high-resistance graft shows less arterialization and more of a venous quality, and clamping induces fewer reductions in P2 pressure, which is already low owing to the pressure gradient across the stenotic segments of the AV conduit.

Comparable effects of stenosis on the pressure gradient across either the arterial or the venous anastomosis have been reported—a stenosis at any site will be evidenced by an increased pressure gradient across the lesion. In addition, normally the pressure within a shunt is less than 50% that measured with the shunt temporarily occluded. When the pressure within the graft is more than 50% of the pressure measured with the graft clamped, analogous to the phenomenon demonstrated in Figure 5-4, poor subsequent patency is observed.[100]

Systemic Hemodynamic Effects of Chronic AVS

All AVFs increase cardiac output, and as flow increases with chronicity, so does total cardiac output. In general, the percentage of cardiac output devoted to the remainder of the peripheral circulation other than the fistula circuit falls modestly after opening a fistula (5%–10%, depending on the organ bed) but, with time, returns close to original levels. Studies in chronic hemodialysis patients show that, on the average, temporary occlusion of forearm AVFs and shunts lowers cardiac output 8% to 13%,[101,102] indicating that a comparable proportion of cardiac output passes through the access. Part of the response to the increased cardiac output induced by AVF flow is increased plasma volume. In experimental animals, the increase in plasma volume is mediated in part by increased elaboration of atrial natriuretic peptide stimulated by increased right atrial pressure.[103] The decrease in cardiac output resulting from temporary AVF occlusion is due to reduction of left ventricular stroke volume more than pulse rate.[51] Patients with high-flow brachial and femoral shunts, in which flows can exceed 2 L/min, have greater risk of cardiac complications. Coronary flow may be reduced because of steal to the fistula despite increased myocardial oxygen requirements from increased cardiac work. Preexisting coronary artery disease and other factors such as anemia and fluid overload also contribute to fistula-induced cardiac failure. Congestive failure may occur when fistula flow increases cardiac output as little as 20%.[50]

Recently, an increased propensity for hemodialysis patients to develop pulmonary hypertension has been recognized. High pulmonary artery pressures (PAP) are more common in hemodialysis patients than in controls—in one study, 48% of the hemodialysis patients were found to have PAP greater than 36 mm Hg by Doppler echocardiography methods.[104]

There is a positive correlation between cardiac output and PAP in hemodialysis patients, and those with pulmonary hypertension tend to have higher access flows. Temporary or permanent occlusion of dialysis access leads to a fall in both cardiac output and PAP. Some data implicate alterations in thromboxane, endothelin, and nitric oxide metabolism to contribute to the development of pulmonary hypertension by increasing pulmonary artery resistance, but it seems likely that the primary factor is increased pulmonary artery blood flow resulting from access construction.[105-107]

Patients with large aortocaval fistulas have several prominent and interesting findings. The overall setting is that of high-output cardiac failure, with tachycardia, lowered diastolic pressure, increased pulse pressure, and cardiac flow murmurs sustained in systole and diastole. The heart enlarges and both ventricles may hypertrophy. Central and peripheral venous pressures are markedly elevated, and peripheral veins such as the femoral may have pressures as high as 60 mm Hg. Measurable peripheral resistance is low. Arterial pressure distal to the fistula is lower than proximal blood pressure, and this may manifest as claudication or limb-threatening ischemia. The shift of blood into the cava may cause venous hypertension with arterial pulsations in the peripheral veins. Raised caval pressure interferes with hepatic and portal venous flow, leading to hepatomegaly and ascites. Below the fistula, marked edema of the scrotum and lower extremities develops.[108] The constellation of lower extremity edema and ischemia in conjunction with pulsatile dilatation of the superficial abdominal veins is pathognomonic of large aortocaval fistula and is present in over 50% of patients. Caval hypertension may also lead to gastrointestinal bleeding as well as hematuria. Renal filtration may be significantly decreased as a result of renal vein hypertension.[109]

Effect of AVS on Lower Extremity Bypass Grafts

Do AVFs promote better graft patency when deliberately constructed as part of lower extremity arterial bypass?

Most authors have recommended ligation of AVFs when found with in situ saphenous bypasses, based on the belief that they interfere with limb salvage.[95,110,111] Several groups of investigators have suggested that graft patency is improved when such fistulas are fashioned at or beyond the distal anastomosis of infrainguinal bypasses.[112-114] It is to be expected that construction of AVFs improves bypass patency, because flows will necessarily be higher when fistulas are present. Flow through the distal anastomosis, however, should be reduced or even directed retrograde, leading to less distal perfusion than would otherwise be achieved; decreased pressures in the distal vascular bed have been observed.[115] On a theoretical basis, then, incorporation of an AVF into a bypass should cause less improvement in distal ischemia than would otherwise occur, and may actually accentuate ischemia, despite improved flow maintaining graft patency.[116] Our own experience with acute intraoperative measurements using transit-time ultrasound during saphenous vein in situ bypass is that as fistulas are identified and ligated, total graft flow decreases but flow directed through the distal anastomosis increases.

Perhaps the alleged benefit of supplemental AVFs in lower extremity bypass is related to stimulation of arterial collateral flow. Presumably, if the AVFs are small, they may stimulate improved collateral supply to the distal vascular bed without excessive steal, and this may be of benefit, particularly after the AVF closes. One confounding factor in evaluating the merit of deliberate AVF construction is the use of this technique with prosthetic grafts. With PTFE, vein patches at the distal anastomosis have been reported to improve graft patency, with the explanation for this effect being that interposition of vein between PTFE and arterial intima inhibits myointimal hyperplasia.[117] If construction of a vein patch and fistula at the distal anastomosis improves patency, is this a consequence of increased flow or amelioration of myointimal hyperplasia? In the absence of more conclusive clinical data regarding the effect of distal AVFs on limb salvage procedures, the technique should be regarded as one of potential but unproven value. The possibility that effective tissue perfusion results from retrograde venous flow with AVFs has been put forward, but only scant experimental data exist to support the conjecture.[118]

Hemodynamic Differences Between Shunts and Fistulas

All else being equal, shunts with anastomoses identical in dimensions to a single fistula opening should have lower flow as the resistance of the bridge limb becomes a factor. Circuit modeling suggests that flow is restricted unless the diameter of the bridge is much larger than the PA diameter. Clinical studies, however, show that satisfactory flows are achieved with prosthetic bridge shunts both 6 and 8 mm diameter; with either diameter, flow rates can be so high that revision to prevent steal and heart failure is occasionally required.[119]

The pressure gradient across a true fistula rapidly dissipates with distance, as does the gradient across a bridge, in which the arterial pressure at the inflow anastomosis rapidly falls to venous levels before emptying into the outflow veins.[120] Increasing both the length of the bridge and the curvature should increase the resistance to blood flow as a consequence of standard hemodynamic principles. Clinical studies with hemodialysis patients, however, show these effects to be apparently negligible, and loop grafts have been reported both to give higher flows[91] or comparable flows[22,89] with those of straight shunt grafts. It has been proposed that looped shunt grafts minimize steal because the angle of the arterial anastomosis streamlines flow and provides a baffle to inhibit reflux from the DA into the bridge communication. No specific data confirm this conjecture, but the more salient physiologic principle—that larger anastomoses promote higher flows (and more retrograde flow through the DA) when other factors are constant—has been confirmed with loop grafts in the femoral system of the dog.[120]

Secondary Effects of AVFs

Fistulas in the extremities lead to alterations in skin temperatures. The temperature gradient may be as high as 3°C between the two upper extremities in chronic hemodialysis patients. This effect is due to warming from increased flow of arterial blood through the extremity directly into the superficial veins, with thermography showing the maximum warming to be in the skin directly overlying the AVF. Immediately after access construction, the hand may be cool owing to decreased peripheral flow, but as arterial collaterals develop, temperatures rise, although they may remain permanently low compared with those in the contralateral hand. The greater the gradient in temperature between the hand and the proximal upper extremity, or between hands, the more likely a significant steal is present.[19, 38,121-123]

Bone growth has been observed to be increased in the presence of congenital AV malformations, and experimental studies in animals have shown long bone growth to be stimulated by AVFs.[124-126] Clinical interventions with this technique were somewhat successful, but the uncertain nature of the underlying physiologic principle and complications such as edema and distal ulceration (presumably from venous stasis or tissue hypoxia) have apparently led to its abandonment.[127,128]

Somewhat paradoxically, given the problems of arterial ischemia and venous stasis associated with hemodialysis access AVFs, wounds near AVFs have been reported to demonstrate enhanced healing, although the effect is not seen distally on involved extremities.[129] Similarly, fractures near AVFs but not distally have increased rates of healing.[121]

As a consequence of decreased flow distal to an AVF, oxygen extraction in the PVB increases, which is manifested as an increased AV oxygen-content difference when blood from the distal bed is sampled with the fistula open. This effect is less pronounced as the fistula matures because of increased arterial collateral supply to the PVB. The overall oxygen consumption of limbs bearing AVFs cannot usually be distinguished from that of normal contralateral limbs.[130]

Tissue P_{O_2} and cellular enzyme activity related to oxygen metabolism are altered in muscle distal to chronic high-flow extremity AVFs.[56] The oxygen content of blood taken from the PV of an AVF is increased compared witho normal venous blood because of the arterial admixture.

REFERENCES

1. Holman E. The physiology of an arteriovenous fistula. *Arch Surg.* 1923;7:64.
2. Holman E. The anatomic and physiologic effects of an arteriovenous fistula. *Surgery.* 1940;8:362.
3. Holman E. Clinical and experimental observations on arteriovenous fistulae. *Ann Surg.* 1940;112:840-878.
4. Holman E. Problems in the dynamics of blood flow: conditions controlling collateral circulation in the presence of an arteriovenous fistula, following the ligation of an artery. *Surgery.* 1949;26:889-917.
5. Holman E. The vicissitudes of an idea. The significance of total blood volume in the story of arteriovenous fistula. *Rev Surg.* 1963;20: 153-174.
6. Holman E, Taylor G. Problems in the dynamics of blood flow. II. Pressure relations at the site of an arteriovenous fistula. *Angiology.* 1952;3:415-430.
7. Wong V, Ward R, Taylor J, Selvakumar S, How TV, Bakran A. Factors associated with early failure of arteriovenous fistulae for haemodialysis access. *Eur J Vasc Endovasc Surg.* 1996;12:207-213.
8. Brescia MJ, Cimino JE, Appel K, Hurwich BJ. Chronic hemodialysis using venipuncture and a surgically created arteriovenous fistula. *N Engl J Med.* 1966;275:1089-1092.
9. Wedgwood KR, Wiggins PA, Guillou PJ. A prospective study of end-to-side versus side-to-side arteriovenous fistulas for haemodialysis. *Br J Surg.* 1984;71:640-642.
10. Ramacciotti E, Galego SJ, Gomes M, Goldenberg S, De Oliveira Gomes P, Pinto Ortiz J. Fistula size and hemodynamics: an experimental model in canine femoral arteriovenous fistulas. *J Vasc Access.* 2007;8:33-43.
11. Hobson RW 2nd, Croom RD 3rd, Swan KG. Hemodynamics of the distal arteriovenous fistula in venous reconstruction. *J Surg Res.* 1973;14:483-489.
12. Reilly DT, Wood RFM, Bell PRF. Arteriovenous fistulas for dialysis: blood flow, viscosity, and long term patency. *World J Surg.* 1982;6: 628-633.
13. Schenk WG Jr, Bahn RA, Cordell AR, Stephens JG. The regional hemodynamics of experimental acute arteriovenous fistulas. *Surg Gynecol Obstet.* 1957;105:733-740.
14. Ingebrigtsen R, Wehn PS: Local blood pressure and direction of flow in experimental arteriovenous fistulae. *Acta Chir Scand.* 1960;120:142-150.
15. Johnson G Jr, Dart CH Jr, Peters RM, Steele F. The importance of venous circulation in arteriovenous fistula. *Surg Gynecol Obstet.* 1966;123:995-1000.
16. Lough FC, Giordano JM, Hobson RW Jr. Regional hemodynamics of large and small femoral arteriovenous fistulas in dogs. *Surgery.* 1976;79:346-349.
17. Schenk WG Jr, Martin JW, Leslie MB, Portin BA. The regional hemodynamics of chronic experimental arteriovenous fistulas, *Surg Gynecol Obstet.* 1960;110:44-56.
18. Sivanesan S, How T, Bakran A. Characterizing flow distributions in AV fistulae for haemodialysis access. *Nephrol Dial Transplant.* 1998;13:3108-3110.
19. Ingebrigtsen R, Krog J, Lerand S. Circulation distal to experimental arterio-venous fistulas of the extremities. *Acta Chir Scand.* 1963;125: 308-317.
20. Alfrey AC, Lueker R, Goss JE, Vogel JH, Faris TD, Holmes JH. Control of arteriovenous shunt flow. *JAMA.* 1970;214:884-888.
21. Oates CP, Williams ED, McHugh MI: The use of Diasonics DRF400 duplex ultrasound scanner to measure volume flow in arteriovenous fistulae in patients undergoing haemodialysis: an analysis of the measurement uncertainties. *Ultrasound Med Biol.* 1990;16:571-579.
22. Johnson CP, Zhu YR, Matt C, Pelz C, Roza AM, Adams MB. Prognostic value of intraoperative blood flow measurements in vascular access surgery. *Surgery.* 1998;124:729-737.
23. Wang E, Schneditz D, Nepomuceno C. Predictive value of access blood flow in detecting access thrombosis. *ASAIO J.* 1998;44:M555-M558.
24. Lindsay R, Blake PG, Malek P, Posen G, Martin B, Bradfield E. Hemodialysis access blood flow rates can be measured by a differential conductivity technique and are predictive of access clotting. *Am J Kidney Dis.* 1997;30:475-482.
25. Oudenhoven L, Pattynama PM, De Roos A, Seeverens HJ, Rebergen SA, Chang PC. Magnetic resonance, a new method for measuring blood flow in hemodialysis fistulae. *Kidney Int.* 1994;45:884-889.

26. Bosman P, Boereboom FT, Bakker CJ, et al. Access flow measurements in hemodialysis patients: in vivo validation of an ultrasound dilution technique. *J Am Soc Nephrol.* 1996;7:966-999.

27. Köksoy C, Kuzu A, Erden I, Türkçapar AG, Düzgün I, Anadol E. Predictive value of colour Doppler ultrasonography in detecting failure of vascular access grafts. *Br J Surg.* 1995;82:50-52.

28. Windus DW, Andraen J, Vanderson R, Jendrisak MD, Picus D, Delmez JA. Optimization of high efficiency hemodialysis by detection and correction of fistula dysfunction. *Kidney Int.* 1990;38:337-341.

29. Lin CH, Chua CH, Chiang SS, Liou JY, Hung HF, Chang CH. Correlation of intraoperative blood flow measurement with autogenous arteriovenous fistula outcome. *J Vasc Surg.* 2008;48:167-172. Epub 2008; May 23.

30. Back RB, et al. Expected flow parameters within hemodialysis access and selection for remedial intervention of nonmaturing conduits. *Vasc Endovasc Surg.* 2008;42:150.

31. Haimov M, Baez A, Neff M, Slifkin R. Complications of arteriovenous fistulas for hemodialysis. *Arch Surg.* 1975;110:708-712.

32. Kwun KB, et al. Hemodynamic evaluation of angioaccess procedures for hemodialysis. *Vasc Surg.* 1979;13:170.

33. Forsberg L, Holmin T, Listedt E. Quantitative Doppler and ultrasound measurements in surgically prepared arteriovenous fistulas of the arm. *Acta Radiol Diagn (Stockh).* 1980;21:769-771.

34. Levinson JA, et al. Pulsed Doppler: determination of diameter, blood flow velocity, and volumetric flow of brachial artery in man. *Cardiovasc Res.* 1981;15:164.

35. Finlay DE, Longley DG, Forshager MC, Letourneau JG. Duplex and color Doppler sonography of hemodialysis arteriovenous fistulas and grafts. *Radiographics.* 1993;13:983-989.

36. Shu MCS, Noon GP, Hwang NHC. Flow profiles and wall shear stress distribution at a hemodialysis venous anastomosis: preliminary study. *Biorheology.* 1987;24:723-735.

37. Van Tricht I, De Wachter D, Tordoir J, Verdonck P. Comparison of the hemodynamics in 6 mm and 4-7 mm hemodialyslis grafts by means of CFD. *J Biomech.* 2006;39:226-236.

38. Ene-Iordache B, Masconi L, Remuzzi G, Remuzzi A. Computational fluid dynamics of a vascular access case for hemodialysis. *J Biomech Eng.* 2001;123:284-292.

39. Ringdén O, Fagrell B, Friman L, Lundgren G. Subcutaneous arteriovenous fistulas for dialysis with special emphasis on vascular insufficiency. *Scand J Urol Nephrol.* 1976;10:73-79.

40. Abbott JA, Campbell M, Bussell JA, Lim RC. Blood flow in end-to-side arteriovenous fistulas and saphenous vein grafts. *Kidney Int.* 1973;3: 342-344.

41. Bussell JA, Abbott JA, Lim RC. Radial steal syndrome with arteriovenous fistula for hemodialysis. *Ann Intern Med.* 1971;75:387-394.

42. Jendrisak MD, Anderson CB. Vascular access in patients with arterial insufficiency. *Ann Surg.* 1990;212:187-193.

43. Mattson WJ. Recognition and treatment of vascular steal secondary to hemodialysis prostheses. *Am J Surg.* 1987;154:198-201.

44. Avitsian R, Abdelmalak B, Saad S, Xu M, O'Hara J Jr. Upper extremity arteriovenous fistula does not affect pulse oximetry readings. *Nephrology (Carlton).* 2006;11:410-412.

45. Lin G, Kais H, Halpern Z, et al. Pulse oxymetry evaluation of oxygen saturaion in the upper extremity with an arteriovenous fistula before and during hemodialysis. *Am J Kidney Dis.* 1997;29:230-232.

46. Crowe CP, Schenk WG Jr. Massive experimental arteriovenous fistulas. *J Trauma.* 1963;3:13-21.

47. Frank CW, Wang HH, Lammerant J, Miller R, Wegria R. An experimental study of the immediate hemodynamic adjustments to acute arteriovenous fistulae of various sizes. *J Clin Invest.* 1955;34:722-731.

48. Leslie MB, Portin BA, Schenk WG Jr. Cardiac output and postural studies in chronic experimental arteriovenous fistulas. *Arch Surg.* 1960;81:123-128.

49. Van Loo A, Heringman EC. Circulatory changes in the dog produced by acute arteriovenous fistula. *Am J Physiol.* 1949;158:103-112.

50. Anderson CB, Codd JR, Graff RA, Groce MA, Harter HR, Newton WT. Cardiac failure and upper extremity arteriovenous fistulas. *Arch Intern Med.* 1976;136:292-297.

51. Fee HJ, Levisman J, Doud RB, Golding AL. High-output congestive failure from femoral arteriovenous shunts for vascular access. *Ann Surg.* 1976;183:321-323.

52. Guyton AC, Sagawa K. Compensations of cardiac output and other circulatory functions in areflexic dogs with large A-V fistulas. *Am J Physiol.* 1961;200:1157-1163.

53. Epstein FH, Ferguson TB. The effect on the formation of an arteriovenous fistula upon blood volume. *J Clin Invest.* 1955;34:434-438.

54. Hilton JG, Kanter DM, Hays DR, et al. The effect of acute arteriovenous fistula on renal functions. *J Clin Invest.* 1955;34:732-736.

55. Mandin H. Mechanism of natriuresis after closure of chronic arteriovenous shunts. *J Clin Invest.* 1973;52:2225-2233.

56. Marinescu V, Pausescu E, Făgărăsanu D, Dincă A. Metabolic factors in the cardiac insufficiency of arteriovenous fistula. *Ann Surg.* 1966;164: 1027-1033.

57. Weber TR, Jewertz BL, Stanley JC, Lindenauer SM, Fry WJ.: Renal effects of acute infrarenal aortocaval fistula. *J Surg Res.* 1978;25: 482-487.

58. Iwashima Y, Horio T, Takami Y, et al: Effects of the creation of arteriovenous fistula for hemodialysis on cardiac function and natriuretic peptide levels in CRF. *Am J Kidney Dis.* 2002;40:974-982.

59. Darling RC, Linton RR. Aneurysm of the abdominal aorta with rupture into the inferior vena cava. *N Engl J Med.* 1962;267:974-982.

60. Jarstfer BS, Rich NM. The challenge of arteriovenous fistula formation following disc surgery: a collective review. *J Trauma.* 1976; 16:726-733.

61. Syme J. Case of spontaneous varicose aneurysm. *Edinb Med Surg J.* 1831;36:1045.

62. Smith RA, Stehbens WE, Weber P. Hemodynamically-induced increase in soluble collagen in the anastomosed veins of experimental arteriovenous fistulae. *Atherosclerosis.* 1976;23:429-436.

63. Ingebrigtsen R, Fönstelien E, Solberg LA: Measurement of forces producing longitudinal stretching of the arterial wall, examined in the artery proximal to an arteriovenous fistula. *Acta Chir Scand.* 1970;136: 569-573.

64. Sho E, Nanjo H, Sho M, et al. Arterial enlargement, tortuosity, and intimal thickening in response to sequential exposure to high and low wall shear stress. *Vasc Surg.* 2004;39:601-612.

65. Ene-Iordache B, Mosconi L, Antega L, et al. Radial artery remodeling in response to shear stress increase within arteriovenous fistula for hemodialysis access. *Endothelium.* 2003;10:95-102.

66. Dammers R, Tordoir JH, Welten RJ, Kitslaar PJ, Hoeks AP. The effect of chronic flow changes on brachial artery diameter and shear stress in arteriovenous fistulas for hemodialysis. *Int J Artif Organs.* 2002;25: 124-128.

67. Tronc F, Warsef M, Esposito B, Henrion D, Glagov S, Tedgui A. Role of NO in flow-induced remodeling of the rabbit common carotid artery. *Arterioscler Thromb Vasc Biol.* 1996;16:1256-1262.

68. Guzman RJ, Abe K, Zarins CK. Flow-induced arterial enlargement is inhibited by suppression of nitric oxide synthase activity in vivo. *Surgery.* 1997;122:273-279.

69. Abbruzzese T, Guzman RJ, Martin RL, Yee C, Zarins CK, Dalman RL. Matrix metalloproteinase inhibition limits arterial enlargement in a rodent arteriovenous fistula model. *Surgery.* 1998;124:328-334.

70. Girerd X, London G, Boutouyrie P, Mourad JJ, Safar M, Laurent S. Remodeling of the radial artery in response to a chronic increase in shear stress. *Hypertension.* 1996;27:799-803.

71. Stehbens WE. Blood vessel changes in chronic experimental arteriovenous fistulas. *Surg Gynecol Obstet.* 1968;127:327-338.

72. Stehbens WE, Karmody AM. Venous atherosclerosis associated with arteriovenous fistulas for hemodialysis. *Arch Surg.* 1975;110: 176-180.

73. Bandyk DF. Essentials of graft surveillance. *Semin Vasc Surg.* 1993;93: 92-102.

74. Hofstra L, Bergmans DC, Leunissen KM, et al. Anastomotic intimal hyperplasia in prosthetic arteriovenous fistulas for hemodialysis is associated with initial high flow velocity and not with mismatch in elastic properties. *J Am Soc Nephrol.* 1995;6:1625-1633.

75. Sho M, Sho E, Singh TM, et al. Subnormal shear stress-induced intimal thickening requires medial smooth muscle cell proliferation and migration. *Exp Mol Pathol.* 2002;72:150-160.

76. Krishnamoorthy MK, Banerjee RK, Wang Y, et al. Hemodynamic wall shear stress profiles influence the magnitude and pattern of stenosis in a pig AV fistula. *Kidney Int.* 2008;74:1410-1419.

77. Moran MR, et al. Hand exercise effect on maturation and blood flow of dialysis arteriovenous fistulas ultrasound study. *Angiology.* 1984; 55:641.

78. Moran MR, et al. Flow of dialysis fistulas. *Nephron.* 1985;40:63.

79. Anderson CB, Etheredge EE, Hurter HR, Graff RJ, Codd JE, Newton WT. Local blood flow characteristics of arteriovenous fistulas in the forearm for dialysis. *Surg Gynecol Obstet.* 1977;144:531-533.

80. Hadjiyannakis EJ. Distal flow internal arteriovenous fistula. *Am J Surg.* 1973;126:122-123.

81. Patel KR, Chan FA, Batista RJ, Clauss RH. True venous aneurysms and arterial "steal" secondary to arteriovenous fistulae for dialysis. *J Cardivasc Surg (Torino).* 1992;33:185-188.

82. Knox RC, Berman SS, Hughes JD, Gentile AT, Mills JL. Distal revascularization-interval ligation: a durable and effective treatment for ischemic steal slyndrome after hemodialysis access. *J Vasc Surg.* 2002;36:250-255.

83. Sessa C, Riehl G, Porcu P, et al. Treatment of hand ischemia following angioaccess surgery using the distal revascularization intervalligation technique with reservation of vascular access: description of an 18-case series. *Ann Vasc Surg.* 2004;18:685-694.

84. Rivers SP, Scher LA, Veith FJ. Correction of steal syndrome secondary to hemodialysis access fistulas: a simplified quantitative technique. *Surgery.* 1992;112:593-597.

85. Delpin EAS. Swelling of the hand after arteriovenous fistulas for hemodialysis. *Am J Surg.* 1976;132:373-376.

86. Beathard GA, Settle SM, Shields MW. Salvage of the nonfunctioning arteriovenous fistula. *Am J Kidney Dis.* 1999;33:910-916.

87. Miller GA. Percutaneous management of steal syndrome. Abstracts, Vieth Symposium; New York, NY; November 21, 2008.

88. Owens ML, Bower RW. Physiologic consequences of arteriovenous fistulas. In Wilson SE (ed). *Vascular Access Surgery.* 2nd ed. St. Louis: CV Mosby; 1988.

89. Anderson CB, Etheridge EE, Harter HR, Codd JE, Graff RJ, Newton WT. Blood flow measurements in arteriovenous dialysis fistulas. *Surgery.* 1977;81:459-461.

90. Levy BI, Bourquelot P, Ponsin JE. Noninvasive and invasive blood flowmetry in hemodialyzed patients with high blood flow fistulas. *ASAIO Trans.* 1984;30:335-337

91. Rittgers SE, Garcia-Valdez C, McCormick JT, Posner MD. Noninvasive blood flow measurements in expanded polytetrafluoroethylene grafts for hemodialysis access. *J Vasc Surg.* 1986;3:635-642.

92. Neyra NR, Ikizler TA, May RE, et al. Change in access blood flow over time predicts vascular access thrombosis. *Kidney Int.* 1998;54:1714-1719.

93. Bouthier JD, Levenson JA, Simon AC, Bariety JM, Bourquelot PE, Safar ME. A noninvasive determination of fistula blood flow in dialysis patients. *Artif Organs.* 1983;7:404-409.

94. Sivanesan S, How TV, Bakran A. Site of stenosis in AV fistulae for haemodialysis access. *Nephrol Dial Transplant.* 1999;14:118-120.

95. Bandyk DF, Kaebnick J, Bergamini TM, Moldenhauer P, Towne JB. Hemodynamics of in situ saphenous vein arterial bypass. *Arch Surg.* 1988;123:477-482.

96. Anderson CB, Groce MA. Banding of arteriovenous dialysis fistulas to correct high output cardiac failure. *Surgery.* 1975;78:552-554.

97. Wijnen E, Essers S, van Meijel G, et al. Comparison between two online reversed line position hemodialysis vascular access flow measurement techniques: saline dilution and thermodilution. *ASAIO J* 2006;52:410-415.

98. Válek M, Lepot F, Dusilová-Sulková S, Polakovic V. Physiologic variability of vascular access blood flow for hemodialysis. *Blood Purif.* 2008;26:468-472. Epub 2008;September 22.

99. Bui TD, Gordon IL, Paraphar A, Vo D, Wilson SE. Resistance within hemodialysis shunts predicts patency. *Vasc Endovasc Surg.* 2006;40:295-302.

100. Sullivan KL, Besarab A, Bonn J, Shapiro MJ, Gardiner GA Jr, Moutz MJ. Hemodynamics of failing dialysis grafts. *Radiology.* 1993;186:867-872.

101. Chandraratna PAN. Determination of contribution of arteriovenous fistula to total cardiac output by Doppler computer. *Nephrol Dial Transplant.* 1984;41:251-254.

102. Johnson G Jr, Blythe WB. Hemodynamic effects of arteriovenous shunts used for hemodialysis. *Ann Surg.* 1970;171:715-723.

103. Huang M, Hester RL, Guyton AC, Norman RA Jr. Hemodunamic changes in rats after opening an arteriovenous fistula. *Am J Physiol.* 1992;262:H846-H851.

104. Nakhoul F, Yigla M, Gilman R, Reusner SA, Abassi Z. The pathogenesis of pulmonary hypertension in haemodialysis patients via arteriovenous access. *Nephrol Dial Transplant.* 2005;20:1686-1692.

105. Abassi Z, Nakhoul F, Khankin E, Reisner SA, Yigla M. Pulmonary hypertension in chronic dialysis patients with arteriovenous fistula: pathogenesis and therapeutic prospective. *Curr Opin Nephrol Hypertens.* 2006;15:353-360.

106. Abdelwhab S, Elshinnawy S. Pulmonary hypertension in chronic renal failure patients. *Am J Nephrol.* 2008;28:990-997.

107. Yigla M, Nakhoul F, Sabag A, et al. Pulmonary hypertension in patients with end-stage renal disease. *Chest.* 2003;123:1577-1582.

108. Länne T, Bergqvist D. Aortocaval fistulas associated with ruptured abdominal aortic aneurysm. *Eur J Surg.* 1992;158:457-465.

109. Thompson RW, Yee LF, Natuzzi ES, Stoney RJ. Aorta-left renal vein fistula syndrome caused by rupture of a juxtarenal abdominal aortic aneurysm. *J Vasc Surg.* 1993;93:310-315.

110. Rordain P, Jensen LP, Schroeder T, Lorentzen JE, Bagi P. The effect of arteriovenous fistulas on in situ saphenous vein bypasses. *Ann Vasc Surg.* 1991;5(5):419-423.

111. Shearman CP, Gannon MX, Gwynn BR, Simms MK. A clinical method for the detection of arteriovenous fistulas during in situ great saphenous vein bypass. *J Vasc Surg.* 1986;4:578-581.

112. Calligaro KD, Ascer E, Torres M, Veith FJ. The effect of adjunctive arteriovenous fistula on prosthetic graft patency: a controlled study in a canine model. *J Cardiovasc Surg (Torino).* 1990;31:646-650.

113. Jacobs MJ, Reul GJ, Greforic ID, et al. Creation of a distal arteriovenous fistula improves microcirculatory hemodynamics of prosthetic graft bypass in secondary limb salvage procedures. *J Vasc Surg.* 1993;18:1-8.

114. Paty PS, Shah DM, Saifi J, et al. Remote distal arteriovenous fistula to improve infrapopliteal bypass patency. *J Vasc Surg.* 1990;11:171-177.

115. Kallakuri S, Ascher E, Hingorani A, Jacob T, Salles-Cunha C. Hemodynamics of intrapopliteal PTFE bypasses and adjunctive arteriovenous fistulas. *Cardiovasc Surg* 2003;11:125-129.

116. Neufang A, Espinola-Klein C, Dorweiler B, et al. Questionable value of adjuvant arteriovenous fistula in pedal bypass at high risk for early failure. *Ann Vasc Surg.* 2008;22:379-387. Epub 2008; March 24.

117. Taylor RS, Loh A, McFarland RJ, Cox M, Chester JF. Improved technique for polytetrafluoroethylene bypass grafting: long-term results using anastomotic vein patches. *Br J Surg.* 1992;79:348-354.

118. Suzuki Y, Suzuki K, Ishikawa K. Direct monitoring of the microcirculation in experimental venous flaps with afferent arteriovenous fistulas. *Br J Plast Surg.* 1994;47:554-559.

119. Rosental JJ, Bell DD, Gaspar MR, Movius HJ, Lemire GG. Prevention of high flow problems of arteriovenous grafts. *Am J Surg.* 1980;140:231-233.

120. Lavigne JE, Messina LM, GOlding MR, Kerr JC, Hobson RW 2nd, Swan KG. Fistula size and hemodynamic events within and about canine femoral arteriovenous fistulas. *J Thorac Cardiovasc Surg.* 1977;74:551-556.

121. Henrie JN, Johnson EW Jr, Wakin KG, Orvis AL. The influence of experimental arteriovenous fistula on the healing of fractures and on blood flow distal to the fistula. *Surg Gynecol Obstet.* 1959;108:591-599.

122. Jamison JP, Wallace WFM. The pattern of venous drainage of surgically created side-to-side arteriovenous fistulae in the forearm. *Clin Sci Mol Med.* 1976;50:37-41.

123. Wallace WFM, Jameson JP. Effect of a surgically created side-to-side arteriovenous fistula on heat elimination from the human hand and forearm: evidence for a critical role of venous resistance in determining fistula flow. *Clin Sci Mol Med.* 1978;55:349-353.

124. Callum KG, Kinmonth JB. The effect of arterio-venous fistula on the lymphatics. *Lymphology.* 1973;6:121-126.

125. Horton BT. Hemihypertrophy of extremities associated with congenital arteriovenous fistula. *JAMA.* 1932;98:373.

126. Janes JM, Musgrove JE. Effect of arteriovenous fistula on growth of bone: preliminary report. *Mayo Clin Proc.* 1949;24:405-408.

127. Kinmonth JB, Negus D. Arterio-venous fistulae in the management of lower limb discrepancy. *J Cardiovasc Surg (Torino).* 1974;15:447-453.

128. Petty W, Winter RB, Felder D; Arteriovenous fistula for treatment of discrepancy in leg length; *J Bone Joint Surg Am.* 1974;56:581-586.

129. Matsubayashi S. Wound healing accelerated by the creation of an arteriovenous fistula [in Japanese]. *Sekei Gaka.* 1974;22:104-109.

130. Solti F, Soltész L, Bodor E. Haemodynamic changes of systemic and limb circulation in extremital arteriovenous fistula. *Angiologia.* 1972;9:69-80.

CHAPTER 6

Thrombophilia as a Cause of Recurrent Vascular Access Thrombosis in Hemodialysis Patients

Khushboo Kaushal and Samuel Eric Wilson

According to the U.S. Renal Data System *2008 Annual Data Report*, the incidence of end-stage renal disease (ESRD) patients in North America has experienced a fourfold increase since 1980.[1] At its peak in 2001, there were approximately 140 hemodialysis patients per 100,000 North Americans. With these trends, it is calculated that there will be about 2.24 million ESRD patients in the United States by 2030. Vascular access–related complications account for 14% to 17% of hospitalizations per year for dialysis patients and annual costs of approximately $1 billion in the United States.[2] The most common and expensive hemodialysis complication is vascular access thrombosis.[3] Patients maintained by chronic hemodialysis also are susceptible to multiple thrombotic complications such as ischemic heart disease and cerebral strokes, in addition to vascular access thrombosis.[4-6] Casserly and Dember,[7] as well as Paulson,[8] have suggested that thrombophilia might be a cause of dialysis access thrombosis in many ESRD patients. Thrombophilia is a result of factors that are acquired, genetically determined, or a combination of both, and leads to a predisposition to thrombosis.[9] This chapter examines coagulation abnormalities in ESRD patients, focusing on thrombophilia and management of the hypercoagulable state of ESRD patients.

Coagulation Abnormalities in ESRD

Paradoxically, hemodialysis patients are at elevated risk for bleeding or thromboses.[10] The more common coagulation abnormality is a hemorrhagic tendency caused by the platelet dysfunction of uremia.[11] Indeed, it is this coagulation abnormality that allows arteriovenous fistulas and grafts to function in ESRD patients, whereas in patients with normal clotting function, these would thrombose.

Insufficient knowledge about the association between renal insufficiency and inflammatory and procoagulant markers led Shlipak and coworkers in 2003[12] to evaluate eight inflammatory and procoagulant factors (C-reactive protein, fibrinogen, interleukin-6, intercellular adhesion molecule-1, factor VII, factor VIII, plasmin-antiplasmin, and D-dimer) using data from the prospective, multicenter Cardiovascular Health Study. Their study revealed that renal insufficiency had an independent correlation with increases in inflammatory and procoagulant biomarkers, which may promote atherosclerosis and thrombosis in ESRD patients. Increases in these biomarkers were a result of increased production, decreased renal clearance, or a combination of the two.

These biochemical changes in hemodialysis patients lead to chronic activation of coagulation and result in a hypercoagulable state.[13] ESRD patients have higher levels of particular markers of coagulation activation, such as prothrombin fragment 1+2 and thrombin.[4] Furthermore, Hafner and colleagues[14] suggested that the levels of the thrombin-antithrombin complex are associated with thrombosis of the extracorporeal hemodialysis circuit while the patient is undergoing hemodialysis. In addition to high levels of coagulation activators, these patients also have lower levels of endogenous anticoagulants such as protein C, protein S, and antithrombin III.[15,16]

Diabetic and nondiabetic ESRD patients have elevated procoagulatory activity, as indicated by increased platelet aggregation, increased D-dimer concentration, von Willebrand factor antigen, and platelet factor 4.[17] Ambühl and associates[18] found elevated D-dimer levels, indicating that accelerated thrombin formation and unimpaired fibrinolytic activity contribute to development of the hypercoagulable state. They demonstrated that ESRD patients are in a procoagulable state and hemodialysis further stimulates coagulatory activity. Previous studies showed that human recombinant erythropoietin (rhEPO) has an overall procoagulatory effect because it influences blood coagulation and fibrinolysis.[19,20] Ambühl and associates[18] confirmed these findings and also found that higher doses of erythropoietin were correlated with smaller amounts of prothrombin fragments.

Vascular endothelium actively participates in hemostasis. Variations in the morphology of the blood flow and vessel wall in the arteriovenous fistula (AVF) may disrupt hemostasis.[21,22] Erdem and coworkers[4] investigated the molecular markers that activate and/or inhibit coagulation and fibrinolysis in patients with ESRD and assessed the effects AVF may have on endothelial surfaces and hemostasis. For ESRD patients, the results showed activated coagulation markers and fibrinolysis in the systemic circulation.

These findings suggest that turbulent flow of an AVF may be a factor that independently influences the coagulation and fibrinolytic cascades.

Calciphylaxis, a rare complication that occurs in approximately 1% of dialysis patients per year, causes ischemic skin lesions such as ulcers and/or gangrene that may require amputation and serious infections that may result in death.[23,24] Mehta and colleagues[25] identified protein C deficiency as a factor in the pathophysiology that induced a hypercoagulable state, thereby leading to thrombosis in vessels. Clinicians are aware of the difficulty of establishing satisfactory vascular access in these patients.

Thrombophilia as a Cause of Access Failure in Hemodialysis Patients

Although a direct cause and effect in vascular access thrombosis has not been proved, it is clear that changes in hemostatic plasma protein enzymes may establish hypercoagulable states in patients on hemodialysis.[26-30] Nampoory and associates[31] investigated changes in hemostatic risk factors that may contribute to hypercoagulability in patients on dialysis and, hypothesizing that renal transplantation would be a highly effective treatment in patients with ESRD, examined the biologic effect renal transplantation had on hypercoagulability. The results of the blood coagulation studies showed the presence of lupus anticoagulant in 5.6%, anticardiolipin antibody immunoglobulin G in 3.9% and immunoglobulin M (IgM) in 5.3%, activated protein C resistance in 20.5%, and deficiencies in protein S, activated protein C, and antithrombin III in 32.1%, 24.4%, and 19.2%, respectively. In comparison with patients who did not experience vascular access thrombosis, those who had these access complications had significantly abnormal levels of lupus anticoagulant, activated protein C, protein S, and activated protein C resistance. It is noteworthy that renal transplantation appeared to correct these levels.

Knoll and coworkers' large and comprehensive, case-controlled study[3] assessed the association between thrombophilic disorders and dialysis access thrombosis. They measured concentrations of factor V Leiden, prothrombin gene mutation, factor XIII genotype, methylenetetrahydrofolate reductase genotype, lupus anticoagulant, anticardiolipin antibody, factor VIII, homocysteine, and lipoprotein in hemodialysis patients. The most common genetic determinants were point mutations in the factor V and prothrombin genes.[32,33] This study demonstrated that the presence of thrombophilia increased the risk for dialysis access thrombosis and, further, that each additional thrombophilic factor increased the likelihood of access thrombosis almost twofold. Conversely, Danis and colleagues[34] examined the role thrombophilia may have in primary and secondary AVF failure and, finding no significant differences in the thrombophilic factors, did not recommend routine testing.

O'Shea and associates[35] found antibodies associated with thrombosis and increased concentrations of factor VIII and fibrinogen, especially in patients with recurring vascular access thrombosis. LeSar and coworkers' study[36] revealed a high correlation (81.8%) between thrombotic complications and hypercoagulability, leading these authors to

suggest that hypercoagulability is a major causative factor in multiple polytetrafluoroethylene (PTFE) graft thromboses that develop independent from anatomic causes. Documentation of a hypercoagulable state in the ESRD patient with repeated access thrombosis, in the absence of anatomic abnormalities or extrinsic factors (eg, compression), naturally leads one to consider therapeutic anticoagulation measures.

Management of the Hypercoagulable ESRD Patient

Recognizing that fistula thrombosis may arise from both anatomic and nonanatomic causes, one should consider that hypercoagulable states might be a cause of vascular access thrombosis in selected patients in whom no anatomic abnormality can be found.[35] As we have discussed, previous studies suggest that inflammatory and procoagulant responses to infection, and subsequent chronic inflammation, may contribute to a hypercoagulable state.[37,38] With aggressive antithrombotic therapy, such as warfarin or low-molecular-weight heparin, even if successful in decreasing the frequency of vascular access failure, it is important to weigh the known risk that use of warfarin sodium in ESRD patients elevates hemorrhagic complications.[35] In short, antithrombotic agents might have the potential to increase vascular access graft patency[35] but at the cost of an increase in the likelihood of serious hemorrhagic complications.[36,39,40]

A variety of factors such as stenosis of the graft-venous anastomosis in 34% to 63% of events[41,42] are more frequent causes of thrombosis than the presence of high antiphospholipid antibody[28,43] or thrombosis arising from external factors such as compression.[42,44] Better understanding of the pathogenesis of thrombosis will allow for more efficient treatment and the opportunity to prevent recurring complications.[36] Diseases that cause hypercoagulability and their complications include antiphospholipid syndrome, antithrombin III deficiency, protein S deficiency, protein C deficiency, activated protein C resistance, and erythropoietin.[36,45-50] In patients with antiphospholipid syndromes, Rosove and Brewer[51] and Khamashta and colleagues[52] found that the incidence of thrombotic events is decreased with warfarin therapies of intermediate to high intensity.

In view of the important role platelets have in thrombus formation, several antiplatelet agents, such as aspirin and clopidogrel, have been used to prevent perioperative and longer-term thrombosis. The simultaneous use of two antiplatelet agents has been found to increase platelet inhibition because the two agents bind to different receptors.[53] A number of antiplatelet agents such as aspirin, thienopyridines, and glycoprotein IIb/IIIa inhibitors that are currently recommended by the American College of Chest Physicians is shown in Table 6-1.[54] Most surgeons recommend discontinuing clopidogrel before surgery, but for certain operations, the incidence of thrombotic complications is substantially increased if clopidogrel is prematurely discontinued before surgery.[55,56] Lo and associates,[13] in their guide to management of thromboembolism in hemodialysis patients, noted that trials of anticoagulants have not shown a benefit for prevention of access thrombosis.

Table 6–1

Principal Indications for Oral Antiplatelet Agents

Clinical Setting	Recommendation[a]	Level of Evidence[b]
Stable CAD	Aspirin (75-162 mg/day) Aspirin continued indefinitely	1A 2C
Stable CAD with risk profile indicating increased risk for ACS	Long-term clopidogrel plus aspirin	2C
Non–ST-segment ACS	Aspirin (75-162 mg/day) continued lifelong Clopidogrel (75 mg/day) for 12 mo	1A 1A/1B
Stable patient after placement of BMS	Clopidogrel (75 mg/day) for 4 weeks	1A
Stable patient after placement of DES	Clopidogrel (75 mg/day) for 12 mo	1C
Atrial fibrillation	Age <65 yr and without risk factors:[d] aspirin (325 mg) Age 65-75 yr without risk factors:[d] aspirin or warfarin	1B 1A
Secondary prevention when cerebrovascular disease	Either aspirin (50-325 mg) or aspirin (25 mg) + controlled-release dipyridamole (200 mg twice a day) or clopidogrel (if warfarin not indicated for CAD)	1A
Carotid endarterectomy	Aspirin (75-325 mg), started preoperatively (at the expense of increased bleeding risk)	1A
Chronic peripheral arterial disease	Aspirin at a dose depending on the presence of CAD or cerebrovascular disease	1A
Primary prevention (coronary events)	Intermediate risk: aspirin (75-162 mg)	2A

[a]Clopidogrel was given as clopidogrel bisulfate.

[b]Grade 1 recommendations are strong and indicate that the benefits do or do not outweigh the risks, costs, and burden. Grade 2 suggests that the patient's values may lead to other choices. Level of evidence is indicated by decreasing order as A, B, or C.[18]

[c]Established risk factors for stroke in patients with atrial fibrillation (apart from age) include a history of stroke, transient ischemic attack, or systemic embolus: left ventricular dysfunction; hypertension; and diabetes mellitus.[18]

ACS, acute coronary syndrome; BMS, bare-metal stent; CAD, coronary artery disease; DES, drug-eluting stent.

Derived from the recommendations of the American College of Chest Physicians;[17] reproduced with permission from the *Canadian Journal of Anaesthesia*;[18] from O'Riordan JM, Margey RJ, Blake G, O'Connell PR. Antiplatelet agents in the perioperative period. *Arch Surg.* 2009;144:69-76.

Kaufman and coworkers[57] reinforced this notion with a study of combinations of 75 mg of clopidogrel and 325 mg of aspirin that did not reduce prosthetic access thrombosis, but increased the likelihood of bleeding in the clopidogrel group. In another study, Crowther and colleagues[58] showed that warfarin increased major bleeding events in hemodialysis patients and 75 mg of clopidogrel did not confer benefits for autogenous access.

After this selective review of literature that is often conflicting, we are unable to make a definite evidence-based recommendation on the use of anticoagulants to prevent access thrombosis. It seems prudent, however, to consider low-dose warfarin or antiplatelet agents in ESRD patients who suffer repetitive thrombosis of "life-line" access sites. Precautions must be taken—monitoring of coagulation tests and avoidance of trauma—to minimize bleeding.

Conclusion

Thrombosis is one of the most common complications of vascular access, deserving further attention directed toward understanding of the multiple etiologies and the contribution of thrombophilia to recurrent, otherwise unexplainable access clotting. The ideal approach to decreasing the morbidity and costs of access thrombosis may be a combination of preventing endothelial and fibromuscular hyperplasia of outflow stenosis along with correction of hypercoaguability.[16,36]

REFERENCES

1. U.S. Renal Data System. *USRDS 2008 Annual Data Report: Atlas of End-Stage Renal Disease in the United States.* Bethesda, MD: National Institutes of Health, 2008. Available at http://www.usrds.org/adr.htm
2. U.S. Renal Data System. The economic cost of ESRD, vascular access procedures, and Medicare spending for alternative modalities of treatment. *Am J Kidney Dis.* 1997;30:S160-S177.
3. Knoll GA, Wells PS, Young D. Thrombophilia and the risk for hemodialysis vascular access thrombosis. *J Am Soc Nephrol.* 2005;16:1108-1114.
4. Erdem Y, Haznedaroglu IC, Celik I, et al. Coagulation, fibrinolysis and fibrinolysis inhibitors in haemodialysis patients: Contribution of arteriovenous fistula. *Nephrol Dial Transplant.* 1996;11:1299-1305.
5. Linder A, Charra B, Sherrad DJ, et al. Accelerated atherosclerosis in prolonged maintenance hemodialysis. *N Engl J Med.* 1974;290:697-702.
6. Ansari A, Kaupke CJ, Vaziri ND, Miller R, Barbari A. Cardiac pathology in patients with end-stage renal disease maintained on haemodialysis. *Int J Artif Organs.* 1993;16:31-36.
7. Casserly LF, Dember LM. Thrombosis in end-stage renal disease. *Semin Dial.* 2003;16:245-256.

8. Paulson WD. Prediction of hemodialysis synthetic graft thrombosis: can we identify factors that impair validity of the dysfunction hypothesis? *Am J Kidney Dis.* 2000;35:973-975.

9. Tripodi A, Mannucci PM. Laboratory investigation of thrombophilia. *Clin Chem.* 2001;47:1597-1606.

10. Tang SCW, Lai KN. Physiologic inhibitors of coagulation in patients on chronic hemodialysis. *Hemodialysis Int.* 2003;7(3):232-238.

11. Ho SJ, Gemmel R, Brighton A. Platelet function testing in uraemic patients. *Hematology.* 2008;13:49-58.

12. Shlipak MG, Fried LF, Crump C, et al. Elevations of inflammatory and procoagulant biomarkers in elderly persons with renal insufficiency. *Circulation* 2003;107:87-92.

13. Lo DS, Rabbat CG, Clase CM. Thromboembolism and anticoagulant management in hemodialysis patients: a practical guide to clinical management. *Thromb Res.* 2006;118:385-396.

14. Hafner G, Klingel R, Wandel E, et al. Laboratory control of minimal heparinization during hemodialysis in patients with a risk of hemorrhage. *Blood Coagul Fibrinolysis.* 1994;5:221-226.

15. Lai KN, Yin JA, Yuen PM, Li PK. Protein C, protein S, and antithrombin III levels in patients on continuous ambulatory peritoneal dialysis and hemodialysis. *Nephron.* 1990;56:271-276.

16. Nakamura Y, Chida Y, Tomura S. Enhanced coagulation—fibrinolysis in patients on regular hemodialysis treatment. *Nephron.* 1991;58:201-204.

17. Gordge MP, Leaker BR, Rylance PB, Neild GH. Haemostatic activation and proteinuria as factors in the progression of chronic renal failure. *Nephrol Dial Transplant.* 1991;6:21-26.

18. Ambühl P, Wüthrich R, Korte W, Schmid L, Krapf R. Plasma hypercoagulability in haemodialysis patient: impact of dialysis and anticoagulation. *Nephrol Dial Transplant.* 1997;12:2355-2364.

19. Taylor JE, Belch JJF, McLaren M, Henderson IS, Stewart WK. Effect of erythropoietin therapy and withdrawal on blood coagulation and fibrinolysis in hemodialysis patients. *Kidney Int.* 1993;44:182-190.

20. Huraib S, al-Momen AK, Gader AM, Mitwalli A, Sulimani F, Abu-Aisha H. Effect of recombinant human erythropoietin (rhEPO) on the hemostatic system on chronic hemodialysis patients. *Clin Nephrol.* 1991;36:252-257.

21. Remuzzi G, Cavenaghi A, Mecca G, Donati M, DeGaetano G. Prostacyclin-like activity and bleeding in renal failure. *Lancet.* 1977;2:1195-1197.

22. Remuzzi G, Perico N, Zoja C, Coma D, Macconi D, Vigano D. Role of endothelium derived nitric oxide in the bleeding tendency of uremia. *J Clin Invest.* 1990;86:1768-1771.

23. Levin A, Mehta R, Goldstein MB. Mathematical formulation to help identify the patient at risk of ischemic tissue necrosis—a potentially lethal complication of chronic renal failure. *Am J Nephrol.* 1993;13:448-453.

24. Budisavljevic MN, Cheek D, Ploth DW. Calciphylaxis in chronic renal failure. *J Am Soc Nephrol.* 1996;7:978-982.

25. Mehta RL, Scott G, Sloand JA, Francis CW. Skin necrosis associated with acquired protein C deficiency in patients with renal failure and calciphylaxis. *Am J Med.* 1990;88:252-257

26. Födinger M, Mannhalter C, Pabinger I, et al. Resistance to activated protein C (APC): mutation at Arg506 of coagulation factor V and vascular access thrombosis in haemodialysis patients. *Nephrol Dial Transplant.* 1996;11:668-672.

27. Prieto LN, Suki WN. Frequent hemodialysis graft thrombosis: association with antiphospholipid antibodies. *Am J Kidney Dis.* 1994;23:587-590.

28. Brunet P, Aillaud M, Marco MS, et al. Antiphospholipids in hemodialysis patients: relationship between lupus anticoagulant and thrombosis. *Kidney Int.* 1995;48:794-800.

29. Sallam S, Wafa E, El-Gayar A, Sobh M, Salama O. Anticardiolipin antibodies in children on chronic haemodialysis. *Nephrol Dial Transplant.* 1994;9:1292-1294.

30. Prakash RM, Miller CC, Suki WN. Anticardiolipin antibody in patients on maintenance hemodialysis and its association with recurrent arteriovenous graft thrombosis. *Am J Kidney Dis.* 1995;26:347-352.

31. Nampoory MRN, Das KC, Johny KV, et al. Hypercoagulability, a serious problem in patients with ESRD on maintenance hemodialysis, and its correction after kidney transplantation. *Am J Kidney Dis.* 2003;42:797-805.

32. Bertina RM, Rosendaal FR. Venous thrombosis—the interaction of genes and environment. *N Engl J Med.* 1998;338:1840-1841.

33. Girndt M, Heine GH, Ulrich C, Köhler H. Gene polymorphism association studies in dialysis: vascular access. *Semin Dial.* 2007;20:63-67.

34. Danis R, Ozmen S, Akin D, et al. Thrombophilias and arteriovenous fistula dysfunction in maintenance hemodialysis. *J Thromb Thrombolysis* 2009;27:307-315.

35. O'Shea SI, Lawson JH, Reddan D, Murphy M, Ortel TL. Hypercoagulable states and antithrombotic strategies in recurrent vascular access site thrombosis. *J Vasc Surg.* 2003;38:541-548.

36. LeSar CJ, Merrick HW, Smith MR. Thrombotic complications resulting from hypercoagulable states in chronic hemodialysis vascular access. *J Am Coll Surg.* 1999;189:73-79.

37. Esmon CT, Taylor FB, Snow TR. Inflammation and coagulation: linked processes potentially regulated through a common pathway mediated by protein C. *Thromb Haemost.* 1991;66:160-165.

38. Jurado R, Ribeiro M. Possible role of systemic inflammatory reaction in vascular access thrombosis. *South Med J.* 1999;92:877-881.

39. Hirsh J, Warkentin TE, Shaughnessy SG, et al. Heparin and low-molecular-weight heparin: mechanisms of action, pharmacokinetics, dosing, monitoring, efficacy, and safety. *Chest.* 2001;119(1 suppl):64S-94S.

40. Gerlach AT, Pickworth KK, Seth SK, Tanna SB, Barnes JF. Enoxaparin and bleeding complications: a review in patients with and without renal insufficiency. *Pharmacotherapy.* 2000;20:771-775.

41. Munda R, First MR, Alexander JW, Linnemann CC Jr, Fidler JP, Kittur D. Polytetrafluoroethylene graft survival in hemodialysis. *JAMA.* 1983;249:219-222.

42. Raju S. PTFE grafts for hemodialysis access: techniques for insertion and management of complications. *Ann Surg.* 1987;206:666-673.

43. Prakash R, Miller CC III, Suki WN. Anticardiolipin antibody in patients on maintenance hemodialysis and its association with recurrent arteriovenous graft thrombosis. *Am J Kidney Dis.* 1995;26:347-352.

44. Palder SB, Kirkman RL, Whittemore AD, Hakim RM, Lazarus JM, Tilney NL. Vascular access for hemodialysis: patency rates and results of revision. *Ann Surg.* 1985;202:235-239.

45. Bick RL, Baker WF. Antiphospholipid and thrombosis syndromes. *Semin Thromb Hemost.* 1994;20:3-15.

46. Bayston TA, Lane DA. Antithrombin: molecular basis of deficiency. *Thromb Hemost.* 1997;78:339-343.

47. Schwarz HP, Fischer M, Hopmeier P, Batard MA, Griffin JH. Plasma protein S deficiency in familial thrombotic disease. *Blood.* 1984;64:1297-1300.

48. Clouse LH, Comp PC. The regulation of hemostasis: the protein C system. *N Engl J Med.* 1986;314:1298-1304.

49. Svensson PJ, Dahlback B. Resistance to activated protein C as a basis for venous thrombosis. *N Engl J Med.* 1994;330:517-522.

50. Shen L, Dahlback B. Factor V and protein S as synergistic cofactors to activated protein C in degradation of factor VIIIa. *J Biol Chem.* 1994;269:18735-18738.

51. Rosove MH, Brewer PM. Antiphospholipid thrombosis: clinical course after the first thrombotic event in 70 patients. *Ann Intern Med.* 1992;117:303-308.

52. Khamashta MA, Cuadrado MJ, Mujic F, Taub NA, Hunt BJ, Hughes GR. The management of thrombosis in the antiphospholipid-antibody syndrome. *N Engl J Med.* 1995;332:993-997.

53. Ibanez B, Vilahur G, Badimon JJ. Pharmacology of thienopyridines: rationale for dual pathway inhibition. *Eur Heart J Suppl.* 2006;8(suppl G):G3-G9.

54. O'Riordan JM, Margey RJ, Blake G, O'Connell PR. Antiplatelet agents in the perioperative period. *Arch Surg.* 2009;144:69-76.

55. Kaluza GL, Joseph J, Lee JR, Raizner ME, Raizner AE. Catastrophic outcomes of noncardiac surgery soon after coronary stenting. *J Am Coll Cardiol.* 2000;35:1288-1294.

56. Wilson SH, Fasseas P, Orford JL, et al. Clinical outcome of patients undergoing non-cardiac surgery in the two months following coronary stenting. *J Am Coll Cardiol.* 2003;42:234-240.

57. Kaufman JS, O'Connor TZ, Zhang JH, et al. Randomized controlled trial of clopidogrel plus aspirin to prevent hemodialysis access graft thrombosis. *J Am Soc Nephrol.* 2003;14:2313-2321.

58. Crowther MA, Clase CM, Margetts PJ, et al. Low-intensity warfarin is ineffective for the prevention of PTFE graft failure in patients on hemodialysis: a randomized controlled trial. *J Am Soc Nephrol.* 2002;13:2331-2337.

CHAPTER 7

Biologic Properties of Venous Access Devices

Peter D. Peng, Louis F. D'Amelio, and Ralph S. Greco

Advances in the field of venous access have paved the way for clinical progress in monitoring, resuscitation, nutritional support, cancer therapy, hemodialysis, and radiologic diagnosis. Rather than acting only as passive conduits, venous access devices elicit active responses from both the host and the endogenous microflora of the host.[1,2] These responses are implicated in the most common complications of venous access: infection, inflammation (phlebitis), and thrombosis. Recent studies comparing surface modified catheters have confirmed the ability of this technology to ameliorate pathologic responses. This chapter examines the properties of biomaterials commonly used in venous access surgery and the host and microbial responses to these materials.

Biomaterials Used in Venous Access Surgery

The ideal biomaterial for venous access would not promote microbial adhesion, activate the coagulation cascade, or cause an inflammatory response with deleterious local or systemic consequences. Catheter technology improvement has been an active area of research; however, the ideal material does not yet exist. All biomaterials in clinical use elicit host responses that are largely dependent on their individual macromolecular structures.[1] Besides the chemical structure, the physical characteristics of biomaterials affect their suitability for use in venous access. Advances in catheter technology focus on the chemical and physical factors affecting host response.

These factors include charge, hydrophilicity, and pliability. A negative electrical surface charge is hypothetically advantageous for several reasons. Most bacteria preferentially adhere to positively charged surfaces.[3] In addition, a negative surface charge more closely mimics the characteristics of host endothelium and may diminish local platelet aggregation.[4] Hydrophilic catheters might absorb tissue fluid and exhibit changes in consistency or diameter.[5] An excessively stiff catheter might predispose the device to technical complications at the time of insertion or cause late endothelial damage with activation of the coagulation cascade. Pliable biomaterials pose technical difficulty in catheter insertion and may be prone to late kinking. To a large extent, therefore, the ultimate choice of biomaterial for a specific venous access device hinges on the intended clinical site and duration of use.

Polyurethanes

Polyurethanes are synthesized from monomers containing urethane groups through a process known as *step-growth polymerization*. In this process, terminal functional groups are reacted sequentially to growing polymer chains.[6] This process allows flexibility in molecular design so that desired physical and chemical properties can be achieved. Of all the biomaterials used in venous access surgery, only polyurethane block copolymers approach the complexity of biologic macromolecules.

Polyurethanes were first developed by Otto Bayer in Germany in 1937.[7] Initially patented in 1960 by DuPont, Biomer was the first polyurethane used as a biomaterial by Pierce in 1967. Its clinical applications include ventricular assist devices and total artificial hearts.[8] Other polyurethane compounds are in widespread use as angiography catheters. Venous applications include acute single-lumen and multilumen central venous catheters as well as pulmonary artery catheters.

Polyurethane is relatively hydrophobic, although it shows slight softening when placed intravascularly. This property provides relative stiffness to facilitate insertion but still maintains some degree of local endothelial protection while the catheter is indwelling.[9] The polyurethane surface is smooth in comparison with other biomaterials when viewed under scanning electron microscopy. This property is thought to contribute to a lack of thrombogenicity relative to other commonly used materials, such as polytetrafluoroethylene (PTFE) and polyvinyl chloride (PVC). Polyurethane also causes less of an inflammatory reaction than these other biomaterials.[10]

Polyethylene

Polyethylene, one of the simplest of plastics, was first synthesized in 1939. As early as 1947, its relative biocompatibility was recognized. Clinical application of this compound, however, did not occur until 1964, when Tsulukidze attempted to use polyethylene shells as artificial urinary bladders.[7] This polymer is synthesized of ethylene monomers linked together with varying degrees of branching. Low-density polyethylene, a highly branched macromolecule, forms a relatively pliable biomaterial that is used in the production of peripheral and central venous catheters. More linear ethylene polymers, high-density polyethylene and ultrahigh-molecular-weight polyethylene, are used in reconstructive plastic surgery and joint replacement, respectively.[11-13]

Polyethylene is relatively hydrophobic and smooth under scanning electron microscopy, with a pore density of approximately 10 μm.[6] The linear high-density polyethylene polymers used in plastic surgery are relatively inert and cause little foreign body reaction.[14] In contrast, the low-density polymers used for intravenous access cause a substantial chronic inflammatory reaction with activation of macrophages and giant cells.[2] For this reason, the use of polyethylene for venous access has been limited to acute catheters.

PVC

PVC is a long-chain thermoplastic polymer. It is synthesized by the sequential addition of monomers to an active center bearing a free radical through a process known as *addition polymerization*. In its native state, it is rigid, brittle, and unsuitable as a material for venous access.[6] A variety of additives collectively termed *plasticizers* has been added to PVC to render it more flexible for clinical use.[15] PVC catheters are used for pulmonary artery monitoring and diagnostic radiologic applications. PVC catheters have been shown to cause platelet activation and surface fibrinogen adsorption.[16] These undesirable biologic properties have been attributed to the plasticizers, which might also migrate to surrounding tissues with prolonged catheterization and promote an acute inflammatory response. Clinical studies have demonstrated a higher incidence of phlebitic and thrombotic complications with the use of PVC catheters.[17] For these reasons, PVC has not had widespread use as an implantable biomaterial for long-term venous access.

PTFE

PTFE is a linear thermoplastic polymer composed only of carbon, oxygen, and fluorine atoms. It is chemically inert and has no known solvent. PTFE was patented by DuPont in 1937 and first used in consumer products under the brand name Teflon in the 1950s. PTFE first had medical application as an orbital floor prosthesis in 1956. In 1969, William Gore patented a method of stretching PTFE into an expanded form (ePTFE), which was commercially marketed as Gore-Tex as an insulator for camping gear. Gore fortuitously introduced Dr. Ben Eisman to Gore-Tex on a 1971 ski trip.[7] Eisman went on to study the properties of this material as a vascular prosthesis in a pig model. It has subsequently had widespread clinical application as a midsized and large vessel arterial prosthesis and as an arteriovenous conduit for hemodialysis.

PTFE is strongly hydrophobic and has a pore size in its various formulations of 20 to 100 μm. Chronic implantation leads to an inflammatory response in which early giant cell and histiocytic infiltration is followed by chronic fibrosis.[18] On an acute basis, PTFE catheters are used for peripheral intravenous access and as catheter introducers. PTFE is most commonly used for venous access as an arteriovenous hemodialysis conduit. PTFE arteriovenous fistulas have a 3-year patency rate of 70% to 80%.[19] Late thrombosis is a

result of an inflammatory response at the host-biomaterial interface that culminates in the clinical phenomenon of neointimal hyperplasia.[18] The cellular mechanisms underlying this process are described in detail later in the chapter.

Silicone Elastomer

Silicone elastomer (Silastic) is by far the most common biomaterial used for chronic indwelling vascular catheters. This material was developed in the 1930s at Corning Glass and had its first practical application as a synthetic rubber during World War II. Its first biologic application was as baby bottle nipples.[7] In 1955, Holter developed a ventriculoperitoneal shunt made of silicone; DeNiola implanted silicone rubber tubing as a urethral prosthesis in 1959.[7]

Silastic, like all elastomers, exhibits impact resistance and elasticity. These physical properties make direct insertion technically difficult; most Silastic catheters are inserted over guidewires or through introducer sheaths. This flexibility also renders Silastic unsuitable for pressure monitoring or peripheral intravenous use. However, Silastic demonstrates significant advantages, because it is hydrophobic and relatively nonthrombogenic.[20,21] Proteins adsorbed to the surface are structurally unaltered; platelet activation and subsequent thrombogenesis are minimized. It is one of the least immunoreactive biomaterials in clinical use.[17] All of these properties are favorable for the long-term intravascular implantation of Silastic.

Infection and Biomaterials Used for Venous Access

Up to 6% of catheters used for long-term venous access become infected.[22] A number of host and microbial factors contribute to the pathogenesis of such infections. Biomaterial infections are caused by smaller bacterial inocula than other clinical infectious processes. Normal flora or opportunistic pathogens become virulent in the presence of an intravascular foreign body. The biomaterial acts as a substratum to facilitate microbial adhesion. An immunocompetent, fibroinflammatory zone is established at the host-biomaterial interface.[23] The biomaterial itself may also alter the host humoral and cellular immune responses. Bacterial exopolysaccharides form a film that provides a ready supply of energy and nutrients. Microbes preferentially adhere to these biofilm surfaces as a survival strategy. Almost all microbes use this mechanism in both natural environments and human disease states.[24-26]

Inanimate biomaterial surfaces provide an ideal environment for the propagation of biofilm and the proliferation of microbes. Infections of intravascular catheters persist until removal of this ideal bacterial environment.

Bacterial adhesion was first recognized as a phenomenon with relevance to human disease in 1908 when Guyot demonstrated microbial adhesion to human erythrocytes. Fifty years later, electron microscopy was used to demonstrate the fimbrias on *Escherichia coli* responsible for adhesion.[27] The clinical significance of the bacterial inoculum relative to biomaterials was first studied in the context of suture material. In 1957, Elek and Cohen[28] demonstrated that an inoculum of as little as 100 *Staphylococcus aureus* organisms could produce infection in the presence of a silk suture.

Through the next 2 decades, a number of researchers gained insight into microbial adhesion to biomaterials. In 1972, Bayston and Penny[29] noted excessive bacterial production of a mucoid material as a factor in the colonization of ventriculoperitoneal shunts.

Divalent actions, particularly Ca^{2+} and Mg^{2+}, were shown to be necessary for microbial adhesion. In 1976, Gristina and colleagues[30] reported that biomaterial surface effects resulted in differential bacterial adhesion; they noted that even inert biomaterials were not immune from bacterial ingrowth.

Later work from this group helped characterize the polysaccharide biofilm responsible for adhesion.[31] Subsequent investigators documented biofilm-mediated adhesion by *Staphylococcus epidermidis* on plastic intravascular catheters.[32] This documentation correlated with the clinical finding that *S. epidermidis* causes most infections of transcutaneous polymeric devices.

The polysaccharide slime, or *biofilm*, produced by microbes contributes to pathogenicity in several ways. It is characterized by a complex of hydrated acidic glycoproteins and polysaccharides. Biofilm blunts the effect of antibiotic therapy on the microbe; it also masks bacterial antigenicity.[33,34] Host neutrophil mechanisms (phagocytosis) become ineffective.[24] Transcutaneous catheter placement results in early biofilm formation. In one study, 81% of 68 percutaneous central venous catheters developed evidence of biofilm formation.[33] Many catheters had biofilm within 24 hours of insertion. Organisms most frequently cultured were cocci of skin origin. Blood cultures drawn through the catheter and entrance site cultures were frequently negative, whereas cultures obtained by sonication or scraping of the catheter were frequently positive.[33]

Catheter-related bloodstream infections (CRBSI) are defined as bloodstream infections resulting from infected vascular access devices or contaminated infusate. Signs of infection must be accompanied by concordant microorganism growth from a peripheral blood culture and a culture from the vascular access device, either blood drawn from the catheter or cultured catheter internal/external surface organisms. Other sources of sepsis with the same organism must be absent. The formation of biofilm clearly does not necessarily correlate with clinical catheter sepsis.[35] A number of other host factors mitigate the transition from biofilm colonization to frank catheter infection. The immune status of the host is first and foremost among these. Patients with defects of humoral- or cell-mediated immunity are more prone to intravascular device–related infection. Virulence of the organism, in part mediated by mechanisms of adhesion, also plays a role. The nature of the biomaterial itself may facilitate or hinder bacterial adhesion. In 1983, Sheth and associates[36] demonstrated that adhesion of coagulase-negative staphylococci to PVC catheters was greater than that to PTFE catheters. Other groups subsequently documented that bacteria preferentially adhere to polyethylene compared with PTFE and siliconized steel.[3] Finally, Ludwicka and coworkeres[37] studied the adhesion of five strains of *S. epidermidis* to 10 different synthetic polymers and found that adhesion increased with increasing contact angle and decreasing surface tension. This group was among the

first to modify the host-biomaterial interface to diminish bacterial adhesion. They found that increasing the negative surface charge and hydrophilicity of the surface diminished the adhesion of staphylococci. Over the next 2 decades, a number of efforts have focused on biomaterial surface modification to favorably alter the host-biomaterial interface.

Modification of the biomaterial surface to diminish bacterial adhesion and reduce clinical infection can be accomplished in one of two basic ways: (1) directly altering the intrinsic physical or chemical properties of the biomaterial and (2) binding antimicrobial agents to the surface of intravascular prosthesis. This second approach is attractive because there are a number of readily available antimicrobial agents that can bind to a biomaterial, resulting in higher drug concentration at the host-biomaterial interface with lower systemic concentrations. The differential drug concentrations increase local efficacy while minimizing potential systemic toxicity. A number of factors, however, complicate biomaterial-mediated drug delivery. To achieve a therapeutic effect, drug concentrations must be maintained for a clinically appropriate time interval; thus factors affecting the half-life of local drug elution are important. Polymer characteristics, the chemical structure of the drug, and the nature of the drug-prosthesis bond all affect drug delivery.[38]

Relatively porous biomaterials such as PTFE present a large surface area for drug binding. In contrast, polymers with a tight molecular structure, such as polyethylene, present very little area for potential drug adsorption.[23] Hydrophobic interactions of the drug and biomaterial also assume importance. Relatively hydrophilic drugs, such as penicillins, cephalosporins, and aminoglycosides, rapidly wash out into the bloodstream. In contrast, relatively hydrophobic antibiotics, including teicoplanin and the fluoroquinolones, can be retained on prosthetic surfaces for some time.[39] Practical considerations also include the stability of the antibiotic-biomaterial bond in common commercial sterilization processes. Ethylene oxide deactivates penicillins but not aminoglycosides. Quantification of both the amounts of bound drug and the rate of elution can be difficult. In vitro measurements with relatively inefficient eluants such as saline do not reliably mimic the in vivo rate of drug elution.

Drugs may be bound to a prosthesis in one of four ways:

1. Incorporation into the bulk phase of the polymer. This approach is limited by the technical complexity of the synthetic processes. Bayston and colleagues[40] developed an in vitro model of clindamycin and rifampin incorporated into silicone that showed antimicrobial activity over 28 days.

2. Covalent binding of drugs or macromolecules to the biomaterial. This approach has the advantage of eliminating elution of the drug. Catheters covalently coated with antithrombin-heparin have undergone preclinical studies that demonstrate improved antithrombogenicity when compared witho uncoated or heparin-coated catheters.[41]

3. Incorporation of the drug into a macromolecule coating added to the catheter surface. Collagen, glucosaminoglycankeratin, cyanoacrylate, and fibrin glue have been used to bind antibiotics.[12,42,43] Rifampin has been bound

to collagen-sealed polyethylene terephthalate (Dacron) arterial prostheses.[44]

4. Adsorption onto biomaterial surfaces either passively or in the presence of surfactant. The applicability of the latter approach was first demonstrated in the 1960s, when Gott and associates[45] first bound heparin to polymer surfaces that had been pretreated with the positively charged quaternary ammonium compound benzalkonium. Many antibiotics have negative surface charges similar to that of heparin. This finding led to the binding of antibiotic molecules to the surface of biomaterials.[46-48] Benzalkonium or TDMAC is adsorbed to catheter surfaces, resulting in positively charged surfactants that can serve to attract negatively charged antibiotic molecules. The antibiotic is eluted in a controlled manner over time with high local and low systemic concentrations.

Early studies by Kamal and colleagues,[49] reported a randomized, controlled clinical trial of antibiotic-bonded intravenous and arterial catheters in intensive care unit patients. Eighty-five arterial and 93 central venous catheters were pretreated with TDMAC and subsequently immersed in the anionic antibiotic cefazolin. All catheters in this study were left in place for 7 days or less. The rate of catheter-related infections diminished from 14% to 2%; this effect was more striking for arterial than for venous catheters. The most common infecting organism was *S. epidermidis*. These authors concluded that antibiotic binding is an efficient, safe, and cost-effective method of reducing intravascular catheter infection in intensive care unit patients.

More recent studies with minocycline/rifampin antibiotic-coated catheters have also demonstrated improved infection profiles. Using tridodecylmethyl–ammonium chloride–mediated coating of minocycline and rifampin, Raad and coworkers[50] demonstrated a significant reduction in risk of catheter-related colonization and bloodstream infections through a randomized, double-blinded trial. Subsequent clinical studies have repeated and confirmed the clinical efficacy of minocycline/rifampin-coated catheters in decreasing the incidence of catheter-associated bloodstream infections.[51]

Metal ions or metal ions in complexes have been used for centuries to disinfect fluids, solids, and tissues. The biocidal effect of silver, with its broad spectrum of activity, including bacterial, fungal, and viral agents, is particularly well known. Silver ions have an affinity to sulfhydryl groups in enzyme systems of the cell wall, through which they interfere with transmembrane energy transfer and electron transport of bacterial organisms. Silver ions also block the respiratory chain of microorganisms reversibly in low concentrations and irreversibly in high concentrations. Binding to the DNA of bacteria and fungi increases the stability of the bacterial double helix and thus inhibits proliferation. There is no cross-resistance with antibiotics and no induction of microbial resistance by silver ions. New technology combines metallic silver in submicron particles in polyurethane. Polyurethane is hydrophilic, and the interaction of electrolyte solutions with the impregnated silver releases bactericidal concentrations of silver ions locally over prolonged periods. Clinical trials demonstrated that silver/chlorhexidine antiseptic-impregnated catheters are associated with lower CRBSI rates.[52]

With technologic advances resulting in multiple antimicrobial catheters, several studies have attempted to compare surface-modified catheters in clinical trials. In 1999, Darouiche and associates[53] reported a comparison of minocycline/rifampin-coated versus chlorhexidine/silver sulfadiazine–coated polyurethane triple-lumen catheters. Through a prospective, randomized and multi-institutional trial, they found that minocyclin/rifampin-coated catheters were one third as likely to be colonized and one twelfth as likely to be associated with bloodstream infectionsas catheters impregnated with chlorhexidine/silver sulfadiazine.[53] However the comparison utilized minocycline/rifampin catheters coated both internally and externally, whereas the chlorhexidine/silver sulfadiazine catheters were only externally coated. A second-generation chlorhexidine/silver sulfadiazine catheter has been engineered with a higher concentration of antiseptic both externally and internally; clinical studies are awaited.[54]

Microscopic particles of silver, platinum, and carbon have been combined with polyurethane to engineer a catheter affecting continuous release of silver ions both internally and externally.[55] Through the process of iontophoresis, carbon facilitates a redox reaction between silver and platinum, resulting in sustained release of silver ions. When Fraenkel and associates[56] completed a prospective, randomized trial comparing silver-platinum-carbon–impregnated catheters with minocycline/rifampin-coated catheters, the minocycline/rifampin catheters were associated with a slightly lower bacterial colonization rate; however, there was no significant difference in CRBSIs.[56]

Antibiotic coating has also been demonstrated to decrease bloodstream infection in long-term catheters. A prospective, randomized trial with minocycline/rifampin-coated long-term silicone central venous catheters showed that these significantly decreased rates of CRBSI when compared with untreated catheters.[57] In addition, when compared with tunneling, a study demonstrated equal rates of colonization between tunneled untreated catheters and minocycline/rifampin-treated untunneled catheters.[58]

The prevalence of skin flora as pathogens in infected transcutaneous venous access devices has led some groups to look into exit site modification as an alternate approach to infection prophylaxis. Regular protocols for exit site care, including topical antimicrobial agents, help diminish infection rates.[59] Most commercially marketed long-term central venous catheters have Dacron cuffs to promote fibroblast ingrowth at the exit site. Insertion techniques that are commonly used involve the construction of a subcutaneous tunnel to distance the exit site and the point of vascular entry. In a study of central venous catheter infections in patients with acquired immunodeficiency syndrome, Stanley and coworkers[60] showed that the infection-free interval was prolonged in patients with tunneled rather than percutaneous catheter entry.

Attempts to inhibit biofilm formation have also focused on the addition of silver-impregnated cuffs to the exit site.[61,62] Exit site modification with silver-impregnated collagen catheter cuffs has been studied.. The collagen-based cuff serves as a framework for fibroblast ingrowth and provides a physical barrier to bacterial migration, whereas the silver ions eluted by the cuff are bactericidal. Maki and associates[62] showed a significant decrease in the number of colonized catheter tips and the incidence of clinical catheter sepsis with silver-impregnated cuffs. When such catheters were changed over guidewires, there was no reduction in the incidence of colonization; however, this finding is not surprising in view of the fact that a guidewire change merely passes a new catheter through pre-existing biofilm.

Clinical results with silver-impregnated cuffs have not been uniform. Groeger and coworkers[63] performed a prospective, randomized evaluation of silver subcutaneous cuffs in tunneled central venous catheters in adult cancer patients. They randomized 200 patients to receive either a 10-Fr dual-lumen, tunneled, cuffed Silastic central venous catheter or the same catheter with a proximal silver-impregnated cuff. Regression analysis of infection-free intervals showed no difference over the lifetime of the catheters. There were no differences in the incidence of systemic bacteremia, fungemia, or tunnel infections between the two groups. The spectra of causative microorganisms in catheter infections were similar.

In addition to exit site modification, exit site elimination by subcutaneously implanted venous access devices has been useful. Commercially available implantable catheters include the Mediport and Port-a-Cath devices. Both have Silastic intravascular catheters connected to subcutaneous ports. These have the advantage of not having an exit site with the resultant risk of biofilm propagation. Ingram and colleagues,[64] from the Hospital for Sick Children in Toronto, reported their experience with long-term venous access in pediatric patients. The use of implantable ports reduced the incidence of infectious episodes sixfold compared with transcutaneous catheters. In addition, subcutaneously implanted ports allow normal activity and require no care on the part of the patient. Mirro and associates[65] reported a similar experience with 93 ports and 146 Broviac catheters in pediatric oncology patients. Ports remained free of infection longer than did catheters. Most infections occurred within the first 100 days after implantation.

Pegues and colleagues[66] duplicated the findings of these two groups in the adult cancer population. Their retrospective study of implanted and transcutaneous central venous catheters showed a fourfold reduction in the incidence of infection per unit of time. They observed that transcutaneous catheters were used more often in terminally ill patients but noted that infection rates were unchanged on stratification of patients by life span. Mueller and coworkers,[67] from the National Institutes of Health, reported conflicting results. In a prospective, randomized study of 100 cancer patients with transcutaneous and subcutaneous Silastic central venous catheters, they noted no difference between the groups in the incidence of infection. In summary, subcutaneous implantation of long-term central venous access devices eliminates the exit site with its potential for biofilm propagation. Strategies to prevent infectious catheter complications are summarized in Table 7-1.

Venous Access Devices and Acute Inflammation

The interface of catheter biomaterial and venous endothelium initiates an acute inflammatory response of varying

Table 7-1
Strategies to Prevent Catheter Infection

Strategy	Example
Exit site modification	Topical antibiotics, silver cuffs, subcutaneous tunnels
Exit site elimination	Port-a-Cath, Mediport
Bulk phase drug binding	Gelseal Dacron prosthesis
Surfactant-mediated drug binding	Bioguard catheters

degrees.[68] The magnitude of this response depends on a number of factors. Local endothelial damage with exposure of the basement membrane, macromolecular structure of the catheter, and the presence and nature of the infusate have all been implicated. By definition, implantation or percutaneous placement of a venous access device involves the creation of a wound. The level of the inflammatory response and the clinical sequelae also depend on the magnitude of this wound. The inflammatory response to a catheter biomaterial may culminate in the clinical entity of thrombophlebitis. Alternatively, inflammation at the host-biomaterial interface may result in neointimal hyperplasia in PTFE conduits used for hemodialysis access.[5] Resultant local turbulence or stasis, particularly at the venous anastomosis, activates the coagulation cascade with ultimate thrombosis.

Inflammation has traditionally been classified as acute or chronic but in reality represents a continuum of host response. With the insertion of a venous access device, local endothelial disruption occurs with concomitant exposure of circulating platelets to basement membrane proteins. Platelet aggregation and activation ensue. Chemotactic factors and proteases released by activated platelets recruit neutrophils and activate the complement cascade by the alternate pathway. Neutrophils in turn release lysosomal enzymes and oxygen free radicals that perpetuate and intensify the local inflammatory response.

Neutrophil interaction with vascular endothelium is dependent on serial mechanisms of adhesion. Soon after catheter insertion and endothelial injury, neutrophil adhesion initiates via a rolling process. Rolling adhesion is mediated by a neutrophil cell surface molecule known as L-selectin (CD62L) that binds to E- and P-selectin ligands on the vascular endothelium.[69,70] After the initial rolling adhesion, the neutrophil sheds its L-selectin. Surface expression of the adhesion heterodimer CD11b-CD 18 (Mac-1) occurs. This molecule is responsible for more stable binding of the neutrophil to the endothelial cell ligand intracellular adhesion molecule-1 (ICAM-1; CD54). ICAM-1 is a transmembrane immunoglobulin whose baseline production is increased by chemotactic peptides, complement, and leukotriene B_4.[1,13,71,72] After neutrophil-endothelial adhesion is firmly established by the Mac-1–ICAM-1 interaction, neutrophil migration to the site of inflammation occurs via a poorly understood mechanism. At the zone of injury, neutrophils release lysosomal proteases and free radicals and phagocytose nonviable tissue

Table 7-2

Neutrophil Products

Category	Example
Reactive oxygen species	Hydrogen peroxide, superoxide anion
Proteases	Collagenase, elastase
Arachidonic acid metabolites	Leukotriene B$_4$, prostaglandins
Miscellaneous	Platelet-activating factor

(Table 7-2). Attempts may be made to phagocytose the catheter, although this is not usually possible because of the macromolecular structure of the biomaterial. This frustrated phagocytosis perpetuates the inflammatory response.[13,73] The duration and degree of this process vary with different biomaterials.

The acute inflammatory response may resolve spontaneously or progress to a phase of chronic inflammation. In this instance, infiltration of macrophages, lymphocytes, and plasma cells ensues. Many of the chemotactic factors that initially attract neutrophils also attract monocytes. At the site of endothelial injury, monocytes differentiate into macrophages.[74] Products of activated macrophages result in the proliferation of T and B lymphocytes. Activated macrophages also secrete peptide growth factors that stimulate growth of fibroblasts, smooth muscle cells, and endothelial cells at the site of injury.

Macrophage products in chronic inflammation also include proteases, coagulation proteins, complement components, and leukotrienes (Table 7-3). The ultimate outcome of catheter-induced inflammatory processes depends in large part on the balance of macrophage activation products.

Catheter-related thrombophlebitis has been associated with a number of clinical variables. It has been known since the 1960s that the incidence of phlebitis increases over time.[75] With current biomaterials, phlebitis rarely occurs in catheters left in situ less than 24 hours. The nature of the infusate affects the inflammatory response. With peripheral intravenous nutrition, lowering carbohydrate, electrolyte, and amino acid concentrations while disproportionately increasing lipid has been shown to have a protective effect on the endothelium.[76] Heparin is traditionally used as a flush for intermittently accessed peripheral intravenous cannulas with the intent of diminishing inflammation and thrombosis.

However, several studies do not support this practice. Ashton and associates[77] randomized patients with intermittent peripheral infusion devices to receive 0.9% saline or traditional dilute heparin injections for catheter maintenance. There was no difference in the incidence of phlebitis or catheter patency between the two groups. Tuten and Gueldner[78] found similar results in 77 hospitalized patients with 114 intermittent-infusion devices.

In-line filters decrease the effect of infusate on venous inflammation and consequently phlebitis and thrombosis by excluding large microparticle load. Both Bivins and coworkers[79] and Falchuk and colleagues[80] demonstrated significant reductions in phlebitis in patients with in-line filters. Presumably, microaggregates that instituted an endothelial inflammatory response were removed before infusion.

The role of catheter biomaterial in the clinical incidence of thrombophlebitis has also been studied. Madan and associates[76] randomized into two groups 50 patients receiving identical peripheral intravenous nutritional solutions. All patients received a standard central formulation of 1250 mOsm/kg via peripheral vein. Such hyperosmotic solutions are irritating to venous endothelium and promote thrombophlebitis. Short PTFE catheters were used in 23 patients. Twenty-seven patients received fine-bore silicone catheters. The mean duration of infusion was 5 days in each group. Thrombophlebitis developed in all patients in the PTFE group but in only 2 (7%) of the silicone group. The authors concluded that the catheter biomaterial was more important in the genesis of thrombophlebitis than was the composition of the infusate.

Elastomer hydrogels are used in the manufacture of peripheral catheters. These cross-linked hydrophilic polymers absorb water into their lattice structures. These

Table 7-3

Macrophage Products

Type	Example
Coagulation factors	Prothrombin, factors V, VII, IX, and X
Complement components	C1,3,4,5: C3b inactivator, properdin
Cytoldnes	TNF, IL-1
Arachidonic acid metabolites	LTB$_4$, PGE$_2$, TXA$_2$, prostacyclin, PGF$_{2\alpha}$
Enzymes	Acid phosphatase, collagenase, elastase, lysozyme
Enzyme inhibitors	α_1-Antitrypsin, α_1-macroglobulin, lipocortin
Oxygen metabolites	Hydrogen peroxide, superoxide anion, hydroxyl ion
Growth factors	TGF-β_2, platelet-derived growth factor

TNF, tumor necrosis factor; IL-1, interleukin-1; LTB$_4$, leukotriene B$_4$; TXA$_2$, thromboxane A$_2$; PGF$_{2\alpha}$, prostaglandin F$_{2\alpha}$; TGF, transforming growth factor β_2.

catheters soften and expand on introduction into the vascular system. Early problems with a lack of mechanical strength have been overcome by using hydrogels as a surface coating on stiff polymers or by combining them with more rigid hydrophilic monomers.[81] One clinical study of elastomer hydrogel peripheral catheters for long-term home feeding showed a low incidence of phlebitis with extended dwell times.[5] This study used historical controls. Larsson and coworkers[17] studied hydrogel, PTFE, and polyurethane catheters. They found uniform evidence of thrombophlebitis with all three catheter types at 72 hours. Characteristics of the inflammatory response (predominant cell type, clinical appearance) varied among the three materials.

Simple factors such as catheter site influence the clinical incidence of thrombophlebitis. Swanson and Aldrete[82] demonstrated that catheters subjected to motion near joint surfaces were more likely to induce phlebitis than were those placed on a flat portion of the extremity. Presumably, motion at the joint is transmitted to the catheter with resultant endothelial abrasion and activation of the inflammatory cascade.

Thrombosis

The insertion of a venous access device activates the coagulation cascade.[83] As previously discussed, endothelial injury leads to platelet activation and aggregation. Even in the absence of significant endothelial injury, however, biomaterials exposed to blood initiate a thrombotic reaction. Mechanisms of biomaterial-induced thrombosis are summarized in Table 7-4.

Within seconds of exposure to blood, all known biomaterials accumulate a protein layer on the exposed surface.[16] The nature of this protein layer determines the subsequent course of events. Proteins containing the amino acid sequence RGD (arginine-glycine-aspartate) readily bind to the glycoprotein IIb/IIIa receptor of platelets.[84] Proteins bearing this sequence include fibrinogen, fibronectin, vitronectin, immunoglobulin G (IgG), and von Willebrand's factor. Binding of the glycoprotein IIb/IIIa receptor to a surface protein requires the presence of calcium and normal pH. The mere presence of an RGD-containing protein on a biomaterial surface does not ensure platelet adhesion. Some RGD-containing proteins undergo conformational changes on biomaterial surfaces; these changes can inhibit platelet adhesion, which occurs with fibrinogen.[85] It has been suggested that "prepassivating" biomaterials with conforma-

tionally changed fibrinogen might be one strategy to decrease thrombogenicity.[86]

An alternate approach to surface modification is adsorption of proteins not containing RGD to the biomaterial surface.[35,87] Albumin does not contain the RGD sequence and is an obvious choice because of its high plasma concentrations. To prevent thrombosis at the host-biomaterial interface, albumin must cover virtually the entire exposed surface. Coverage of as little as 2% of the biomaterial surface with RGD-containing proteins has been shown to be sufficient for platelet activation.[88]

In addition to platelet adhesion and activation, biomaterial surfaces cause contact activation of the coagulation cascade. Factor XII (Hageman factor) adheres to negatively charged surfaces and undergoes autoactivation. Activated factor XII converts factor XI to factor XIa, which then enters the intrinsic coagulation pathway with the ultimate formation of fibrin.[87] The contact activation system is multifaceted. Biomaterial surfaces in contact with blood also result in activation of the bradykinin and kallikrein pathways.[73]

A number of investigators have studied catheter characteristics related to thrombosis. Early studies of angiography catheters showed that PTFE was more thrombogenic than polyethylene or polyurethane.[17,82] Later studies that incorporated electron microscopy showed greater thrombus formation on polyurethane than on polyethylene surfaces.[89] The intuitive notion that thrombosis increases with increasing duration of cannulation has been confirmed by several authors.[20] For a given biomaterial, thrombogenicity also increases with the surface area in contact with the bloodstream. Manufacturing techniques used with any given biomaterial also affect the clotting response. Schwarzmann and Sefrin[90] studied two types of polyurethane catheters in a rabbit model. Despite identical compounds, they found many production-related qualitative differences in catheter morphology by scanning electron microscopy.

Surface modification has been used for several decades in an effort to diminish the thrombogenicity of biomaterials used for venous access. Two basic approaches have been used. The first of these is surface pretreatment with plasma proteins not containing RGD, such as albumin.[6,34] This approach is complicated by the rapid desorption of the protein on exposure to the bloodstream. A variety of intermediate compounds have been used to limit this process. Eberhart and colleagues[91] covalently bound alkyl chains to biopolymer surfaces. These surfaces were then able to bind serum albumin on implantation in a dog model and proved to be relatively thromboresistant. Ryu and coworkers[87] used hexamethylene diisocyanate to produce an albumin-immobilized polyurethane surface. This biomaterial was then applied in a rabbit ex vivo arterial shunt. Compared with untreated polyurethane, the albumin-adsorbed surface showed increased hydrophilicity and less fibrinogen adsorption, platelet adhesion, platelet activation, and thrombus formation. Albumin-polyurethane shunts remained unclotted to 150 minutes of ex vivo occlusion, compared with only 50 minutes for untreated polyurethane. Amiji and Park[14] reported polyethylene oxide to be an alternate hydrophilic polymer capable of reducing the thrombogenicity of biomaterials. This neutral synthetic polymer afforded

Table 7-4

Catheter-Related Thrombosis

Event	Outcome
Adsorption of fibrinogen, vitronectin	Platelet activation
Contact activation of coagulation cascade	Thrombin generation
Complement activation	Leukocyte recruitment

resistance to plasma protein adsorption and platelet adhesion predominantly via a steric repulsion mechanism.

Prosthesis-mediated drug delivery provides a second mechanism of surface modification. Gott and associates[45] first reported graphite-benzalkonium-heparin coating of polymer tubing in 1963. This coating was used clinically in aortic surgery as an intraoperative shunt to avoid the consequences of systemic anticoagulation. Heparin-bound angiography catheters were soon introduced into clinical practice.[78] Heparin-coated cardiopulmonary bypass circuits were developed in an attempt to ameliorate activation of the clotting and fibrinolytic cascades during cardiac procedures. Pradhan and colleagues[4] found that such circuits did not reduce pulmonary neutrophil sequestration, retinal microembolism, or postoperative blood loss.

Attempts at biomaterial-based drug delivery continue. Freeman AJ et al.[61] reported a heparin-TDMAC-glutaraldehyde treatment process that extended duration of patency in a chronically cannulated rat model. Both the luminal and the extraluminal surfaces of the catheter were treated with surfactant and heparin. Harvey and colleagues[38] used TDMAC as an intermediate to bind tissue plasminogen activator (tPA) to polyurethane, Dacron, Silastic, PTFE, and polyethylene.

tPA elution from these biomaterials in human plasma followed a biphasic pattern. An initial drop in the amount of surface-bound drug in the 1st hour was followed by a slower, exponential release with a half-life of 75 hours. Prostheses containing bound tPA showed persistent fibrinolytic activity in vitro. In a subsequent study from the same laboratory, Kim and associates[15] bound the prostacyclin analogue iloprost to catheter surfaces. Biphasic drug elution was again observed. Prostheses with bound iloprost completely inhibited adenosine diphosphate-induced platelet aggregation. These investigators concluded that surfactant-treated prostheses provided a reliable slow-release drug delivery system with the potential to reduce device-related thrombosis. Clinical attempts at prosthesis-mediated anticoagulant delivery have met with limited success outside the angiography suite, and most of these attempts have used catheters with surface-bound heparin. However, recent preclinical trials with antithombin-heparin complexes covalently bound to polyurethane catheters suggest an improved thrombogenicity profile when compared with heparin binding alone; these antithrombin/heparin-bound catheters may show clinical promise.[92]

Concluding Remarks

Biomaterials used in venous access surgery elicit a wide spectrum of responses. Many of the host responses are beneficial and represent attempts at healing of the host-biomaterial interface. Deleterious host responses initiate thrombosis or inflammation that may ultimately lead to failure of the access device. Intravascular biomaterials also present a favorable environment for microbial adhesion and proliferation. Infection, phlebitis, and thrombosis continue to be considerable clinical problems. The search for the ultimate biocompatible material continues. Any attempt at surface or host response modification must take into account its effect on both the beneficial and the detrimental aspects of the host-biomaterial interaction. Measures that reduce the inflammatory response may concomitantly inhibit local healing and antimicrobial responses.

Promising avenues in the search for the ideal vascular catheter include new biomaterials, prosthesis-mediated drug delivery, and selective modulation of the host response. As the mechanisms involved in host-catheter interactions become clarified at the molecular level, the ideal hemocompatible vascular access device will come closer to reality.

REFERENCES

1. Djeu JY, Matsushima K, Oppenheim JJ, Shiotsuki K, Blanchard DK. Functional activation of human neutrophils by recombinant monocyte-derived neutrophil chemotactic factor. *J Immunol.* 1990;144:2205-2210.
2. Terkeltaub RA, Ginsberg MH. Platelets in response to injury. In Clark RAF (ed). *The Molecular and Cellular Biology of Wound Repair.* 2nd ed. New York: Plenum Press; 1996:3-9.
3. Ashkenazi S, Weiss E, Drucker MM. Bacterial adherence to intravenous catheters and needles and its influence by cannula type and bacterial surface hydrophobicity. *J Lab Clin Med.* 1986;107:136-140.
4. Pradhan MJ, Fleming JS, Mkere UU, Arnold J, Wildlevuur CR, Taylor KM. clinical experience with heparin-coated cardiopulmonary bypass circuits. *Perfusion.* 1991;6:235-242.
5. Crocker KS, Devereaux GB, Ashmore DL, Coker MH. Clinical evaluation of elastomeric hydrogel peripheral catheters during home infusion therapy. *J Intraven Nurs.* 1990;13:89-97.
6. Marchant RE, Wang I. Physical and chemical aspects of biomaterials used in humans. In Greco RS (ed). *Implantation Biology: The Host Response and Biomedical Materials.* Boca Raton, FL: CRC Press; 1994.
7. Friedman D, et al. Biomaterials: an historic perspective. In Greco RS (ed). *Implantation Biology: The Host Response and Biomedical Materials.* Boca Raton, FL: CRC Press; 1994.
8. Norman J, Duncan JM, Frazier OH, et al. Intracorporeal (abdominal) left ventricular assist devices or partial artificial hearts: a five-year clinical experience. *Arch Surg.* 1981;116:1441-1445.
9. Sheppeck RA, LoGerfo FW. Blood and biomaterials. In Greco RS (ed). *Implantation Biology: The Host Response and Biomedical Materials.* Boca Raton, FL: CRC Press; 1994.
10. Krause T, Robertson FM, Liesch JB, Wasserman AJ, Greco RS. Differential production of interleukin 1 on the surface of biomaterials. *Arch Surg.* 1990;125:1158-1160.
11. Berghaus A. Porous polyethylene in reconstructive head and neck surgery. *Arch Otolaryngol.* 1985;111:154-160.
12. Moore WS, Chvapil M, Seiffert G, Keown K. Development of an infection-resistant vascular prosthesis. *Arch Surg.* 1981;116:1403-1407.
13. Schmaier AH, et al. Contact activation and its abnormalities. In Colman RW (ed). *Hemostasis and Thrombosis.* 5th ed. Philadelphia: JB Lippincott; 2005:107-130.
14. Amiji M, Park K. Surface modification of polymeric biomaterials with poly(ethylene oxide), albumin, and heparin for reduced thrombogenicity. *J Biomater Sci Polym Ed.* 1993;4:217-234.
15. Kim SW, Petersen RV, Lee ES. Effect of phthalate plasticizer on blood compatibility of polyvinyl chloride. *J Pharm Sci.* 1976;65:670-673.
16. Baier RE, Dutton RC. Initial events in interaction of blood with a foreign surface. *J Biomed Mater Res.* 1969;3:191-206.
17. Larsson N, Stenberg K, Linder LE, Curelaru I. Cannula thrombophlebitis: a study in volunteers comparing polytetrafluoroethylene, polyurethane, and polyamide-ether-elastomer cannulae. *Acta Anaesthesiol Scand.* 1989;33:223-231.
18. Clowes AW, Kirkman TR, Clowes MM. Mechanisms of arterial graft failure. II. Chronic endothelial and smooth muscle cell proliferation in healing polytetrafluoroethylene prostheses. *J Vasc Surg.* 1986;3:877-884.
19. Palder SB, Kirkman RL, Whittemore AD, Hakim RM, Lazarus JM, Tilney NL. Vascular access for hemodialysis. Patency rates and results of revision. *Ann Surg.* 1985;202:235-239.
20. Braley S. The chemistry and properties of medical grade silicone rubber. *J Macromol Sci Chem.* 1970;23:529-544.

21. Habal MB. The biologic basis for the clinical application of the silicones. *Arch Surg.* 1984;119:843-848.
22. Bernard RW, Stahl WM, Chase RM Jr. Subclavian vein catheterizations: a prospective study. II. Infectious complications. *Ann Surg.* 1971;173:191-200.
23. Gristina AG, et al. Bacteria and biomaterials. In Greco RS (ed). *Implantation Biology: The Host Response and Biomedical Materials.* Boca Raton, FL: CRC Press; 1994.
24. Costerton JW. The role of bacterial exopolysaccharides in nature and disease. *Dev Indiv Microbiol.* 1964;26:249-261.
25. Costerton JW, et al. The bacterial glycocalyx in nature and disease. *Annu Rev Microbiol.* 1981;35:299-324.
26. Jones HC, Roth IL, Sanders WM 3rd. Electron microscopy study of a slime layer. *J Bacteriol.* 1969;99:316-325.
27. Duguid JP, Smith IW, Dempster G, Edmunds PN. Non-flagellar filamentous appendages (fimbriae) and hemagglutinating activity in *Bacterium coli. J Pathol Bacteriol.* 1955;70:335-348.
28. Elek SD, Cohen PE. The virulence of *Staphylococcus pyogenes* for man: a study of the problems of wound infection. *Br J Exp Pathol.* 1957;38:573-586.
29. Bayston R, Penny SR. Excessive production of mucoid substances in *Staphylococcus* SIIA: A possible factor in the colonisation of Holter shunts. *Dev Med Child Neurol Suppl.* 1972;14:25-28.
30. Gristina AG, Rovere GD, Shoji H, Nicastro JF. An in vitro study of bacterial response to inert and reactive metals and to methylmethacrylate. *J Biomed Mater Res.* 1976;10:273-281.
31. Gristina AG, Casterton JW, Leale E, et al. Bacterial colonization of biomaterials: clinical and laboratory studies. *Orthop Trans.* 1980;4:383.
32. Christensen GD, Simpson WA, Bisno AL, Beachey EH. Adherence of slime-producing strains of *Staphylococcus epidermidis* to smooth surfaces. *Infect Immun.* 1982;37:318-326.
33. Passerini L, Lam K, Costerton JW, King EG. Biofilms on indwelling vascular catheters. *Crit Care Med.* 1992;20:665-673.
34. Peters G, Locci R, Pulverer G. Adherence and growth of coagulase-negative staphylococci on surfaces of intravenous catheters. *J Infect Dis.* 1982;146:479-482.
35. Maki DG, Weise CE, Sarafin HW. A semiquantitative culture method for identifying intravenous-catheter-related infection. *N Engl J Med.* 1977;296:1305-1309.
36. Sheth NK, Rose HD, Franson TR, Buckmire FL, Sohnle PG. In vitro quantitative adherence of bacteria to intravascular catheters. *J Surg Res.* 1983;34:213-218.
37. Ludwicka A, Jansen B, Wadström T, Pulverer G. Attachment of staphylococci to various synthetic polymers. *Zentralbl Bakteriol Mikrobiol Hyg [A].* 1984;256:479-489.
38. Harvey RA, Kim HC, Pincus J, Trooskin SZ, Wilcox JN, Greco RS. Binding of tissue plasminogen activator to vascular grafts. *Thromb Haemost.* 1989;61:131-136.
39. Jansen B, Jansen S, Peters G, Pulverer G. In-vitro efficacy of a central venous catheter ("Hydrocath") loaded with teicoplanin to prevent bacterial colonization. *J Hosp Infect.* 1992;22:93-107.
40. Bayston R, Grove N, Siegel J, Lawellin D, Barsham S. Prevention of hydrocephalus shunt catheter colonization in vitro by impregnation with antimicrobials. *J Neurol Neurosurg Psychiatry.* 1989;52:605-609.
41. Dougherty SH, Simmons RL. Infections in bionic man: the pathobiology of infections in prosthetic devices—part I. *Curr Probl Surg.* 1982;19:217-264.
42. Ney AL, Kelly PH, Tsukayama DT, Bubrick MP. Fibrin glue-antibiotic suspension in the prevention of prosthetic graft infection. *J Trauma.* 1990;30:1000-1005.
43. Sobinsky KR, Flanigan DP. Antibiotic bonding to polytetrafluoroethylene via glucosaminoglycan-keratin luminal coating. *Surgery.* 1986;100:629-634.
44. Strachen CJ, Newsom SW, Ashton TR. The clinical use of an antibiotic-bonded graft. *Euro J Vasc Surg.* 1991;5:627-632.
45. Gott VL, Whiffen JD, Dutton RC. Heparin bonding on colloidal graphite surfaces. *Science.* 1963;142:1297-1298.
46. Greco RS, et al. Prevention of graft infection by antibiotic bonding. *Surg Forum.* 1980;31:29.
47. Jagpal R, Greco RS. Studies of a graphite-benzalkonium-oxacillin surface. *Am Surg.* 1979;45:774-779.
48. Powell TW, Burnham SJ, Johnson G Jr. A passive system using rifampin to create an infection-resistant vascular prosthesis. *Surgery.* 1983;94:765-769.
49. Kamal GD, Pfaller MA, Rempe LE, Jebson PJ. Reduced intravascular catheter infection by antibiotic bonding. *JAMA.* 1991;265:2364-2368.
50. Raad I, Darouiche R, Dupuis J, et al: Central venous catheters coated with minocycline and rifampin for the prevention of catheter-related colonization and bloodstream infections. A randomized, double-blind trial. *Ann Intern Med.* 1997;127:267-274.
51. Chatzinikolaou I, Finkel K, Hanna H, et al. Antibiotic-coated hemodialysis catheters for the prevention of vascular catheter-related infections: a prospective, randomized study. *Am J Med.* 2003;115:352-357.
52. Maki DG, Stolz SM, Wheeler S, Mermel LA. Prevention of central venous catheter-related bloodstream infection by use of an antiseptic-impregnated catheter. A randomized, controlled trial. *Ann Intern Med.* 1997;127:257-266.
53. Darouiche RO, Raad II, Heard SO, et al. A comparison of two antimicrobial-impregnated central venous catheters. *N Engl J Med.* 1999;340:1-8.
54. Bassetti S, Hu J, D'Agostino RB Jr, Sheretz RJ. Prolonged antimicrobial activity of a catheter containing chlorhexidine-silver sulfadiazine extends protection against catheter infections in vivo. *Antimicrob Agents Chemother.* 2003;45:1535-1538.
55. Guggenbichler JP, Böswald M, Lugauer S, Krall T. A new technology of microdispersed silver in polyurethane induces antimicrobial activity in central venous catheters. *Infection.* 1999;27(suppl 1):S16-S23.
56. Fraenkel D, Rickard C, Thomas P, Faoagali J, George N, Ware R. A prospective, randomized trial of rifampin-minocycline-coated and silver-platinum-carbon-impregnated central venous catheters. *Crit Care Med.* 2006;34:668-675.
57. Hanna H, Benjamin R, Chatzinikolaou I, et al: Long-term silicone central venous catheters impregnated with minocycline and rifampin decrease rates of catheter-related bloodstream infection in cancer patients: a prospective randomized clinical trial. *J Clin Oncol.* 2004;22:3163-3171.
58. Darouiche RO, Berger DH, Khardori N, et al. Comparison of antimicrobial impregnation with tunneling of long-term central venous catheters: a randomized controlled trial. *Ann Surg.* 2005;242:193-200.
59. Maki DG, Ringer M, Alvarado CJ. Prospective randomised trial of povidone-iodine, alcohol, and chlorhexidine for prevention of infection associated with central venous and arterial catheters. *Lancet.* 1991;338:339-343.
60. Stanley HD, Charlebois E, Harb G, Jacobson MA. Central venous catheter infections in AIDS patients receiving treatment for cytomegalovirus disease. *J Acquir Immune Defic Syndr* 1994;7:272-278.
61. Freeman AJ, Gardner CJ, Dodds MG. An improved method for bonding heparin to intravascular cannulae. *J Pharmacol Methods.* 1990;24:7-11.
62. Maki DG, Cobb L, Garman JK, Shapiro JM, Ringer M, Helgerson RB. An attachable silver-impregnated cuff for prevention of infection with central venous catheters: A prospective randomized multicenter trial. *Am J Med.* 1988;85:307-314.
63. Groeger JS, Lucas AB, Coit D, et al. A prospective, randomized evaluation of the effect of silver-impregnated subcutaneous cuffs for preventing tunneled chronic venous access catheter infections in cancer patients. *Ann Surg.* 1993;218:206-210.
64. Ingram J, Weitzman S, Greenberg ML, Parkin P, Filler R. Complications of indwelling venous access lines in the pediatric hematology patient: A prospective comparison of external venous catheters and subcutaneous ports. *Am J Pediatr Hematol Oncol.* 1991;13:130-136.
65. Mirro J Jr, Rao BN, Kumar M, et al. A comparison of placement techniques and complications of externalized catheters and implantable port use in children with cancer. *J Pediatr Surg.* 1990;25:120-124.
66. Pegues D, Axelrod P, McClarren C, et al. Comparison of infections in Hickman and implanted port catheters in adult solid tumor patients. *J Surg Oncol.* 1992;49:156-162.
67. Mueller BU, Skelton J, Callender DP, et al: A prospective randomized trial comparing the infectious and noninfectious complications of an externalized catheter versus a subcutaneously implanted device in cancer patients. *J Clin Oncol.* 1992;10:1943-1948.
68. Shankar R, Greisler HP. Inflammation and biomaterials. In Greco RS (ed). *Implantation Biology: The Host Response and Biomedical Materials.* Boca Raton, FL: CRC Press; 1994.
69. Picker LJ, Warnock RA, Burns AR, Doerschuk CM, Berg EL, Butcher EC. The neutrophil selectin LECAM-1 presents carbohydrate ligands to the vascular selectins ELAM-1 and GMP-140. *Cell.* 1991;66:921-933.
70. von Andrian UH, Chambers JD, McEvoy LM, Bargatze RF, Arfors KE, Butcher EC. Two-step model of leukocyte-endothelial interactions in inflammation: distinct roles for LECAM-1 and the leukocyte beta 2 integrins in vivo. *Proc Natl Acad Sci U S A.* 1991;88:7538-7542.

71. Dustin ML, Rothlein R, Bhan AK, Dinarello CA, Springer TA. Induction by I1-1 and interferon, tissue distribution, biochemistry, and function of a natural adherence molecule (ICAM-1). *J Immunol.* 1986; 137:245-254.

72. Ford-Hutchinson AW, Bray MA, Doig MV, Shipley ME, Smith MJ. Leukotriene B, a potent chemokinetic and aggregating substance released from polymorphonuclear leukocytes. *Nature.* 1980;286: 264-265.

73. Scarborough DE, Mason RG, Dalldorf FG, Brinkhous KM. Morphologic manifestations of blood-solid interfacial interactions. *Lab Invest.* 1969;20:164-169.

74. Margiotta MS, et al. Integrins, adhesion molecules, and biomaterials. In Greco RS (ed). *Implantation Biology: The Host Response and Biomedical Materials.* Boca Raton, FL: CRC Press, 1994.

75. Cheney FW, Lincoln JR. Phlebitis from plastic intravenous catheters. *Anesthesiology.* 1964;25:650-652.

76. Madan M, Alexander DJ, McMahon MJ. Influence of catheter type on occurrence of thrombophlebitis during peripheral intravenous nutrition. *Lancet.* 1992;339:101-103.

77. Ashton J, Gibson V, Summers S. Effects of heparin versus saline solution on intermittent infusion device irrigation. *Heart Lung.* 1990;19: 608-612.

78. Tuten SH, Gueldner SH. Efficacy of sodium chloride versus dilute heparin for maintenance of peripheral intermittent intravenous devices. *Appl Nurs Res.* 1991;4:63-71.

79. Bivins BA, Rapp RP, DeLuca PP, McKean H, Griffen WO Jr. Final inline filtration: A means of decreasing the incidence of infusion phlebitis. *Surgery.* 1979;85:388-394.

80. Falchuk KH, Peterson L, McNeil BJ. Microparticulate-induced phlebitis. *N Engl J Med.* 1985;212:78-82.

81. Gibbons DF. Biomedical materials. *Annu Rev Biophys Bioeng.* 1975;4: 367-375.

82. Swanson JT, Aldrete JA. Thrombophlebitis after intravenous infusion. *Rocky Mt Med J* 1969;4:48-51.

83. Spilezewski KL, Anderson JM, Schaap RN, Solomon DD. In vivo biocompatibility of catheter materials. *Biomaterials.* 1988;9:253-256.

84. Salzman EW, Lindon J, McManama G, Ware JA. Role of fibrinogen in activation of platelets by artificial surfaces. *Ann N Y Acad Sci.* 1987; 516:184-195.

85. Shiba E, Lindon JN, Kushner L, et al. Antibody-detectable changes in fibrinogen adsorption affecting platelet activation on polymer surfaces. *Am J Physiol.* 1991;260(5 pt 1):C965-C974.

86. Chinn BS, et al. Postadsorptive transitions in fibrinogen adsorbed to Biomer: changes in baboon platelet adhesion, antibody binding, and sodium dodecyl sulfate elutability. *J Biomed Mater Res.* 1991;25:535.

87. Ryu G, Han D, Kim Y, Min B. Albumin-immobilized polyurethane and its blood compatibility. *ASAIO J.* 1992;38:M644-M648.

88. Park K, Mao FW, Park H. The minimum surface fibrinogen concentration necessary for platelet activation on dimethyldichlorosilane-coated glass. *J Biomed Mater Res.* 1991;25:407-420.

89. Snyderman R, Gewurz H, Mergenhagen SE. Interactions of the complement system with endotoxin lipopolysaccharide: generation of a factor chemotactic for polymorphonuclear leukocytes. *J Exp Med.* 1968;128:259-275.

90. Schwarzmann G, Sefrin P. Thrombogenicity of central venous catheters: comparison of two polyurethane catheters [in German]. *Infusionsther Transfusionsmed.* 1993;20:148-156.

91. Eberhart RC, Munro MS, Frautschi JR, et al: Influence of endogenous albumin binding on blood-biomaterial interactions. *Ann NY Acad Sci.* 1987;516:78-95.

92. Du YJ, Klement P, Berry LR, Tressel P, Chan AK. In vivo rabbit acute model tests of polyurethane catheters coated with a novel antithrombin-heparin covalent complex. *Thromb Haemost.* 2005;94: 366-372.

CHAPTER 8

Biologic Response to Prosthetic Dialysis Grafts

Rodney A. White and Khushboo Kaushal

Prosthetic materials used for vascular access grafts continue to have an important role in the growing population of patients with end-stage renal disease who require chronic hemodialysis. Commonly, either inadequate vessels preclude the construction of or early failure complicates the use of radiocephalic (Brescia-Cimino)[1] or other autologous arteriovenous (AV) fistulas and necessitates the use of alternative biologic or synthetic conduits as interposition or bridge AV shunts. Proposed secondary AV access conduits have included autogenous veins in 1969,[2] bovine carotid artery xenografts in 1972,[3] polyethylene terephthalate (Dacron) grafts in 1972,[4] expanded polytetrafluoroethylene (PTFE) grafts in 1973,[5] and umbilical vein allografts in 1976.[6] These alternative conduits are less than ideal. Small-diameter (6-mm) Dacron grafts are plagued by high thrombosis rates in both arterial reconstruction and AV access applications. Eliminating these complications has become the focus of more recent studies, with tissue-engineered grafts potentially reducing the difficulties associated with small-diameter grafts.[7] Interposition AV grafts have widely varying reported 1-year patency rates ranging from 40% to 80%.[8] Use of autogenous vein requires more extensive harvesting and interposition or transposition of saphenous or basilic vein lengths for AV access. Despite their reasonably successful results and advantage of not inducing immediate rejection, homologous saphenous veins may contribute to allosensitization.[9] Preserved collagen grafts, such as human umbilical vein and bovine carotid artery, poorly tolerate repeated needle punctures and are prone to focal pseudoaneurysmal degeneration. The use of human umbilical veins may result in additional difficulties from the differences in wall thickness between the patient's vessels and the umbilical veins.[10] PTFE (Teflon) is the most commonly used material for conduits for secondary AV access and has similar rates of infection as the other prosthetic grafts. Overall patency rates and salvage rates of infected prostheses, however, are higher for PTFE bridge grafts than for bovine xenografts.

Prosthetic materials must possess a number of characteristics to function optimally as an AV access graft. The luminal flow surface of the graft must be relatively thromboresistant. The prosthetic wall should be rapidly incorporated by adjacent tissues to prevent accumulation of blood or serum around the graft and potential bacterial contamination and proliferation. The graft material must have adequate mechanical strength to prevent aneurysmal degeneration, to withstand repeated large-bore needle punctures, and to rapidly seal and heal at the puncture sites. AV grafts should be large enough in diameter to maintain high flow rates (~400 mL/min) for hemodialysis and to be easily palpated for puncture. AV grafts must be flexible enough for loop constructions. Further evaluation of the early and late mechanisms responsible for AV graft failure will enable better understanding of blood- and tissue-material interactions and ultimately lead to the development of improved prosthetic devices. Much effort is currently focused on preventing myointimal hyperplasia at the venous outflow.

Prosthetic Devices and the Blood-Material Interface

Thrombosis is the most common mode of failure of AV access grafts. Early graft occlusion is relatively uncommon and is due to unmitigated thrombus formation at the biomaterial surface leading to luminal obstruction. Blood hypercoagulability or low graft flow rates due to intravascular volume contraction in the dialysis patient are often contributing factors in the absence of technical errors during access construction. Thrombosis of vascular access grafts long after implantation is initiated by a pseudointimal layer lining the flow surface of the biomaterial that is devoid of endothelial cell covering and therefore rendered relatively thrombogenic. The amount and, possibly, the character of early thrombus formation on the graft surface immediately after implantation and the biomaterial type and structure (porosity and surface roughness) may affect the thickness and cellular and molecular composition, as well as the endothelialization of the pseudointimal layer that later develops. The thrombogenic potential of a vascular prosthesis at early and late follow-up intervals may thus be related.

The thrombotic process at the vascular prosthetic surface is affected mainly by the site and geometry of the constructed interposition graft, the rate of blood flow, and the critical surface tension. In high-flow applications without significantly disturbed flow patterns, many materials are acceptable as short-term blood-compatible surfaces (Fig. 8-1). At low flow rates or with highly disturbed flow

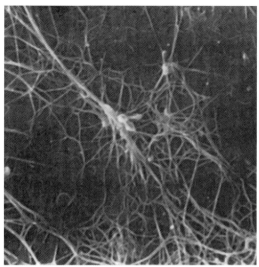

Figure 8-1.
Limited fibrin and platelet adhesion to a relatively thromboresistant smooth surface in a high blood flow area (original magnification × 4000).

patterns near the prosthetic surface, such as at anastomoses where flow separation, reattachment, and recirculation regions may exist, thrombotic and embolic complications limit the applicability of many materials.[11] Critical surface tensions of 20 to 30 dynes/cm are the least thrombogenic[12]; values above and below this range accentuate thrombus formation (Fig. 8-2). The roughness of a material increases the critical surface tension. An attempt is made to approximate the critical surface tension of autogenous vessels, which is 25 dynes/cm.

Early thrombogenicity of a vascular prosthesis is influenced by the chemical composition of the flow surface. Fourier transform infrared spectroscopy/attenuated total reflectance (FTIR/ATR) and electron spectroscopy for chemical analysis (ESCA) have been used to study the chemical and morphologic structures of the surface before and after implantation.[13] Labeling of specific protein fractions, electrophoresis of eluted proteins, and postimplantation FTIR/ATR or ESCA evaluations are three techniques that have been used to assess specific protein deposition.[14,15] Routine histologic staining methods and scanning electron micrographs have failed to quantify cellular responses to flow surfaces, although histologic and immunochemical techniques may demonstrate different cell populations and identify cellular activation.[16]

Protein Adsorption

After implantation and exposure to flowing blood, the luminal surface of a vascular prosthesis is immediately coated with a layer of serum proteins. In vitro flow studies using human whole blood and various vascular graft materials have shown that the amount of protein adsorbed to the surface is not strictly a function of the plasma concentration of the protein.[17] This finding suggests an active process whereby selective adsorption of proteins is dictated by specific affinities to a polymer surface. Dependence of protein adsorption on exposed charges at the biomaterial surface has been implicated in the observed selective binding affinities. To this end, ultrathin graphite (carbon) coatings have been applied to vascular grafts without changing their material properties (eg, surface roughness, porosity). Carbon coating adds an electronegative charge to the graft surface and theoretically repels circulating procoagulant proteins and platelets.[18] Mixed results of improved patency with graphite-coated grafts in animals have been reported.[19]

Preliminary evidence suggests that surfaces that preferentially adsorb albumin are less thrombogenic than surfaces that adsorb fibrinogen or immunoglobulin G (IgG).[20] These three proteins also adsorb to graft surfaces in vitro in greater quantities than other plasma proteins.[17] Adsorbed immunoglobulins may be able to activate circulating leukocytes, especially monocytes or macrophages, and to initiate inflammatory response at the graft surface. Fibronectin, factor VIII, and Hageman factor (factor XII) have been found to adsorb to surfaces in lesser amounts.[17] Hageman factor and factor VIII are active participants in the intrinsic clotting cascade. Hageman factor can also activate complement, as well as kallikrein and kinin, pathways stimulating local inflammatory responses. Factor VIII and its von Willebrand factor (vWF) moiety serve as an attachment site for platelets through membrane vWF receptors.

Vascular endothelial cells, which are known to produce vWF, regulate adhesion of plasma proteins and platelets particularly with their ability to prevent aggregation of platelets.[21] Anticoagulant factors such as thrombomodulin, adenosine diphosphate, and heparin-like glycosaminoglycans are present in the membranes of vascular endothelial cells, with heparin-like glycosaminoglycans having a critical role in the activity of antithrombin III. Vascular endothelial cells express a tissue factor, which is also known as factor III or thromboplastin. Conditions that elicit thrombosis may increase expression of tissue factor and decrease the rate of gene expression of anticoagulants

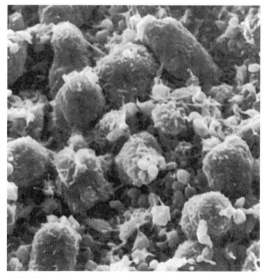

Figure 8-2.
Dense accumulation of platelets, fibrin, and white blood cells on a thrombogenic vascular surface (original magnification × 4000).

such as thrombomodulin. Tissue factor combines with factor VII/VIIa and activates factor IX and factor X, and the active form of factor X cleaves prothrombin to produce thrombin. To regulate this activity and inhibit factor X, tissue factor pathway inhibitor binds to the tissue factor/factor VIIa complex.

Fibronectins, a group of high-molecular-weight glycoproteins, have been implicated in a variety of cell interactions with collagen and fibrin, including promotion of platelet adhesion.[22] Fibronectin binds covalently to fibrin through the action of factor XIII and is thought to enhance thrombogenicity of synthetic surfaces. Platelet-fibrin mesh on synthetic surfaces is coated with fibronectin, suggesting that fibrin strands formed during clotting are probably fibrin-fibronectin copolymers. Blood cells other than platelets found in thrombi have no fibronectin on their surfaces.

Platelet Deposition

Early platelet adhesion, either directly to biomaterial surface or via adsorbed plasma proteins such as factor VIII, fibronectin, or fibrin, leads to thrombus deposition along a vascular graft. Initial adhesion of platelets to synthetic surfaces appears to be independent of specific platelet integrin receptors (glycoproteins Ic/IIa and IIb/IIIa) that are known to mediate adhesion on damaged subendothelium.[23] These integrin receptors are important for subsequent platelet spreading and surface activation (via pseudopod formation) and for further attachment of platelets (and other blood elements) to propagating thrombus along the synthetic material. Platelet transport to the biomaterial surface and deposition is dependent on the relative magnitudes of several governing forces. High flow rates and disturbed blood flow patterns along the vascular graft resulting in flow separation, reattachment, and recirculation regions will deliver greater numbers of platelets to the material surface with time. Platelets and leukocytes are damaged and activated by higher shear stresses as well, thus favoring their attachment.[24,25] Initial adherence of platelets requires that the electrochemical binding force between platelet membrane and biomaterial surface be greater than the shear (drag) force generated on the platelet by local blood flow favoring detachment from the wall. Higher blood flow rates, although favoring increased platelet transport to the biomaterial surface, paradoxically tend to dislodge adherent platelets by generating higher shear forces at the wall. Net platelet aggregation and thrombus formation reflect some balance between adhesive forces and the local flow field conditions.

Longer-term thrombotic complications of vascular prostheses involve platelet accumulation on nonendothelialized pseudointima that covers the synthetic graft. Small-diameter arterial grafts placed in dogs and evaluated before pseudointimal endothelialization (earlier than 1 mo) show greatest platelet deposition on Dacron prostheses, less deposition on PTFE, and least deposition on carotid autografts, paralleling a trend toward lower patency rates with Dacron.[26] Platelet deposition was seen to decrease during the 1st week after implantation in both synthetic grafts but to increase again at 3 weeks in Dacron grafts (Fig. 8-3). These observations were attributed to progressively thicker pseudointima in Dacron grafts containing greater amounts of thrombogenic collagen. Platelet deposition diminished

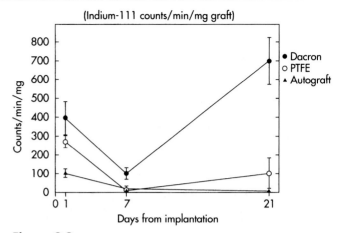

Figure 8-3.
Midgraft platelet accumulation in polyethylene terephthalate (Dacron), polytetrafluoroethylene (PTFE), and autograft segments implanted in canine carotid arteries. (From Seeger JM, Borgeson M, Lawson G. Pseudointimal thrombogenicity changes in small arterial grafts. *Surgery.* 1990;107:620-626.)

with time at anastomotic regions of synthetic grafts, correlating with an observed ingrowth of luminal cells resembling endothelial cells at these sites. Furthermore, Wyers and coworkers[27] demonstrated that covalently binding hirudin, which is an anticoagulant found in the salivary glands of leeches, to the surface of Dacron further reduces thrombus formation in comparison with Dacron by itself.

In general, antiplatelet drugs decrease the amount of platelet damage at a given shear rate but do not prevent platelet damage.[28] Aspirin and dipyridamole decrease platelet aggregation and survival time.[29,30] Antiplatelet agents are effective in reducing platelet deposition in synthetic vascular grafts.[31] Heparin has little effect on platelet function but limits thrombus propagation. A number of investigators are dispersing pharmacologic agents or their analogues in polymers in an attempt to control the protein and cellular responses to vascular prosthetic surfaces. For example, Aldenhoff and colleagues[32] developed a novel prototype of coiled tubes with larger diameters than those of coiled metallic guidewires and found that the presence of immobilized heparin within the coating of the inner surface of the tubes minimized thrombin formation.

Biomaterial Properties That Affect Thrombogenicity

The surface properties of a biomaterial will influence its relative thrombogenicity as a vascular graft. Crystalline polymers are more active with respect to platelet retention and activation than are their amorphous or noncrystalline counterparts. Hydrophilic surfaces lacking ionic charge and lacking strong hydrogen-bonding groups are desirable for minimizing platelet activation. These observations have prompted the suggestion that the chemical structure of blood flow surfaces be random, amorphous, and perhaps of a mobile nature, with nothing in excess on the surface.[20] Hoffman and associates[33] demonstrated the importance of surface chemistry on diminishing Dacron graft thrombogenicity by applying a thin surface coating of tetrafluoroethylene via gas discharge without changes in porosity, compliance, or surface topography.

Porosity and roughness of the luminal surface also influence graft thrombogenicity. Campbell and coworkers[34] evaluated the effect of pore size on the patency of 4-mm internal diameter PTFE prostheses in dogs and found that grafts with pore sizes less than 22 μm maintain the best patency. PTFE prostheses with pore sizes greater than 22 μm had progressively thicker pseudointimal development as the pore size increased, which led to ultimate occlusion. PTFE prostheses with pore sizes greater than 110 μm were excessively thrombogenic and rapidly occluded on implantation. Similarly, canine small-diameter arterial polyurethane or silicone rubber grafts with pore sizes of 60 to 120 μm are more thrombogenic than grafts with pore sizes of 20 to 30 μm.[35]

Merrill[36] studied the effects of roughness of a surface on thrombogenicity. He showed that surface defects of 0.1 μm stimulate protein adhesion and that defects of 10 to 100 μm also promote adhesion of cells. Rough areas on a surface are sites where entrapped air initiates protein and cellular adhesion.[37]

Gas denucleations of PTFE grafts to remove potentially thrombogenic trapped air bubbles have successfully reduced acute thrombosis and increased patency in small-diameter reconstructions in dogs.[38] Didisheim and colleagues[39] studied the effect of roughness on the thrombogenicity of PTFE surfaces, using smooth expanded PTFE compared with textured PTFE felt. The surfaces were otherwise identical except for slightly higher bulk crystallinity in the felt. They demonstrated increased thrombogenicity in the rougher felt materials by reactivity to vWF, total protein adsorption, and platelet and leukocyte adhesion. Smooth, porous coatings have been applied to the luminal surfaces of various arterial prostheses in dogs, improving the thromboresistance by decreasing the surface roughness yet preserving wall porosity.[40]

Healing Responses and Pathologic Features of Expanded PTFE

Expanded PTFE, discovered in 1938, is the preferred synthetic graft for AV dialysis access and smaller-diameter arterial reconstructions in the absence of adequate autogenous vein. PTFE is a chemically inert, high-molecular-weight synthetic carbon and fluorine polymer fabricated by an extrusion process into porous tubes or sheets, often known by the DuPont brand name Teflon. Porosity of the graft material can be altered by mechanical stretching at construction to form various solid node and interconnecting fibril configurations (Fig. 8-4). Standard PTFE vascular grafts have fibril length and internodal distances of 20 to 30 μm. The node-fibril structure occupies 15% to 20% of the total material volume, leaving 80% to 85% porous volume for tissue ingrowth. PTFE grafts are relatively thromboresistant and hydrophobic by virtue of an electronegative surface potential (−17 μV). Early clinical prototypes of tubular PTFE graft had a wall thickness of 0.5 mm but were subject to circumferential creep and aneurysmal dilatation. Now, PTFE vascular grafts are reinforced with an external porous PTFE wrapping or have greater wall thickness and improved circumferential strength. Reinforced PTFE grafts exhibit high tensile strength and minimal deformation under axial and circumferential loading.

Graft Healing

The implantation of a synthetic vascular prosthesis generates a chronic inflammatory reaction in the perigraft tissues. The cellular response is primarily mononuclear with aggregation of macrophages and lymphocytes. Increased local vascularity allows fibroblast proliferation and collagen deposition along the outer surface of the biomaterial. Porous grafts undergo tissue incorporation via penetration and ingrowth of fibrous components within 1 month after

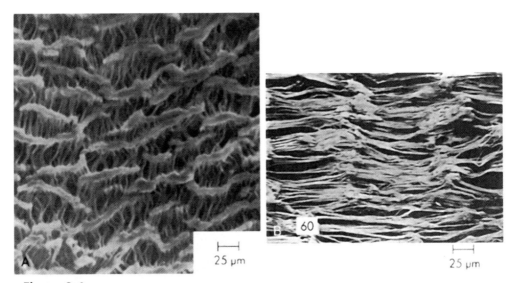

Figure 8-4.
Scanning electron micrographs of luminal surfaces of polytetrafluoroethylene prostheses. *A,* Fibril length (pore size) of 30 μm. *B,* Fibril length of 60 μm. (*A* and *B,* From Hirabayashi K, Saitoh E, Ijima H, Takenawa T, Kodama M, Hori M. Influence of fibril length upon ePTFE graft healing and host modification of the implant. *J Biomed Mater Res.* 1992;26:1433-1447.)

implantation in the absence of local infection, perigraft hematoma formation, and extensive lymphatic or serous fluid accumulation. Fibrous tissue ingrowth provides vascularity and the cellular substrates for an organized pseudointimal layer composed ideally of smooth muscle cells, fibroblasts, extracellular matrix, fibrin, and blood-borne cells. The transport of nutrients via diffusion from the vessel lumen can maintain a viable pseudointima only up to 500 µm in thickness.[41] Connective tissue penetration is not essential for the genesis of a pseudointima, but connective tissue support is critical to its long-term existence. This assertion is based on the observation that a pseudointima is not formed in areas where tissue incorporation is completely absent, although it is frequently present in areas where adjacent connective tissue is minimal.[38] Ultimately, healing of porous prostheses decreases the susceptibility to infection, anchors the graft to prevent kinking and perigraft fluid collection, and improves flow surface endothelialization.[42]

In contrast to grafts in various experimental animals in which luminal healing and endothelialization are more complete, both PTFE and Dacron vascular grafts implanted in humans have limited inner capsules predominantly composed of fibrin and devoid of endothelial and smooth muscle cells.[43,44] Endothelialization of the luminal surface in humans occurs only 1 to 2 cm into the graft from the anastomotic site. These endothelial cells are thought to be derived from adjacent, native arterial endothelium. In the animal models in which endothelialization of Dacron and nonreinforced, high-porosity PTFE grafts occurs, transmural capillaries are seen to accompany fibrous tissue ingrowth through the biomaterial wall. This capillary ingrowth has been proposed as the source of midgraft endothelial cells.[45] Capillary ingrowth in Dacron and reinforced PTFE grafts in humans is limited and does not provide for a complete luminal endothelial lining.[44,46]

Porosity

The effect of graft porosity on vascular healing has been studied in small–internal diameter (6-mm) PTFE conduits with sometimes conflicting results. Campbell and coworkers[34] performed extensive testing of various modifications of PTFE and concluded that pore size (fibril length) of 20 to 30 µm was optimal for use as a vascular prosthesis. Larger luminal pores (≥110 µm) were associated with lower patency rates. Improved healing characterized by better perigraft tissue ingrowth and complete endothelialization of neointimal layers has been noted in baboon,[47] canine,[19] and rat[48] models using high-porosity (60-µm), nonreinforced (unwrapped) PTFE grafts.

In baboons, endothelial cells are derived from penetrating capillaries and, by 2 weeks after implantation, completely cover a thin neointima of uniform thickness lining the graft. Neointimal thickening parallels smooth muscle cell proliferation beneath the endothelial lining and is thought to be regulated by factors from cells within the vessel wall and not from adherent platelets.[49] Nonreinforced, lower-porosity (10- and 30-µm) PTFE grafts in baboons developed endothelial cell coverage only at anastomotic sites. Smaller pores in the biomaterial are thought to limit the ingrowth of supporting connective tissue and capillaries along the graft. Despite early complete endothelial cell coverage, 90-µm-pore PTFE grafts develop later

neointimal instability with focal endothelial loss and platelet adherence.

Akers and associates[19] have shown improved patency up to 4 months in addition to better healing with nonreinforced 60-µm PTFE grafts compared with standard reinforced 30-µm prostheses in canines. High-porosity (60-µm) PTFE grafts with a reinforcing porous wrapping to prevent circumferential creep and aneurysmal dilatation have been implanted as above-knee femoropopliteal bypasses in humans.[46] Limited histologic inspection of these grafts revealed partial capillary ingrowth and lack of endothelial or smooth muscle cells along the luminal surface. These findings and quantitative indium-111 platelet uptake were similar to those in standard reinforced 30-µm grafts used as controls in these patients. The authors concluded that failure of PTFE endothelialization is a result of inadequate angiogenesis in humans or retardation of capillary ingrowth by the reinforcing wrap.

The relation between specific vascular tissue response and the pore size of a vascular graft may be independent of the biomaterial. Studies with replamineform vascular prostheses, which were fabricated by reproducing the uniform, microporous configuration of different pore size calcium carbonate templates, have permitted independent assessment of the effect of pore size and biomaterial on tissue incorporation.[50] These studies have shown that silicone rubber and polyurethane vascular prostheses with pore sizes of less than 15 µm exhibit minimal tissue ingrowth, that prostheses with pore sizes between 15 and 45 µm are incorporated with fibrohistiocytic cellular elements, and that prostheses with pore sizes greater than 45 µm are incorporated with organized fibrous tissue[35] (Fig. 8-5). The effect of pore size on the type of tissue ingrowth is also evident in Dacron and PTFE vascular grafts.[51] The larger void spaces in knitted fabrics become infiltrated with fibrous tissue, whereas the smaller interstices in the filamentous velours have a reactive fibrohistiocytic appearance. The expanded PTFE materials used clinically as vascular grafts have fibril lengths of 20 to 30 µm and become infiltrated with fibrohistiocytic cellular elements (see Fig. 8-5).

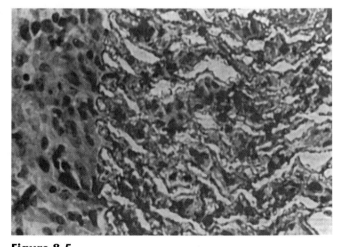

Figure 8-5.
Fibrohistiocytic cellular incorporation of a PTFE prosthesis (original magnification × 100). (From White RA. The effect of porosity and biomaterial on the healing and long-term mechanical properties of vascular prostheses. *ASAIO Trans.* 1988;11:95-100.)

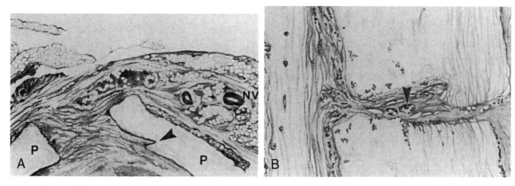

Figure 8-6.
Connective tissue ingrowth filling needle puncture holes *(arrow)* of PTFE dialysis grafts. *A,* Disrupted graft wall. *P,* Puncture site. *B,* Neocapillary *(arrow)* formation in puncture tract. (*A* and *B,* From Delorme JM, Guidoin R, Canizales S, et al. Vascular access for hemodialysis: pathologic features of surgically excised ePTFE grafts. *Ann Vasc Surg.* 1992;6:517-524.)

Fibrohistiocytic cells from porous implants with 20- to 30-μm pores have high total protein production with approximately 10% being type I and type III collagen.[52] Type III collagen is associated with organs that have elastic properties, such as dermis, cardiovascular, and gastrointestinal systems. In contrast, knitted Dacron and 60- to 120-μm porous silicone rubber and polyurethane prostheses contain 50% to 60% of the total protein content as type I collagen, the primary constituent of relatively stiff fibrous tissue.[52]

Healing of prostheses with stiff fibrous tissue has the potential for long-term contracture and strangulation of ingrowing capillaries. In contrast, fibrohistiocytic ingrowth appears to have lower mechanical strength and may be more elastic, related to the type III collagen component. By fabricating vascular prostheses with a pore size less than 45 μm, it may be possible to avoid the long-term complications of prosthetic stiffening and tissue cicatrization, in addition to attaining viable tissue incorporation and maintaining compliance.

Consequences of Dialysis Cannulation

Repeated needle punctures of PTFE AV grafts, although necessary for hemodialysis, pose a continuing threat to the long-term integrity of the conduit wall. Thrombi rapidly fill the track left by needle punctures through PTFE grafts. Fibrous tissue ingrowth then fills the needle puncture holes and typically blends with the fibrous capsule surrounding the graft. Capillary formation within the fibrous tissue that fills the needle holes occurs infrequently (Fig. 8-6). In a pathologic analysis of surgically excised AV PTFE graft segments, pseudoaneurysm formation occurred in focal regions subjected to repeated needle interrogation.[44]

The microporous structure of PTFE graft was fragmented by needle punctures with absent fibrous tissue ingrowth and support in these regions (Fig. 8-7). The outer reinforcing wrap of PTFE grafts was commonly detached from the inner wall, also at pseudoaneurysmal sites. In contrast, increasing degrees of encapsulation were observed with longer durations of graft implantation away from sites of repeated venipuncture. Primary wall degeneration such as that which occurs in bovine xenografts and human umbilical vein grafts does not account for pseudoaneurysm formation in PTFE grafts. Pseudoaneurysm formation in regions of repeated needle puncture was attributed to overuse of certain PTFE cannulation sites, use of oversized needles, and use of improper techniques of graft puncture at hemodialysis. Although uncommon, pseudoaneurysms along PTFE grafts generally require local excision and replacement with interposition segments of PTFE.

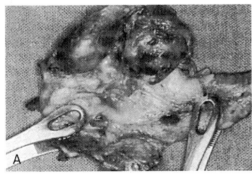
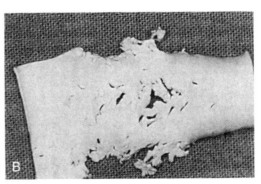

Figure 8-7.
Segment of surgically excised PTFE dialysis graft due to pseudoaneurysm formation (see Fig. 8-6). *A,* Fresh specimen. *B,* Cleaned specimen showing destruction of graft wall. (*A* and *B,* From Delorme JM, Guidoin R, Canizales S, et al. Vascular access for hemodialysis: pathologic features of surgically excised ePTFE grafts. *Ann Vasc Surg.* 1992;6:517-524.)

Repeated needle puncture of PTFE AV grafts also predisposes to other modes of access failure. Accumulation of organized laminated clot at frequently used sites of graft cannulation creates an uneven and relatively thrombogenic flow surface. With regenerative fibrosis at these sites, luminal narrowing may occur, leading to flow-limiting stenosis and graft thrombosis. Leakage of blood into perigraft tissues at the time of needle puncture occurs with most cannulations. Significant perigraft hematomas and seromas can cause mechanical separation of outer fibrous tissue capsules from graft material. Persistent perigraft fluid collections are an ominous precursor for graft thrombosis. Loss of perivascular tissue support leads to sloughing of pseudointimal lining and luminal thrombus deposition. Repetitive needle puncture at the same site will destroy that portion of the PTFE graft wall, and access should be spaced along the length of the graft.

Graft Infection

Perigraft fluid collections also provide a medium for bacterial colonization, with inoculation at the time of graft implantation or percutaneous cannulations for hemodialysis. Clinically significant infection of PTFE grafts is uncommon, however, because it occurs generally at a focal point along the external surface of the graft and requires destruction of the outer fibrous capsule for propagation. In fact, the incidence of PTFE infection correlates with the presence of puncture site hematomas[53] and inversely with the completeness of tissue ingrowth after AV graft insertion.[8,54]

Hematogenous seeding of the luminal flow surface during bacteremic episodes in the host has also been postulated as a potential route of graft infection. In a canine model, the susceptibility of PTFE grafts to infection from a bacteremic source was related to the extent of luminal coverage by pseudointima.[55] Grafts with more complete luminal healing had a lower incidence of infection produced by intravenous injection of *Staphylococcus aureus*. Despite this experimental observation, PTFE vascular grafts in humans demonstrate less pseudointimal healing than in canine models but rarely become infected long after implantation. Several investigators have used PTFE grafts to repair traumatically injured peripheral arteries where bacterial contamination was frequent, and they have not found infection to be a significant problem.[56] Localized PTFE graft infection may be treated with combinations of local drainage, segmental excision and bypass, and intravenous antibiotics. More extensive infections or anastomotic involvement predisposes PTFE grafts to thrombosis and requires excision and access placement at a remote site.

Hemodynamic Considerations and Graft Function

Relatively high blood flow rates are required in an AV conduit to perform adequate hemodialysis and to prevent thrombosis. For optimal function in the upper extremity, blood flow rates for either AV fistulas or interposition grafts are roughly an order of magnitude ($\times 10$) greater than flow in the native radial or brachial arteries. High flow rates are maintained by low conduit resistance and outflow into the compliant, high-capacitance venous system. In a newly placed AV conduit, the controlling resistance is dependent on conduit diameter and the shortest cross-sectional dimension at the arterial end-to-side anastomosis. Most end-to-side anastomoses are elliptical in cross section, with the short axis aligned in a transverse direction on the artery. When this short-axis dimension and the conduit diameter are greater than 75% of the inflow artery diameter, resistance in the AV conduit is minimized and neither larger anastomoses nor wider conduits will further increase flow. Conduit flow therefore depends on the size of the inflow artery and not on the diameter or length of routinely constructed fistulas or grafts.

Luminal Surface Response to Graft Flow

Evidence in experimental animals supports the concept of blood flow rate (and mean wall shear stress) regulation of neointimal or pseudointimal thickness within vascular grafts. Kohler and coworkers[57] have shown that high rates of blood flow (and shear stress) inhibit neointimal thickening in a flow switch model of PTFE grafts placed in baboons. Nonreinforced, 60-μm-pore PTFE bypass grafts were placed in an aortoiliac position and subjected to high flow rates, initially using a distal AV fistula, which provides low peripheral resistance. Neointimal hyperplasia was studied in the midgraft section away from disturbed flow present in the anastomotic regions. Neointima was seen to thicken dramatically when grafts were returned to normal flow conditions after ligation of the distal fistula. Smooth muscle cell proliferation and extracellular matrix accumulation accounted for the neointimal thickening in this model and were hypothesized to occur via endothelial cell modulation along the graft luminal surface.[58] These observations parallel those seen in experimental models of atherosclerosis in which the arterial wall can alter its luminal diameter via changes in intimal thickness to maintain mean wall shear stress within a specific physiologic range.[59]

If wall shear stress does play a role in the regulation of neointimal or pseudointimal thickness, an optimal graft diameter may exist. A vascular graft too small in diameter will limit flow, whereas a graft too large in diameter will ultimately thrombose.[60] Using carotid and femoral arterial interposition grafts of reinforced, 30-μm-pore PTFE in dogs, Binn and colleagues[61] demonstrated that various prosthetic diameters yield differing pseudointimal thicknesses and associated patency rates. Grafts of diameters less than those of native arteries (3-mm PTFE) had high initial mean wall shear stresses (41 dynes/cm^2), and all thrombosed by 15 weeks. Grafts of 6-mm (approximately isodiametric) and 8-mm (oversize) diameters had approximately 75% patency rates at 15 weeks. However, midgraft pseudointimal (no endothelial coverage) and anastomotic neointimal (endothelialized) thicknesses were greater in 8-mm than in 6-mm diameter grafts and at the lower-flow femoral position. Mean wall shear stress in the grafts was seen to inversely correspond to the thickness of neointimal and pseudointimal layers present. Although not statistically significant, the change in wall shear stress in the larger grafts from implantation to 15 weeks tended toward increasing shear stress to a normal level by intimal thickening. Wall shear stress in native canine arteries ranged from

14 to 27 dynes/cm^2. These values are similar to those found in other experiments with animals in which shear stress–luminal diameter regulation was observed.

These results support the concept of an optimal graft diameter for which intimal thickening is minimized and patency rates maximized. Because the pseudointimal lining of the PTFE grafts was not endothelialized in dogs, these cells may not be necessary for transduction of wall shear stress and regulation of intimal thickening. By purely mechanical means, blood flow rate and corresponding wall shear stress along the graft can dictate both the net balance between platelet aggregation and dislodgment from the luminal surface and, ultimately, pseudointimal thickness. Low flow rates and wall shear stresses will favor platelet deposition, whereas greatly elevated shear stresses (≥70 dynes/cm^2) cause increases in thrombus area and height because of platelet activation at these shear levels.[62]

AV PTFE grafts used in the upper extremity have inner diameters of 6 or 7 mm, and their performance as dialysis access depends on blood flow rate. Flow rates of 500 to 1000 mL/min provide for optimal function and patency.[63] Graft flow of less than 300 mL/min after implantation predisposes the patient to thrombosis. Flow rates averaging more than 1500 mL/min long after implantation may cause high-output cardiac failure or arterial steal from the distal arm by excessive shunting.[64] A tapered 4-mm (arterial) to 7-mm (venous) PTFE graft has been studied in elderly persons and in patients with high-flow complications, and it generally limits flow to no greater than 1000 mL/min with acceptable patency rates.[65,66] In comparison, flow rates in PTFE femoropopliteal arterial bypass grafts are at least two to three times lower than similar-diameter AV conduits because of higher outflow resistance in the commonly diseased, lower leg arterial tree. Pseudointimal linings of 0.5 to 1.0 mm are common along PTFE dialysis grafts. Without changes in arterial inflow or development of venous outflow obstruction (ie, at the same graft flow rate), a cross-sectional decrease in lumen caused by pseudointimal thickening increases blood velocity and wall shear stresses along the graft. Quantification of this phenomenon and its influence on graft function has not been addressed in AV conduits.

Venous Anastomotic Intimal Hyperplasia

In the absence of uncommon causes for graft failure, such as pseudoaneurysm formation, prosthetic infection, early thrombosis caused by technical error during implantation, and hypercoagulability or low flow states, late thrombosis remains the common final mechanism of failure. Simple thrombogenicity of the graft luminal surface does not appear to account for most delayed failures, however. Hyperplastic neointimal thickening occurs at all anastomoses between prosthetic graft and native vessels and at anastomoses involving autogenous vein or other arterial substitutes. This hyperplastic response is characterized by a ringlike area of cellular and matrix proliferation of the intima and neointima predominantly at the distal venous end-to-side anastomosis of the dialysis graft and in the outflow veins. Progressive stenosis of the anastomotic region or outflow veins by neointimal hyperplasia can increase resistance to flow and reduce blood velocity and flow rate through the graft. Below some critical level of blood flow,

velocity thrombus formation may be favored along the vascular graft, leading to total occlusion.[13,67] The localized nature of anastomotic hyperplasia has led to speculation on the causative roles of foreign body reaction to anastomotic suture and graft materials, pulsatile wall stresses associated with anastomotic compliance mismatch, and flow disturbances at anastomoses.

The role of flow disturbances in anastomotic intimal thickening has been studied primarily in Dacron and PTFE arterial bypass grafts in dogs, with comparison with the flow patterns detailed in plastic models of various anastomotic configurations.[68,69] The development of secondary, disturbed flow patterns at vessel branches, including separated flow regions, is dependent on branch or anastomosis geometry, Reynolds' number, and the ratio of flow division between run-off vessels.[70,71] With higher flow rates and associated Reynolds' numbers characterizing AV grafts compared with femoropopliteal arterial bypasses, the magnitude of expected flow disturbances is likely to be greater. However, degrees of anastomotic hyperplasia have not been well quantified and compared in AV and arterial bypass grafts. Further, the development of anastomotic hyperplasia was poorly correlated with the presence or absence of flow separation in canine arterial bypass grafts.[72] Intimal thickening along the graft-vessel suture line is believed to represent response to foreign body or vascular healing and to not be flow dependent.[68] Controversy exists over the distribution of neointimal hyperplasia around the anastomosis and correlation to local low[68] and high[73] wall shear stress regions. The contributions of mechanical and hemodynamic forces to biologic responses are not easily distinguished from healing and thrombogenic reactions to vascular grafts. The roles of flow disturbance and compliance mismatch in anastomotic hyperplasia remain inferential at the present time.

Present Status and Future Developments

Grafts of organic and semi-organic compositions are seen to have better results in comparison with synthetic grafts with lower incidence of infection and steal syndrome and greater likelihood of preserving patients' vessels.[10] Despite these advantages, both synthetic and biologic grafts used for AV dialysis access have patency rates that are worse than those reported for similar-diameter prostheses used for above-knee, femoropopliteal arterial bypasses. Even with relatively high flow conditions in the AV position, which lessen blood stasis and thrombus formation, the choice of conduit for hemodialysis plays a major role in graft failure. Overall secondary patency rates for PTFE bridge grafts are close to those for functioning autogenous AV fistulas and generally better than those for bovine carotid artery xenografts.[74] Also, the initial functional patency of PTFE grafts is close to 100%, whereas only about 50% of constructed autogenous AV fistulas function satisfactorily for hemodialysis. Neither patient nor surgeon is happy with a futile operation. PTFE grafts, however, require more frequent revision than mature AV fistulas, and cumulative patency declines with increasing numbers of surgical interventions. Using an aggressive salvage approach to malfunctioning grafts, Sicard and associates[74] demonstrated a 50% patency rate at 2 years in PTFE conduits requiring up to three revisions. Standard revisions to extend graft longevity, including thrombectomy, excision, segmental bypass or patching of anastomotic stenosis, and replacement of pseudoaneurysmal regions, have been augmented by the use of combined conduit thrombolysis and balloon angioplasty of stenotic sites. Preliminary comparative data suggest that surgical correction may provide longer secondary patency than that of thrombolysis and angioplasty.

Bovine heterografts have been reexamined in several studies. Bacchini and coworkers[75] explored differences in the survival of varying prosthetic grafts through a comparison of PTFE grafts and bovine vein grafts. Bovine vein grafts demonstrated better survival, which may be attributed to its unique properties, such as increased viscoelastic compliance and increased biocompatibility, that do not result in neointimal hyperplasia. These results indicate that bovine vein grafts may be critical in reducing venous run-off stenosis particularly among end-stage renal disease patients who are at escalated risk. Additional studies by Katzman and colleagues[76] reveal that bovine mesenteric vein, a more recently developed prosthetic graft, has shown reduced incidence of thrombosis, infection, and reoperation, and increased patency in comparison with synthetic grafts.

There clearly remains a need for improved graft performance. Further understanding of the basic mechanisms of blood- and tissue-biomaterial interactions at the molecular, cellular, and biomechanical levels is required. This advance necessitates a multidisciplinary research effort. No animal species is accepted as appropriate for predicting the overall human response to cardiovascular prostheses. In addition, long-term animal implant studies have prohibitive expense and do not provide rapid enough evaluation of new materials. However, reliable, cost-effective methods to test and predict clinical performance of vascular biomaterials have yet to be developed.

Two basic directions exist for the development of thromboresistant biomaterials for vascular prostheses. One approach is to develop new thromboresistant materials, which are either smooth and remain passive to blood components or microporous and accumulate a limited protein and cellular layer and, ideally, endothelialize. In humans, present vascular prostheses do not endothelialize, owing to either low porosity without necessary capillary penetration or high porosity with eventual development of pseudointimal instability.

A second approach involves endothelial cell seeding of the luminal surface of existing synthetic vascular grafts to potentially improve early thromboresistance and long-term patency. Existing seeding techniques are limited by inefficient harvesting of endothelial cells and poor attachment and proliferation of cells on the prosthetic surface. Treatment of prosthetic grafts with extracellular matrix components such as fibronectin, laminin, gelatin, elastin, or RGD (arginine-glycine-aspartate) containing peptide (cell integrin receptor for laminin and fibronectin) has been shown to substantially increase endothelial cell attachment and proliferation in vitro.[77] Preliminary in vivo results in dogs, using fibrous polyurethane grafts coated with gelatin and fibronectin and seeded with subcultured autogenous endothelial cells, have been promising but required

antiplatelet medications to achieve optimal patency.[78] Further detailed investigations are needed to determine what combinations and concentrations of matrix proteins provide for ideal endothelial function on seeded vascular prostheses.

Repeated needle puncture of AV grafts, although necessary for frequent hemodialysis, contributes significantly to failure due to thrombosis, pseudoaneurysm formation, and graft infection. In an attempt to prevent puncture site leakage and to provide a conduit for immediate access, Schanzer and colleagues[79] developed a coaxial PTFE graft in which the space formed between the two layers of PTFE is filled with a silicone rubber sealant. The aim is to prevent pseudoaneurysm formation and significant perigraft hematomas. Patency rates of these grafts in dogs were equivalent to those for standard PTFE grafts. Bacterial infections of PTFE grafts are uncommon but are associated with higher risk of thrombosis and generally require surgical intervention. Continued efforts are directed toward the development of antibiotic-impregnated vascular grafts to ideally prevent incipient graft infection and improve management of established infections.[80] Various methods have been used to bond antibiotics to both Dacron and PTFE vascular grafts, with mixed results in animal models. Further clinical evaluations are required.

Several recent studies are focusing on the use of vascular endothelial cells from various sources in order to develop improved prosthetics such as omental fat cells, endothelial progenitor cells, and mesenchymal stem cells.[21,81] Whereas the source of the endothelial cells is not entirely determined, studies have shown that synthetic grafts have fewer advantages in comparison with grafts that are tissue engineered. Xue and associates[7] further explain that tissue-engineered grafts may be the much-needed solution that eliminates the complications associated with small-diameter vascular grafts. It is anticipated that such a graft may be "constructed by culturing blood vessel cells on biological/synthetic scaffolds in bioreactors with optimal hemodynamic and biomechanical conditions and supplemented with spatially and temporally controlled 3-dimensional delivery of bioactive agents, the use of genetic engineering techniques, or both."

Progressive neointimal hyperplasia at anastomoses between native vessel and all biologic and synthetic conduits is responsible for the majority of late graft failures by thrombosis. Although the biomechanical and hemodynamic influences on this phenomenon are not well understood, considerable experimental evidence exists describing the complex cellular and biochemical interactions responsible for producing the pathologic lesion. Various growth factors produced by endothelial and smooth muscle cells, macrophages, and platelets appear to be key modulators in neointimal development.[82] The role that synthetic graft material itself plays in anastomotic hyperplasia remains unknown.

REFERENCES

1. Brescia MJ, Cimino JE, Appel K, Hurwich BJ. Chronic hemodialysis using venipuncture and a surgically created arteriovenous fistula. N Engl J Med. 1966;275:1089-1092.
2. May J, Tiller D, Johnson J, Stewart J, Sheil AG. Saphenous-vein arteriovenous fistula in regular dialysis treatment. N Engl J Med. 1969;280:770.

3. Chinitz JL, Yokoyama T, Bower R, Swartz C. Self-healing prosthesis for arteriovenous fistula in man. *Trans Am Soc Artif Intern Organs.* 1972;18:452-457.

4. Dunn I, Frumkin E, Forte R, Requena R, Levowitz BS. Dacron velour vascular prosthesis for hemodialysis. *Proc Clin Dial Transplant Forum.* 1972;2:85.

5. Volder JG, Kirkham RL, Kolff WJ. A-V shunts created in new ways. *Trans Am Soc Artif Intern Organs.* 1973;19:38-42.

6. Dardik H, Ibrahim IM, Dardik I. Arteriovenous fistulas constructed with modified human umbilical cord vein graft. *Arch Surg.* 1976; 111:60-62.

7. Xue L, Greisler HP. Biomaterials in the development and future of vascular grafts. *J Vasc Surg.* 2003;37:472-480.

8. Morgan AP. The problem of dialysis interface. *Arch Surg.* 1977; 112:239.

9. Benedetto B, Lipkowitz G, Madden R, et al. Use of cryopreserved cadaveric vein allografts for hemodialysis access precludes kidney transplantation because of allosensitization. *J Vasc Surg.* 2001;34: 139-142.

10. Berardinelli L. Grafts and graft materials as vascular substitutes for hemodialysis access construction. *Eur J Vasc Endovasc Surg.* 2006;32:203-211.

11. Anderson GH, Hellums JD, Moake JL, Alfrey CP Jr. Platelet lysis and aggregation in shearfields. *Blood Cells.* 1978;4:499-511.

12. Baier RE, Akers CK. Blood surface interactions: recognized factors and unsettled quesitons. *Trans Am Soc Artif Intern Organs.* 1978;24: 770-773.

13. Bandyk DF, Cato RF, Towne JB. A low flow velocity predicts failure of femoropopliteal and femorotibial bypass grafts. *Surgery.* 1985;98: 799-809.

14. Lyman DJ, Knutson K, McNeil B, Shibatani K. The effect of chemical structure and surface properties of synthetic polymers on the coagulation of blood. IV. The relation between polymer morphology and protein absorption. *Trans Am Soc Artif Intern Organs.* 1975;21:49-54.

15. Weathersby PK, Horbett TA, Hoffman AS. A new method for analysis of the absorbed plasma protein layer on biomaterial surface. *Trans Am Soc Artif Intern Organs.* 1976;22:242-252.

16. Sun NCJ (ed). *Hematology: An Atlas and Diagnostic Guide.* Philadelphia: WB Saunders; 1983.

17. Pankowsky DA, Ziats NP, Topham NS, Ratnoff OD, Anderson JM. Morphologic characteristics of adsorbed human plasma proteins on vascular graft biomaterials. *J Vasc Surg.* 1990;11:599-606.

18. Sawyer PN, Pate JW. Bio-electric phenomena as an etiologic factor in intravascular thrombosis. *Am J Physiol.* 1953;175:103-107.

19. Akers DL, Du YH, Kempczinski RF. The effect of carbon coating and porosity on early patency of expanded polytetrafluoroethylene grafts: An experimental study. *J Vasc Surg.* 1993;18:10-15.

20. Andrade J, Coleman DL, Didisheim P, Hanson SR, Mason R, Merrill E. Blood-materials interactions—20 years of frustration. *Trans Am Soc Artif Intern Organs.* 1981;27:659-662.

21. Sarkar S, Sales KM, Hamilton G, Seifalian AM. Addressing thrombogenicity in vascular graft construction. *J Biomed Mater Res B Appl Biomater.* 2007;82:100-108.

22. Grinnell F. *Blood material interactions: adsorption of fibronectin.* Summary of the Devices and Technology Branch Contractors Meeting, December 1982. Bethesda, MD: National Heart, Lung and Blood Institute; 1984. NIH Publication No. 84-1651.

23. Goodman SL, Cooper SL, Albrecht RM. Integrin receptors and platelet adhesion to synthetic surfaces. *J Biomed Mater Res.* 1993;27:683-695.

24. Dewitz TS, McIntire LV, Martin RR, Sybers HD. Enzyme release and morphological changes in leukocytes induced by mechanical trauma. *Blood Cells.* 1979;5:499-512.

25. Stevens DE, Joist JH, Sutera SP. The role of platelet prostaglandin synthesis in shear-induced platelet aggregation, release and lysis. *Blood.* 1980;56:753-758.

26. Seeger JM, Borgeson M, Lawson G. Pseudointimal thrombogenicity changes in small arterial grafts. *Surgery.* 1990;107:620-626.

27. Wyers MC, Phaneuf MD, Rzucidlo EM, Contreras MA, LoGerfo FW, Quist WC. In vivo assessment of a novel dacron surface with covalently bound recombinant hirudin. *Cardiovasc Pathol.* 1999;8:153-159.

28. Harwick RA, Hellums JD, Moake JL, Peterson DM, Alfrey CP. Effects of antiplatelet agents on platelets exposed to shear stress. *Trans Am Soc Artif Intern Organs.* 1980;26:179-184.

29. Fuster V, Chesebro JH. 10. Antithrombotic therapy: role of platelet-inhibitor drugs. II. Pharmacologic effects of platelet-inhibitor drugs. *Mayo Clin Proc.* 1981;56:185-195.

30. Moncada S, Korbut R. Dipyridamole and other phosphodiesterase inhibitors act as antithrombotic agents by potentiating endogenous prostacyclin. *Lancet.* 1978;1:1286-1289.

31. Oblath RW, Buckley FO Jr, Green RM, Schwartz SI, DeWeese JA. Prevention of platelet aggregation and adherence to prosthetic vascular grafts by aspirin and dipyridamole. *Surgery.* 1978;84:37-44.

32. Aldenhoff YBJ, Knetsch ML, Hanssen JH, Lindhout T, Wielders SJ, Koole LH. Coils and tubes releasing heparin. Studies on a new vascular graft prototype. *Biomaterials.* 2004;25:3125-3133.

33. Hoffman AS, Ratner BD, Horbett TA, Hanson SR. The importance of vascular graft surface composition as demonstrated by a new gas discharge treatment for small diameter grafts. In Kambic HE, Kantorwitz A, Sung P (eds). *Vascular Graft Update: Safety and Performance.* Philadelphia: American Society for Testing and Materials Publications; 1986:STP 898.

34. Campbell CD, Goldfarb D, Roe R. A small arterial substitute: expanded microporous polytetrafluoroethylene: patency versus porosity. *Ann Surg.* 1975;82:138-143.

35. White RA. Evaluation of small diameter graft parameters using replamineform vascular prostheses. In Wright CB (ed). *Vascular Grafting.* Littleton, MA: John Wright; 1983.

36. Merrill EFW. Distinction and correspondence among surfaces contacting blood. *Ann N Y Acad Sci.* 1987;516:196-203.

37. Ward CA, Koheil A, Johnson WR, Madras PN. Reduction of complement activation from biomaterials by removal of air nuclei from the surface roughness. *J Biomed Mater Res.* 1984;18:255-269.

38. Vann RD, Ritter EF, Plunkett MD, et al. Patency and blood flow in gas denucleated arterial prostheses. *J Biomed Mater Res.* 1993;27:493-498.

39. Didisheim P, Tirrell MV, Lyons CS, Stropp JQ, Dewanjee MK. Relative role of surface chemistry and surface texture in blood-material interactions. *Trans Am Soc Artif Intern Organs.* 1983;29:169-176.

40. White RA, Shors E, Miranda RM, et al. Microporous flow surface variation and short term thrombogenicity in dogs. *Biomaterials.* 1982;3:145-139.

41. Wesolowski SA. Foundations of modern vascular grafts. In Sawyer PN (ed). *Vascular Grafts.* New York: Appleton-Century-Crofts; 1978.

42. Moore WS, Malone JM. Vascular repair. In Hunt TK, Dumphy JE (eds). *Fundamentals of Wound Management.* New York: Appleton-Century-Crofts; 1979.

43. Berger K, Sauvage LR, Rao AM, Wood SJ. Healing of arterial prosthesis in man: its incompleteness. *Ann Surg.* 1972;175:118-127.

44. Delorme JM, Guidoin R, Canizales S, et al. Vascular access for hemodialysis: pathologic features of surgically excised ePTFE grafts. *Ann Vasc Surg.* 1992;6:517-524.

45. Clowes AW, Kirkman TR, Reidy MA. Mechanisms of arterial graft healing. Rapid transmural capillary ingrowth provides a source of intimal endothelium and smooth muscle in porous PTFE prostheses. *Am J Pathol.* 1986;123:220-230.

46. Kohler TR, Stratton JR, Kirkman TR, Johansen KH, Zierler BK, Clowes AW. Conventional versus high-porosity polytetrafluoroethylene grafts: clinical evaluation. *Surgery.* 1992;112:901-907.

47. Golden MA, Hanson SR, Kirkman TR, Schneider PA, Clowes AW. Healing of polytetrafluoroethylene arterial grafts is influenced by graft porosity. *J Vasc Surg.* 1990;11:838-844.

48. Hirabayashi K, Saitoh E, Ijima H, Takenawa T, Kodama M, Hori M. Influence of fibril length upon ePTFE graft healing and host modification of the implant. *J Biomed Mater Res.* 1992;26:1433-1447.

49. Golden MA, Au YP, Kenagy RD, Clowes AW. Growth factor gene expression by intimal cells in healing polytetrafluoroethylene grafts. *J Vasc Surg.* 1990;11:580-585.

50. White RA, White EW, Hanson EL, Rohner RF, Webb WR. Preliminary report: evaluation of tissue ingrowth into experimental replamineform vascular prostheses. *Surgery.* 1976;79:229-232.

51. White RA. The effect of porosity and biomaterial on the healing and long-term mechanical properties of vascular prostheses. *ASAIO Trans.* 1988;11:95-100.

52. Long J, Tan E, Uitto J, et al. Implant microstructure and collagen synthesis. *Trans Am Soc Artif Intern Organs.* 1982;28:195-199.

53. Connolly JE, Brownell DA, Levine EF, McCart PM. Complications of renal dialysis access procedures. *Arch Surg.* 1984;119:1325-1328.

54. Bhat DJ, Tellis VA, Kohlberg WI, Driscoll B, Veith FJ. Management of sepsis involving expanded PTFE grafts for hemodialysis access. *Surgery.* 1980;87:445-450.

55. Malone JM, Moore WS, Campagna G, Bean B. Bacteremic infectability of vascular grafts: the influence of pseudointimal integrity and duration of graft function. *Surgery.* 1975;78:211-216.

56. Vaughan GD, Mattox KL, Feliciano DV, Beall AC Jr, DeBakey ME. Surgical experience with expanded polytetrafluoroethylene (PTFE) as a replacement graft for traumatized vessels. *J Trauma.* 1979;19: 403-408.

57. Kohler TR, Kirkman TR, Kraiss LW, Zierler BK, Clowes AW. Increased blood flow inhibits neointimal hyperplasia in endothelialized vascular grafts. *Circ Res.* 1991;69:1557-1565.

58. Geary RL, Kohler TR, Vergel S, Kirkman TR, Clowes AW. Time course of flow-induced smooth muscle cell proliferation and intimal thickening in endothelialized baboon vascular grafts. *Circ Res.* 1993; 74:14-23.

59. Zarins CK, Zatina MA, Giddens DP, Ku DN, Glagov S. Shear stress regulation of artery lumen diameter in experimental atherogenesis. *J Vasc Surg.* 1987;5:413-420.

60. Sanders RJ, Kempczinski RF, Hammond W, DiClementi D. The significance of graft diameter. *Surgery.* 1980;88:856-866.

61. Binn RL, Ku DN, Stewart MT, Ansley JP, Coyle KA. Optimal graft diameter: effect of wall shear stress on vascular healing. *J Vasc Surg.* 1989;10:326-337.

62. Sakariassen KS, Baumgartner HR. Axial dependence of platelet-collagen interactions in flowing blood. *Arteriosclerosis.* 1989;9:33-42.

63. Vanderwerf BA, Williams T, Koep LJ. Hemodynamics of arteriovenous fistulas. In Koofstra G, Jorning PJG (eds). *Access Surgery.* Ridgeway, NJ: George A. Bogden & Son; 1983.

64. Anderson CB, Codd JR, Graff RA, Groce MA, Harter HR, Newton WT. Cardiac failure and upper extremity arteriovenous dialysis fistulas. *Arch Intern Med.* 1976;136:292-297.

65. Hinsdale JG, Lipkowitz GS, Hoover EL. Vascular access for hemodialysis in the elderly: results and perspectives in a geriatric population. *Dial Transplant.* 1985;14:560-565.

66. Rosental JJ, Bell DD, Gaspar MR, Movius HJ, Lemire GG. Prevention of high flow problems of arteriovenous grafts: development of a new tapered graft. *Am J Surg.* 1980;140:231-233.

67. Sauvage LR, Berger KE, Mansfield PB, Wood SJ, Smith JC, Overton JB. Future directions in the development of arterial prostheses for small and medium caliber arteries. *Surg Clin North Am.* 1974; 54:213-228.

68. Bassiouny HS, White S, Glagov S, Choi E, Giddens DP, Zarins CK. Anastomotic intimal hyperplasia: mechanical injury or flow induced. *J Vasc Surg.* 1992;15:708-716.

69. Crawshaw HM, Quist WC, Serallach E, Valeri CR, LoGerfo FW. Flow disturbance at the distal end-to-side anastomosis. Effect of patency of the proximal outflow segment and angle of anastomosis. *Arch Surg.* 1980;115:1280-1284.

70. Back MR, Cho YI, Crawford DW, Back LH. Fluid particle motion and Lagrangian velocities for pulsatile flow through a femoral artery branch model. *J Biomech Eng.* 1987;109:94-101.

71. Cho YI, Back LH, Crawford DW. Experimental investigation of branch flow ratio, angle, and Reynolds' number effects on the pressure and flow fields in arterial branch models. *J Biomech Eng.* 1985;107: 257-267.

72. LoGerfo FW, Quist WC, Nowak MD, Crawshaw HM, Haudenschild CC. Downstream anastomotic hyperplasia. A mechanism of failure in Dacron arterial grafts. *Ann Surg.* 1983;1197:479-483.

73. Shu MCS, Noon GP, Hwang NHC. Flow profiles and wall shear stress distribution at a hemodialysis venous anastomosis: preliminary study. *Biorheology.* 1987;24:723-735.

74. Sicard GA, Allen BT, Anderson CB. PTFE grafts for vascular access. In Sommer BG, Henry ML (eds). *Vascular Access for Hemodialysis.* New York: Pluribus Press; 1989.

75. Bacchini G, Del Vecchio L, Andrulli S, Pontoriero G, Locatelli F. Survival of prosthetic grafts of different materials after impairment of a native arteriovenous fistula in hemodialysis patients. *ASAIO J.* 2001;47:30-33.

76. Katzman HE, Glickman MH, Schild AF, Fujitani RM, Lawson JH. Multicenter evaluation of the bovine mesenteric vein bioprostheses for hemodialysis access in patients with an earlier failed prosthetic graft. *J Am Coll Surg.* 2005;201:223-230.

77. Sank A, Rostami K, Weaver F, et al. New evidence and new hope concerning endothelial seeding of vascular grafts. *Am J Surg.* 1992;164: 199-204.

78. Hess F, Steeghs S, Jerusalem R, et al. Patency and morphology of fibrous polyurethane vascular prostheses implanted in the femoral artery of dogs after seeding with subcultivated endothelial cells. *Eur J Vasc Surg.* 1993;7:402-408.

79. Schanzer H, Martinelli GP, Bock G, Peirce EC 2nd. A self-healing dialysis prosthesis. Coaxial double PTFE-silicone graft. *Ann Surg.* 1986;204:574-579.

80. Gelabert HA, Colburn MD. Development and results of antibiotic-impregnated vascular grafts. In Moore WS, Gelabert HA (eds). *Antibiotic-Impregnated Vascular Grafts.* Austin,, TX: RG Landis; 1992.

81. Alobaid N, Salacinski HJ, Sales KM, et al. Nanocomposite containing bioactive peptides promote endothelialisation by circulating progenitor cells: an in vitro evaluation. *Eur J Vasc Endovasc Surg.* 2006;81: 76-83.

82. Greisler H. Vascular graft healing: interfacial phenomena. In Greisler H (ed). *New Biologic and Synthetic Vascular Prostheses.* Austin, TX: RG Landis; 1991.

CHAPTER 9

Strategies to Reduce Intimal Hyperplasia in Dialysis Access Grafts

Ted R. Kohler

As noted in prior chapters, narrowing of the distal anastomosis by intimal hyperplasia is the main cause of prosthetic access graft failure. This process can also affect autogenous vein fistulas, causing narrowing at either the anastomoses, sites of injury, or areas of stasis or turbulence, such as valve cusps. In every case, intimal hyperplasia likely results as a response to injury. As with other healing processes in the body, this response involves thrombosis and development of scar by migration, proliferation, and matrix production of mesenchymal cells. The biology of this process has been studied extensively in animal models. This chapter discusses four animal models that are particularly relevant to dialysis access failure: carotid balloon injury in the rat, arterialized vein grafts in rabbits, polytetrafluorethylene (PTFE) grafts in baboons, and dialysis access failure in sheep. We review what these models convey about dialysis access failure, examine the ways access failure is unique, and finally, explore possible ways to reduce or eliminate this problem.

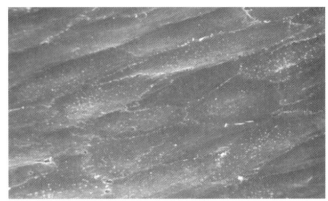

Figure 9-1.

A scanning electron micrograph of surface endothelium shows a confluent, nonthrombogenic monolayer (no platelets attached). These cells are responsive to flow and align with their long axis along the line of shear (*left* to *right* in this photograph).

The Response to Injury: The Rat Carotid Model

The rat carotid injury model, developed and extensively described by Clowes and coworkers,[1] consists of injury to the artery by three passages of an overinflated balloon catheter. This entirely disrupts the endothelium, breaks the internal elastic lamina, and kills approximately 25% of the medial smooth muscle cells. The injury most closely resembles that of angioplasty or endarterectomy, but the biologic responses to the injury are undoubtedly similar in many respects to those that follow other types of injury such as vein bypass grafting, chronic indwelling catheters, and injury to the vein at the distal anastomoses of synthetic access grafts.

Loss of endothelium triggers a cascade of events. The vessel may actively narrow due to release of vasoconstrictors such as serotonin, fibrinogen, adenosine diphosphate, and von Willebrand factor and loss of the normal production of vasodilators, such as nitric oxide. Normal endothelium is a confluent monolayer that prevents formation of thrombosis on the lumen by many mechanisms including the presence of thrombomodulin, prostacyclin, and heparan sulfate at the surface (Fig. 9-1). Thrombomodulin binds thrombin, and this complex activates protein C,

which in turn activates protein S, which is also bound to the surface. Protein S inactivates factor Va. After injury, this thromboresistant layer is lost, exposing highly thrombogenic collagen and elastin. Despite this, only a thin layer of platelets adheres and aggregates at the injured surface during the first 24 hours after injury. After 24 hours, the lumen surface passivates by the adsorption of plasma proteins, such as albumen, and platelet activity decreases.

Activated platelets release cytokines that are growth factors and chemoattractants for smooth muscle cells. These include platelet-derived growth factor (PDGF), transforming growth factor beta, and epidermal growth factor. Studies in animals given additional PDGF or given factors blocking this cytokine have demonstrated that its primary role is to stimulate smooth muscle cell *migration* into the intima. *Proliferation* occurs even in thrombocytopenic animals, but fewer cells migrate into the intima.

Normal endothelium is quiescent owing to cell-cell contact. At the boundary of the injury, where this contact is lost, the endothelium begins to proliferate and re-endothelialize the lumen. This process also occurs wherever a side branch comes off the vessel. Healthy endothelium from branch vessels proliferates and migrates onto the surface of the injured parent vessel. Endothelial regrowth is a limited process, at least in rodents, and stops at about 6 weeks, regardless of whether or not the surface is completely repopulated. If there are frequent branches, as in the aorta, the entire denuded segment can re-endothelialize. The carotid artery does not completely heal in the rat because there are no side branches. The midportion of the artery remains denuded of endothelium and instead has surface smooth muscle cells, which also provide a nonthrombogenic surface and have the appearance of endothelial cells under light microscopy, although immunohistochemistry shows them to be positive for actin and negative for endothelial markers such as von Willebrand factor. Addition of basic fibroblast growth factor can stimulate the endothelium to continue proliferation until re-endothelialization is complete.

The content of DNA in the media is reduced by about 25% after this injury, indicating a loss of a similar percentage of smooth muscle cells, which are the predominant cell type in this layer. These cells are normally quiescent with less than a tenth of a percent proliferating at any time. Within 24 hours of injury, 20% to 40% of the remaining viable smooth muscle cells enter the synthetic phase of the cell cycle and proliferate for 1 to 2 weeks (Fig. 9-2). Following the progress of labeled proliferating cells demonstrates that the smooth muscle cells either begin proliferation immediately after injury or remain quiescent throughout the healing process. Studies using basic fibroblast growth factor and its inhibitor reveal that proliferation is largely a response to release of this growth factor, which is not normally excreted, from injured smooth muscle cells and is thus an autocrine event. It is now apparent that mesenchymal cells in the adventitia also participate in the formation of intimal hyperplasia.[2] Many of these cells, as well as medial smooth muscle cells, migrate across the damaged internal elastic lamina to the luminal surface where proliferation continues, forming a lesion of intimal hyperplasia, sometimes referred to as *neointima*. The adventitia itself may participate in scarring and constriction, causing luminal narrowing, often referred to as *negative remodeling*.

Although proliferation has essentially ceased by 2 weeks, the neointima continues to thicken owing to deposition of matrix components, collagen and elastin, by the smooth muscle cells for as long as 12 weeks after injury. These cells change phenotype from the contractile state of quiescent medial cells to the synthetic state associated with proliferating cells and cells that produce matrix. As seen in Figure 9-3, there is considerable additional intimal thickening due to this process, which also results in decreased cell density in the neointima. Mature neointima contains approximately one-third smooth muscle cells by volume; the remainder is matrix.

The Rabbit Model of Vein Graft Hyperplasia

Vascular wall thickening caused by increased tension and stress is a universal response seen both during development (eg, when the aorta is subjected to systolic pressure after birth) and in mature arteries (eg, in the case of hyperten-

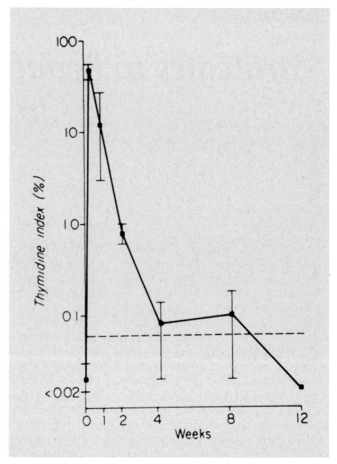

Figure 9-2.
Smooth muscle cell proliferation as measured by the percentage of cells that take up tritiated thymidine, which is incorporated into DNA of cell in the S phase of the cell cycle. (From Clowes AW, Reidy MA, Clowes MM. Mechanisms of stenosis after arterial injury. *Lab Invest.* 1983;49:208-215, with permission.)

sion). Veins placed in the arterial circulation also thicken. This is a partially a response to injury during surgery, which results in loss of luminal endothelium and damage to the media, and to increased wall stress caused by exposure to arterial pressure. In the rabbit model, when the thin-walled jugular vein is placed in the carotid artery, the wall thickens first by proliferation of smooth muscle cells and then by their production of matrix components (Fig. 9-4). The final result is very similar to that of intimal hyperplasia following injury of the rat carotid artery. Vein wall thickening was noted early on and referred to as *arterialization* of the vein when Carrel and Guthrie[3] first used the saphenous vein as an arterial bypass. This process is a likely cause of some of the vein wall thickening seen in access grafts and fistulas. If a dialysis access graft has nonstenotic, high-capacity venous outflow, the pressure within the graft will be nearly at venous levels by the time flow reaches the vein. Therefore, increase in wall tension due to increased pressure may not play a prominent role. However, if stenosis develops in the outflow, pressure upstream from the stenosis rises to arterial levels and may then cause increased wall tension and compensatory thickening.

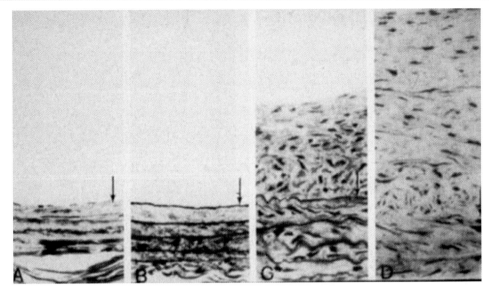

Figure 9-3.
A, Composite photomicrograph of a normal rat carotid artery. *B,* A similar artery immediately after balloon injury. Note the edema. *C,* The surface consists of exposed internal elastic lamina), 2 weeks after injury. Note neointima with dense cellularity. *D,* Twelve weeks after injury. Note continued thickening due to matrix deposition, causing decreased cellular density. (*A-D,* From Clowes AW, Reidy MA, Clowes MM. Mechanisms of stenosis after arterial injury. *Lab Invest.* 1983;49:208-215. with permission.)

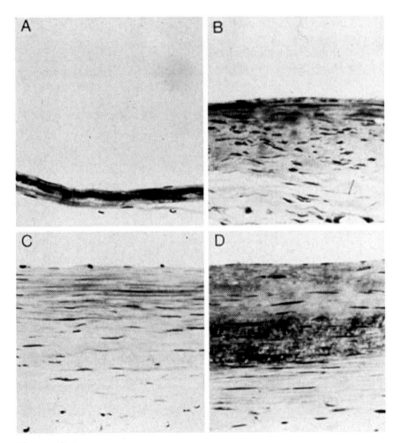

Figure 9-4.
A rabbit vein graft prior to implantation. *A,* Note the wall is only a few cells thick. *B,* Two weeks after implantation. The wall is markedly thickened. *C,* A month after implantation. Cells are now concentrically arranged rather than randomly situated. *D,* A year after implantation degenerative changes are occurring.

Intimal Hyperplasia in High-Porosity PTFE Grafts in Baboons

Porosity of extruded PTFE grafts are composed of solid, disklike nodes held together by a dense meshwork of thin fibrils. Porosity is assessed by measurement of the average internodal distance (IND). Standard grafts have an IND of 20 to 30 μm. They develop a neointima for a centimeter or two adjacent to the anastomoses where tissue can grow onto the graft from adjacent vessels, but the remainder of the luminal surface is covered with a pseudointima composed mainly of fibrin. In contrast, experimental PTFE grafts with an IND of 60 μm placed in the aortoiliac position in juvenile baboons can heal throughout the graft by the ingrowth of capillaries from the surrounding granulation tissue growing across the wall. On reaching the surface, these capillaries spread and the endothelium coalesces to form a complete monolayer (Fig. 9-5). Mesenchymal cells derived from pericytes grow in underneath the endothelium to form a neointima of uniform thickness throughout the graft (Fig. 9-6). The neointima does not thicken enough to cause significant narrowing of the lumen, even after several months. Immunohistochemistry reveals the surface to be populated by endothelial cells, the underlying cells to be actin positive, consistent with smooth muscle, and the graft matrix to be rich in macrophages.

Unfortunately, clinical trials with this material used as femoropopliteal grafts did not demonstrate improved healing as measured by the uptake of indium-labeled platelets. However, this model is useful for studying the effect of flow on growth of the neointima of these grafts. If a femoral arteriovenous anastomosis is made below the grafts, increasing

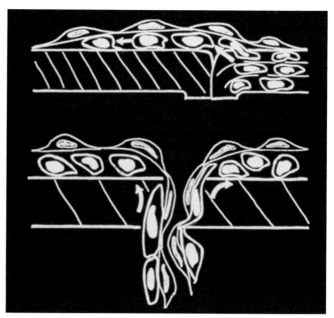

Figure 9-5.

Cartoon demonstrates the difference in healing of standard polytetrafluorethylene (PTFE; *top*) versus the more porous, 60-μm internodal distance material *(bottom),* which allows transmural ingrowth of capillaries, which spread and coalesce after reaching the surface. (From Clowes AW, Reidy MA, Clowes MM. Mechanisms of stenosis after arterial injury. *Lab Invest.* 1983;49:208-215, with permission.)

flow on one side and not on the other, a complete neointima still forms, but is dramatically thinner than on the side

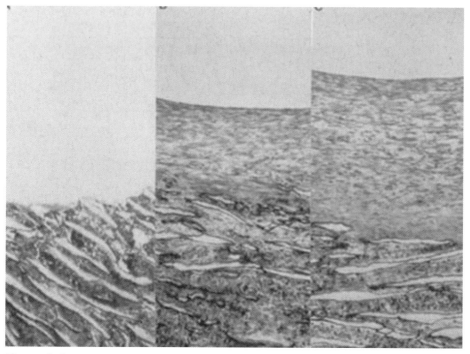

Figure 9-6.

A 60-μm PTFE graft from the aortoiliac position in the baboon. There is a thin endothelialized surface at 2 weeks *(left),* a thickened neointima at 2 weeks *(center)* and more thickening at 4 weeks *(right).* (From Clowes AW, Reidy MA, Clowes MM. Mechanisms of stenosis after arterial injury. *Lab Invest.* 1983;49:208-215, with permission.)

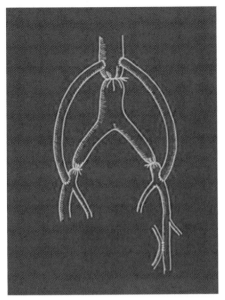 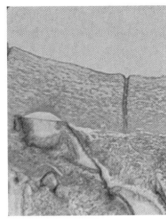 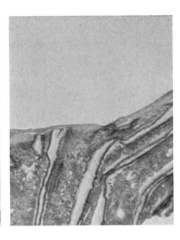

Standard Flow   Fistula Flow

Figure 9-7.
The baboon model to test fistula flow in PTFE grafts (cartoon on *left* shows femoral fistula on the animal's *left* side). The neointima is much thicker on the normal flow side *(left photomicrograph)* than the fistula side *(right photomicrograph)*. (From Kohler TR, Kirkman TR, Kraiss LW, Zierler BK, Clowes AW. Increased blood flow inhibits neointimal hyperplasia in endothelialized vascular grafts. *Circ Res.* 1991;69:1557-1565, with permission.)

with normal flow (Fig. 9-7).[4] Further, if grafts are allowed to heal for a month before the fistula is constructed, the neointima thins in response to the increase in flow. Conversely, if flow is normalized on the fistula side after the neointima has formed, it becomes thicker. These responses are mediated by the endothelium, which acts as the biotransducer to convert changes in shear forces into biochemical signals that affect changes in the blood vessel wall. Thinning of the neointima is associated with increased activity of inducible nitric oxide synthase.

Increased shear causes increased production of nitric oxide, which induces vasodilatation by relaxation of smooth muscle cells. Thus, when flow increases, the blood vessel dilates until shear at the luminal surface returns to normal levels. Acutely, this allows vessels to meet demands of tissues whose arteriolar beds have reduced resistance due to increased oxygen demand as seen, for example, in muscles during exercise. If demand stays high, the wall of the vessel alters its structure to adjust to the new diameter. The opposite occurs when flow is reduced. This process occurs during development as arteries grow to the appropriate size to accommodate the tissues they supply, which may be either growing or atrophying. This principle was demonstrated in an elegant experiment by Langille and associates,[5] who showed that ligation of the external carotid artery of the rabbit reduces flow in the common carotid artery by about 30%. In response, the common carotid diameter decreases until wall shear is normalized. Initially, this is an active process that can be reversed by application of local vasodilators. After several weeks, however, the vessel wall adapts to the reduced flow and application of vasodilators has a minimal effect. A similar phenomenon occurs when flow is increased: arteries dilate until wall shear is normalized. This occurs in growth and development as well as in mature arteries. Arteries supplying fistulas enlarge over time (Fig. 9-8). A similar mechanism is likely to be at work

in the neointima of baboon PTFE grafts responding to alterations in flow.

Flow also affects development of intimal hyperplasia in the rat carotid injury model. Wall thickening in response to injury is increased if flow is reduced by ligation of the external carotid artery.[6] Similarly, when there is curvature of a vein graft, hyperplasia of the wall is increased on the inner curvature, where shear is low, and decreased on the outer wall, where shear is greater.[7] Although the mechanisms may be quite different, wall thickening due to early

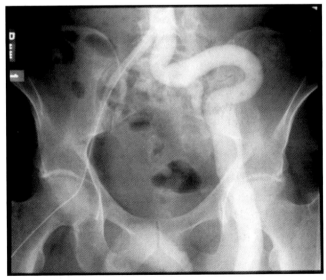

Figure 9-8.
This patient had a left femoral arteriovenous fistula for several decades after a shrapnel injury in the Vietnam War. The iliac artery supplying the fistula and the iliac vein draining it enlarged severalfold over the years owing to increased flow.

atherosclerosis tends to occur in regions of low or oscillating flow, such as the lateral wall of the carotid bulb and the upstream side of the orifice of lumbar branches from the aorta. The question then becomes: If increased shear is associated with decreased wall thickening in all of these other situations, why is neointimal hyperplasia so robust at the venous end of access grafts where flow is high?

A Sheep Model of Intimal Hyperplasia in PTFE Access Grafts

Many models of graft access failure have been developed to study the problem of access failure in dogs, pigs, and sheep, among other species. We used a model of access failure in PTFE grafts in sheep because their vessels are similar in size to those in humans and can accommodate standard clinic grafts, their coagulation system is similar to that in humans, they are docile enough to undergo dialysis, and there is an established model of uremia in sheep, which was developed to study erythropoietin therapy. We placed standard dialysis access PTFE grafts between the carotid artery and the jugular vein in the neck. This allowed ready access to the grafts for determination of patency by palpation for a thrill or Doppler. As in clinical grafts, neointimal hyperplasia was minimal at the arterial end, whereas the venous end rapidly developed intimal hyperplasia, which caused graft failure after only 8 weeks. Histology of the lesions was very similar to that in clinical grafts. As in human grafts, angiogenesis is a prominent feature producing abundant, large vessels in the neointima, which is composed of actin-positive cells with some macrophages.[8,9] Cellular proliferation is abundant, particularly in association with the neovasculature and inflammatory cells. As in clinical grafts, calcification occurs and even bone formation was noted in some specimens. This model has been useful both for exploring why PTFE access grafts develop hyperplasia at the venous anastomoses and for testing methods to improve graft patency.

Preliminary studies with PTFE of various internodal distances demonstrate that the nodal structure is very important for full incorporation and graft healing. Nodes that are too far apart do not produce a stable neointima. This was also observed in the baboon studies, where 90-μm IND grafts initially formed a neointima, but it was not stable. Similarly, ingrowth cannot occur if the nodes are packed too densely. The ideal IND appears to be 60 μm. The density of the fibrils between nodes might also be important, but this has been difficult to study.

Potential Causes of Intimal Hyperplasia at the Venous Anastomosis

There are many differences between the distal anastomosis of interposition arterial grafts and that of dialysis access grafts that could be responsible for accelerated hyperplasia (Table 9-1). Flow in access grafts is manyfold higher than in arterial grafts. This high flow causes increased shear in the vein, particularly on the segment of vein wall directly opposite the anastomosis. Conversely, there is low flow at

Table 9–1
Unique Features of Access Grafts That May Contribute to Intimal Hyperplasia

- High flow
- Turbulence
- Wall vibration
- Anastomosis to thin-walled vein
- Repeated puncture
- Receives blood with activated platelet products
- Patients have uremia

the heel of the anastomosis, and there might even be stagnant flow in the upstream segment of the vein because competent venous values might obstruct reverse flow. This might lead to thrombus, which would then organize and initiate intimal hyperplasia. Normal venous endothelium is subjected to relatively constant and low shear, which differs from the turbulence and high shear at venous anastomoses. This cell layer is very sensitive to changes in shear and may respond to abnormal levels with a response to injury, including modulating from an antiproliferative, antithrombogenic state to a mitogenic state and a procoagulant surface.

Wall vibration (which is what causes the audible bruit and palpable thrill over these sites) may also produce mechanical injury to the vein wall. Veins, particularly in the upper extremity, normally are subjected to low pressure and therefore are thin walled and less able to handle these mechanical stresses. Puncture of the access grafts produces direct injury. Puncture sites of PTFE grafts heal by thrombus formation at the puncture site. The thrombus becomes organized by ingrowth first of macrophages then granulation tissue with microvessels and, finally, becomes a lesion of intimal hyperplasia on the luminal surface of the graft. Repeated puncture eventually causes mechanical breakdown of the graft material and pseudoaneurysm formation.

Thrombus at puncture sites of both native and synthetic grafts causes release of cytokines from activated platelets and formation of coagulation factors, such as thrombin, that not only contribute to the local formation of neointimal hyperplasia but also are carried downstream where they may act on the vein wall to enhance wall thickening in this region as well. Similar factors released during the passage of blood through the dialysis apparatus enter the graft and venous drainage system. Finally, uremic plasma has factors that are mitogenic and may be responsible for an increased propensity to intimal hyperplasia. These factors may also be responsible for intimal hyperplasia that occurs in veins downstream from the access graft. Hemodynamics likely play a role in these distant lesions as well because they commonly occur in specific sites, such as the most distal aspect of the cephalic vein where it turns down into the deep system, the subclavian vein, and at valves, possibly due to stagnant flow in the cusps (Fig. 9-9).

These various mechanisms of inducing intimal hyperplasia are ongoing in dialysis access grafts. This is unlike the model of injury in the rat carotid model or the clinical situation of arterial angioplasty or bypass in which the

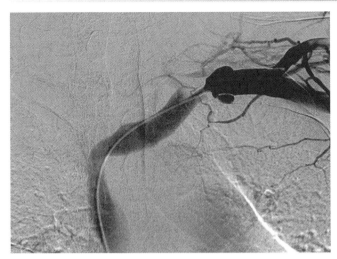

Figure 9-9.
A subclavian vein thrombosis at the site of a valve.

Table 9–2

Potential Graft Modification to Reduce Intimal Hyperplasia

- **Geometry (reduce turbulence)**
  - Taper
  - Cuff
- **Porosity (promote incorporation, healing)**
  - Increased (allow capillary ingrowth)
  - Gradient (better incorporation)
- **Surface (reduce thrombogenicity)**
  - Carbon coating
  - Endothelial cells
- **Compliance**
- **Pharmacology**
  - Local or systemic
  - Antithrombotic/antiplatelet
  - Antiproliferative
  - Genetically modified cells

vascular wall can stabilize after recovering from injury. Therapy for access graft hyperplasia must therefore address the ongoing nature of the injury process.

Compliance mismatch between the PTFE graft and the more compliant vein is also a possible mechanism for graft failure. In arterial grafts, interposition of a segment of vein between the artery and the PTFE can improve patency, particularly in bypasses to tibial-level arteries. Similar strategies in PTFE grafts involve elimination of the mechanical connection of graft to vein (see later).

Potential Graft Modifications to Reduce Intimal Hyperplasia

Fistula First

The Kidney Disease Outcomes Quality Initiative (K/DOQI) guidelines[10] and the Fistula First campaign emphasize the importance of using native vein fistulas whenever possible rather than synthetic grafts, owing to their superior performance (see Chapter 11). As a result of these initiatives, the rate of native fistula construction has markedly increased in the United States, which has traditionally lagged far behind Europe in this regard. PTFE grafts have been favored for their ease of placement, ease of use, reduced waiting time prior to use, and more favorable reimbursement patterns for the procedures to place them. They are much simpler to place and easier on the patients than basilic vein transpositions in the upper arm, which is the most frequent last option for a native fistula before using PTFE. Although most studies show superiority of native fistulas, PTFE patency has approached that of native fistulas in some trials.[11] Some reports question the use of more difficult vein fistulas like the basilica transposition rather than PTFE, particularly in certain groups, such as the elderly, who may do just as well with PTFE as with native fistulas. Others have suggested that a forearm PTFE brachiobasilic loop fistula can be used before a basilic vein transposition and may allow maturation of the basilic vein in the upper arm for immediate use when the PTFE fails. The issue of

forearm PTFE versus upper arm basilic vein transposition fistula was addressed in a trial from the Netherlands of 105 patients who could not have a radiocephalic or brachiocephalic fistula. Subjects were randomized to a PTFE forearm loop graft or a basilic vein transposition fistula.[12] Those in the latter group had better one-year primary patency (47% vs 22%) and primary-assisted patency (87% vs 71%), similar one-year secondary patency (89% vs 85%), and fewer complications (1.6 versus 2.7 per patient year). If the problem of venous intimal hyperplasia could be cured, or at least reduced, PTFE would be an acceptable alternative to native fistulas. We explore many of the possible graft modifications that may limit hyperplasia (Table 9-2). Even if stenosis could be eliminated, there would remain the increased risk of infection with prosthetic grafts, but this problem is much less common than loss of patency, and it is also being addressed with graft modifications (eg, silver impregnation, incorporation of antibiotics on the surface). Use of cryopreserved vein is one method to address the problem of infection, because this material is thought to be less prone to infection than PTFE in patients who have had multiple graft infections. These grafts are disadvantaged owing to high cost and may not have as good long-term function as native fistulas or PTFE. Clearly, more work is needed in this area.

Graft Geometry

The amount of shear and turbulence at the venous end of the access graft can be altered by the configuration of the graft. Creating a narrower arterial anastomosis can reduce flow to make less mechanical injury while still maintaining adequate flow for dialysis. Studies that used dogs revealed that a graft with a narrowed diameter at the arterial anastomosis produced less venous intimal hyperplasia than a graft with a normal arterial diameter and tapered venous end.[13] Tapered grafts are now routinely available for clinical use. They typically have a 4-mm arterial end. This segment needs to be only a centimeter or so long to provide the desired reduction in flow. The graft then expands to a 7-mm length for the remainder of the body. This configuration also has the theoretical advantage of reducing the incidence of steal phenomenon, which is caused by excessive graft flow. Although these considerations are compelling from a clinician's perspective, to date clinical trials have not demonstrated dramatic improvements.

Another method of improving flow characteristics at the venous anastomosis is to make a hooded graft. The expanded hood is sewn to the venous anastomosis and theoretically produces more laminar flow patterns and therefore less turbulence and endothelial damage. Small trials in our sheep model with this configuration did not lead to reduction in venous hyperplasia, but clinical trials have shown some potential benefit.[14] These grafts require a fairly good–sized vein to accommodate the hooded configuration, a fact that must be taken into consideration because it could lead to bias in clinical studies. Similar configurations are used for femorotibial bypass grafts with some suggestive trials of clinical utility.[15]

Eliminating the Venous Anastomosis

The venous anastomosis can be eliminated if the PTFE graft is inserted through a side hole into a large vein. One small clinical series suggested that this technique can improve patency.[16] Another approach is attaching the access graft to a central catheter inserted through the jugular vein into the superior vena cava. One such device has recently been approved for clinical use (Fig. 9-10). Early experience with this device suggests that, whereas patency rates are not different than those for standard PTFE grafts, infection

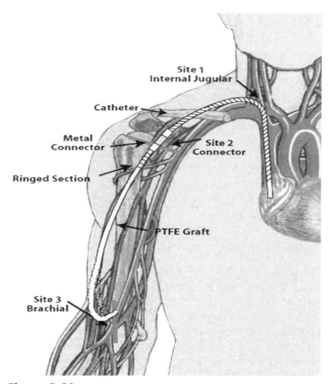

Figure 9-10.
The HeRO device, which is a combination of PTFE access graft in the upper arm connected to a central venous catheter for outflow.

rates are lower. This approach allows creation of an access graft in patients who have no useable upper extremity veins and may be beneficial for those who have had frequent infections.

Graft Porosity

The importance of the IND of PTFE grafts has been discussed earlier. Theoretically, a well-incorporated graft that develops a complete endothelial lining would have a lessened tendency to thrombosis and may not develop such robust thickening at the venous anastomosis. Sixty-micron IND grafts in the sheep access model did not endothelialize (unpublished data). This may be related to the high flow, species difference, or nodal architecture, which needs to be strictly engineered for uniformity. We are currently working on biologic methods to enhance the ability of neovasculature to cross the graft wall by adding a particular combination of matrix molecules and growth factors. IND can be made to vary across the wall of the graft. This could be advantageous if a different porosity were needed for optimal ingrowth of granulation tissue into the wall of the graft for "incorporation," which helps prevent seroma formation, hemorrhage outside the graft, and infection, whereas a lower porosity is optimal for the luminal surface.

Surface Manipulations

The PTFE surface can be altered to reduce thrombogenicity or infection. Currently, carbon-coated grafts are available, and some clinical trials suggest that these have similar or marginally better patency rates.[17,18] We have studied silicon coating at the venous end of the graft and other lipid coatings, none of which has been beneficial in the sheep model. More sophisticated methods are available to bond specific molecules to the graft surface. For example, the surface could be made with attachment sites for circulating progenitor cells, which could endothelialize the surface. Cell seeding and sodding have been used for arterial grafts with some modest clinical benefit,[19] but these have not been tried in dialysis access grafts, nor are they very practical for this application. The high flow in these grafts could make it more difficult to maintain an endothelial lining derived from cell cultures.

Reduction of Intimal Hyperplasia by Other Means

Investigation of the causes of intimal hyperplasia has allowed the development of potential mechanisms to reduce the cellular proliferative response that is responsible for it. As with restenosis after coronary bypass or peripheral angioplasty or bypass, various therapies have been tried to reduce smooth muscle cell proliferation. In our sheep model, we investigated high-intensity, focused ultrasound application to the venous anastomosis. This is attractive because it could be applied externally during regular dialysis sessions. Unfortunately, we did not see any benefit in our animal studies (unpublished data). Brachytherapy is also attractive in that it could be applied regularly and externally. In coronary stents, brachytherapy suffered from

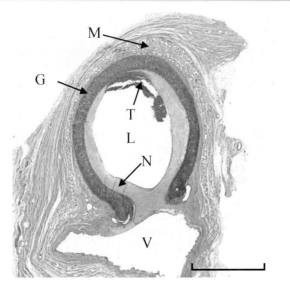

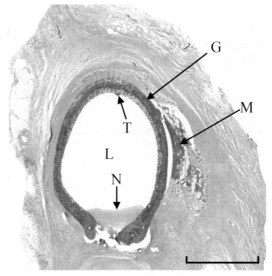

0 Dose Mesh Control   1.2 µg/mm2 Paclitaxel Mesh

Figure 9-11.
Experimental PTFE grafts near the venous anastomosis in sheep with a paclitaxel wrap. Neointimal thickening is much greater on the *left (control side)* than on the *right (drug side)*. *M,* Mesh; *G,* graft; *T,* thrombus; *L,* lumen; *N,* neointima, *V,* vein. (From Kohler TR, Toleikis PM, Gravett DM, Avelar RL. Inhibition of neointimal hyperplasia in a sheep model of dialysis access failure with the bioabsorbable Vascular Wrap paclitaxel-eluting mesh. *J Vasc Surg.* 2007;45: 1029-1038, with permission.)

shoulder stenosis that occurred at either end of the segment being treated where radiation doses were below therapeutic levels and actually increased intimal thickening.

Many drugs have been used in attempts to reduce intimal hyperplasia. Systemic administration of drugs such as steroids or anticoagulants is not desirable owing to potential toxicity. Local therapies can be delivered either directly at the time of graft implantation, within the graft itself, or by application using specialized delivery catheters placed endovascularly. One obvious choice of therapy is paclitaxel, which is one of the drugs shown to reduce restenosis when applied to drug eluting coronary stents. This drug can be delivered locally using a drug-eluting wrap around the venous anastomosis at the time of surgery. The drug can be eluted over days or weeks to prevent cellular proliferation and reduce inflammation in the early period. Reducing early injury response may significantly improve patency, even if chronic injury eventually causes intimal hyperplasia. We tested such a drug-eluting wrap in the sheep model and found reduced intimal hyperplasia and less inflammation at 1 month (Fig. 9-11).[20] Unfortunately, in clinical trials, infection was significantly more common in the grafts with drug-eluting wrap.

Earlier in the chapter, we discussed how important a healthy endothelium is for normal vascular wall structure and function. These cells regulate structure and function of the vascular wall through the production of a number of cytokines and other molecules, such as nitric oxide. Nugent and coworkers[11] showed that many of the benefits of normal endothelium can be derived from endothelial cells grown in culture and placed around the vessel in a Gelfoam matrix.[21] These allogeneic cells create no immune response in this environment and have reduced intimal hyperplasia in a

porcine arteriovenous fistula model and carotid injury model. Clinical trials are under way with this product.

Future Directions

This chapter has presented a brief summary of the problem of dialysis access graft failure and a few approaches to therapy. It is by no means an exhaustive list of the possible ways to approach this problem. As our understanding of the biology becomes more sophisticated, other therapies will emerge. For example, it is possible to use genetic manipulation to modify local cells to produce proteins that may reduce thrombosis (such as tissue plasminogen activator), enhance angiogenesis (vascular endothelial growth factor), or limit neointimal growth (nitric oxide synthase). Use of appropriate promoter regions enables turning gene production on or off by systemic administration of triggering drugs, such as tetracycline for promoter regions sensitive to it. Very few advances have been made toward construction of a more durable vascular access device over the last two decades. It is anticipated that a breakthrough will come with our improved understanding of the fundamental causes of access failure.

REFERENCES

1. Clowes AW, Reidy MA, Clowes MM. Mechanisms of stenosis after arterial injury. *Lab Invest.* 1983;49:208-215.
2. Roy-Chaudhury P, Sukhatme VP, Cheung AK. Hemodialysis access dysfunction: a cellular and molecular viewpoint. *J Am Soc Nephrol.* 2006;17:1112-1127.
3. Carrel A, Guthrie CC. Uniterminal and biterminal venous transplantations. *Surg Gynecol Obstet.* 1906;2:66-286.

4. Kohler TR, Kirkman TR, Kraiss LW, Zierler BK, Clowes AW. Increased blood flow inhibits neointimal hyperplasia in endothelialized vascular grafts. *Circ Res.* 1991;69:1557-1565.

5. Langille BL, O'Donnell F. Reductions in arterial diameter produced by chronic decreases in blood flow are endothelium-dependent. *Science.* 1986; 231:405-407.

6. Kohler TR, Jawien A. Flow affects development of intimal hyperplasia following arterial injury in rats. *Arterioscler Thromb.* 1992;12: 963-971.

7. Rittgers SE, Karayannacos PE, Guy JF, et al. Velocity distribution nd intimal proliferation in autologous vein grafts in dogs. *Circ Res.* 1978;42:792-801.

8. Rekhter MD, Nicholls SC, Ferguson M, Gordon D. Cell proliferation in human arteriovenous fistulas used for hemodialysis. *Arterioscler Thromb.* 1993;13:609-617.

9. Kohler TR, Kirkman TR. Dialysis access failure: a sheep model of rapid stenosis. *J Vasc Surg.* 30:744-751, 1999.

10. National Kidney Foundation. K/DOQI clinical practice guidelines for vascular access, 2000. *Am J Kidney Dis.* 2001;37(suppl 1):S137-S181.

11. Palder SB, Kirkman RL, Whittemore AD, Hakim RM, Lazarus JM, Tilney NL. Vascular access for hemodialysis. Patency rates and results of revision. *Ann Surg.* 1985;202(2):235-239.

12. Keuter XH, De Smet AA, Kessels AG, van der Sande FM, Welten RJ, Tordoir JH. A randomized multicenter study of the outcome of brachial-basilic arteriovenous fistula and prosthetic brachial-antecubital forearm loop as vascular access for hemodialysis. *J Vasc Surg.* 2008;47(2):395-401.

13. Fillinger MF, Reinitz ER, Schwartz RA, et al. Graft geometry and venous intimal-medial hyperplasia in arteriovenous loop grafts. *J Vasc Surg.* 1990;11:556-566.

14. Sorom AJ, Hughes CB, McCarthy JT, et al. Prospective, randomized evaluation of a cuffed expanded polytetrafluoroethylene graft for hemodialysis vascular access. *Surgery.* 2002;132:135-140.

15. Oderich GS, Panneton JM, Yagubyan M, Bower TC, Hofer J, Noel AA, Sullivan T, Kalra M, Cherry KJ Jr, Gloviczki P. Comparison of pre-cuffed and vein-cuffed expanded polytetrafluoroethylene grafts for infragenicular arterial reconstructions: a case-matched study. Ann Vasc Surg. 2005 Jan;19(1):49-55.

16. Coulson AS. Modification of venous end of dialysis drafts. *Dial Transplant.* 2000;29(1):10-18.

17. Bacourt F. Prospective randomized study of carbon-impregnated polytetrafluoroethylene grafts for below-knee popliteal and distal bypass: results at 2 years. The Association Universitaire de Recherche en Chirurgie. Ann Vasc Surg. 1997;11(6):596-603.

18. Kapfer X, Meichelboeck W, Groegler FM. Comparison of carbon-impregnated and standard ePTFE prostheses in extra-anatomical anterior tibial artery bypass: a prospective randomized multicenter study. *Eur J Vasc Endovasc Surg.* 2006;32(2):155-168.

19. Bordenave L, Fernandez P, Rémy-Zolghadri M, Villars S, Daculsi R, Midy D. In vitro endothelialized ePTFE prostheses: clinical update 20 years after the first realization. *Clin Hemorheol Microcirc.* 2005;33(3):227-234.

20. Kohler TR, Toleikis PM, Gravett DM, Avelar RL. Inhibition of neointimal hyperplasia in a sheep model of dialysis access failure with the bioabsorbable Vascular Wrap paclitaxel-eluting mesh. *J Vasc Surg.* 2007;45:1029-1038.

21. Nugent HM, Groothuis A, Seifert P, et al. Perivascular endothelial implants inhibit intimal hyperplasia in a model of arteriovenous fistulae: a safety and efficacy study in the pig. *J Vasc Res.* 2002;39: 524-533

VASCULAR ACCESS FOR HEMODIALYSIS

Epidemiology and Pathophysiology of Chronic Renal Failure and Guidelines for Initiation of Hemodialysis

Nosratola D. Vaziri, Cyril H. Barton, and Ashish Kalthia

Epidemiology of Chronic Renal Failure

The incidence of end-stage renal disease (ESRD) in the United States has increased substantially since the mid-1990s owing to the type 2 diabetes epidemic. According to the data recently published by the U.S. Renal Data System (USRDS), 104,364 new adult individuals reached ESRD and the population of patients receiving renal replacement therapies rose to over 472,000 in 2004.[1] Among patients receiving renal replacement therapy in the United States at that time, 335,963 patients were maintained on dialysis therapy and 136,136 patients had undergone renal transplantation. During this period, the prevalence of hemodialysis modality rose from approximately 61% to 65.6% whereas chronic peritoneal dialysis fell from 7.3% to 5.5% and renal transplantation remained virtually unchanged at approximately 29%.

The population of elderly ESRD patients, 65 years of age or older, has dramatically increased since the mid-1990s, representing over 50% of the incident ESRD population. The adjusted incident rate of ESRD is approximately four-fold higher among African Americans and Native American than in the Caucasian population.

Diabetes is the most common cause of ESRD, accounting for close to 50% of all cases, reflecting the explosive rise in the prevalence of type 2 diabetes in the United States. The second most common cause of ESRD is hypertension, which accounts for approximately 20% of all cases. It is of note that the impact of diabetes is far greater among Native Americans and that of hypertension is much larger among African Americans than those reported in the general population. Atherosclerotic renal vascular disease, also known as ischemic nephropathy, has emerged as an increasing cause of ESRD. This process results in chronic progressive ischemia leading to insidious loss of renal function and structure. Although the precise prevalence of ischemic nephropathy in ESRD population is unknown, its rising incidence reflects the increasing age and rising burden of atherosclerosis in the U.S. population.

The most common cause of death in patients with ESRD is cardiovascular disease, followed by infection, stroke, and malignancies. The annual USRDS publication and the USRDS website (www.usrds.org) provide additional epidemiologic information.[1]

Renal Replacement Therapies

Prior to the advent and widespread availability of various renal replacement therapies, death was an inevitable consequence of ESRD. However, death as a direct cause of renal failure can be prevented with the use of these modalities, which include various hemodialysis and peritoneal dialysis modalities as well as renal transplantation. In addition to their use in the treatment of renal failure, hemodialysis and peritoneal dialysis techniques are occasionally used in the treatment of certain types of poisoning, severe acid-base and electrolyte disorders, and severe diuretic-resistant hypervolemia.

An important distinction between successful renal transplantation and chronic dialysis is that the former provides a natural replacement for both excretory and endocrine functions of the kidney. In contrast, various dialysis modalities partially replace the excretory function of the kidney, which is responsible for the elimination of endogenous metabolic waste products, exogenous drugs and toxins, hydrogen ions, and surplus water, minerals, and electrolytes and for the generation of bicarbonate. Therefore, the use of dialysis therapies can provide satisfactory control of azotemia and fluid, electrolyte, and acid-base disorders but fails to correct deficiencies of the renal hormones in patients with ESRD. Fortunately, two of the important hormones of renal origin (erythropoietin, an essential factor for erythropoiesis, and calcitriol, a vital factor for calcium homeostasis and bone metabolism) are available for clinical use in patients with chronic kidney disease. The routine use of erythropoietin, calcitriol, and newer vitamin D analogues has helped to ameliorate ESRD-associated anemia and osteodystrophy, which are among the disabling complications of chronic renal failure. An additional distinction between dialysis and native or transplant kidney is that dialysis indiscriminantly removes not only the endogenous and exogenous waste products but also many important water-soluble molecules including amino acids, vitamins, and other products.

In contrast, once filtered in the glomeruli, the useful molecules are reabsorbed by the renal tubules, a capability that has not yet been incorporated into the existing dialysis technologies. This deficiency is partly overcome by routine prescription of high-potency vitamin preparations in all dialysis-dependent patients. In addition, interaction of blood with the dialyzer membrane, dialysis lines, and roller pump and influx of impurities from dialysate to the blood compartment can have adverse consequences. Finally, the intermittent nature of hemodialysis procedures results in wide fluctuations in body fluid volume and composition, which can cause biologic stress. Despite these and other shortcomings, dialysis modalities can prevent death and sustain life indefinitely despite lack of a functioning kidney. In this context, dialysis fulfills the unique designation as a true artificial kidney, the like of which does not yet exist for the other vital organs.

Decisions concerning the timing of the initiation of dialysis are based on careful monitoring and evaluation of various clinical and biochemical features of renal failure; a brief overview of the main clinical and biochemical manifestations of chronic renal failure is provided here.

Biochemical and Clinical Features of Chronic Renal Failure

Biochemical Abnormalities

The most conspicuous biochemical abnormalities observed in patients with advanced renal failure include azotemia (elevation of plasma urea, creatinine, and other nitrogenous end products), hyperkalemia, hyperphosphatemia, hypocalcemia, and high anion gap metabolic acidosis.[2-4] In addition, advanced chronic kidney disease results in oxidative stress, inflammation, and profound dysregulation of lipid metabolism, which together contribute to progressive cardiovascular disease and other adverse outcomes in this population.[5-8]

Clinical Features

Accumulation of endogenous and exogenous waste products, fluid–electrolyte–acid-base disorders, hormonal abnormalities, oxidative stress, inflammation, and dyslipidemia in advanced renal failure result in a complex multisystem dysfunction affecting nearly all organ systems. These abnormalities are briefly outlined later.

Cardiovascular Features

Numerous cardiovascular complications occur in patients with renal failure. The most common cardiovascular complications of advanced renal failure are hypertension and hypervolemia, which can lead to congestive heart failure and pulmonary edema, requiring urgent dialysis.[9] When present for extended periods, hypertension, hypervolemia, and anemia lead to left ventricular hypertrophy.[10,11] Another serious cardiac complication of renal failure is uremic pericarditis, which can result in pericardial tamponade.[12] The diagnosis of uremic pericarditis necessitates rapid initiation of intense dialysis without systemic heparinization (to avoid pericardial hemorrhage and tamponade). In addition, chronic renal failure due to all causes, particularly diabetes, is associated with accelerated arteriosclerosis, atherosclerosis, and ischemic cardiovascular disease.[9] Oxidative stress, inflammation, dyslipidemia, vascular calcification, hypertension, and insulin resistance, which are common features of advanced chronic kidney disease, are the driving force behind the atherogenic diathesis in this population.[5-8]

Neurologic Features

Both central nervous system and peripheral nerves are adversely affected by uremia.[13] The most common manifestations of uremic brain dysfunction are impaired cognitive function, reversal of sleep pattern, depression, myoclonus, asterixis, restless leg syndrome, uncontrollable twitching, and an abnormal electroencephalogram.[13-15] However, severe uremia and hypertension can result in either uremic or hypertensive encephalopathy, or both, presenting with seizures, coma, and even death.[13,15] The presence of encephalopathy represents a clear indication for the prompt initiation of dialysis.

Advanced uremia can cause an asymmetrical distal sensory and motor neuropathy that occurs earlier and with greater severity in diabetic than in nondiabetic patients. Sensory involvement is more pronounced and usually presents as a burning sensation, prickling, or dysesthesias. Symptoms of motor nerve involvement, such as foot or hand drop, are relatively rare, particularly in nondiabetic patients. Uremic neuropathy is frequently associated with abnormal nerve conduction patterns. The presence of peripheral neuropathy calls for the early initiation of adequate dialysis.

Hematologic Abnormalities

One of the disabling consequences of renal failure is severe anemia, which is primarily due to deficiency of erythropoietin, a renal hormone necessary for proliferation and differentiation of erythroid progenitor cells in the bone marrow.[16] In addition to erythropoietin deficiency, impaired iron utilization and shortened erythrocyte life span, which are caused by the associated oxidative stress and inflammation, contribute to anemia of renal failure. The presence of severe erythropoietin-resistant anemia (in the absence of other known causes of anemia) signifies the need for the initiation of dialysis. The advent and widespread use of recombinant erythropoietin and intravenous iron preparations have greatly facilitated management of anemia in patients with chronic kidney disease. However, owing its nonerythropoietic actions, administration of erythropoietin, particularly when given at high doses, causes hypertension and promotes vascular access thrombosis and stenosis.[17]

The other important hematologic complication of uremia is platelet dysfunction, which can lead to prolongation of bleeding time and hemorrhage.[18] Accumulation of uremic toxins and impaired calcium signaling have been implicated in the pathogenesis of uremic platelet dysfunction.[18-20] When present, severe platelet dysfunction and bleeding diathesis calls for the early initiation of dialysis, which can improve platelet function by reducing azotemia.

Several medications have been used in the management of uremic bleeding, including erythropoietin, 1-deamino-8-D-arginine vasopressin (DDAVP), and estrogen. In addition, by improving calcium signaling, enhancing platelet–vessel wall interaction, and increasing platelet production, erythropoietin improves uremic bleeding diathesis.[19,21]

DDAVP enhances platelet adhesion by increasing the release of von Willebrand factor (vWF) and simultaneously raising expression of vWF receptors on the platelets, which rapidly improve uremic platelet dysfunction and bleeding diathesis.[22] When administered intravenously (0.3 μg/50 mL normal saline over 30 min), DDAVP has a more rapid onset of action (1 hr) than when administered via the intranasal or subcutaneous routes (2 hr). The effect of intravenous DDAVP lasts for approximately 4 to 8 hours. One of the drawbacks of DDAVP therapy is the development of tachyphylaxis.

Oral, intravenous, and topical estrogen preparations are also effective in the management of uremic bleeding tendency.[23] The intravenous administration of conjugated estrogens (0.6 mg/kg/day for 5 days) improves uremic bleeding within approximately 6 hours, but 6 days of therapy is required for the maximal effect. Topical estrogen (estradiol patch, 50–100 μg applied every 3.5 days) and oral conjugated estrogens (50 mg/day) are also effective, but the onset of their action is delayed by 24 to 48 hours and 3 to 5 days, respectively. As with intravenous conjugated estrogen, the maximum effect of the latter products occurs within 5 to 7 days of treatment.

Packed red blood cell transfusion or cryoprecipitate infusion has also been used for rapid correction of uremic bleeding. The reader is referred to reviews for further details on the pathophysiology and management of uremic bleeding.[18,24]

Gastrointestinal Abnormalities

The most common gastrointestinal complications of uremia include anorexia, nausea, and vomiting.[25] In addition, gastritis and peptic ulcer disease are more common in patients with ESRD than in the general population. Stomatitis, enterocolitis leading to diarrhea, and even dysentery can occur with severe uncontrolled uremia. The latter disorders are often associated with mucosal ulcerations, which are thought to be caused by the release of ammonia from hydrolysis of urea, which is present at high concentrations in the saliva, gastric, and intestinal secretions in uremic patients. The occurrence of gastrointestinal manifestations points to the need for early initiation of dialysis therapy.

Immunologic Abnormalities

Both cell-mediated and humoral immunity are depressed in uremia.[25] This can, in part, account for the high incidence of infection and impaired response to vaccination in patients with ESRD. In fact, infection is the second most common cause of death in this patient population. Depressed cell-mediated immunity of uremia is marked by T-cell lymphopenia, reduced CD4/CD8 cell ratio, deficient T-cell response to antigens, and defective antigen presentation by monocytes, as well as impaired granulocyte/monocyte function.[26-29] Impaired humoral immunity in ESRD is evidenced by depressed antibody response to various vaccines, such as hepatitis B, pneumococcal, and influenza vaccines. Paradoxically, the chronic kidney disease–induced adaptive immune deficiency is associated with systemic inflammation stemming from activation of innate immunity.[30,31]

Endocrine Abnormalities

Uremia is accompanied by diffuse abnormalities of the endocrine function. The most significant feature of uremic endocrinopathy is depressed calcitriol production, leading to hypocalcemia. This, together with phosphate retention, results in secondary hyperparathyroidism leading to osteodystrophy and soft tissue and vascular calcification.[32,33] In addition, ESRD results in insulin resistance leading to glucose intolerance and impaired hypothalamic-pituitary-gonadal axis, resulting in amenorrhea and sexual dysfunction.[34,35] Although patients with ESRD are clinically euthyroid, they frequently exhibit reduced thyroxin (T_4) levels and impaired T_4 to triiodothyronine (T_3) conversion capacity.[36] Chronic renal failure results in diminished clearance, elevated plasma level, and resistance to the action of growth hormone. In fact, the rise in production of insulin-like growth factor in response to growth hormone is impaired in ESRD. Furthermore, the nocturnal surge in melatonin production and release by the pineal gland that is central to normal sleep pattern is defective in renal failure.[37] Thus, ESRD leads to a profound and diffuse dysregulation of multiple facets of the endocrine system.

Dermatologic Abnormalities

ESRD is frequently associated with a variety of dermatologic disorders. One of the most common cutaneous manifestations of uremia is the diffuse brown pigmentation of the skin, which is attributed to deposition of urochrome. Another characteristic abnormality is the so-called half-and-half nail, in which the proximal half of the nail is white and the distal half is brown. Dryness of the skin is extremely common in patients with ESRD and is occasionally associated with frank scaling, lichenification, and pruritus.

Pruritus is a relatively common complication of ESRD and can be highly disruptive, leading to widespread excoriation and secondary infections.[38] The severity of itching can intensify with heat and emotional stress. Pruritus in patients with ESRD is frequently associated with a high calcium × phosphate product (≥77 mg/dL) and dry skin. Adequate dialysis, hyperphosphatemia control, application of skin-moisturizing lotions, use of light garments, and avoidance of heat are sometimes helpful in mitigating the severity of pruritus. In addition, ultraviolet B radiation therapy and certain medications, such as the narcotic antagonist naltrexone, activated charcoal, cholestyramine, antihistamines, and ondansetron, have had varying results. In patients with severe secondary hyperparathyroidism, parathyroidectomy usually alleviates the symptoms.

Rarely, bullous eruptions occur in light-exposed areas and mimic porphyria cutanea tarda in patients with ESRD.[39] The bullas can be variably filled with serous or sanguineous fluids and frequently take weeks to months to heal. This condition has been attributed to the retention of photosensitizing uroporphyrins and iron overload and reportedly improves with the reduction of tissue iron stores by administration of erythropoietin.

Guidelines for Initiation of Hemodialysis

The U.S. Health Care Financing Administration (HCFA) monitors the decision to start dialysis therapy and oversees payment for chronic dialysis in association with regional networks. The guidelines for the initiation of dialysis are based primarily on the serum creatinine concentration or creatinine clearance, either measured (ie, by 24-hr urine collection) or estimated (ie, using the Cockcroft-Gault or Modification of Diet in Renal Disease [MDRD] formulas)[40] (see website: www.hcfa.gov). According to HCFA guidelines, dialysis may be initiated when the creatinine clearance falls to or below 10 mL/min for nondiabetic patients. Diabetic patients may initiate dialysis once the creatinine clearance falls below 15 mL/min, because they typically exhibit uremic signs and symptoms earlier than nondiabetic patients. Patients with uremic symptoms may be initiated on chronic dialysis earlier if the physician provides justification and the request is approved. If the request is not approved, payments for chronic dialysis services are denied.

In 1997, the National Kidney Foundation (NKF) published clinical practice guidelines for the initiation of dialysis.[41] The criteria used by the NKF take into consideration measurements of urea clearance and markers of malnutrition in addition to clinical signs and symptoms of uremia.[41] Other clinical practice guidelines for the initiation of dialysis have also been proposed.[42]

Conditions considered to be absolute indications for the initiation of maintenance dialysis include uremic encephalopathy, peripheral neuropathy, uremic pericarditis, fluid overload refractory to diuretics, severe hyperkalemia, metabolic acidosis, accelerated hypertension, persistent nausea and vomiting, uremic bleeding, and severe azotemia (serum creatinine >12 mg/dL or blood urea nitrogen >100 mg/dL) (Table 10-1).[43] Relative indications include anorexia, decreased ability to concentrate or to perform cognitive tasks, depression, anemia refractory to erythropoietin administration, uremic pruritus refractory to conservative therapies, and restless leg syndrome.[43]

Although these general guidelines are useful, it may be desirable to initiate chronic dialysis at an earlier stage, before the onset of malnutrition syndrome or other severe uremic complications.[44]

Vascular Access Recommendations

The NKF first published clinical practice guidelines for vascular access in 1997 and most recently in 2006.[45] According to these guidelines, surgical referral for the placement of vascular access (preferably an arteriovenous fistula) should occur when the patient's creatinine clearance falls below 25 mL/min, the serum creatinine rises above 4 mg/dL, or within 1 year of the anticipated need for

Table 10–1
Indications for Initiation of Hemodialysis in Chronic Renal Failure
Clearance-Based Criteria
Creatinine clearance < 10 mL/min
Creatinine clearance < 15 mL/min if diabetic
Creatinine clearance above these levels with appropriate documentation of conditions necessitating earlier dialysis
Non–Clearance-Based Criteria
Absolute indications
Uremic encephalopathy
Uremic neuropathy
Pericarditis
Severe fluid overload/pulmonary edema refractory to diuretics
Accelerated hypertension unresponsive to medications
Pericarditis
Significant uremic bleeding
Persistent nausea and vomiting
Serum creatinine > 12 mg/dL
Blood urea nitrogen > 100 mg/dL
Relative indications
Decreased attention span; poor cognition
Depression
Anorexia
Anemia unresponsive to erythropoietin
Pruritus
Restless leg syndrome

dialysis. An arteriovenous graft should be used when arteriovenous fistula creation is not feasible. These guidelines underscore the need for early referral to a nephrologist in order to determine the anticipated need for dialysis and for the provision of other pre-ESRD care.[44] When patients are either identified or referred late, however, dialysis may need to be started immediately. In these situations, insertion of a tunneled hemodialysis catheter is indicated. In such circumstances, creation of a permanent vascular access should occur either simultaneously or shortly thereafter. These and other clinical practice guidelines are periodically reviewed and updated. The reader is referred to the NKF-Kidney Disease Outcomes Quality Initiative (K/DOQI) website (www.kidney.org/professionals/doqi/index.cfm) to keep abreast of these developments.

REFERENCES

1. U.S. Renal Data System. *USRDS 2006 Annual Data Report.* Bethesda, MD: National Institutes of Health, National Institute of Diabetes and Digestive and Kidney Diseases, April 2006. Available at http://www.usrds.org/adr.htm

2. Winearls CG. Chronic renal failure and the uremic syndrome. In Johnson RJ, Feehally J (eds). *Comprehensive Clinical Nephrology.* London: Mosby; 2000.

3. Kemper MJ, Harps E, Müller-Wiefel DE. Hyperkalemia: therapeutic options in acute and chronic renal failure. *Clin Nephrol.* 1996;46:67-69.

4. Alpern RJ, Sakhaee K. The clinical spectrum of chronic metabolic acidosis: homeostatic mechanisms produce significant morbidity. *Am J Kidney Dis.* 1997;29:291-302.

5. Vaziri ND. Oxidative stress in uremia: nature, mechanisms, and potential consequences. *Semin Nephrol.* 2004;24:469-473.
6. Stenvinkel P. Inflammation in end-stage renal disease: the hidden enemy. *Nephrology (Carlton).* 2006;11:36-41.
7. Kaysen GA. Inflammation: cause of vascular disease and malnutrition in dialysis patients. *Semin Nephrol.* 2004;24:431-436.
8. Vaziri ND. Dyslipidemia of chronic renal failure: the nature, mechanisms, and potential consequences. *Am J Physiol Renal Physiol.* 2006;290:F262-F272.
9. Levin A, Foley RN. Cardiovascular disease in chronic renal insufficiency. *Am J Kidney Dis.* 2000;36(6 suppl 3):S24-S30.
10. Amann K, Rychlik I, Miltenberger-Milteny G, Ritz E. Left ventricular hypertrophy in renal failure. *Kidney Int Suppl.* 1998;68:S78-S85.
11. Levin A, Singer J, Thompson CR, Ross H, Lewis M. Prevalent left ventricular hypertrophy in the predialysis population: identifying opportunities for intervention. *Am J Kidney Dis.* 1996;27:347-354.
12. Alpert MA, Ravenscraft MD. Pericardial involvement in end-stage renal disease. *Am J Med Sci.* 2003;325:228-236.
13. Burn DJ, Bates D. Neurology and the kidney. *J Neurol Neurosurg Psychiatry.* 1998;65:810-821.
14. Tan EK, Ondo W. Restless legs syndrome: clinical features and treatment. *Am J Med Sci.* 2000;319:397-403.
15. Moe SM, Sprague SM. Uremic encephalopathy. *Clin Nephrol.* 1994;42:251-256.
16. Kausz AT, Obrador GT, Pereira BJ. Anemia management in patients with chronic renal insufficiency. *Am J Kidney Dis.* 2000;36(6 suppl 3):S39-S51.
17. Vaziri ND. Anemia and anemia correction: surrogate markers or causes of morbidity in chronic kidney disease? *Nature Clin Pract Nephrol.* 2008;4:436-445.
18. Weigert AL, Schafer AI. Uremic bleeding: pathogenesis and therapy. *Am J Med Sci.* 1998;316:94-104.
19. Zhou XJ, Vaziri ND. Defective calcium signaling in uremic platelets and its amelioration with long-term erythropoietin therapy. *Nephrol Dial Transpl.* 2002;17:992-997.
20. Vaziri ND, Zhou XJ, Naqvi F, et al. Role of nitric oxide resistance in erythropoietin-induced hypertension in rats with chronic renal failure. *Am J Physiol.* 1996;271(1 pt 1):E113-E122.
21. Kaupke CJ, Butler GC, Vaziri ND. Effect of recombinant human erythropoietin on platelet production in dialysis patients. *J Am Soc Nephrol.* 1993;3:1672-1679.
22. Chen KS, Huang CC, Leu ML, Deng P, Lo SK. Hemostatic and fibrinolytic response to desmopressin in uremic patient. *Blood Purif.* 1997;15:84-91.
23. Salvati F, Liani M, Golato M. Long-term therapy for uremic bleeding: effects of conjugate estrogens on the expression of platelet surface receptors for von Willebrand factor and fibrinogen (GPIb and GPIIb/IIIa glycoproteins). *Int J Artif Organs.* 1997;20:184-185.
24. Noris M, Remuzzi G. Uremic bleeding: closing the circle after 30 years of controversies? *Blood.* 1999;94:2569-2574.

25. Etemad B. Gastrointestinal complications of renal failure. *Gastroenterol Clin North Am.* 1998;27:875-892.
26. Cohen G, Haag-Weber M, Horl WH. Immune dysfunction in uremia. *Kidney Int Suppl.* 1997;62:S79-S82.
27. Descamps-Latscha B, Chatenoud L. T cells and B cells in chronic renal failure. *Semin Nephrol.* 1996;16:183-191.
28. Kato S, Chmielewski M, Honda H, et al. Aspects of immune dysfunction in end-stage renal disease. *Clin J Am Soc Nephrol.* 2008;3:1526-1533.
29. Yoon JW, Gollapudi S, Pahl MV, Vaziri ND. Naïve and central memory T-cell lymphopenia in end-stage renal disease. *Kidney Int.* 2006;70:371-376.
30. Yoon JW, Pahl MV, Vaziri ND. Spontaneous leukocyte activation and oxygen-free radical generation in end-stage renal disease. *Kidney Int.* 2007;71:167-172.
31. Stenvinkel P. Inflammation in end-stage renal disease—a fire that burns within. *Contrib Nephrol.* 2005;149:185-199.
32. Slatopolsky E, Brown A, Dusso A. Calcium, phosphorus and vitamin D disorders in uremia. *Contrib Nephrol.* 2005;149:261-271.
33. Ritz E, Schömig M, Bommer J. Osteodystrophy in the millennium. *Kidney Int Suppl.* 1999;73:S94-S98.
34. Alvestrand A. Carbohydrate and insulin metabolism in renal failure. *Kidney Int Suppl.* 1997;62:S48-S52.
35. Palmer BF. Sexual dysfunction in uremia. *J Am Soc Nephrol.* 1999;10:1381-1388.
36. Lim VS. Renal failure and thyroid function. *Int J Artif Organs.* 1986;9:385-386.
37. Vaziri ND, Oveisi F, Reyes GA, Zhou XJ. Dysregulation of melatonin metabolism in chronic renal insufficiency: role of erythropoietin deficiency anemia. *Kidney Int.* 1996;50:653-656.
38. Schwartz IF, Iaina A. Management of uremic pruritus. *Semin Dial.* 2000;13:177-180.
39. Peces R, Enríquez de Salamanca R, Fontanellas A, et al: Successful treatment of hemodialysis-related porphyria cutanea tarda with erythropoietin. *Nephrol Dial Transplant.* 1994;9:433-435.
40. Cockcroft DW, Gault MH. Prediction of creatinine clearance from serum creatinine. *Nephron.* 1976;16:31-41.
41. National Kidney Foundation. *NKF-DOQI Clinical Practice Guidelines for Peritoneal Dialysis Adequacy.* New York: National Kidney Foundation; 1997:17-22.
42. Churchill DN, Blake PG, Jindal KK, Toffelmire EB, Goldstein MB. Clinical practice guidelines for initiation of dialysis. *J Am Soc Nephrol.* 1999;10(suppl 13):S289-S291.
43. Hakim RM, Lazarus JM. Initiation of dialysis. *J Am Soc Nephrol.* 1995;6:1319-1328.
44. Obrador GT, Pereira BJG. Early referral to the nephrologist and timely initiation of renal replacement therapy: a paradigm shift in the management of patients with chronic renal failure. *Am J Kidney Dis.* 1998;31:398-417.
45. National Kidney Foundation. *NKF-DOQI Clinical Practice Guidelines for Vascular Access.* New York: National Kidney Foundation; 1997.

CHAPTER 11

Autologous Arteriovenous Fistulas: Direct Radiocephalic Anastomosis for Hemodialysis Access

Samuel Eric Wilson

Increasing numbers of patients require long-term vascular access for hemodialysis. A conservative estimate by the 2008 U.S. Renal Data System report shows almost 400,000 patients with end-stage renal disease (ESRD) maintained on dialysis in 2006.[1] The majority of patients beginning dialysis are now older than 60 years of age, have diabetes, or both.

The necessity of reliable vascular access is paramount and has resulted in many surgeons and patients spending frustrated hours during either the construction or the management of subsequent complications of the various methods of providing vascular access. Despite advances made in the development of graft materials and indwelling silicone elastomer (Silastic) catheters, the autogenous radiocephalic fistula first described in 1966[2] continues to be regarded as the ideal form of access when this anastomosis can be constructed. The reasons for this preference include factors such as superior long-term patency rates, lower incidence and ease of managing infectious complications, and relatively few other complications such as aneurysm formation.[3]

Even with the generally accepted advantages of direct autogenous fistulas for dialysis, some dialysis centers in North America use this method in a minority of patients for reasons such as urgency of dialysis and poor-quality vessels (particularly in the elderly and the diabetic populations). A report on 1266 permanent vascular access procedures described only 104 patients (8.2%) as having primary autogenous fistulas constructed, but, beginning in the 1990s, use of autogenous fistulas often exceeds 50% in dialysis patients.[4,5] In most European and Japanese centers, the majority of permanent vascular access procedures uses autogenous techniques.[6] The Kidney Disease Outcomes Quality Initiative (K/DOQI) guidelines, developed under the sponsorship of the National Kidney Foundation, emphasize the enduring value of the autogenous arteriovenous (AV) anastomosis and recommend that approximately 60% of hemodialysis patients have this vascular access.

The first part of this chapter discusses the techniques used in constructing a radiocephalic fistula, and in the second part, some of the other autogenous fistulas commonly constructed are reviewed. Complications and their management are described.

Preparation and Planning

The surgical construction of an AV fistula requires careful planning, timing, and selection of the operative site and meticulous technique. Patients with progressive renal failure who are being observed in an ESRD clinic should have an AV fistula created in anticipation of the start of maintenance dialysis. However, should renal failure occur more acutely, urgent dialysis may be carried out using a temporary percutaneous central venous cannula, an AV graft, or peritoneal dialysis. If a central venous cannula is used, it is preferable to use the internal jugular vein and to avoid leaving the cannula in longer than 4 to 6 weeks in an effort to decrease the incidence of central vein thrombosis, which will make permanent access difficult.

The very ill patient with uremia may benefit from several acute hemodialysis treatments using a temporary form of access before operation for a forearm fistula. During this preparatory period, it is important that clear instructions be given to the patient and to other attending staff that under no circumstances should the cephalic vein at the wrist and forearm be used for venipuncture or intravenous infusion. It has been the practice of some dialysis units not to permit phlebotomy of any forearm or wrist veins because permanent damage may be caused to these valuable lifelines.

An AV fistula is planned when the serum creatinine clearance exceeds 4 mg/dL or with a creatinine clearance between 15 to 20 mL/min. Arterialization of these fistulas occurs over the subsequent maturation period (4–6 wk). During this time, it is unwise to puncture even a dilated vein, because early on, this vessel is thin walled and hematomas form easily. Some physicians encourage arterialization of the cephalic vein by regular, vigorous exercising of the forearm muscles. Patients are encouraged to regularly squeeze a rubber ball or engage in other, similar exercise.

Before surgery, thorough examine both arms. Keep the patient warm. Carefully palpate the arterial pulses throughout both arms. Apply a sphygmomanometer cuff to the upper arm and inflate it to a pressure below the systolic pressure, allowing the veins to be studied. Use Doppler ultrasound to determine their patency and diameter (vein mapping study).

To facilitate extremity use, especially in patients who are being trained for regular home hemodialysis, it is preferable to use the nondominant arm. The ulnar artery and basilic vein in the nondominant arm may also be used, but cannulation is more difficult. An anatomic prerequisite is that the chosen vein should have a continuous prograde run. Proximal obstruction to flow will initiate retrograde flow with distal congestion and arm edema. Once the choice of anastomosis has been made, mark the veins and their tributaries along their length at the surgical site. This practice simplifies the planning of an adequate incision, and should the fistula fail at surgery, facilitates the location of another anastomotic site.

Local, monitored anesthesia is usually very satisfactory. One percent xylocaine *without* epinephrine is infiltrated. Alternatively, an axillary block provides excellent regional anesthesia and promotes vasodilatation. In an uncooperative patient or a child, general anesthesia will be required to allow careful and meticulous dissection and anastomosis. If the patient is on dialysis, a small, temporary fluid infusion may facilitate function of the new fistula. It is essential to avoid hypotension because this may initiate fistula thrombosis.

Surgical Technique

The surgeon should be comfortably seated with adequate lighting; magnifying glasses are very helpful for a precise vein-to-artery anastomosis. Various techniques for forearm fistulas have evolved since the Brescia et al. description of 1966.[2] Methods that have proved to be successful are described here.

Autogenous Radiocephalic Fistula

Make an oblique or a longitudinal incision overlying the selected anastomotic site (Fig. 11-1). Locate the cephalic vein, and isolate a segment 3 to 5 centimeters in length from the surrounding subcutaneous and areolar tissue (Fig. 11-2). Ligate and divide venous tributaries to improve mobility of the vein. Remove adventitial bands during dissection to avoid kinking and segmental stenosis. Attention is now focused on the radial artery. Make an incision in the fascia of the forearm. The fascial fibers run transversely, and the radial artery along with its venae comitantes is carefully exposed. The radial artery is carefully mobilized, with ligation of the muscular branches and isolation of the artery from the venae comitantes. The origins of some of its fine branches require ligation or a touch with the electrocautery.

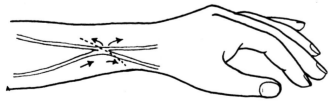

Figure 11-1.
An oblique incision is made crossing the cephalic vein and radial artery for construction of a side-to-side radiocephalic fistula. An end of the cephalic vein to the side of radial artery is the preferred construction.

Inadvertent tearing of these branches causes periarterial hemorrhage, but pressure with a gauze swab controls it. A cephalic vein of not less than 3 mm diameter and a radial artery of 2 mm are required.

Electrocautery of these small side branches using a fine, smooth-tipped forceps applied a few millimeters from the radial artery wall is very helpful. Gentle handling is essential in mobilization of both artery and vein. If the radial artery goes into spasm, papaverine may be applied topically to the periarterial sheath, using a blunt needle, before starting the dissection.

Use small-angled instruments to elevate the vessels; a sling made of very fine Silastic provides good vascular control and retracts the artery and vein without trauma. An end of vein–to–side of artery is the preferred anastomosis. Adequately mobilized lengths of the two vessels are necessary so that the anastomosis can be made without tension. It is important that there be no angulation or kinking. Divide the distal cephalic vein and mobilize its proximal segment until there is sufficient length to approximate to the radial artery in an end-to-side fashion. Take care to not twist the vein axis; the application of dots of indelible ink on the superior surface aids in avoidance of this.

Four different anastomotic connections of artery and vein have been used, each with advantages and disadvantages (Fig. 11-3), but end-to-side anastomosis results in the highest fistula flows. Today, most surgeons *prefer the end-to-side, vein-to-artery anastomosis*, which, if constructed properly, decreases turbulence and results in the highest proximal venous flow with minimal distal venous hypertension.[7] A bifurcation of the cephalic vein is often present and offers an opportunity for a patulous anastomosis (Fig. 11-2 A, B, C).

In construction of the end vein–to–side artery anastomosis, use a double-armed, monofilament, 6-0 polypropylene suture. Start suturing on the posterior wall at the end of the venotomy, and place the knot on the outside. Continue suturing along the back wall from the inside and complete the anastomosis by approximating the anterior layers. At this stage, wash the lumina of the artery and vein with heparinized saline to remove any clot, and before placing the final suture, pass a blunt-ended probe or an arterial dilator proximally and distally to ensure that there is no stenosis. One has to be careful that spiral rotation of either vessel has not occurred. To this end, leaving one of the lateral branches in situ is useful.

Remove the distal arterial clamp first. Then open the proximal radial artery. Light compression with a hemostatic pledget is often necessary to stop immediate anastomotic bleeding. Maintain compression for precisely 5 minutes, and if bleeding is still present, use an interrupted 6-0 suture to gain control.

If a side-to-side anastomosis is to be performed, place the artery and vein in juxtaposition. Proximal and distal control of these vessels is achieved with atraumatic vascular clamps or Silastic slings. Make a longitudinal venotomy measuring about 8 to 12 mm in length, and place fine traction sutures to eliminate intimal damage from the forceps. If valves are present at the venotomy site, remove these with fine scissors.

At the completion of a fistula, a thrill is palpable. Palpable pulsation and the absence of a thrill or bruit indicate

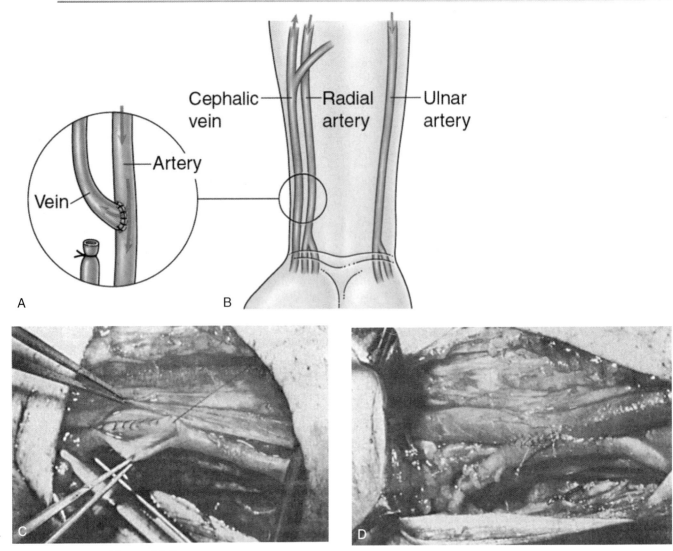

Figure 11-2.
Construction of a side-to-side arteriovenous fistula. *A, B,* Anastomosis in progress with posterior wall completed. *C,* Completed anastomosis shows engorgement of cephalic vein. *D,* The preferred construction is the end cephalic vein to side radial artery.

outflow obstruction and may herald impending thrombosis. When inadequate flow exists, it is useful to probe the proximal vein with a small catheter to evaluate the possibility of stricture. If a stricture is suspected, obtain an estimate of its functional significance by partially withdrawing the catheter and rapidly injecting 20 to 30 mL of saline; ordinarily there is no detectable resistance to flow. If inadequate flow is due to spasm, it is usually eliminated by the rapid injection of saline. If a stricture is suspected, an on-table venogram can be obtained and balloon angioplasty performed. Occasionally, it is necessary to cut down on the site of the stricture and to repair it directly. On rare occasions, the vein must be abandoned, and another vein or even another site is used for construction of the fistula.

If an obstruction is found in the proximal vein, insert a small catheter via the opened anastomosis and flush the vein with heparinized saline. Inflation and withdrawal of an embolectomy catheter balloon should be avoided if possible because this may result in damage to the valves and to the venous endothelium.[8]

If good pulsation is present, a thrill is absent, and the venogram shows no obstruction, the fistula may be left with the anticipation of a bruit appearing at a later time.

After the operation, keep the hand elevated. Cover the incision with a light gauze, and loosely apply a dressing. Take blood pressure readings on the opposite arm. Cannulation of the fistula may be attempted after 4 weeks if sufficient dilatation has occurred.

If the radiocephalic AV fistula at the wrist is not possible, the next consideration is evaluation of the radial artery and cephalic vein in the mid-forearm, an excellent secondary site.

Brachiocephalic AV Fistula

When construction of a fistula at the wrist is not possible, anastomosis of the cephalic vein and brachial artery imme-

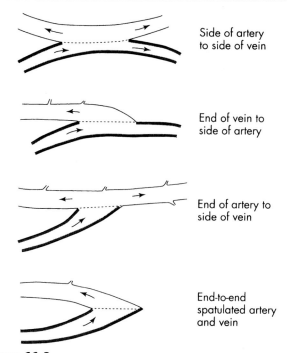

Side of artery
to side of vein

End of vein to
side of artery

End of artery to
side of vein

End-to-end
spatulated artery
and vein

Figure 11-3.
Four different anastomoses commonly constructed between the radial artery and the cephalic vein.

diately proximal to the antecubital crease will provide satisfactory access.[9] In thin patients, the cephalic vein is usually visible between the elbow and the shoulder and can be used for cannulation for dialysis. Make a transverse incision proximal to the cubital fossa. Mobilize the brachial artery until it reaches the bifurcation at the level of the bicipital tendon. It is often necessary to partially divide the bicipital aponeurosis. The median nerve lies medial and posterior to the artery and should be carefully protected. The anastomosis is similar to that described for the end vein–to–side artery radiocephalic fistula, but the arteriotomy should be limited to approximately 3 to 5 mm to minimize the incidence of steal syndrome. On occasion, the radial artery may be satisfactory for arterial inflow. The antecubital vein, if of sufficient size, may be used instead of the cephalic vein. The incidence of late steal syndrome is higher with autogenous proximal brachiocephalic fistulas.

Basilic Vein–to–Radial Artery Fistula

Mobilization of the basilic vein in the forearm and anastomosis of its end to the radial artery also may be used to provide access for hemodialysis.[10] Mobilize the basilic vein along the ulnar border of the forearm to about the middle of the forearm. Prepare a subcutaneous tunnel between the vein and the radial artery. Then anastomose these vessels, with attachment of the vein end to the side of the radial artery. This technique of fistula formation may be used in patients who have an obliterated cephalic vein or distal radial artery. It is possible to anastomose the basilic vein to the ulnar artery; however, if there has been a previous radiocephalic fistula in that arm, there is the danger that circulation in the hand will be compromised. Creating a fis-

tula that leaves the basilic vein in situ presents an awkward position for cannulation.

Symptomatic steal is unusual with this end basilic vein–to–side radial artery fistula, and there is no significant effect on cardiac output. The fistula is not recommended as a primary procedure, but it does provide a means for creating vascular access in patients in whom other convenient sites for construction of a vascular access have been exhausted.

The transposed basilic vein fistula in the brachium is described in Chapter 13.

Other forearm autogenous AV access configurations include vein transposition and anastomosis to the ulnar artery, but I find the mid forearm end cephalic vein to radial artery the most useful.

Complications

Failure

The most frequently reported complication is that of early failure, with a reported incidence of up to 27%.[3] Because the autogenous fistula remains patent with lower flow rates, the access may be considered patent, but it is not functional (ie, <400 mL/min flow). With increased emphasis on construction of autogenous fistulas since the K/DOQI guidelines were established, it is likely only 50% of autogenous AV fistulas become functional. Failure might be a result of postoperative thrombosis, or it might be failure to mature and achieve an adequate flow rate to maintain dialysis. An inadequate flow rate may be caused by technical problems in construction of the anastomosis, a sclerotic vein segment in the forearm due to previous venipuncture or indwelling catheters, inadequate venous size or poor venous run-off, calcification of the arterial wall leading to poor flow, or hypotension, which may be associated with hypovolemia during dialysis. The tendency to thrombose is increased particularly in diabetic patients (possibly related to an increased tendency for platelet aggregation[11]). The increasing use of erythropoietin has also been suggested to increase the risk of fistula thrombosis,[12] but in practice, this does not appear to present a major problem. Once successful, long-term patency of the AV fistula is good and has been reported as approximately 75% to 80% at 3 years.[3]

When thrombosis is suspected by clinical evaluation, further assessment can be made by angiography or with color Doppler ultrasound. The advantages of Doppler ultrasound are that it is noninvasive and may differentiate nonthrombotic stenosis from partial thrombosis.[13] Surgical thrombectomy is achieved by making a small venotomy and using a Fogarty balloon catheter to remove the thrombus. A more proximal fistula can be constructed in the case of a distal narrowing. Endovascular techniques are useful in salvage of the failing fistula.

Aneurysm

Both true aneurysm and pseudoaneurysm formation may occur at the puncture sites made by dialysis cannulas (Fig. 11-4), but the incidence is lower than that in prosthetic grafts. In one study, an incidence of 2% was reported compared with 10% for polytetrafluoroethylene (PTFE) grafts.[14] If aneurysms are large enough to be cosmetically disfiguring,

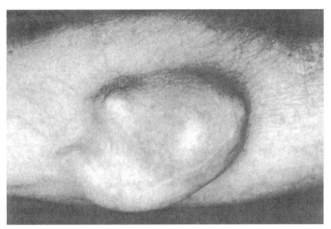

Figure 11-4.
Pseudoaneurysm at the antecubital fossa.

to thrombose, or to cause skin thinning and breakdown of skin, they can be repaired with resection and either end-to-end anastomosis or placement of a short segment of PTFE graft to allow continued functioning of the AV fistula.[15] A covered stent graft is another option.

Infection

Infection of autogenous fistulas is rare compared with that in prosthetic grafts.[14] Patients present with fever, erythema, tenderness, and complications such as thrombosis or pseudoaneurysm formation.[16,17] The most common infecting bacterium is *Staphylococcus aureus*, although other bacteria such as streptococci and Gram-negative bacilli may be implicated. Compared with prosthetic grafts, the fistula is more likely to be salvaged with systemic antibiotics, local drainage, and revision as necessary.

Ischemic Changes

Steal symptoms may occur in about 4% of patients with autogenous fistulas.[14] The incidence is higher in diabetic patients, in elderly patients with atherosclerotic disease, and in antecubital fistulas compared with wrist fistulas. The symptoms may manifest only during dialysis and, in some patients, may be managed by careful observation and pain control.[18] At worst, gangrene of the extremities (Fig. 11-5) may occur, requiring amputation.[19] Correction of steal phenomenon is detailed in Chapter 22. Digital gangrene in an extremity with an AV fistula may not be due to arterial steal but rather to the severe vascular disease of the patient with ESRD.

Venous Hypertension

A venous hypertension syndrome may develop (Fig. 11-6) in which the hand distal to the fistula becomes swollen and uncomfortable with thickening of the skin and hyperpigmentation.[20,21] In its most advanced form, this syndrome may result in ulceration of the distal extremities or even the development of pseudo–Kaposi's sarcoma,[22] a non-neoplastic process characterized by the development of purpuric lesions on the extremities. Venous hypertension may be

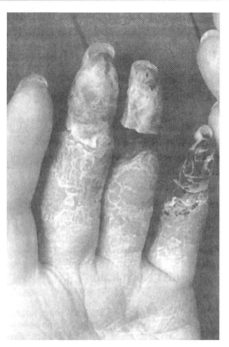

Figure 11-5.
Gangrenous changes in the digits after the placement of a fistula.

avoided by forming an end-to-side or end-to-end anastomosis. Ligation of the enlarged venous tributaries causing the hypertension of the distal digits may relieve symptoms while preserving the fistula.

The increasing use of central venous catheters for dialysis has led to an increased incidence of subclavian vein thrombosis or stenosis. The subsequent placement of a fistula may lead to massive arm edema caused by venous hypertension and, in women, ipsilateral breast enlarge-

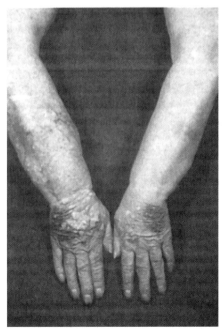

Figure 11-6.
Venous hypertension syndrome in the arm, distal to the fistula.

ment.[23] Subclavian vein thrombolysis and angioplasty with stenting may allow continued use of the fistula. This complication may also be lessened by using the internal jugular vein for central line placement.

Neuropathy

Ischemic neuropathy[24] is unusual with the radiocephalic fistula and is seen mainly in diabetic patients with preexisting atherosclerotic disease and in those with proximal fistulas. It is characterized by the onset of severe, acute, painful weakness of the distal extremity, with wrist drop and minimal wrist flexion. This development is probably due to peripheral nerve ischemia, and if recognized early, fistula interception may preserve neurologic function.

Cardiovascular Complications

High-output cardiac failure is a rare complication, which occurs particularly in patients who display a combination of low hematocrit and cardiomyopathy from diabetes, in the presence of a high-flow fistula.[25] Treatment usually involves interrupting the fistula, although banding may be attempted.[26]

Conclusion

The demand for permanent durable vascular access is high. Primary autogenous fistulas continue to provide the best form of access, with a lower complication rate than the alternatives. With early planning, preservation of arm veins, and careful postoperative management, the autogenous fistula can be the first choice of vascular access for the hemodialysis patient.

REFERENCES

1. U.S. Renal Data System. *2008 Annual Report: Atlas of Chronic Kidney Disease and End-Stage Renal Disease in the United States.* Bethesda, MD: National Institutes of Health, 2008. Available at http://www.usrds.org/.
2. Brescia M, Cimino JE, Appel K, Hurwich BJ. Chronic hemodialysis using venipuncture and a surgically created arteriovenous fistula. *N Engl J Med.* 1966;275:1089-1092.
3. Winsett OE, Wolma FJ. Complications of vascular access for hemodialysis. *South Med J.* 1985;78:513-517.
4. Connolly JE, Brownell DA, Levine EF, McCart PM. Complications of renal dialysis access procedures. *Arch Surg.* 1984;119:1325-1328.
5. Glazer S, Diesto J, Crooks P, et al. Going beyond the Kidney Disease Outcomes Quality Initiative: hemodialysis access experience at Kaiser Permanente Southern California. *Ann Vasc Surg.* 2006;20:75-82.
6. Burger H, Kootstra G, de Charro F, Leffers P. A survey of vascular access for hemodialysis in the Netherlands. *Nephrol Dial Transplant.* 1991;6:5-10.
7. Karmody AM, Lempert N. "Smooth loop" arteriovenous fistulas for haemodialysis. *Surgery.* 1974;75:238-242.
8. Siegal B. Improving the patency of arteriovenous fistulas. *Surg Gynecol Obstet.* 1977;144:82-83.
9. Nguyen TH, Bui TD, Gordon IL, Wilson SE. Functional patency of autogenous AV fistulas for hemodialysis. *J Vasc Access.* 2007;8:275-280.
10. LoGerfo FW, Menzoian JO, Kumaki DJ, Idelson BA. Transposed basilic vein-brachial arteriovenous fistula: a reliable secondary-access procedure. *Arch Surg.* 1978;113:1008-1010.
11. Gensini GF, Abbate R, Favilla S, Neri Serneri GG. Changes of platelet function and blood clotting in diabetes mellitus. *Thromb Haemost.* 1979;42:983-993.
12. Canadian Erythropoietin Study Group. Association between recombinant human erythropoietin and quality of life and exercise capacity of patients receiving hemodialysis. *BMJ.* 1990;300:573-578.
13. Nonnast-Daniel B, Martin RP, Lindert O, et al. Colour Doppler ultrasound assessment of arteriovenous hemodialysis fistulas. *Lancet.* 1992;339:143-145.
14. Suding P, Wilson SE. Strategies for management of ischemic steal syndrome. *Semin Vasc Surg.* 2007;20:184-188.
15. Patel K, Chan FA, Batista RJ, Clauss RH. True venous aneurysms and arterial "steal" secondary to arteriovenous fistulae for dialysis. *J Cardiovasc Surg.* 1992;33:185-188.
16. Fong IW, Capellan JM, Simbul M, Angel J. Infection of arterio-venous fistulas created for chronic haemodialysis. *Scand J Infect Dis.* 1993;25:215-220.
17. Padberg FT Jr, Lee BC, Curl GR. Hemoaccess site infection. *Surg Gynecol Obstet.* 1992;174:103-108.
18. Rivers SP, Scher LA, Veith FJ. Correction of steal syndrome secondary to hemodialysis access fistulas: a simplified quantitive technique. *Surgery.* 1992;112:593-597.
19. Mactier RA, Stewart WK, Parham DM, Tainsh JA. Acral gangrene attributed to calcific azotemic arteriopathy and the steal effect of an arteriovenous fistula. *Nephron.* 1990;54:347-350.
20. Deshmukh N, Reppert M. Venous ulceration of the hand secondary to a Cimino fistula. *Mil Med.* 1993;158:752-753.
21. Irvine C, Holt P. Hand venous hypertension complicating arteriovenous fistula construction for hemodialysis. *Clin Exp Dermatol.* 1989;14:289-290.
22. Bogaert AM, Vanholder R, De Roose J, et al. Pseudo-Kaposi's sarcoma as a complication of Cimino-Brescia arteriovenous fistulas in hemodialysis patients. *Nephron.* 1987;46:170-173.
23. Gadallah MF, el-Shahawy MA, Campese VM. Unilateral breast enlargement secondary to hemodialysis arteriovenous fistula and subclavian vein occlusion. *Nephron.* 1993;63:351-353.
24. Riggs JE, Moss AH, Labosky DA, Liput JH, Morgan JJ, Gutmann L. Upper extremity ischemic monomelic neuropathy: a complication of vascular access procedures in uremic diabetic patients. *Neurology.* 1989;39:997-998.
25. Lala MSA. Problems and prospect of internal arteriovenous fistula for dialysis. *Angiology.* 1985;36:27-32.
26. Anderson CB, Groce MA. Banding of arteriovenous fistulas to correct high-output cardiac failure. *Surgery.* 1975;78:552-554.

CHAPTER 12

Autogenous Vein for Fistulas and Interposition Grafts

Geoffrey H. White and Michael S. Hayashi

The 2008 annual report by the U.S. Renal Data System found nearly half a million Americans living with end-stage renal disease.[1] The National Kidney Foundation Kidney Dialysis Outcomes Quality Initiative (K/DOQI) guidelines for clinical practice favor the use of an arteriovenous (AV) fistula for hemodialysis access. Autogenous AV fistulas are well known to offer longer patency, fewer infectious complications, and a decreased need for secondary interventions compared with other forms of hemodialysis access. The Dialysis Outcomes and Practice Patterns Study (DOPPS), however, has demonstrated that the United States uses far fewer AV fistulas for dialysis access compared with our international counterparts in Europe and Japan.[2] This discrepancy appears to arise from the preferences of local dialysis centers, the practice of individual surgeons, as well as the timing of referral to a surgeon before the impending need for hemodialysis. For new dialysis patients, 25% in Europe versus 46% in the United States do not have permanently placed access sites before starting hemodialysis.[3]

Surgery at "high-volume" centers (>30 procedures/yr) is associated with a threefold increased likelihood of constructing an AV fistula.[4] Construction of a radiocephalic fistula at the wrist is firmly established as the procedure of choice for hemodialysis access. After a period of maturation, the arterialized vein typically has a dilated, thickened wall that is suitable for the repeated trauma of routine hemodialysis and is relatively resistant to thrombosis. Patient characteristics of female sex, African American race, and diabetes have been found to increase the rates of primary access failure for autogenous fistulas by 18%, 14%, and 10%, respectively. Age as an independent risk factor does not affect patency, but a history of failed access incurs an 81% increased risk of a functioning failure.[5] Under the best circumstances, autogenous fistulas may have a 2-year patency as high as 60% to 70% compared with a 40% patency for the best prosthetic grafts.[6,7] Infection rarely occurs in the autogenous construction, and the peripheral position of the fistula allows easy access and patient comfort during dialysis.

Alternatives to the radiocephalic fistula at the wrist are considered when the patient's anatomy is unsuitable for construction or as a secondary procedure after the original fistula has occluded. These various alternative sites in the upper extremity are detailed in Table 12-1. Common sites

include the brachiobasilic, brachiocephalic, and the brachial artery–median antecubital vein fistulas. These have been found to offer a primary patency rate of approximately 50% and an assisted primary patency rate of 74% at 12 months. On average, these are ready for access within 1 to 3 months, with longer times to usage for brachiobasilic fistulas, which are transposed at a second operation.[8]

Prosthetic material is also widely used for constructing AV grafts for hemodialysis access. Grafts are advantageous in that they require less time until maturation and provide ease of cannulation. Onet review, however, showed that they carry a 41% greater risk of primary failure compared with autogenous fistulas with a 2-year patency of 24.6% versus 39.8% for autogenous fistulas.[5] These substitutes for autogenous access are also associated with a 20% incidence of infectious complications, as well as seroma formation, unpredictable inflammatory reactions, pseudoaneurysm formation, steal syndrome, and neurologic deficits.[9-13] When complications necessitate removal of the graft, extensive

Table 12–1

Access Configurations for Forearm Autogenous Accesses

Autogenous posterior radial branch–cephalic direct wrist access (snuffbox)

Autogenous radial-cephalic direct wrist access (Brescia-Cimino-Appel)

Autogenous radial-cephalic forearm transposition

Autogenous brachial (or proximal radial)–cephalic forearm looped transposition

Autogenous radial-basilic forearm transposition

Autogenous ulnar-basilic forearm transposition

Autogenous brachial (or proximal radial)–basilic forearm looped transposition

Autogenous radial-antecubital forearm greater saphenous translocation

Autogenous brachial (or proximal radial)–antecubital forearm looped greater saphenous translocation

Modified from Sidawy AN, Spergel LM, Besarab A, et al. The Society for Vascular Surgery: clinical practice guidelines for the surgical placement and maintenance of arteriovenous hemodialysis access. *J Vasc Surg.* 2008;48:19S-20S.

tissue thickening and fibrosis can render dissection difficult and tedious. Occasionally, with anastomotic disruption caused by infection, ligation of the supply artery may also be required and in rare instances lead to limb amputation.[14]

AV Fistulas

Radiocephalic (Brescia-Cimino-Appel) AV Fistula

The techniques of construction and various configurations of the Brescia-Cimino-Appel radiocephalic fistula at the wrist are discussed in detail in Chapter 11. The end of vein–to–side of artery configuration has patency rates that are equivalent to those of the side-to-side anastomosis, with less incidence of venous hypertension and hyperemia of the hand.[15,16] Alternative sites for a direct AV fistula are used less commonly because of the more difficult exposure of vessels and necessity for extensive mobilization of the vein for some of these procedures. Nevertheless, these sites may provide satisfactory long-term use, so the operative time and dissection may more than repay the effort.

Snuffbox Fistula

A radiocephalic fistula may be fashioned in the anatomic snuffbox between the tendons of the extensor pollicis longus and brevis (Fig. 12-1). The cephalic vein runs directly over the artery at this point and requires minimal mobilization. The principal advantages for this technique are that the proximity of the vessels in this area reduces angulation of the anastomosis and preserves construction of a radiocephalic fistula for a later date, if necessary.[17,18] This procedure, however, calls for an anastomosis where the vessels are of narrow caliber, leaving little room for technical error and requires greater experience. We reserve this technique for the few young, muscular, usually men, who have a wide vein and easily palpable distal radial artery. Long-term patency is similar to that of the Brescia-Cimino fistula if the vessels are suitable for construction.[19]

Ulnar Artery–to–Basilic Vein Fistula

An ulnar artery–to–basilic vein fistula may be fashioned by anastomosis at the wrist or proximally in the forearm.[20] The technique is not used often because the vessels tend to be

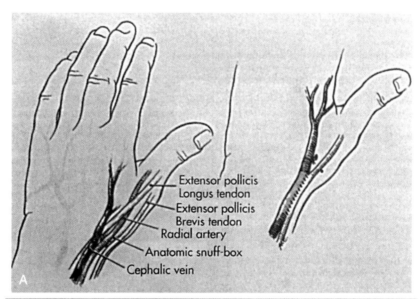

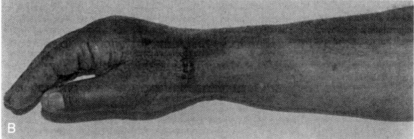

Figure 12-1.
Snuffbox fistula. *A,* This distal fistula is formed between the tendons of the extensor pollicis longus and brevis, where the radial artery and cephalic vein run in close proximity. *B,* The incision for this procedure may be transverse (as shown) or longitudinal. (*A,* From Mehigan JT, McAlexander RA. Snuffbox arteriovenous fistula for hemodialysis. *Am J Surg.* 1982;143:252-253.)

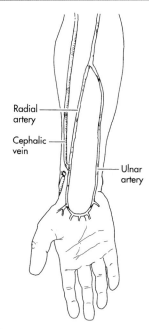

Figure 12-2.
End of the cephalic vein anastomosed to the side of the radial artery at a site superior to the usual location of the radiocephalic fistula. This technique can be useful if the distal radial artery is small or the cephalic vein at the wrist is thrombosed.

deeper, the basilic vein is often not well developed, and access to this vein for subsequent puncture is difficult because of its position on the medial side of the arm. Extensive mobilization and repositioning of the basilic vein may allow easier positioning of the arm for access. In select patients, however, this fistula can be very useful with acceptable long-term patency.

Proximal Forearm Fistula

A radiocephalic fistula may also be performed in the mid forearm, especially after a previous fistula at the wrist has dilated the veins at this position.[21] This procedure is most conveniently performed by anastomosis in the end of the mobilized cephalic vein to the side of the radial artery (Fig. 12-2). The median antecubital vein may also be joined end of vein to side of proximal radial artery. "Reverse

fistulas" have also been described with an anastomosis near the elbow, ligation of the proximal veins as needed, and destruction of valves within the distal veins.[22,23] A variation of this technique has been used successfully by Jennings[24] who achieved a primary patency of 91% and an overall assisted patency of 97% at 11 months, exceeding that of patients receiving a radialcephalic fistula. Venous hypertension in the hand remains a concern with this method.

Vein Transposition Procedures

Occasionally, the native AV fistula will fail to mature and require a second operation. A transposed AV fistula can be constructed to decrease this nonmaturation rate from 26.7% to 4.7% with a 76% 1-year patency as reported by Choi and coworkers.[25] Although offering a more easily identifiable access site, this maneuver requires careful attention to prevent kinks or twists in the vein during translocation and is subject to seroma formation around the subcutaneous tunnel.[25]

The basilic vein within the forearm or upper arm may be transposed after dissection and mobilization to place it superficially in a more favorable anterolateral location on the upper arm (Fig. 12-3). Thus, anastomosis to the radial artery in the forearm can create transposed vein access that is similar in configuration to the Brescia-Cimino-Appel fistula.[26] Disadvantages are the extensive dissection required and the fragility of this vein.

The brachiobasilic fistula within the upper arm requires mobilization of the basilic vein from its deep course, where it has been protected from damage by previous venipuncture, followed by repositioning in the superficial subcutaneous tunnel toward the lateral side of the arm (Figs. 12-4 to 12-6).[27] Use of this technique provides an excellent alternative for patients without favorable vasculature in the forearm, given its 2-year patency rate of greater than 60%.[28] This method is considered in more detail in Chapter 13.

The saphenous vein loop fistula within the upper thigh is a vein transposition procedure used infrequently. The saphenous vein is mobilized down to the knee without being detached at the saphenofemoral junction and is then repositioned in the subcutaneous plane in a gentle curve

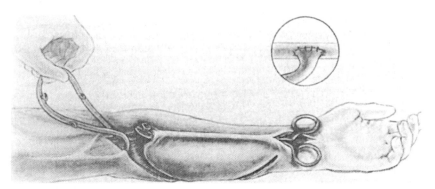

Figure 12-3.
Radiobasilic fistula in the forearm, with transposition of the vein to the anterolateral aspect. (From Patrick W, May J. Basilic vein transposition. *Am J Surg.* 1982;143:254.)

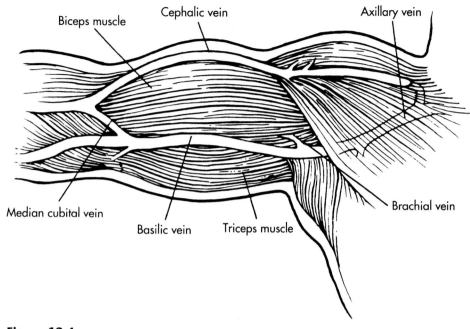

Figure 12-4.
The basilic vein has a constant location in the groove between the biceps and the triceps muscles. (From Criado E, Marston WA, Keagy BA. *Surg Rounds.* 1993;16:17.)

and anastomosed onto the superficial femoral artery. Contamination and infections are more frequent in the leg, and needle puncture is uncomfortable.[29] For these reasons, this technique is reserved for patients who have exhausted access in the upper extremities.

Use of Saphenous Vein for Interposition Grafts

Autogenous saphenous vein interposition grafts are used infrequently in the United States, but there is more experience with this technique in Australia, Europe, and

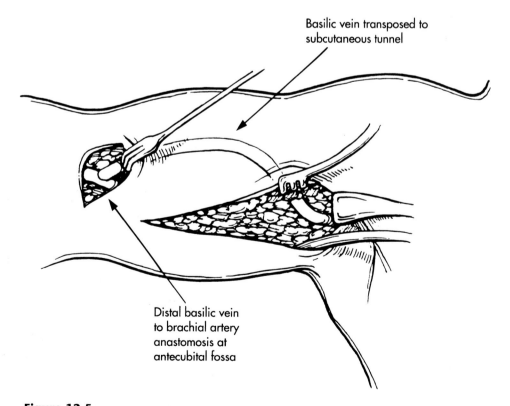

Figure 12-5.
Placement of the incisions and the subcutaneous tunnel, to which the basilic vein is transposed. (From Criado E, Marston WA, Heagy BA. *Surg Rounds.* 1993;16:17.)

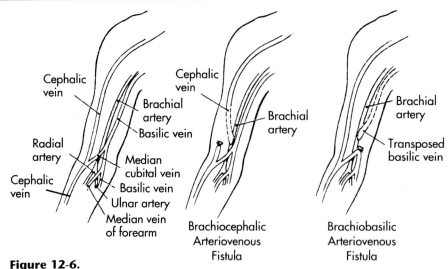

Figure 12-6.
Brachiocephalic and brachiobasilic fistulas in the upper arm. The brachiobasilic fistula requires mobilization and transposition of the vein to an accessible, subcutaneous plane. (From Cantelmo NL, Logerfo VW, Menzoian JO: Brachiobasilic and brachiocephalic fistulas as secondary angioaccess routes. *Surg Gynecol Obstet.* 1982;155:545.)

Japan. May and colleagues[29] first described this procedure in 1969 as a forearm loop fistula between the brachial vessels. Alternatively, the autogenous vein may also be used as a straight forearm graft, as an upper arm brachioaxillary conduit, or in the leg between the femoral vessels.[30-32]

Saphenous vein interposition grafts have a reported 70% 18-month patency and a long-term cumulative patency of 66% and 40% at 2 and 3 years, respectively.[33,34] Other studies published in the 1980s reported patency of 40% to 60% extending into the 5- to 8-year range.[31,35]

In contrast, others have found that these grafts are prone to thrombosis with technical difficulty and stenosis at the curvature of the graft playing an important role.[30,35]

The surgical technique involves one surgeon removing as atraumatically as possible an adequate length of vein from the thigh while a second surgeon exposes the relevant forearm artery (brachial or radial) and vein. The prepared saphenous vein is tunneled subcutaneously in the forearm or brachium in a looped or straight manner, and the ends are anastomosed end-to-side to the prepared artery and vein (Fig. 12-7). A period of 3 to 4 weeks of maturation is advantageous; an alternative temporary access technique is used during this interval.

In a large series of vascular access procedures in which the use of saphenous vein and polytetrafluoroethylene (PTFE) grafts were compared, May and associates[36] reported similar patency rates of approximately 70% at 18 months for each material. The prosthetic graft group, however, had significantly more secondary complications, with infection and distal ischemia being twice as common. Long-term cumulative patency rates of 66% at 2 years and 40% at 3 years were obtained with saphenous vein.[37] Other series have demonstrated similar satisfactory results;

Lornoy and coworkers[35] reported a cumulative patency rate of 58% at 5 years and 38% at 8 years for 20 patients with saphenous AV grafts in the arm, and Valenta and colleagues[31] achieved a cumulative patency rate of 62% at 6 years, with one graft still functional after more than 1000 dialyses over 10 years. In contrast, Haimov and associates[30] found that the forearm loop had a marked tendency to thrombosis, with only 7% of grafts patent at 24 months compared with 75% at the same interval for the straight vein graft. Technical factors such as the curvature of the graft may be important stenosis of a segment of graft, when it occurs, is often localized to the curve.[35]

Intraoperative measurement of blood flow through the graft has not proved to be useful as an indicator of long-term patency, and renal transplantation does not increase the occlusion rate.[37]

Stenosis may occur at needle puncture sites, causing decreased flow and high venous resistance during dialysis; it has been corrected with percutaneous balloon angioplasty[38] (Fig. 12-8) or replacement of the affected segment.[35] Infection is uncommon and is more easily treated than is infection of a prosthetic graft.[37]

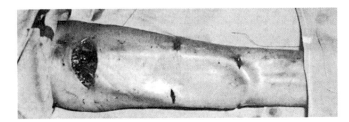

Figure 12-7.
Forearm saphenous vein loop anastomosed to the brachial artery and antecubital vein at the cubital fossa.

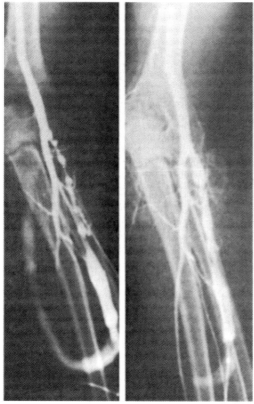

Figure 12-8.
Angiograms demonstrate multiple stenotic lesions within a forearm saphenous vein loop and the appearance after dilation by percutaneous, transluminal balloon angioplasty.

Conclusion

The relative failure of prosthetic graft materials to provide complication-free, long-term access in patients who require secondary procedures for hemodialysis has led to a reappraisal of their use.[39] There is a strong case for using the patient's own vessels wherever possible,[40] with AV prosthetic grafts being reserved until all convenient sites for direct autogenous fistula have been exhausted.[28] The conclusions of the 18-center Canadian Hemodialysis Morbidity Study group support this approach; they found that "the probability for hospitalization for any cause was greater for patients with grafts for vascular access than for those with fistulae."[41]

An autogenous fistula should be constructed whenever feasible for long-term access to hemodialysis for patients with end-stage renal disease. There are numerous autogenous options for delivering access through the forearm and brachium, which require ingenuity in design and adaptability to anatomic variations by the surgeon for each patient. Ideally, this access should be established well before, at least 3 months, the start of dialysis. Unfortunately, many patients are referred with a temporary catheter already in place or have significant upper extremity edema in part due to their impending need for dialysis. In addition, the multiple hospitalizations associated with comorbid conditions takes its toll on the superficial veins of the upper extremity that are

subjected to recurrent venipuncture. Prosthetic grafts should be reserved for those patients whose native vasculature or body habitus precludes construction of an autogenous access. Knowledge of the alternative techniques discussed in this section provides the access surgeon with a larger range of possibilities from which to choose an appropriate autogenous fistula for the individual patient.

REFERENCES

1. U.S. Renal Data System. 2008 *Annual Report: Atlas of Chronic Kidney Disease and End-Stage Renal Disease in the United States.* Bethesda, MD: National Institutes of Health, 2008. Available at http://www.usrds.org/.
2. Rayner HC, Pisoni RL, Brown WW, Disney A, Saito A, Pisoni RL. Vascular access results from the Dialysis Outcomes and Practice Patterns Study (DOPPS): performance against Kidney Disease Outcomes Quality Initiative (K/DOQI) Clinical Practice Guidelines. *Am J Kidney Dis.* 2004;44(5 suppl 2):22-26.
3. Pisoni RL, Young EW, Dykstra DM, et al. Vascular access use in Europe and the United States: results from the DOPPS. *Kidney Int.* 2002;61: 305-316.
4. O'Hare AM, Dudley RA, Hynes DM, et al. Impact of surgeon and surgical center characteristics on choice of permanent vascular access. *Kidney Int.* 2003;64:681-689.
5. Gibson KD, Gillen DL, Caps MT, Kohler TR, Sherrard DJ, Stehman-Breen CO. Vascular access survival and incidence of revisions: a comparison of prosthetic grafts, simple autogenous fistulas, and venous transposition fistulas from the United States Renal Data System Dialysis Morbidity and Mortality Study. *J Vasc Surg.* 2001;34:694-700
6. Wilson SE, Stabile BE, Williams RA, Owens ML. Current status of vascular access techniques. *Surg Clin North Am.* 1982;62:531-551.
7. Munda R, First MR, Alexander JW, Linnemann CC Jr, Fidler JP, Kittur D. Polytetrafluoroethylene graft survival in hemodialysis. *JAMA.* 1983; 249:219-222.
8. Fitzgerald JT, Schanzer A, Chin AI, McVicar JP, Perez RV, Troppmann C. Outcomes of upper arm arteriovenous fistulas for maintenance hemodialysis access. *Arch Surg.* 2004;139:201-208.
9. Guillou PJ, Levison SH, Kester RC. The complications of arteriovenous grafts for vascular access. *Br J Surg.* 1980;67:517.
10. Tellis VA, Kohlberg WI, Bhat DJ, Driscoll B, Veith FJ. Expanded polytetrafluoroethylene graft fistula for chronic haemodialysis. *Ann Surg.* 1979;189:101-105.
11. Bhat DJ, Tellis VA, Kohlberg WI, Driscoll B, Veith FJ. Management of sepsis involving expanded polytetrafluoroethylene grafts for hemodialysis. *Surgery.* 1980;87:445-450.
12. Bolton W, Cannon JA. Seroma formation associated with PTFE vascular grafts used as arteriovenous fistulae. *Dial Transplant.* 1981;10:60.
13. Mennes PA, Gilula LA, Anderson CB, Etheredge EE, Weerts C, Harter HR. Complications associated with arteriovenous fistulas in patients undergoing chronic hemodialysis. *Arch Intern Med.* 1978;138: 1117-1121.
14. Morgan AP, Knight DC, Tilney NL, Lazarus JM. Femoral triangle sepsis in dialysis patients: frequency, management, and outcome. *Ann Surg.* 1980;191:460-464.
15. Haimov M. Vascular access for hemodialysis. *Surg Gynecol Obstet.* 1975;141:619-625.
16. Wedgwood KR, Wiggins PA, Guillou PJ. A prospective study of end-to-side vs. side-to-side arteriovenous fistulas for haemodialysis. *Br J Surg.* 1984;61:640-642.
17. Mehigan JT, McAlexander RA. Snuffbox arteriovenous fistula for hemodialysis. *Am J Surg.* 1982;143:252-253.
18. Bogers AJ, Daatselaar DD, Rijksen JF. Anatomical snuffbox vs. radial styloid process as the location of choice for hemodialysis arteriovenous fistula: a retrospective analysis. *Vasc Surg.* 1985;19:405-407.
19. Harder F, Landmann J. Trends in access surgery for hemodialysis. *Surg Annu.* 1984;16:135-149.
20. Hanson JS, Carmody M, Keogh B, O'Dwyer WF. Access to circulation by permanent arteriovenous fistula in regular dialysis treatment. *Br Med J.* 1967;4:586-589.
21. Giacchino JL, Geis WP, Buckingham JM, Vertuno LL, Bansal VK. Vascular access: long-term results, new techniques. *Arch Surgl* 1979;114:403-409.

22. Geis WP, Giacchino JL, Iwatsuki S, Vaz AJ, Hano JE, Ing TS. The reverse fistula for vascular access. *Surg Gynecol Obstet.* 1977;145: 901-904.

23. Parvin SD, James MR, Veitch PS, Bell PR. Brachiodistal vein arteriovenous fistula with valve destruction as a secondary access procedure for haemodialysis. *Br J Surg.* 1984;71:323-324.

24. Jennings WC. Creating arteriovenous fistulas in 132 consecutive patients. Exploiting the proximal radial artery arteriovenous fistula: reliable, safe, and simple forearm and upper arm hemodialysis access. *Arch Surg.* 2006;141:27-32.

25. Choi HM, Lal BK, Cerveira JJ, et al. Durability and cumulative functional patency of transposed and nontransposed arteriovenous fistulas. *J Vasc Surg.* 2003;38:1206-1212

26. Patrick W, May J. Basilic vein transposition. *Am J Surg.* 1982;143:254.

27. Dagher F, Gelber R, Ramos E, Sadler J. The use of basilic vein and brachial artery as an A-V fistula for long-term hemodialysis. *J Surg Res.* 1976;20:373-376.

28. Cantelmo NL, LoGerfo FW, Menzoian JO. Brachiobasilic and brachiocephalic fistulas as secondary angioaccess routes. *Surg Gynecol Obstet.* 1982;155:545-548.

29. May J, Tiller D, Johnson J, Stewart J, Sheil AG. Saphenous-vein arteriovenous fistula in regular dialysis treatment. *N Engl J Med.* 1969;280:770.

30. Haimov M, Burrows L, Baez A, Neff M, Slifkin R. Alternatives for vascular access for hemodialysis: experience with autogenous saphenous vein autografts and bovine heterografts. *Surgery.* 1974;75:447-452.

31. Valenta J, Bílek J, Simána J, Opatrný K. [Secondary access routes for hemodialysis.] *Rozhl Chir.* 1989;68:42-48.

32. Hibbard AD. Brachiobasilic fistula with autogenous basilic vein: surgical technique and pilot study. *Aust N Z J Surg.* 1991;61:631-635.

33. May J, Harris J, Patrick W. Polytetrafluoroethylene (PTFE) grafts for haemodialysis: patency and complications compared with those of saphenous vein grafts. *Aust N Z J Surg.* 1979;49:639-642.

34. May J, Harris J, Fletcher J.: Long-term results of saphenous vein graft arteriovenous fistulas. *Am J Surg.* 1980;140:387-390.

35. Lornoy W, Becaus I, Gillardin JP, et al: Autogenous saphenous vein AV fistulae for haemodialysis: eight years' experience with 30 patients. *Proc Eur Dial Transplant Assoc.* 1983;19:227-233.

36. May J, Harris J, Patrick W. Polytetrafluoroethylene grafts for hemodialysis: patency and complications compared with those of saphenous vein grafts. *Aust N Z J Surg.* 1979;49:639-642.

37. May J, Harris J, Fletcher J. Long-term results of saphenous vein graft arteriovenous fistulas. *Am J Surg.* 1980;140:387-390.

38. Lawrence PF, Miller FJ, Mineaud E. Balloon catheter dilatation in patients with failing arteriovenous fistulas. *Surgery.* 1981;89:439-442.

39. Hamill FS, et al. A critical reappraisal of the changing approaches to vascular access for chronic hemodialysis. *Dial Transplant.* 1980; 9:325.

40. Reilly DT, Wood, RFM, Bell PRF. Prospective study of dialysis fistulas: problem patients and their treatment. *Br J Surg.* 1982;69:54-553.

41. Churchill DN, Taylor DW, Cook RJ, et al: Canadian Hemodialysis Morbidity Study. *Am J Kidney Dis.* 1992;19:214-234.

CHAPTER 13

Basilic Vein Transposition: A Modern Autogenous Vascular Access for Hemodialysis

Clarence E. Foster III and Merisa Piper

When comparing 1995 with 2005, the prevalence of end-stage renal disease (ERSD) in the United States increased 1.4 times.[1] This increase is expected to continue and is predicted to result in the cost of caring for patients with ESRD to escalate to $53 billion in the year 2020.[1] In the management of patients with ESRD, vascular access greatly influences both cost and morbidity.

It is well recognized that arteriovenous fistulas (AVFs) outperform arteriovenous grafts (AVGs) and central venous catheters when contrasting the morbidity and mortality results of vascular access choices.[2] Brachial artery–to–basilic vein arterial vein fistula (BBAVF) transposition is a suitable and superior alternative for vascular access when compared with AVG.[3] BBAVF transposition is a frequently overlooked method of arteriovenous (AV) access that has a superior patency in comparison with that of bridge fistulas using polytetrafluoroethylene (PTFE) (AVGs).[4,5] BBAVF was first described by Cascardo and associates[6] and Dagher and colleagues[7,8] in the 1970s. The fistula is composed of the deep basilic vein, which is mobilized to a more superficial position (*transposed*). The basilic vein is often pristine because it has not been accessible to routine venipuncture for peripheral access and phlebotomy. The construction of this AVF requires more dissection and time than do other access options. However, there are clear benefits to the use of the BBAVF transposition. The long-term patency is good, native fistulas have fewer complications than do artificial conduits, and the fistula can often be constructed in patients who are not otherwise candidates for bridge fistulas (AVGs). In addition, if the BBAVF transposition fails, the ipsilateral axillary vein is still available for construction of an upper arm AV graft between the brachial artery and the axillary vein, making this an important option in the progressive choices for vascular access, as advocated by Santoro and Cambria.[9]

Preoperative Evaluation

The basilic vein is a superficial vein in the medial forearm that extends to the wrist and, although often visible in thin patients, the course is deeper in the brachium (Fig. 13-1). Preoperative evaluation of the basilic vein requires a careful physical examination. In addition, preoperative vascular ultrasound or venography of the basilic vein has an important role in assessing the caliber and character of this vein as well as in the subsequent strategy as to whether the procedure will be staged or a single operation.[10]

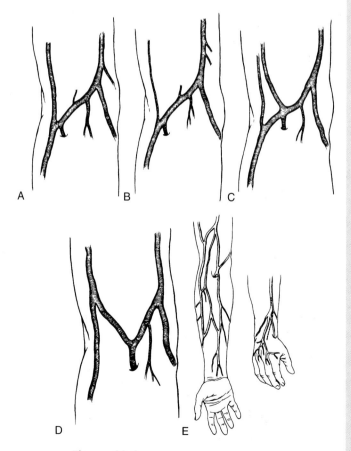

Figure 13-1.
A–E, Superficial venous anatomy of the arm.

Preoperative Evaluation and Operative Strategy

All patients should have a thorough evaluation of radial and brachial pulse bilaterally. Some patients are thin and the actual basilic vein can be visualized during this physical examination. Patients with a poor radial pulse or diabetes may be at risk for complications such as ischemia.[11] Accordingly, the arterial assessment in the patient is vital.

Every vascular access patient for whom BBAVF is considered should undergo preoperative duplex ultrasound vein mapping of the upper extremity. The preoperative upper arm vein mapping provides the diameter of the cephalic vein at the antecubital fossa and upper arm cephalic vein. The diameter of the brachial vein and artery at the antecubital fossa is also assessed. The basilic vein is also measured at the distal end near the median cubital vein and in the upper arm. If the patient does not have a suitable cephalic vein at the wrist for a Brescia-Cimino native AVF[12] or at the upper arm for a brachial artery–to–cephalic vein AVF, BBAVF transposition is considered.

A vein that measures 3 mm in diameter on preoperative ultrasound is considered suitable for fistula construction. Arroyo and coworkers[13] described the adequacy of the basilic vein of 2.5 to 4 mm on ultrasound. Patients who had a 2.5- to 4-mm basilic vein underwent a staged procedure to allow time for the vein to enlarge and arterialize before transposition. If the patient had a basilic vein of 4 mm, a single (nonstaged) basilic transposition was performed. Venography is another method for preoperative venous evaluation and is reserved for patients who have had multiple failed access procedures. In general, preoperative venography is unnecessary if any suitable veins are demonstrated on preoperative ultrasound duplex vein mapping.

Surgical Technique

At our institutions, the anesthetic of choice is a regional or local anesthetic agent with intravenous sedation. General anesthesia is also a suitable option if the patient cannot tolerate regional anesthesia. The operation as described by Dagher and colleagues in 1976[7,8] is still current. An incision is made longitudinally over the basilic vein just proximal to the antecubital fossa. In patients who have a vein too deep to visualize, a Doppler probe can be useful. The basilic vein is then mobilized from the median cubital vein to its junction with the upper brachial vein or axillary vein. Several counterincisions are recommended rather than one continuous incision because they are less disfiguring and wound healing is more consistent. Care must be taken to ligate venous tributaries to avoid postoperative bleeding. Some surgeons recommend suture ligature of the tributaries during the mobilization.[7,8] We carefully ligate branches with 3-0 or 4-0 silk ties and have had no problems with this technique. The forearm sensory nerves that cross the basilic vein should be preserved if possible. The medial brachial cutaneous nerves have a very predictable course and can be easily identified as they cross the basilic vein.[14]

Once the vein is fully mobilized, ligate and transect it distally and then flush with heparinized saline (Fig. 13-2). The transected mobilized vein can be used as a guide on the skin to mark the subcutaneous tunnel that will need to be

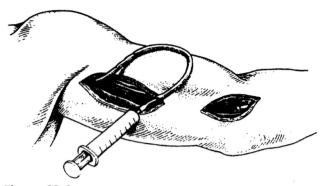

Figure 13-2.
The mobilized basilic vein is flushed with a heparin and saline solution.

anesthetized by infiltration of local anesthetic. The brachial artery is easily isolated through one of the incisions that have been used to mobilize the basilic vein by dividing the brachial fascia to expose the neurovascular bundle. Proximal and distal control of the artery can be achieved using silicone elastomer (Silastic) vessel loops or vascular clamps. Then create a subcutaneous tunnel using a blunt curved tunneling device as used for PTFE grafts (Fig. 13-3). Then pull the vein through the subcutaneous tunnel, with care taken not to twist or angulate the vein. Marking the vein before tunneling helps prevent torsion of the vein. The vein can also be distended with heparinized saline by occluding the outflow to ensure a smooth course within the tunnel. Then incise the distal vein on the dorsal aspect to create a hood for a spatulated anastomosis. Construct an end-to-side anastomosis in the standard manner with 6-0 or 7-0 monofilament nonabsorbable suture.

Results

Patency

Since the 1970s, multiple series have been published on basilic vein transposition (Table 13-1). The median primary patency rate at 12 months is 72% with a range of 35% to 92%, whereas the median secondary rate is 74.6% with a range of 55% to 96% (see Table 13-1).[15] Primary and secondary patency rates at 24 months are 60.4% (28%-86%)

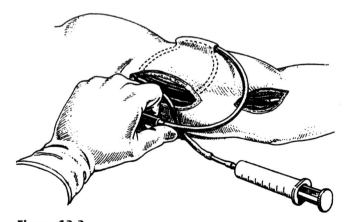

Figure 13-3.
A tunnel is made in the subcutaneous tissue of the brachium.

Table 13–1
Patency Rates and Complications of the Brachial-Basilic Arteriovenous Fistula

Author (yr)	Type of Study	N	Age (yr)	Male	Follow-up (mo)	Primary Patency	Secondary Patency
Dagher (1976)	Retrospective	24	44 (18-73)	13/23	8 (2-15)	92%	—
LoGerfo (1978)	Retrospective	25	—	—	12 (0-19)	85%	—
Barnett (1979)	Prospective nonrandomized	16	(24-83)	—	(0-9)	94%	—
Dagher (1980)	Retrospective	90	16-73	36/81	12 (0-60)	78%	—
Cantelmo (1982)	Retrospective	68	—	—	12	70%	—
					24	66%	—
					36	57.2%	—
Koontz (1983)	Retrospective	12	—	—	12 (1-34)	75%	—
Dagher (1986)	Retrospective	96	—	—		70%	—
Davis (1986)	Retrospective	66	—	—	? (0-24)	83.3%	—
Hibberd (1991)	Prospective nonrandomized	15	54 (43-67)	1/15	12	70%	—
					24	50%	—
Hatjibaloglou (1992)	Retrospective	25	(32-69)	4/22	12 (7-24)	81%	—
Rivers (1993)	Retrospective	65	(10-77)	25/65	12	—	55%
					30	—	49%
Elcheroth (1994)	Retrospective	80	(17-87)	—	12	76.7%	—
					48	49.2	
Coburn (1994)	Retrospective	59	64	30/59	12	90%	90%
					24	86%	86%
Stonebridge (1995)	Retrospective	19	54 (28-73)	—	16 (4-41)	79%	—
El Mallah (1998)	Prospective randomized	40	35	23/40	15 (6-24)	50% IS	—
						80% 2S	—
Butterworth (1998)	Retrospective	23	60 (32-77)	10/30	8 (2-18)	78.3%	
Hakaim (1998)	Retrospective	26	59 (35-85)	16/26	18	79%	—
Matsuura (1998)	Retrospective	30	59	14/30	24	70%	70%
Humphries (1999)	Retrospective	67	(11-73)	33/66	12	84%	—
					36	73%	—
					60	73%	—
					120	52%	—
Murphy (2000)	Retrospective	74	61 (24-94)	29/65	12	—	73%
					24	—	53%
					36	—	43%
Gibson (2001)	Retrospective	181	66	96/181	12	44%	68%
					24	28%	60%
Dahduli (2002)	Retrospective	16	(25-85)		6	85%	
Murphy (2002)	Retrospective	74	60 (14-94)	—	12	68%	75%
				—	24	54%	60%
					36	44%	46%
Tsai (2002)	Prospective	54	61 (31-80)		12	90%	96%
				23/54	24	73%	85%
					36	65%	77%
Hossny (2003)	Retrospective	70	49 (16-98)		26 (4-36)		
	30 TD			27/70	12	—	87%
					24	—	83%
	20 1SE				12	—	90%
					24	—	70%
	20 2SE				12	—	84%
					24	—	68%
Segal (2003)	Retrospective	99	55		12	47%	64%
				46/99	24	41%	58%
Taghizadeh (2003)	Retrospective	75	49 (6-77)		12	92%	66%
				—	24	—	52%
					36	—	43%
Rao (2004)	Retrospective	56	56	30/56	12	35%	47%

TD, transposed; ISE, one-stage elevation; 2SE, two-stage elevation; —, not stated.

Reprinted from the European Journal of Vascular and Endovascular Surgery, Vol. 31, F. P. Dix, Y. Khan, and H. Al-Khaffaf, "The Brachial Artery-Basilic Vein Arterio-Venous Fistula in Vascular Access for Haemodialysis: A Review Paper," p. 74, Jan. (2006), with permission from Elsevier.

and 67.5% (52%-86%), respectively. A study performed by Coburn and Carney[5] compared BBAVF and PTFE grafts, reporting superior primary patency rates at 1 and 2 years for BBAVF (90% and 86%) compared with PTFE (70% and 49%). PTFE grafts have more complications (17% vs. 43%), a higher thrombosis rate (51% vs. 30%), and a higher infection rate (10% vs. 0%).[5,16] Patency at 3 years with PTFE ranges from 50% to 70%.[9]

Hossny[17] evaluated three surgical techniques for superficialization of BBAVFs, including transposition, elevation in one stage, and elevation in two stages of the basilic vein. Secondary patency rates at 1 year (87%, 90%, and 84%) and 2 years (83%, 70%, and 68%) of the transposed, one-stage elevated, and two-stage elevated indicate that transposition may be the best approach, but further studies are warranted. El Mallah[18] evaluated a one-stage versus a two-stage BBAVF procedure in a randomized trial of 40 patients and found primary patency rates at a median of 15 months to be 50% (one stage) and 80% (two stage), suggesting that a staged procedure is beneficial.

Complications

All fistula techniques have complications, including BBAVFs, and certain patient characteristics are associated with more problems and poorer outcomes. Older age, obesity, ipsilateral central venous catheterization, gender, and previous vascular access have been reported as significant factors in access failure by several studies.[19–25] Recognized complications of BBAVF include failure of the fistula to mature,[26] inability to create the fistula,[4,5,27,28] thrombosis (9.7% of patients),[15,17,27–29] bleeding (observed in 3.8% of patients),[15] infection (rate of 3.6%),[15] edema of the forearm and hand (frequently underreported, although a common symptom),[17,27,28,30] steal syndrome (observed in 2.9% of patients),[4,5,15,29,31,32] stenosis (2.3% of patients),[4,15,29,32] and pseudoaneurysm (rate of 1.9%).[15] Other complications that may be observed include pain (not frequently indicated, thus likely not a significant problem), distal embolization (very rare),[31] high-output cardiac failure (high mortality rate but uncommon), ischemic neuropathy (very rare),[33] peripheral nerve compression,[34,35] and lymphatic leak.[17,32,36]

▆ Conclusion

Vascular access for hemodialysis becomes increasingly challenging as patients survive for longer periods on dialysis. To maximize benefit to these patients, surgeons must offer many different access options. The BBAVF transposition allows for the creation of a native fistula while preserving deep brachial venous systems for subsequent placement of forearm or upper arm PTFE AVGs. The patency of the BBAVF transposition is not as high as that of the Brescia-Cimino fistula,[12] which should still be considered the "gold standard" of access. The reported 1-year patency rate is reported to be 60% to 90%. However, patency is sufficiently high to place this type of access before the placement of any prosthetics in the arm because the axillary vein is preserved for subsequent PTFE upper arm graft placement. This access can be used as the initial access procedure in up to 25% of patients.[4]

Recently, several studies have been published that present technical modifications on BBAVF in order to minimize complications. Kapala and associates[37] proposed a modified technique of BBAVF transposition by transecting the vein at its widest point, thus minimizing stenosis, axial torsion, and kinking. Several groups have described endoscopic techniques that result in faster healing times, fewer infections, minimal scarring, and minimal complications.[38–40] Tordoir and colleagues[40] described a video-assisted, minimally invasive endoscopic dissection in which all AVFs could be used successfully with no wound complications.

BBAVF transposition is an important option in the sequential use of different access configurations to maximize the duration of functional hemodialysis access and combat the dilemma of the patient who has no access options remaining. BBAVF is also an excellent option as the initial vascular access for patients who do not have a superficial vein available for an AVF.

REFERENCES

1. U.S. Renal Data System. *2007 Annual Data Report: Atlas of Chronic Kidney Disease and End-Stage Renal Disease in the United States.* Bethesda, MD: National Institutes of Health, 2007. Available at http://www.usrds.org/.
2. Dhingra RK, Young EW, Hulbert-Shearon TE, Leavey SF, Port FK. Type of vascular access and mortality in U.S. hemodialysis patients. *Kidney Int.* 2001;60:1443-1451.
3. Moossavi S, Tuttle AB, Vachharajani TJ, et al. Long-term outcomes of transposed basilic vein arteriovenous fistulae. *Hemodial Int.* 2008;12:80-84.
4. Rivers SP, Scher LA, Sheehan E, Lynn R, Veith FJ. Basilic vein transposition: an underused autologous alternative to prosthetic dialysis angioaccess. *J Vasc Surg.* 1993;18:391-396.
5. Coburn MC, Carney WI. Comparison of basilic vein and polytetrafluoroethylene for brachial arteriovenous fistula. *J Vasc Surg.* 1994;20:896-904.
6. Cascardo S, Acchiardo S, Beven EG, et al. Proximal arteriovenous fistulae for hemodialysis when radial arteries are not available. *Proc Eur Dial Transpl Assoc.* 1970;7:42-46.
7. Dagher F, Gelber R, Ramos E, Sadler J. The use of basilic vein and brachial artery as an A-V fistula for long-term hemodialysis. *J Surg Res.* 1976;20:373-376.
8. Dagher FJ, Gelber GL, Ramos EJ, Sadler JH. Basilic vein to brachial artery fistula: a new access for chronic hemodialysis. *South Med J.* 1976;69:1438-1440.
9. Santoro TD, Cambria RA. PTFE shunts for hemodialysis access: progressive choice of configuration. *Semin Vasc Surg.* 1997;10:166-174.
10. Pasch AR. A two-staged technique for basilic vein transposition. *J Vasc Access.* 2007;8:225-227.
11. Dagher FJ. The upper arm AV hemoaccess: long term follow-up. *J Cardiovasc Surg (Torino).* 1986;27:447-449.
12. Brescia MJ, Cimino JE, Appel K, Hurwich BJ. Chronic hemodialysis using venipuncture and a surgically created arteriovenous fistula. *N Engl J Med.* 1966;275:1089-1092.
13. Arroyo MR, Sideman MJ, Spergel L, Jennings WC. Primary and staged transposition arteriovenous fistulas. *J Vasc Surg.* 2008;47:1279-1283.
14. Race CM, Saldana MJ. Anatomic course of the medial cutaneous nerves of the arm. *J Hand Surg Am.* 1991;16:48-52.
15. Dix FP, Khan Y, al-Khaffaf H. The brachial artery–basilic vein arteriovenous fistula in vascular access for haemodialysis: a review paper. *Eur J Vasc Endovasc Surg.* 2006;31:70-79.
16. Matsuura JH, Rosenthal D, Clark M, et al. Transposed basilic vein versus polytetrafluoroethylene for brachial-axillary arteriovenous fistulas. *Am J Surg.* 1998;176:219-221.
17. Hossny A. Brachiobasilic arteriovenous fistula: different surgical techniques and their effects on fistula patency and dialysis-related complications. *J Vasc Surg.* 2003;37:821-826.
18. El Mallah S. Staged vasilic vein transposition for dialysis angioaccess. *Int Angiol.* 1998;17:65-68.

19. Gibson KD, Caps MT, Gillen DL, Bergelin RO, Primozich J, Strandness DE Jr. Identification of factors predictive of lower extremity vein graft thrombosis. *J Vasc Surg.* 2001;33:24-31.

20. Gibson KD, Caps MT, Kohler TR, et al. Assessment of a policy to reduce placement of prosthetic hemodialysis access. *Kidney Int,* 2001; 59:2335-2345

21. Gibson KD, Gillen DL, Caps MT, Kohler TR, Sherrard DJ, Stehman-Breen CO. Vascular access survival and incidence of revisions: a comparison of prosthetic grafts, simple autogenous fistulas, and venous transposition fistulas from the United States Renal Data System Dialysis Morbidity and Mortality Study. *J Vasc Surg.* 2001;34:694-700.

22. Gibson KD, Stehman-Breen CO, Kohler TR. Use of the vascular diagnostic laboratory in improving the success of angioaccess procedures. *Semin Vasc Surg.* 2001;14:222-226.

23. Woods JD, Port FK. The impact of vascular access for haemodialysis on patient morbidity and mortality. *Nephrol Dial Transplant.* 1997; 12:657-659.

24. Woods JD, Turenne MN, Strawderman RL, et al. Vascular access survival among incident hemodialysis patients in the United States. *Am J Kidney Dis.* 1997;30:50-57.

25. Segal JH, Weitzel WF. Monitoring techniques of vascular access. *Contrib Nephrol.* 2004;142:216-227.

26. Rao RK, Azin GD, Hood DB, et al. Basilic vein transposition fistula: a good option for maintaining hemodialysis access site options? *J Vasc Surg.* 2004;39:1043-1047.

27. Murphy GJ, White SA, Knight AJ, Doughman T, Nicholson ML. Long-term results of arteriovenous fistulas using transposed autologous basilic vein. *Br J Surg.* 2000;87:819-823.

28. Murphy GJ, White SA, Nicholson ML. Vascular access for haemodialysis. *Br J Surg.* 2000;87:1300-1315.

29. Taghizadeh A, Dasgupta P, Khan MS, Taylor J, Koffman G. Long-term outcomes of brachiobasilic transposition fistula for haemodialysis. *Eur J Vasc Endovasc Surg.* 2003;26:670-672.

30. Dagher FJ. Upper arm arteriovenous fistula for chronic hemodialysis: 20 years later. *Transplant Proc.* 1996;28:2325-2327.

31. Dagher FJ, Gelber RL, Reed W. Basilic vein to brachial artery, arteriovenous fistula for long-term hemodialysis: a five year follow-up. *Proc Clin Dial Transplant Forum.* 1980;10:126-129.

32. Butterworth PC Doughman TM, Wheatley TJ, Nicholson ML. Arteriovenous fistula using transposed basilic vein. *Br J Surg.* 1998;85: 653-654.

33. Riggs JEM, Moss AHM, Labosky DAM, Liput JH, Morgan JJ, Gutmann L. Upper extremity ischemic monomelic neuropathy: a complication of vascular access procedures in uremic diabetic patients. *Neurology.* 1989;39:997-998.

34. Barnett SM, Waters WC 3rd, Lowance DC, Rosenbaum BJ. The basilic vein fistula for vascular access. *Trans Am Soc Artif Intern Organs.* 1979; 25:344-346.

35. Reinstein L, Reed WP, Sadler JH, Baugher WH. Peripheral nerve compression by brachial artery–basilic vein vascular access in long-term hemodialysis. *Arch Phys Med Rehabil.* 1984;65:142-144.

36. Tsai YT, Lin SH, Lee GC, Huen GG, Lin YF, Tsai CS. Arteriovenous fistula using transposed basilic vein in chronic hypotensive hemodialysis patients. *Clin Nephrol.* 2002;57:376-380.

37. Kapala A, Szmytkowski J, Stankiewicz W, Dabrowiecki S. A modified technique of delayed basilic transposition—initial results. *Eur J Vasc Endovasc Surg.* 2006;32:316-317.

38. Hayakawa K, Tsuha M, Aoyagi T, et al. New method to create a vascular arteriovenous fistula in the arm with an endoscopic technique. *J Vasc Surg.* 2002;36:635-638.

39. Martinez BD, LeSar CJ, Fogarty TJ, Zarins CK, Hermann G. Transposition of the basilic vein for arteriovenous fistula: an endoscopic approach. *J Am Coll Surg.* 2001;192:233-236.

40. Tordoir JHM, Dammers R, de Brauw M. Video-assisted basilic vein transposition for haemodialysis vascular access: preliminary experience with a new technique. *Nephrol Dial Transplant.* 2001;16:391-394.

CHAPTER 14

Interposition Arteriovenous Grafts (Bridge Fistulas) for Hemodialysis

Samuel Eric Wilson

The patient who has end-stage renal disease will outlive the usefulness of several arteriovenous (AV) fistulas during successful long-term management of chronic renal failure by hemodialysis. Owing to the simplicity of construction, relative freedom from complications, and long life, the autogenous radiocephalic or brachiocephalic fistula remains the first choice for long-term dialysis.[1] The National Kidney Foundation's initiative and the Society for Vascular Surgery have reaffirmed the role of the autogenous AV fistula as the preferred access for hemodialysis.

For a number of sound reasons, fistulas constructed from vascular grafts provide the best second choice for the patient who cannot have a simple autogenous fistula. Prosthetic conduits can be placed from almost any artery to any vein of sufficient size to permit an anastomosis and are readily available "off the shelf" in various lengths, diameters, and configurations.[2] Fistulas constructed from polytetrafluoroethylene (PTFE) are tunneled subcutaneously and easily located for puncture for hemodialysis. With care, early use (within 24 hr) can be accomplished without a higher incidence of complications, so it is technically possible to use the graft for dialysis soon after surgery, thus avoiding the complications of central venous catheters.[3,4]

Most bridge fistulas are established through anastomosis of a prosthetic graft end-to-side to an artery and end-to-side to a vein. In between, the graft runs subcutaneously and allows a 10- to 15-cm span for dialysis access. If the anastomotic sites to the artery and vein are close together, the result is a *loop fistula*, sometimes called a *U fistula*. If the anastomotic sites are some distance apart and most of the length of the graft is used in reaching from artery to vein, the result is a *straight, or slightly curved, bridge graft*. The literature is divided on which configuration stays open longer.[4–8] The differences in results, however, have more to do with venous outflow occlusion, technical problems such as kinking, or the size of the vessels that provide the arterial inflow and venous run-off than with differences relating to graft configuration.

Site

The 1-year actuarial secondary patency rate for bridge fistulas is approximately 70%, with the upper extremity by far the preferred site.[9–11] Nevertheless, several authors have described better patency with bridge fistulas placed in the thigh.[4,11–14] In our experience, this finding was explained by the larger vessels and greater blood flows available in the thigh. The lower incidence of thrombosis in femorosaphenous fistulas, however, is outweighed by the greater infection rate for bridge fistulas placed in the thigh compared with those in the arm. Urinary or fecal incontinence is a relative contraindication because these conditions magnify the risk of infection. Lower extremity AV grafts do leave the patient free to use both hands during dialysis—possibly desirable in those few patients who are on home dialysis. Upper extremity fistulas should be constructed in elderly patients with significant arterial atherosclerosis in the lower extremities and in obese patients in whom perspiration or dermatitis involving the groin folds may increase the likelihood of infection. Some patients express concern that an AV graft in the inner thigh may interfere with sexual function. Overall, over 90% of AV grafts are placed in the arm.

The most advantageous site for a prosthetic AV fistula is the upper arm, using the distal brachial artery for inflow and the proximal brachial or axillary vein for outflow. Several subsequent grafts can be placed in this configuration progressing proximally to the subclavian vein for outflow sites. In the patient older than 65 years, a PTFE graft in the brachioaxillary position has patency equivalent to that of the transposed autogenous AV fistula. Although radial artery–to–antecubital vein interposition grafts are feasible, the surgeon should first evaluate the outflow vein for construction of a brachiocephalic AV fistula.

Graft Materials

Of the many graft materials evaluated for hemodialysis, none is perfect, and modification of existing prosthetics occurs regularly.[15,16] Bovine carotid artery heterografts and expanded PTFE grafts have equivalent 1-year secondary patency rates of approximately 70%.[9–11] Some surgeons consider PTFE more durable and less likely to require reoperation than biologic materials. PTFE is the most commonly used material in the construction of bridge fistulas. At Brigham and Women's Hospital in Boston, Palder and associates[17] found the 3-year patency rate for PTFE to be from 70% to 80%. Results with PTFE exceed by about 15% the patency rates with transposed saphenous vein (Fig. 14-1). Results with external polyethylene terephthalate (Dacron) velour grafts have been encouraging but are

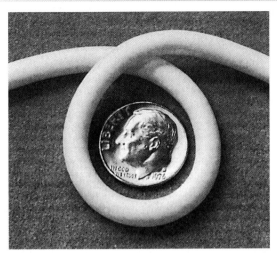

Figure 14-1.
Expanded polytetrafluoroethylene (PTFE), the most commonly used prosthetic material for vascular access surgery, has many advantages: it comes in various diameters, and it is microporous, flexible, easily packaged and stored, and able to withstand repeated needle punctures. (Courtesy Impra, Tempe, AZ.)

limited to a few reports; the grafts are more resistant to needle puncture than are PTFE grafts.[18–20] Human umbilical veins were introduced as another alternative for the bridge fistula.[21] If infection occurs, bacterial enzymes rapidly dissolve the biologic grafts, which are mainly composed of collagen, resulting in early hemorrhage. Synthetic grafts do not break down with infection, although this advantage is small if infection occurs at the anastomotic site where the native vessels may dissolve and bleed. Cryopreserved human saphenous vein grafts have been used in patients with infection, with reported primary and secondary patency rates of 49% and 75%, respectively.[21] PTFE has also been modified to allow fast sealing after removal of the large-bore dialysis needle. Clearly, this characteristic would be valuable in facilitating early puncture after implantation.

Size of Graft

The diameter of the graft in a prosthetic bridge fistula is usually considerably greater than that of the supply artery, so neither the diameter nor the length of the graft material chosen has significant effects on fistula flow (see Chapter 5). Rather, the diameter of the vein and upstream resistance are more important in determining graft flow. Grafts that are 6 mm in diameter usually provide good arterial inflow with few side effects. When choosing a graft, remember that the longer the graft, the larger the diameter necessary to achieve the same flow. This follows naturally from Poiseuille's law. It is interesting to consider why grafts of the same diameter under certain circumstances produce similar flows whether attached to small arm vessels or much larger leg vessels. In the arm, the ratio of the diameter of the graft to the supply artery is large and flow is maximal; in the leg, the ratio is smaller and the graft diameter may offer significant resistance. In the arm, the graft is shorter than in the leg, and resistance due to length is decreased. In brief, the commonly used lengths and diameters limit flow when attached to the larger leg vessels but do not restrict flow when attached to the smaller arm vessels. The result is similar flows from feeding vessels of dissimilar sizes.

Precautions

Thrombosis is best avoided by creating large, oblique or cobra-head venous anastomoses that allow some later narrowing without decreasing flow (Fig. 14-2). Equally important, care must be taken to avoid twisting or kinking of the graft as it is passed through the subcutaneous tunnel or angles to pass from the subcutaneous plane to deeper lying vessels.

Distal ischemia occurs secondary to steal in both the upper[22,23] and the lower[24] extremity as an uncommon complication. On theoretical grounds, fistula resistance is determined by vessel size and graft diameter and length. However, distal tissue perfusion also may be importantly affected by occlusive disease in the proximal artery (eg, common femoral or subclavian artery stenosis), the arterial collaterals (eg, profunda femoris), and the distal vascular bed (eg, popliteal trifurcation or radial and ulnar arteries). If atherosclerosis makes distal perfusion a concern or if collateral arterial inflow is deficient, as occurs in patients with diabetes mellitus, segmental blood pressure, Doppler imaging, or arteriography may be helpful in planning a safe procedure. The "steal" phenomenon is discussed at length in Chapter 22.

An infected graft that causes bacteremia is best removed before attempting to establish another prosthetic AV fistula at another site in the patient. This seems to be the safer course even if the infected fistula can still be used for dialysis and the patient is being treated with antibiotics. The worry is that a critical inoculation of bacteria may enter the bloodstream to contaminate the second graft. Removal of the infected graft will reduce the inoculum of bacteria not only associated with the graft but also on the skin surface. A second graft can probably be implanted safely if the infection is limited to a needle puncture site. *Staphylococcus*

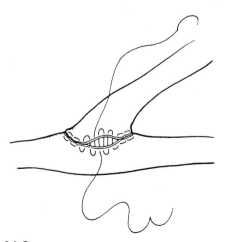

Figure 14-2.
One method of suturing the end of a PTFE graft to the side of an artery, using an everted anastomosis. Note the S-shaped end of the graft. (From Welch GH, Leiberman DP. A modified anastomosis suturing technique for arterial anastomoses with expanded PTFE. *Br J Surg.* 1985;72:498.)

aureus bacteremia should be treated early with antibiotics effective against methicillin-resistant organisms. *S. aureus* bacteremia can cause secondary infections such as endocarditis and metastatic abscess, and antimicrobials are often continued for several weeks.

When graft infection involves the anastomotic site, removal of the graft and repair of the anastomotic site by direct suture is preferable, but in very few advanced infections, it may be necessary to ligate the artery and, sometimes, the vein proximally and distally. If the graft has been anastomosed to the brachial or common femoral arteries where they bifurcate, in unusual circumstances of advanced infection, multivessel ligations may be necessary and distal ischemia is likely. If possible, the surgeon should anticipate this eventuality and attach the graft to an arterial site where ligation is less likely to produce ischemic changes. This precaution is one strong reason to prefer upper extremity sites.

Operations

In the majority of patients, vascular access intervention is done on an outpatient basis.[25] Preoperative testing is kept to a minimum (hematocrit, serum potassium, and electrocardiogram). An access site can usually be established, with the patient recovered and discharged within 4 to 6 hours.

Radial Artery–to–Antecubital Vein Prosthetic Fistula

When the radiocephalic autogenous fistula at the wrist fails or the veins of the forearm are inadequate for the construction of a radiocephalic AV fistula, a prosthesis positioned between the radial artery or brachial artery and an antecubital vein is a consideration for vascular access but still the second choice after an autogenous fistula (Fig. 14-3). The prosthetic forearm AV graft may be used when the radial or brachial artery is patent but there are no satisfactory superficial veins for an AV fistula and a deeper vein is located in the antecubital fossa. I select the upper extremity because of the unlikely incidence of infection, the low risk of hemodynamic complications leading to arterial insufficiency or loss of the extremity, and the ease with which this technique can be performed under local infiltration anesthesia or axillary block. In comparison, the radiocephalic bridge fistula is more technically demanding to construct than the upper arm or thigh fistula, and in our experience, the long-term patency rate is somewhat less than that for the brachioaxillary, femorosaphenous, or femorofemoral AV graft.

My choice of material for the forearm is PTFE because a 6-mm graft fits nicely in this location without kinking, the flow is sufficient for hemodialysis, and PTFE is relatively nonthrombogenic. In the radiocephalic position, I prefer a graft with a diameter of 6 mm, but in a female patient or a patient with small vessels, one may have to use a more proximal arterial site. The likelihood of long-term patency with smaller-diameter grafts is poor, and a small diameter presents a more difficult problem in accurate needle puncture for the hemodialysis staff.

Before surgery, examine the patient's upper extremity is examined and carefully select the positioning of the graft (Figs. 14-4 and 14-5). Palpation of a strong radial pulse is sufficient evidence that the graft will have a successful arterial inflow. An Allen test is performed to ensure adequacy of collateral inflow via the ulnar artery. Even when a radiocephalic AV fistula has failed, the graft can easily originate from the radial artery just proximal to the site of the AV anastomosis. The adequacy of venous run-off is of critical importance; therefore, the antecubital fossa is carefully examined by observation after application of a tourniquet and ultrasound imaging before surgery. My practice is to

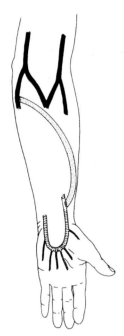

Figure 14-3.
Straight radiobasilic fistula. Any of the antecubital veins may be used for venous anastomosis.

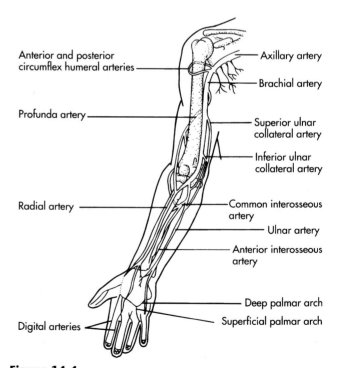

Figure 14-4.
Anatomy of arteries of the arm. (From Snell RS. *Clinical Anatomy for Medical Students.* 2nd ed. Boston: Little, Brown; 1981.)

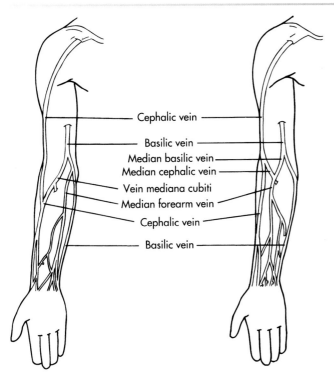

Figure 14-5.
Anatomy of veins of the arm commonly used for vascular access. (From Hollinshead WH. *Anatomy for Surgeons.* Vol 3. 3rd ed. New York: Harper & Row; 1982; with permission of Lippincott-Raven.)

abandon the procedure if a satisfactory vein for anastomosis of the graft cannot be identified; it is often possible to identify a suitably large basilic or brachial vein just distal to the flexion crease at the elbow for insertion of the graft. Doppler ultrasound is routinely used in identifying a suitable vein if doubt remains after a careful physical examination. Forearm grafts do not preclude and indeed may enhance later transposition of the basilic vein in the brachium. If I am unable to find a vein, rather than explore in the hope that a patent vein might be located deep in the subcutaneous tissue, I much prefer to perform another type of AV fistula. Nothing is more demoralizing for the chronic hemodialysis patient than to undergo multiple unsuccessful procedures for vascular access. Indeed, the surgeon who performs fruitless explorations for vessels will soon find that the nephrologists are referring patients to another practitioner.

Technique

Anesthesia is readily obtained by infiltration of 0.5% or 1.0% lidocaine without epinephrine into the area of the volar surface of the distal forearm overlying the course of the radial artery. An axillary block is also a useful method of anesthesia. Both patient and surgeon benefit from standby monitoring by anesthesia personnel. Make a longitudinal incision over the radial artery about 3 cm proximal to the flexion crease of the wrist. Deepen this incision until the radial artery is identified, with care taken to avoid injury to the superficial branch of the radial nerve, which may be identified at this point in dissection. Then mobilize

the artery from the surrounding tissue for a distance of about 2 to 3 cm and isolated with soft silicone elastomer (Silastic) sling. Topical papaverine applied in drops to the surface of the artery will help avert vasospasm. Divide very small side branches, invariably paired, with a quick touch of cautery.

Identify the site of venous anastomosis, having been previously marked, in the antecubital fossa and dissected without the aid of a tourniquet. Careful dissection of the deep brachial veins is required to avoid troublesome bleeding. Make a subcutaneous tunnel along the lateral aspect of the forearm. Make a small 1-cm transverse incision midway between the two incisions so that the graft, when it lies in the tunnel, may be inspected for kinking and tautness. I emphasize the importance of *carrying the graft along the lateral rather than the medial aspect of the forearm.* During dialysis, it is tiresome for the patient to maintain the arm in the position of external rotation necessary for needle puncture of a more medially placed graft.

I often administer 2500 to 3000 units of heparin intravenously to prevent clotting of the blood that enters the prosthesis, but this precaution is not a necessity. After first testing the pressure of the clamp jaws on the dorsum of the surgeon's gloved hand, occlude the radial artery with bulldog clamps. Make an incision in the artery with a No. 11 blade scalpel and tailor it to fit the graft with Potts-Smith or iris scissors.

At this point, the artery may be in spasm, but careful dilation with coronary artery dilators will ensure a lumen of 3 to 4 mm with which to work. If dilation of the artery is not graded slowly with successively larger dilators, the arteriotomy incision may be torn. Trim the vascular graft to size and sutured it to the radial artery with a continuous suture of 5-0 or 6-0 polypropylene or other cardiovascular suture. The graft is not filled with blood after the completion of anastomosis, but place a clamp across the graft near its origin from the radial artery and remove the vascular clamps so that flow is restored to the hand. Now advance the graft through the tunnel, bring it out midway through the small incision, and pass it again to the antecubital fossa. A graft tunneler, such as the Kelly-Wick, is a useful device here. Again bevel the graft, make a venotomy, and complete the anastomosis, again using 5-0 or 6-0 polypropylene suture. Before the last two stitches are inserted, bleed air from the graft by removing the proximal clamp, and flush out any clots that may have formed.

The surgeon now ascertains patency of the vascular construction. With completion of the anastomosis, flow should be apparent through the graft by palpation of a thrill. The pulse at the radial end of the graft should be strong, whereas the pulse at the proximal end will seem weak or absent. This phenomenon should not be a cause for concern because it simply reflects the decrease in pressure as the arterial blood pressure is dissipated into the low-resistance venous system. With partial occlusion of the venous anastomosis, however, the surgeon should be able to distinctly feel a thrill, and with complete occlusion, the pulse is augmented. This is routinely appreciated with practice and is the one reliable physical sign of a well-constructed prosthetic AV fistula. Bleeding from the anastomosis is generally not a problem and is best controlled with pressure. The incisions are closed in two layers, using 4-0 polyglycolic acid (Dexon) suture for the subcutaneous tissue and subcuticular 4-0 Dexon suture for the skin.

Brachial Artery–to–Antecubital Prosthetic Fistula

If it is not possible to use the radial artery for the inflow to a forearm prosthesis, usually because of small size, the next best option is the brachial artery in the antecubital fossa just before it divides into its radial and ulnar branches (Fig. 14-6). Place the incision for this exposure transversely across the antecubital fossa. Identify the brachial artery as it lies just lateral to the brachial tendon. A basilic or deeper brachial vein is satisfactory for the loop fistula. If a patent cephalic vein is greater than 3 mm in diameter, consider a direct end of cephalic vein–to–side of brachial artery autogenous fistula. Again, using local infiltration with 0.5% lidocaine, dissect the tunnel in a U configuration over the forearm. A small 1-cm incision placed about two thirds of the distance between the elbow and the wrist will serve for accurate positioning of the graft. Passing the graft through the tunnel is somewhat more difficult for the loop fistula than it is for a straight graft. In fact, kinking of the graft is a possibility in the apex of the loop. If the tunnel is made sufficiently wide at the U-turn, on distention of the graft with arterial inflow, the kink will usually disappear. Some PTFE grafts are specially constructed to have a center segment externally supported with a spiral ring structure that smoothes the U-turn. Now construct the anastomosis to the vein. Flow through the brachiobasilic loop fistula is usually higher than that for the straight radiobasilic bridge fistula, and a vascular thrill is palpated by the surgeon at the completion of the procedure.

After surgery, no heparin is administered to the patient, and the wound is inspected routinely over the next few postoperative days by dialysis personnel. At this time, in a few patients, one may see some local erythema overlying the graft tunnel. Although I generally treat these patients for suspected cellulitis, in most of the cases, this is not documented on bacteriologic examination, and the cellulitis may be a reaction to the prosthetic material. Although dialysis may be successful within the first 24 hours after implantation, care must be taken with the first needle punctures to avoid perigraft hematoma and thrombosis with proper dialysis technique. Safe use of PTFE grafts within the first 72 postoperative hours has been reported.[26]

Brachioaxillary Prosthetic Fistula (R. Ozeran, MD)

Upper extremity fistulas are particularly well suited for elderly patients who have significant peripheral vascular disease in the lower extremities or who have no antecubital veins. The brachioaxillary prosthetic fistula seems well adapted to these situations and has allowed the fistula to be used within a few days of construction, eliminating the need for a central catheter in patients who require urgent hemodialysis. Further, Cinat and colleagues[24] reported that brachioaxillary AV bridge grafts have a significantly longer patency than do forearm grafts. A comparison of indications for the transposed basilic vein fistula versus the brachioaxillary graft is shown in Table 14-1.

Technique

The fistula is constructed between the brachial artery and the axillary vein (Fig. 14-7). The procedure usually is performed on an outpatient basis with the patient under general anesthesia, but it may be performed using a local or regional block if the condition of the patient so requires.

Make a transverse or longitudinal incision in the low axilla (Fig. 14-8) and carry it down to the axillary vein. The

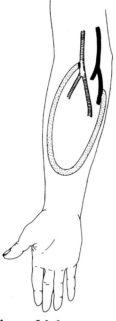

Figure 14-6.
Loop brachiobasilic fistula.

Table 14–1	
Advantages and Disadvantages of Transposed Basilic Vein Versus PTFE Brachioaxillary Graft	
Basilic Vein Transposition	**Brachioaxillary Graft**
Often two operations	One operation
At least 3 months for maturity before dialysis scheduled to start	Can be used for urgent or ongoing dialysis
Avoids central venous catheters	May allow early puncture
Under 65 years	Over 65 years
Basilic vein identified by Duplex scan	Axillosubclavian by vein patency confirmed by Duplex scan
Major complications: hematoma, pseudoaneurysm, fibrosis	Major complication: outflow revision

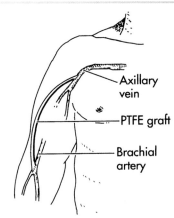

Figure 14-7.
Straight brachioaxillary bridge fistula positioned in an anteromedial tunnel. Placement of the graft over the lateral aspect of the brachium is more conspicuous but allows a longer segment for puncture.

axillary vein is dependably patent and of large caliber. Mobilize the vein, and ligate and divide one or two branches to allow easier access for the anastomosis.

Then dissect a tunnel along the anterior aspect of the brachium and into the axilla using a tunneling device. The patient may be administered heparin (3000-4000 units intravenously), but this is the surgeon's choice.

Use a 6-mm graft. Bevel the upper end, as shown in Figure 14-9. Apply vascular clamps to the axillary vein, and make a longitudinal venotomy. Then suture the graft end-to-side into the vein and bring it down through the tunnel to the brachial wound (Fig. 14-10). Then bevel and suture it into the brachial artery, usually in an anterior position. Make an oblique skin incision over the palpable artery, just above the antecubital fold medial to the biceps muscle. Carry dissection down to the vascular sheath, which is then opened (Fig. 14-11). The artery may be freed to a distance of about 2 to 3 cm in preparation for the anastomosis (Fig. 14-12). Then open the fistula to flow. Usually, 1 to 2 minutes of pressure over the arterial suture line is necessary for

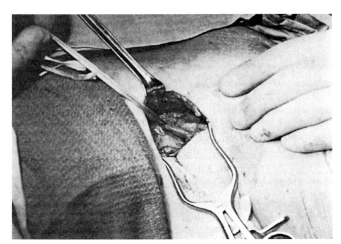

Figure 14-8.
Exposure of axillary vein.

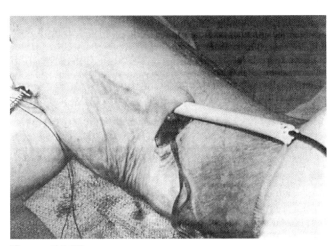

Figure 14-10.
Graft is tunneled along the anterior aspect of the upper arm.

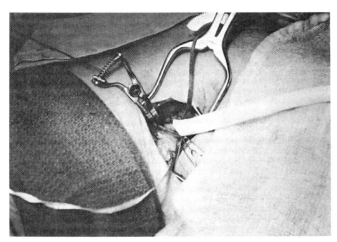

Figure 14-9.
Expanded PTFE graft is beveled and sutured to the vein.

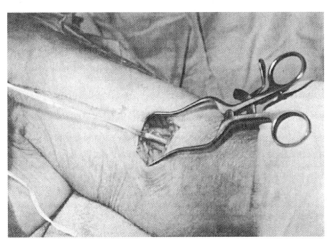

Figure 14-11.
Brachial artery is exposed.

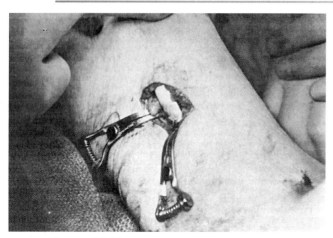

Figure 14-12.
Graft has been sutured to the brachial artery.

cessation of oozing from the suture holes in the graft. Many surgeons prefer to construct the arterial anastomosis first and use the pressurized graft for more accurate positioning. Then suction blood from the graft lumen and complete the venous anastomosis.

Close the incisions in two layers, and apply dressings to the wounds. If necessary, the fistula may be used for dialysis in 24 hours, but it is preferable to wait 1 week or so to allow the tunnel to close around the graft (Fig. 14-13).

Clinical experience with the brachioaxillary prosthetic fistula has been excellent. Early failure or bleeding has been noted in only 5% of patients. Steed and coworkeres[14] reported excellent results with this technique. The success of the brachioaxillary interposition graft has been attributed by Bittner and Weaver[27] to the capacious run-off through the large axillary vein and to a narrow graft-to-vein inflow angle, which may lessen turbulence and neointimal hyperplasia, thereby prolonging long-term patency.

The brachioaxillary prosthetic fistula is an effective access method for hemodialysis, especially in patients whose forearm vessels have already been used or who have poor vessels elsewhere.

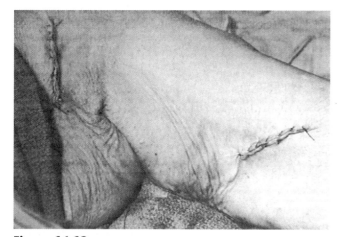

Figure 14-13.
Both skin incisions are closed. It is preferable to wait at least 7 to 10 days before using the graft for hemodialysis, although in an emergency, the graft may be punctured within 24 hours.

Femorosaphenous and Femorofemoral Prosthetic Fistulas (M. Owens, MD)

If the patient's ankle blood pressure is 80% of systemic pressure and the patient does not have leg claudication, it is likely that a thigh fistula will function without causing distal insufficiency symptoms. General, spinal, or local anesthesia may be used. Activity is not restricted postoperatively. Preoperative antibiotics are routine, as is intraoperative systemic heparinization. The arterial anastomosis should be anterolateral on the vessel, and the graft should leave the vessel at an acute angle, as would a branch. Because the femoral vessels lie deep beneath a fascial layer, the graft's limbs are configured to emerge anteriorly toward the surface for about 2 cm before entering the subcutaneous tunnel.

Technique

Place a transverse skin incision in the groin for a loop graft. Make an additional 2 cm longitudinal incision medially on the thigh, two thirds of the distance from the groin to the knee over the course of the superficial femoral artery for a straight graft (Fig. 14-14). In isolating the vessels, considerable care must be taken to not leave torn lymphatic channels, because these may leak or form lymphoceles and contribute to graft infection. If a lymph node is incised, it should be removed in toto. Next create a subdermal tunnel using a curved aneurysm clamp or a tunneler; then pull an umbilical tape or Silastic sling through the tunnel to maintain its location during arterial anastomosis. It is important to make the second incision along the course of the graft to ensure good positioning without kinking. This precaution avoids the trauma that occurs if the tunneler is pushed and driven to extend the full distance. In the latter instance, there is likely to be a considerable amount of postoperative swelling and pain, and the injured tissues are less resistant to infection.

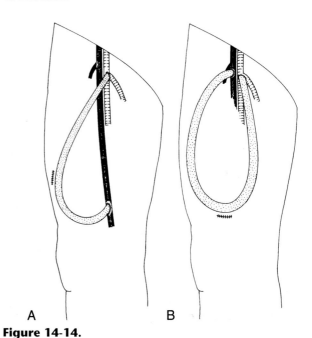

A   B

Figure 14-14.
A, Straight femorosaphenous bridge fistula. B, Loop femorofemoral bridge fistula.

When the arterial anastomosis is completed, allow the graft to fill at arterial pressure. With the graft distended, it is an easy matter to correct any twisting and to pull the graft through the tunnel without twisting or kinking. As the graft is pulled through the tunnel, the force of the pulse is a continuing indicator that the lumen has not been narrowed.

The arterial anastomosis is usually constructed by sewing the end of the graft to the side of the artery. This procedure is done either in the groin incision, where the graft is sewn to the proximal superficial femoral artery for a U configuration, or just above the adductor canal, where the graft is sewn to the distal superficial femoral artery for a slightly curved graft position. The course of the superficial femoral artery can be estimated to follow an imaginary line drawn from the anterior superior iliac spine to the medial condyle of the humerus.

Make the venous anastomosis, similar to the arterial anastomosis, end-to-side to either the saphenous or the femoral vein. Narrowing at the venous anastomosis, even in a vein larger than the conduit, may be a cause of early graft thrombosis.

The diameter and length of the graft have an important effect on the quantity of fistula flow in the lower extremity and hence on the likelihood of high-output failure and distal limb ischemia. We have used grafts of 6 and 8 mm, reserving special graft configurations (step down, taper) for patients in whom we suspect that high fistula flow would be detrimental to cardiac performance or distal blood flow.

We have occasionally ligated the caudal portion of the saphenous vein to prevent retrograde hypertension, but we have not done this when using the femoral vein. Venous hypertension in the lower extremity has not been a problem.

The Step-Graft Technique (J. Rosental, MD)

By the time the vascular surgeon is asked to provide hemodialysis access for the patient with renal failure, it is not unusual, even today, that all superficial veins suitable for autogenous fistula have been damaged by multiple punctures and infusions. Various nonautogenous substitutes have been used, but the most popular graft material is PTFE. This graft is competitive in price with other grafts, such as the bovine heterograft, umbilical vein homograft, or cryopreserved human vein, but it is much easier to handle during the initial implantation and subsequent reoperations.

Choice of Graft Site

The two essential criteria for choosing the graft site are an artery of sufficient size to provide adequate blood flow and patent veins of adequate caliber to provide venous drainage. Dialysis access surgeons agree that the venous end is the most common site for problems that compromise graft function. We have noted that the smaller the venous outflow, the sooner fibrosis, thickening, and occlusion will occur.

We prefer to use the larger veins, such as the axillary or subclavian vein in the upper extremity or the saphenofemoral junction in the thigh. An alternative in the upper extremity is the plexus of veins in the antecubital fossa, where there is a communication among the cephalic vein, the basilic vein, and the deep venous system.

To obtain as many graft sites as possible, we place the initial graft in a peripheral site, such as the forearm, and then as revisions or new grafts are needed, we use the more central veins or arteries.

Careful physical examination is usually all that is needed to establish the adequacy of the antecubital veins. Other noninvasive modalities, such as duplex scanning, are helpful; contrast venography may be necessary at times, when edema of the extremity suggests occlusion of the major venous channels.

The choice of the site of arterial anastomosis is easier. Careful examination of pulses will indicate the most peripheral available location. Noninvasive Doppler evaluation may be helpful in a patient with arterial occlusive disease. A straight graft between the radial artery at the wrist and the veins in the antecubital fossa is the optimum first graft site when an autogenous fistula is not possible.[17]

When the radial artery at the wrist is not adequate, the graft is placed in a loop configuration, with both arterial and venous connections in the antecubital fossa.

Arm grafts are placed in a straight configuration, between the brachial artery at the elbow and the axillary vein in the axilla. Subsequent venous-end revisions can be extended across the shoulder to the proximal axillary artery just below the clavicle or to the internal jugular vein in the supraclavicular fossa.

The thigh provides another anatomic area for graft placement. We make the venous connection to the saphenofemoral junction, with the venotomy extending into the common femoral vein. The arterial end can be near the adductor hiatus if a straight graft configuration is chosen. More often, we have used a loop configuration, with both vascular connections made in the groin. We make the arterial anastomosis to the superficial femoral artery near its origin. In case of infection, the potential problems are much less serious if a suture line in the common femoral artery has been avoided.

Choice of Graft Size: The Step-Graft

It is unusual to have problems of peripheral steal or an excessive workload on the heart when an AV graft is placed in the forearm. Blood flow through forearm grafts is limited by the smaller size of the source artery and the resistance in the effluent venous channels. When more centrally placed, grafts are connected to vessels of much larger flow capacity, and the flow rate then depends on the diameter of the graft.

We have observed flows of 2 to 3 L/min through PTFE grafts of an 8-mm diameter.[28] Flows of less than 1 L/min can be consistently obtained only if the graft diameter at the arterial end is reduced to 4 mm by narrowing the graft with suture for high-flow symptoms or at the time of initial graft insertion. These observations led us to suggest to the graft manufacturers that they develop a stepped graft that has a short 4-mm diameter segment at one arterial end. The body of the graft is 7 mm in diameter, a size that seems optimum for most graft sites in most patients.

In small patients, with small forearm vessels, we have used 6-mm and even 5-mm diameter grafts; flow, under these circumstances, is limited by the host vessels, and excessive flow is seldom a problem.

Method of Graft Insertion

Place most upper extremity grafts with the patient under local or regional block anesthesia, with additional sedation by the anesthesiologist. Thigh grafts require spinal block or general anesthesia and therefore are seldom done as the first procedure.

Always expose the recipient vein first, and confirm its patency and size. It is important to surgically prepare and drape the entire upper extremity, so there is always the option of having the axilla available for an arm graft if intraoperative findings preclude a forearm graft. In an obese or edematous patient, we explore the antecubital fossa if a suitable vein has been identified by preoperative ultrasound evaluation. It is remarkable how often suitable veins are present, protected from damaging venipunctures by the size of the limb. Make the incision along the course of the brachial artery and its bifurcation. Consequently, if the veins are inadequate for a forearm graft, this same incision can be used for the arterial end of an arm graft. If the antecubital veins are satisfactory, construct a forearm graft. If an arm graft is to be placed, expose the axillary vein and then dissect the brachial artery.

Occlude the artery with gentle, atraumatic vascular clamps, and do not remove the clamps until after the venous anastomosis is completed. This maneuver, along with avoidance of systemic heparinization and the use of small-caliber polypropylene suture and small needles, minimizes bleeding from the suture lines.

Bevel the 4-mm segment of the step-graft 45 degrees, and perform the arterial anastomosis. Make a subcutaneous tunnel between the two incisions. Various tunneling devices are available, but we most often use the Hegar cervical dilators, gradually enlarging the tunnel to 8 mm (the outside diameter of the 7-mm PTFE graft). Pass the graft through the tunnel and check for unwanted kinks or angulation. Then complete the venous anastomosis, and establish flow through the graft. If the venous run-off channels offer little resistance, the intensity of the pulse near the venous end of the graft should be slight. Test the adequacy of arterial inflow by temporary occlusion of the graft; the pulsation in the graft should increase to systolic intensity with the next heartbeat. If it takes several heartbeats to reach maximum pulse intensity, this indicates inadequate arterial input, and the graft is unlikely to function.

Irrigate the incisions with antibiotic solution and close with mattress sutures of nonabsorbable material. Ideally, the graft is not to be used until 11 to 14 days after implantation, although often we allow their puncture after 5 to 7 days, and as early as 24 hours if necessary.

PTFE grafts provide an alternative when autogenous venous grafts or fistulas are not possible. The use of the 4- to 7-mm step-graft avoids problems of peripheral steal and high-output failure. Planning for future access is critical, and the axillary of femorosaphenous veins should allow additional graft outflow sites.

Announcement of the Kidney Disease Outcomes Quality Initiatives focused more attention on objective comparison of autogenous fistulas with prosthetic AV fistulas. A meta-analysis of 83 studies, however, was not definitive because 80 were nonrandomized trials.[29] Murad and associates[29] found the autogenous AV fistula to be associated with a significant reduction in risk of death and access infection. However, with regard to other complications, they concluded "that low quality evidence from inconsistent studies with limited protection against bias shows that autogenous access for chronic hemodialysis is superior to prosthetic access."[29] Two recent studies are of note. Kakkos and colleagues[30] found that primary patency of a prosthetic AV graft was equivalent to that of the transposed brachiobasilic autogenous AV fistulas, and with graft surveillance and endovascular treatment, secondary patency rates at 12 and 18 months were also similar. Conversely, Keuter and coworkers,[31] although agreeing with the comparable secondary patency rates between PTFE and brachiobasilic autogenous fistula, found significantly higher primary patency rates at 1 year with the autogenous operation. The answer may be that each construction has a unique application for an individual patient and the fine surgical judgment required in making the decision outweighs standardized directives.

REFERENCES

1. Roon AJ, Moore WS, Goldstone J, Towan H, Campagna G. Comparative surface thrombogenicity of implanted vascular grafts. *J Surg Res*. 1977;22:165-173.
2. Butt KMH, Rao TK, Maki T, et al. Bovine heterograft as a preferential hemodialysis access. *Trans Am Soc Artif Intern Organs*. 1974;20A:339-342.
3. Levowitz BS, Flores L, Dunn I, Frumkin E. Prosthetic arteriovenous fistula for vascular access in hemodialysis. *Am J Surg*. 1976;132:368-372.
4. Owens ML, Stabile BE, Gahr JA, Wilson SE. Vascular grafts for hemodialysis: an evaluation of sites and materials. *Dial Transplant*. 1979;8:521-530.
5. Fee HJ Jr, Golding AL. Lower extremity ischemia after femoral arteriovenous bovine shunts. *Ann Surg*. 1976;183:42-45.
6. Haimov M, Jacobson JH 2nd. Experience with the modified bovine arterial heterograft in peripheral vascular reconstruction and vascular access for hemodialysis. *Ann Surg*. 1974;180:291-295.
7. Haimov M, Burrows L, Baez A, Neff M, Slifkin R. Alternatives for vascular access for hemodialysis: experience with autogenous saphenous vein autografts and bovine heterografts. *Surgery*. 1974;75:447-452.
8. Tellis VA, Kohlberg WI, Bhat DJ, Driscoll B, Veith FJ. Expanded polytetrafluoroethylene graft fistula for chronic hemodialysis. *Ann Surg*. 1979;189:101-105.
9. Burbridge GE, Biggers JA, Remmers AR Jr, Lindley JD, Saries HE, Fish JC. Late complications and results of bovine xenografts. *Trans Am Soc Artif Intern Organs*. 1976;22:377-381.
10. Merickel JH, Anderson RC, Knutson R, Lipschultz ML, Hitchcock CR. Bovine carotid artery shunts in vascular access surgery. Complications in the chronic hemodialysis patient. *Arch Surg*. 1974;109:245-250.
11. Mindich B, Silverman M, Elguezabal A, Flores L, Sheka RP, Levowitz BS. Human umbilical cord vein for vascular replacement: preliminary report and observations. *Surgery*. 1977;81:152-160.
12. Haimov M, Baez A, Neff M, Slifkin R. Complications of arteriovenous fistulas for hemodialysis. *Arch Surg*. 1975;110:708-712.
13. Payne JE, Chatterjee SN, Barbour BH, Berne TV. Vascular access for chronic hemodialysis using modified bovine arterial graft arteriovenous fistula. *Am J Surg*. 1974;128:54-57.
14. Steed DL, McAuley CE, Rault R, Webster MW. Upper arm graft fistula for hemodialysis. *J Vasc Surg*. 1984;1:660-663.
15. Ackman CFD, O'Regan S, Herba MJ, Laplante MP, Lemaitre P, Kaye M. Experience with polytetrafluoroethylene grafts in patients on long-term hemodialysis. *Can J Surg*. 1979;22:152-154.
16. Butler HG 3rd, Baker LD Jr, Johnson JM. Vascular access for chronic hemodialysis: polytetrafluoroethylene (PTFE) versus bovine heterograft. *Am J Surg*. 1977;134:791-793.
17. Palder SB, Kirkman RL, Whittemore AD, Hakim RM, Lazarus JM, Tilney NL. Vascular access for hemodialysis. Patency rates and results of revision. *Ann Surg*. 1985;202:235-239.

18. Burdick JF, Scott W, Cosimi AB. Experience with Dacron graft arteriovenous fistulas for dialysis access. *Ann Surg.* 1978;187:262-266.

19. Hertzer NR, Beven EG. Venous access using the bovine carotid heterograft: techniques, results, and complications in 75 patients. *Arch Surg.* 1978;113:696-700.

20. Pontari MA, McMillen MA. The straight radial-antecubital PTFE angioaccess graft in an era of high-flux dialysis. *Am Surg.* 1991;161:450-453.

21. Matsuura JH, Johansen KH, Rosenthal D, Clark MD, Clarke KA, Kirby LB. Cryopreserved femoral vein grafts for difficult hemodialysis access. *Ann Vasc Surg.* 2000;14:50-55.

22. Bussell JA, Abbott JA, Lim RC. A radial steal syndrome with arteriovenous fistula for hemodialysis: studies in seven patients. *Ann Intern Med.* 1971;75:387-395.

23. Foran RF, Shore EH, Levin PM, Treiman RL. Bovine heterografts for hemodialysis. *West J Med.* 1975;123:269-274.

24. Cinat M, Hopkins J, Wilson SE. A prospective evaluation of PTFE graft patency and surveillance techniques in hemodialysis access. *Ann Vasc Surg.* 1999;13:191-198.

25. Taucher LA. Immediate, safe hemodialysis into arteriovenous fistulas created with a new tunneler. An 11 year experience. *Am J Surg.* 1985;150:212-215.

26. Ryan JJ, Dennis MJ. Radiocephalic fistula in vascular access. *Br J Surg.* 1990;77:1321-1322.

27. Bittner HB, Weaver JP. The brachioaxillary interposition graft as a successful tertiary vascular access procedure for hemodialysis. *Am J Surg.* 1994;176:615-617.

28. Rohr MS, Browder W, Frentz GD, McDonald JC. Arteriovenous fistulas for long-term dialysis. Factors that influence fistula survival. *Arch Surg.* 1978;113:153-155.

29. Murad MH, Elamin MB, Sidawy AN, et al. Autogenous versus prosthetic vascular access for hemodialysis: a systematic review and meta-analysis. *J Vasc Surg.* 2008;48(5 suppl):34S-47S,.

30. Kakkos SK, Andrzejewski T, Haddad JA, et al. Equivalent secondary patency rates of upper extremity Vectra Vascular Access Grafts and transposed brachial-basilic fistulas with aggressive access surveillance and endovascular treatment. *J Vasc Surg.* 2008;47:407-414.

31. Keuter XH, De Smet AA, Kessels AG, van der Sande FM, Welten RJ, Tordoir JH. A randomized multicenter study of the outcome of brachial-basilic arteriovenous fistula and prosthetic brachial-antecubital forearm loop as vascular access for hemodialysis. *J Vasc Surg.* 2007;47:395-401.

CHAPTER 15

New Synthetic Grafts and Early Access

Brian Mailey, Khushboo Kaushal, and Samuel E. Wilson

New Hemodialysis Graft Materials

The U.S. Renal Data System reports approximately one-half million North Americans with end-stage renal disease (ESRD).[1,2] Because not all ESRD patients have vessels suitable for an autogenous vascular access site, research has concentrated on identifying superior graft materials that would allow earlier access and provide longer patency. The current functional 1-year primary patency rate is approximately 50% and approximately 35% at 2 years for access grafts; the secondary patency rates are higher at 1 year.[3–8] The principal benefit of grafts over fistulas are a shorter and more predictable time to initiation of hemodialysis and the ability to place and remove larger-bore needles. The most notable limitations are the lower primary rate and the need for further procedures to achieve acceptable secondary patency rates.

In the United States, most arteriovenous grafts (AVGs) are constructed with expanded polytetrafluoroethylene (PTFE) material.[5] The graft is anastomosed to an artery and a vein, most commonly in the forearm or upper arm, to form a synthetic arteriovenous conduit enabling long-term hemodialysis treatment. Kidney Disease Outcomes Quality Initiative (K/DOQI) guidelines[2] currently recommend that PTFE grafts should not be routinely used until 14 days after placement or longer depending on the amount of time required for resolution of postoperative edema. During this period of early access, the subcutaneous tissue that surrounds the graft is poorly attached (or not attached at all), creating a perigraft space or tunnel into which blood can collect when the dialysis needle is removed and before hemostasis is achieved.[6] New graft development has focused on materials that would be "self-sealing," allowing immediate (or within 24 hr) access after operation and thereby avoiding need for a central venous catheter. A secondary benefit would be less "bleed-through" after dialysis needle removal.

The ideal vascular access graft will be easy to handle (mimicking native vessels), nonthrombogenic (allow endothelialization and prevent neointimal hyperplasia), immunologically inert, resistant to infection and puncture trauma, and able to retain tensile strength and can be manufactured and sold at a reasonable cost. Many have attempted to develop such graft alternatives; however, to date, no prosthetic equivalent to native vessels exists. The two major objectives in current graft research are to prevent intimal hyperplasia and resultant thrombosis and to develop an "early puncture" graft material.

Alternatives to Fistulas

In the search for small-diameter vascular substitutes, alternatives to autogenous fistulas have included autografts (eg, saphenous vein), homografts (eg, cryopreserved human umbilical vein), xenografts (eg, bovine carotid artery), and synthetics (eg, PTFE). The necessary functions of the graft include maintaining flow, sealing after cannulation, and minimizing thrombus formation after access. Currently, PTFE has proved to be the most durable and is the most commonly used graft material. PTFE has become the preferred material because of its ready availability, ease of implantation, fair patency, and complication rates. The reported long-term patency of these synthetic grafts, however, rarely exceeds 50%.[8,9] Most grafts experience myointimal hyperplasia of the venous lumen just distal to the graft vein anastomosis, resulting in progressive stenosis and eventually failure as a result of thrombosis.[10] Most work for improving current AVG materials focuses on decreasing time to first puncture or improving longevity.

Autografts: Saphenous Vein

Autogenous greater saphenous vein would seem to be the obvious conduit for AVG construction with advantages including no antigenicity, low cost, and availability in many patients (see Chapter 12 for discussion). Patency rates for saphenous vein grafts, however, have been inconsistent, with 2-year results as low as 20%. Even with reported higher patency rates (60%-89%, 2 yr), when balanced with drawbacks, including healing of the additional thigh wound, the increased operating time for vein harvesting, and the need to preserve the vein for peripheral vascular or coronary arterial revascularization, attention remains focused on synthetic vascular substitutes.[11]

Homografts and Xenografts: Human and Bovine Vessels

Modern biologic homografts and xenografts (heterografts) have included bovine ureter, bovine carotid artery, bovine mesenteric vein, and cryopreserved human umbilical and greater saphenous vein. Selected reports have shown these biologic materials to have less intimal hyperplasia at the venous anastamosis, a reduced tendency to thrombose, and a lower risk of infection than PTFE.[8,12] Some have reported excellent 2-year cumulative patency rates (<100%) using cryopreserved venous homografts without allograft rejection, but these reports are tempered by subsequent reports with inconsistent patency rates, graft infections, and allograft rupture. A biohybrid with human umbilical vein and Dacron mesh was devised by Dardik and coworkers.[13] Human umbilical vein and other biologic grafts may be subject to pseudoaneurysm formation.[13]

Denatured homologous vein grafts have produced variable overall results with 1-year primary patencies of 30% to 57%.[14] Human umbilical vein was first reported in 1976 as an alternative graft material; however, patency rates were not significantly improved, perigraft fluid collections occurred, and infection could cause breakdown of the umbilical vein.

Moreover, it was difficult to handle because of the disparity in thickness between the umbilical vein wall and the patient's vessels. Homologous saphenous veins have been developed commercially (Vascogref; Varivas; Dardik) and have been reported to be easier to handle and to give excellent results, although cryopreserved cadaveric veins may preclude later kidney transplantation because of allosensitization.[15] Human denatured arterial homografts have also been implanted but have been associated with inflammatory and immunologic interactions and are now not commonly used.[16]

Bovine carotid artery (Artegraft) was first described in 1966 as a conduit and used for hemodialysis access in the early 1970s.[17] Advantages of this graft include its soft, naturally compliant nature and ease of use. Several case series, a large retrospective study, and a prospective, randomized trial compared bovine carotid artery to PTFE grafts;[17–20] the majority of these published reports (including the prospective trial[20]) reported that bovine carotid artery grafts had primary and secondary patency rates equal or inferior to those of PTFE. Since then, long-term patency rates have been mixed, and reports of graft disintegration with infection and aneurysms have emerged.

Developed in the 1990s, bovine mesenteric vein (ProCol; Hancock Jaffe Laboratories, Inc., Irvine, CA) was approved by the U.S. Food and Drug Administration (FDA) in 2003 and was evaluated in a large, nonrandomized, multicenter trial that demonstrated a 2-year primary patency rate of 60%, which was significantly better than their PTFE control arm (43%).[21] Owing to its high elastin content and moderate wall thickness, bovine mesenteric vein has theoretic advantages of compliance and lower rates of structural degeneration (eg, aneurysm formation). ProCol is indicated in patients in whom a previous graft has failed.

Biohybrids

Optimizing tissue-biomaterial interactions offer the possibility that biodegradable polymers can constitute a scaffold to allow tissue ingrowth and leave a vascular conduit entirely of host origin. This tissue-engineering concept has been proposed to obviate the limitations seen in synthetic grafts. Various bioactive substances (eg, heparin; growth factors; carbon) have been integrated onto synthetic grafts (PTFE, Dacron, and polyurethane) to promote endothelialization or to limit intimal hyperplasia.[22] Other biohybrid prostheses using combinations of synthetics and allografts decellularized and chemically cross-linked with gluteraldehyde are currently under investigation.

In part, to facilitate cell repopulation and tissue remodeling, glutaraldehyde is used as a fixative in the preparation of bioprosthetic vascular conduits. The Omniflow II (Bio Nova International, Australia) prosthesis is formed from gluteraldehyde-tanned ovine collagen grown around a polyester mesh. This collagen-encapsulated graft is reported to have reduced thrombogenicity, low rates of infection, and a low incidence of aneurysm formation (patency 71%-77% at 1 yr).[23]

The CryoLife graft (CryoLife, Inc., Kennesaw, Ga) has been used successfully in sites where infection has been a problem. Cryopreserved femoral vein allograft (CryoVein) is another homograft commercially available.

Although selected reports have indicated biologic grafts to be superior to PTFE in patency,[24] the limitations of high cost and reports of aneurysm formation have limited widespread use.[25]

Synthetic Grafts

Dacron

Polyethylene terephthalate or Dacron (DuPont, Inc, Wilmington, Del) was first introduced as a multiple filament polyester in 1939 and used as a vascular graft by Julian in 1957 and DeBakey in 1958. Dacron grafts are manufactured as either a woven or a knitted fabric.[5,7] The woven grafts consist of smaller pores, whereas the knitted grafts are formed by looping fibers together and have larger pores that promote greater tissue ingrowth, more compliance, and radial distensibility.[5,7] Owing to the larger pore sizes, knitted Dacron is treated with albumin (Bard Cardiovascular, Billerica, Mass), gelatin (Vascutek, Renfrewshire, Scotland), or collagen (Boston Scientific, Oakland, NJ) or preclotted during the operation with the patient's blood to prevent seepage. Advantages of Dacron have included its strength and nonbiodegradability. Dacron's limitations include dilation over time (knitted type),[26] kinking, need for preclotting, and inherent thromboenicity. Some modifications (ie, coils or external rings incorporated to minimize graft kinking or mechanical compression) have been employed to obviate some limitations; however, Dacron is now usually reserved for aortic and high-pressure, large-diameter peripheral bypass grafts or aortic endografts rather than hemodialysis vascular access.

Polypropylene

Discovered in the 1950s, polypropylene is a relatively inert, biostable polyester graft with high tensile strength that is known for its crystalline and thermoplastic nature.[6] Its hydrocarbon structure renders it insensitive to hydrolysis but susceptible to oxidation, making the addition of antioxidants necessary (vitamin C, vitamin E, and N-acetylcysteine).[27] Polypropylene has been studied as a vascular prosthesis bypass graft in animal models with good success, and in vivo studies suggest advantages over PTFE or Dacron in small-diameter vascular grafts;[28,29] however, its use has primarily been in other biologic prosthetics (ie, hernia mesh).

Polyurethane

Polyurethane was originally developed commercially in the 1930s for surface coatings and adhesives. More recently, polyurethane has been made into vascular grafts known for elasticity and greater compliance than either PTFE or polyethylene; these properties have been suggested to result in less intimal hyperplasia at the anastomotic site.[22] Polyurethane grafts, approved for use in the United States in December 2000, have been promoted for their self-sealing properties with the advantage of early cannulation over that of conventional PTFE.[30,31] This property allows polyurethane grafts to be used within 24 hours of their placement, thereby providing an immediate vascular access for patients with urgent dialysis needs. A randomized clinical trial confirmed the safety of early cannulation and observed similar primary and cumulative graft patencies with a low infection rate (6%, similar in both groups).[32] A retrospective review in 2007 demonstrated similar thrombosis rates and graft survival rates but substantially higher infection rates with polyurethane grafts versus standard PTFE.[30] Another concern about polyurethane grafts is the potential carcinogenic effect of 2,4-toluene diamine, one of its degradation products. The next generation of polyurethane grafts are carbonate-based with no ester linkages and are hydrolytically and oxidatively stable and more resistant to biodegradation.[33] Also, pilot studies of sirolimus-loaded polyurethane conduits placed as arteriovenous bridge grafts in sheep show less neointimal narrowing.[34]

Expanded PTFE

In 1973, PTFE or Teflon (DuPont, patent 1937) became the first synthetic material introduced specifically for vascular access. Three years after its introduction, PTFE was subsequently modified, making it more microporous to form expanded PTFE.[35] Owing to this increased porosity, PTFE had improved tissue adhesion characteristics and an antithrombotic electronegative luminal surface. PTFE is now the type of synthetic graft most widely used by most vascular surgeons in the United States.[36,37] It is widely available "off the shelf" in various lengths and diameters, has a reasonable patency rate, handles well, does not require preclotting, and is flexible.

PTFE is available in different diameters (4 to 7 mm) with a thickness of approximately 0.50 to 0.60 mm and may be tailored to fit the site needed. Recommended time to first use for dialysis is 14 days, although earlier use is possible with care. Further modifications of standard PTFE have been introduced in an attempt to improve current limitations. PTFE has been modified to improve patency with tapered ends, external support (rings),[38] thinner walls,[39] change in elasticity or shape (straight, looped, or curved) without lasting success; these have all failed to consistently improve patency rates. Other modifications of PTFE (eg, heparin-bonded, carbon-coated, impregnation with growth factors) have recently been introduced. A cuffed venous end of the PTFE conduit has been used in an effort to prevent runoff stenosis.[40] PTFE vascular grafts have been improved

incrementally since they were first introduced but are still considered inferior to the arteriovenous fistula.[41]

The Hemasite (Renal Systems, USA), a transcutaneous button as an external part of a titanium nonthrombogenic tube connected to the side of a PTFE internal bypass graft or the "carbon transcutaneous access device" (DiaTAB, Bentley Laboratories, USA), avoided the need for skin puncture but was at risk for infection with exogenous microorganisms.[42,43]

No significant differences in patency, complications, or cost between the different PTFE grafts have been consistently shown.[44,45]

Problems with PTFE include clotting, infection, and pseudoaneurysms. Thrombosis of the graft is the most common and usually the use-limiting factor. Occlusion of the graft is usually due to myointimal hyperplasia at the venous anastomosis, and thrombosis has been noted as early as 3 months after implantation. Interventions to extend patency, including patch angioplasty, anastomotic revisions, thrombolysis, or balloon angioplasty and stenting, provide an average of 3 to 7 months of additional patency; however, immediate rethrombosis is a frustrating and common occurrence. In addition, infection occurs in a small percentage (<10%) of grafts with some requiring removal.[46] Other complications include vascular access neuropathy, aneurysms, congestive heart failure, vascular insufficiency, seroma formation, and venous hypertension. Factors that have been examined to predict graft failure include venous line pressure, blood flow rates, Duplex imaging, and recirculation values.[47-49]

Overall 12-month patency rates for PTFE bridge grafts are approximately 50% with secondary patency rates of 50% to 96% after either surgical intervention and/or pharmacologic thrombectomy.[50,51] Two-year patency rates are usually 30% to 40%. Surgical outflow revision provides longer patency intervals than those of endovascular repair.

Early Cannulation

Early surgical referral for access placement has been the major achievement of the K/DOQI guidelines; however, a significant number of patients require urgent access. Neither autogenous nor standard prosthetic grafts are intended for immediate use in these patients. Early cannulation may cause hematomas, thrombosis, or wall injury.

When immediate access is required, temporary percutaneous or tunneled and cuffed hemodialysis catheters are inserted. In 2000, approximately 250,000 of these catheters were used annually in the United States,[52] representing additional procedures, costs, and risks for patients. According to the Medicare database, catheters are the initial access in 72% of U.S. ESRD patients.[3,53] In addition, these devices deliver the lowest average flow rates, have a short use-life, and are prone to infections and other complications. Placing a percutaneous catheter in a central vein is the most hazardous type of vascular access and is nothing less than penetrating chest trauma.

Early cannulation of grafts has been proposed to avoid the additional temporary central venous catheters needed for immediate access. Self-sealing grafts have been developed to reduce time to hemostasis and enable earlier cannulation. Since the early 1990s, a number of multicenter clinical trials have been devised to prospectively demonstrate the patency and complication rates as well as their intended use of early cannulation.[54] Results have been mixed, with some reports of early access grafts having a greater incidence of thrombosis, infection, hematoma, bleeding, and swelling. Others, however, obtained success with standard PTFE by slight modifications in implantation (using a smaller tunneling device) and careful hemostasis after needle removal and demonstrated no difference in patency at 12 months compared with later dialysis with standard PTFE grafts punctured at 2 weeks.[55] Most studies have at least demonstrated the feasibility of achieving early access to a newly implanted graft, and some have reported equivalent patency rates as standard grafts. The longer-term loss of patency (often due to the proliferation of intimal tissue at and around the anastomosis) and difficulty encountered in performing revisions of some grafts still remain a concern. Initial graft puncture for hemodialysis may be initiated as early as 24 hours after implantation, provided there are no contraindications to graft puncture (eg, signs of infection, bleeding, swelling or severe edema, hematoma, or absence of thrill).

PTFE Early Access: Diastat, Fusion, Rapidax

In the early 1990s, the Diastat (W.L. Gore & Associates, Inc., Flagstaff, Ariz) graft was developed as a permanent vascular access to allow early cannulation and avoid the need for a temporary dialysis catheter. It was composed of a self-sealing PTFE-silicon graft and plasma tetrafluoroethylene with a thicker-walled mesh cannulation segment in the middle, covered with several layers of PTFE fibers and an outer layer of a thin fenestrated PTFE. The ends were designed to enable standard arterial and venous anastomoses with the cannulation segment designed to promote clotting after cannulation needle removal. Some initial reports had promising results, with early cannulation and patency rates similar to those of standard PTFE.[56,57] Longer-term follow-up, however, showed lower primary and secondary patency rates with significantly higher thromboses and more complications.[58,59]

Fusion

Fusion Vascular Access Grafts (Boston Scientific Co., Natick, Mass) were synthetic vascular grafts constructed of two layers: an inner layer composed of extruded PTFE and an outer layer composed of woven polyester. These two layers are fused together with a middle proprietary polycarbonate-urethane layer (Corethane). The Fusion graft was designed to offer early cannulation within 72 hours of implantation, improved hemostasis at the dialysis puncture site, and improved handling at the anastomosis sites. They were evaluated in a prospective, multicenter, single-arm trial to evaluate the safety and efficacy in patients who require early (≤72 hr) access starting in 2005. This trial was electively suspended in January 2007.

Rapidax

Another self-sealing vascular access graft, Rapidax (Vascutek Co., Scotland), is a triple-layered graft consisting of an internal and external PTFE layer with a proprietary middle elastomeric membrane designed for self-sealing. The inner and outer layers of the grafts are identical to those used in the manufacturing of the PTFE MAXIFLO Wrap grafts. The graft is a permanent vascular access designed for early access with reduced time to hemostasis and similar long-term patency and safety profiles as those of PTFE. Rapidax has been approved for use in Japan, Canada, and Europe since 2005. Manufacturer reports include good clinical success in these grafts implanted in Japan with similar adverse event profiles to other grafts. In the United States, the multicenter, randomized clinical trial comparing Rapidax with the MAXIFLO Wrap graft was suspended in 2009 in part due to study costs and lengthy projected time to complete the large patient enrollment.

Polyurethane Early Access: Vectra

Vectra (Thoratec Laboratories Co., Pleasanton, Calif) is a three-layered polyetherurethan urea vascular access graft blended with silicone and reinforced by spiral polyester fibers with a nonporous layer under the luminal surface; the outer layer is porous, the middle layer is a nonpermeable self-sealable coat, and the inner layer is made of impermeable polyurethane. It has been developed to create a self-sealing vascular access for immediate use and in 2001 received FDA clearance as a vascular access graft designed to allow for hemodialysis use as soon as 24 hours after surgical implantation and allow sealing of the graft after needle puncture.

The graft was constructed to resist kinking, improve hemostasis at the anastomotic suture line, and have better sealing of puncture sites. Some have found patency rates similar to those of PTFE grafts[32]; however, others have noted that the elasticity of the graft (which is designed to prevent stenosis by radial compression by the surrounding tissue) also causes some elongation over time with increased incidence of intimal hyperplasia near the venous anastomosis and kinking. Moreover, early cannulation may damage the graft material, as shown by color Doppler ultrasound.[60,61] Despite this, some have found the graft acceptable, including a multicenter, prospective, randomized, controlled clinical study published in 2001 that found primary and secondary patency rates equivalent to those of PTFE.[32] Vectra is currently the only FDA-approved polyurethane graft available in the United States.[62]

Conclusions

In the United States, approximately 60% of hemodialysis patients have a synthetic graft for vascular access. Research has been directed at development of better conduits with a focus on two areas: early-access/self-sealing material to prevent the need for tunneled catheters and inhibition of myointimal hyperplasia. Evolution in biocompatible surface modifications and controlled-release modalties including impregnation of the graft with antithrombotic pharmaceuticals may improve prosthetics used for vascular access in hemodialysis patients in the future.

REFERENCES

1. U.S. Renal Data System. *2008 Annual Data Report: Atlas of Chronic Kidney Disease and End-Stage Renal Disease in the United States.* Bethesda, MD: National Institutes of Health, 2007. Available at http://www.usrds.org/.

2. III. NKF-K/DOQI Clinical Practice Guidelines for Vascular Access: update 2000. *Am J Kidney Dis.* 2001;37(1 suppl 1):S137-S181.

3. Eggers PW. A quarter century of medicare expenditures for ESRD. *Semin Nephrol.* 2000;20:516-522.

4. Di Giulio S, Meschini L, Triolo G. Dialysis outcome quality initiative (DOQI) guideline for hemodialysis adequacy. *Int J Artif Organs.* 1998;21:757-761.

5. Ku DN, Allen RC (eds). *Vascular Grafts.* Boca Raton, FL: CRC Press; 1995.

6. Hakaim AG, Scott TE. Durability of early prosthetic dialysis graft cannulation: results of a prospective, nonrandomized clinical trial. *J Vasc Surg.* 1997;25:1002-1005.

7. Kannan RY, Salacinski HJ, Butler PE, Hamilton G, Seifalian AM. Current status of prosthetic bypass grafts: a review. *J Biomed Mater Res B Appl Biomater.* 2005;74:570-581.

8. Berardinelli L. Grafts and graft materials as vascular substitutes for haemodialysis access construction. *Eur J Vasc Endovasc Surg.* 2006;32:203-211.

9. Bosman PJ, Blankestijn PJ, van der Graaf Y, Heintjes RJ, Koomans HA, Eikelboom BC. A comparison between PTFE and denatured homologous vein grafts for haemodialysis access: a prospective randomised multicentre trial. The SMASH Study Group. Study of Graft Materials in Access for Haemodialysis. *Eur J Vasc Endovasc Surg.* 1998;16:126-132.

10. Hughes K, Adams FG, Hamilton DN. The radiology of local complications of haemodialysis access devices. *Clin Radiol.* 1980;31:489-496.

11. Bhandari S, Wilkinson A, Sellars L. Saphenous vein forearm grafts and gortex thigh grafts as alternative forms of vascular access. *Clin Nephrol.* 1995;44:325-328.

12. Berardinelli L. The endless history of vascular access: a surgeon's perspective. *J Vasc Access.* 2006;7:103-111.

13. Dardik H, Ibrahim IM, Dardik I. Arteriovenous fistulas constructed with modified human umbilical cord vein graft. *Arch Surg.* 1976;111:60-62.

14. Heintjes RJ, Eikelboom BC, Steijling JJ, et al. The results of denatured homologous vein grafts as conduits for secondary haemodialysis access surgery. *Eur J Vasc Endovasc Surg.* 1995;9:58-63.

15. Benedetto B, Lipkowitz G, Madden R, et al. Use of cryopreserved cadaveric vein allograft for hemodialysis access precludes kidney transplantation because of allosensitization. *J Vasc Surg.* 2001;34:139-142.

16. Abu-Dalu J, Urca I, Zonder HB, Rosenfeld JB. Hemodialysis treatment by means of a cadaver arterial allograft. *Arch Surg.* 1972;105:798-801.

17. Rosenberg N, Martinez A, Sawyer PN, Wesolowski SA, Postlethwait RW, Dillon ML Jr. Tanned collagen arterial prosthesis of bovine carotid origin in man. Preliminary studies of enzyme-treated heterografts. *Ann Surg.* 1966;164:247-256.

18. Lilly L, Nighiem D, Mendez-Picon G, Lee HM. Comparison between bovine heterograft and expanded PTFE grafts for dialysis access. *Am Surg.* 1980;46:694-696.

19. Butler HG 3rd, Baker LD Jr. Johnson JM. Vascular access for chronic hemodialysis: polytetrafluoroethylene (PTFE) versus bovine heterograft. *Am J Surg.* 1977;134:791-793.

20. Hurt AV, Batello-Cruz M, Skipper BJ, Teaf SR, Sterling WA Jr. Bovine carotid artery heterografts versus polytetrafluoroethylene grafts. A prospective, randomized study. *Am J Surg.* 1983;146:844-847.

21. Katzman HE, Glickman MH, Schild AF, Fujitani RM, Lawson JH. Multicenter evaluation of the bovine mesenteric vein bioprostheses for hemodialysis access in patients with an earlier failed prosthetic graft. *J Am Coll Surg.* 2005;201:223-230.

22. Xue L, Greisler HP. Biomaterials in the development and future of vascular grafts. *J Vasc Surg.* 2003;37:472-480.

23. Wang SS, Chu SH. Clinical use of Omniflow vascular graft as arteriovenous bridging graft for hemodialysis. *Artif Organs.* 1996;20:1278-1281.

24. Senkaya I, Aytac II, Eercan AK, Aliosman A, Percin B. The graft selection for haemodialysis. *Vasa.* 2003;32:209-213.

25. Hamilton G, Megerman J, L'Italien GJ, et al. Prediction of aneurysm formation in vascular grafts of biologic origin. *J Vasc Surg.* 1988;7:400-408.

26. Wilson SE, Krug R, Mueller G. Late disruption of Dacron aortic grafts. *Ann Vasc Surg.* 1997;11:383-386.

27. Glowinski J, Glowinski S, Farbiszewski R, Makarewicz-Plonska M, Chwiecko M. Endogenic non-enzymatic antioxidative system of polyester grafts during their healing. *J Cardiovasc Surg (Torino).* 1997;38:465-471.

28. Greisler HP, Tattersall CW, Klosak JJ, Cabusao EA, Garfield JD, Kim DU. Partially bioresorbable vascular grafts in dogs. *Surgery.* 1991;110:645-654; discussion 654-655.

29. Puskas JE, Chen Y. Biomedical application of commercial polymers and novel polyisobutylene-based thermoplastic elastomers for soft tissue replacement. *Biomacromolecules.* 2004;5:1141-1154.

30. Peng CW, Tan SG. Polyurethane grafts: a viable alternative for dialysis arteriovenous access? *Asian Cardiovasc Thorac Ann.* 2003;11:314-38.

31. Maya ID, Weatherspoon J, Young CJ, Barker J, Allon M. Increased risk of infection associated with polyurethane dialysis grafts. *Semin Dial.* 2007;20:616-620.

32. Glickman MH, Stokes GK, Ross JR, et al. Multicenter evaluation of a polyurethane urea vascular access graft as compared with the expanded polytetrafluoroethylene vascular access graft in hemodialysis applications. *J Vasc Surg.* 2001;34:465-472; discussion 472-473.

33. Tanzi MC, Fare S, Petrini P. In vitro stability of polyether and polycarbonate urethanes. *J Biomater Appl.* 2000;14:325-348.

34. Schuman E., Babu J. Sirolimus-loaded polyurethane graft for hemodialysis access in sheep. *Vascular.* 2008;16:269-274.

35. Elliott MP, Gazzaniga AB, Thomas JM, Haiduc NJ, Rosen SM. Use of expanded polytetrafluoroethylene grafts for vascular access in hemodialysis: laboratory and clinical evaluation. *Am Surg.* 1977;43:455-459.

36. Kaplan MS, Mirahmadi KS, Winer RL, Gorman JT, Dabirvaziri N, Rosen SM. Comparison of "PTFE" and bovine grafts for blood access in dialysis patients. *Trans Am Soc Artif Intern Organs.* 1976;22:388-893.

37. Scott EC, Glickman MH. Conduits for hemodialysis access. *Semin Vasc Surg.* 2007;20:158-163.

38. Kao CL, Chang JP. Fully ringed polytetrafluoroethylene graft for vascular access in hemodialysis. *Asian Cardiovasc Thorac Ann.* 2003;11:171-173.

39. Lenz BJ, Veldenz HC, Dennis JW, Khansarinia S, Atteberry LR. A three-year follow-up on standard versus thin wall ePTFE grafts for hemodialysis. *J Vasc Surg.* 1998;28:464-470; discussion 470.

40. Sorom AJ, Hughes CB, McCarthy JT, et al. Prospective, randomized evaluation of a cuffed expanded polytetrafluoroethylene graft for hemodialysis vascular access. *Surgery.* 2002;132:135-140.

41. Scher LA, Katzman HE. Alternative graft materials for hemodialysis access. *Semin Vasc Surg.* 2004;17:19-24.

42. Reed WP, Sadler JH. Experience with a needleless vascular access device (Hemasite) for hemodialysis. *South Med J.* 1984;77:1501-1505.

43. Smits PJ, Slooff MJ, Lichtendahl DH, van der Hem GK. The Biocarbon vascular access device (DiaTAB) for haemodialysis. *Proc Eur Dial Transplant Assoc Eur Ren Assoc.* 1985;21:267-269.

44. Kaufman JL, Garb JL, Berman JA, Rhee SW, Norris MA, Friedmann P. A prospective comparison of two expanded polytetrafluoroethylene grafts for linear forearm hemodialysis access: does the manufacturer matter? *J Am Coll Surg.* 1997;185:74-79.

45. Hurlbert SN, Mattos MA, Henretta JP, et al. Long-term patency rates, complications and cost-effectiveness of polytetrafluoroethylene (PTFE) grafts for hemodialysis access: a prospective study that compares Impra versus Gore-tex grafts. *Cardiovasc Surg.* 1998;6:652-656.

46. Bonomo RA, Rice D, Whalen C, Linn D, Eckstein E, Shlaes DM. Risk factors associated with permanent access-site infections in chronic hemodialysis patients. *Infect Control Hosp Epidemiol.* 1997;18:757-761.

47. Bay WH, Henry ML, Lazarus JM, Lew NL, Ling J, Lowrie EG. Predicting hemodialysis access failure with color flow Doppler ultrasound. *Am J Nephrol.* 1998;18:296-304.

48. May RE, Himmelfarb J, Yenicesu M, et al. Predictive measures of vascular access thrombosis: a prospective study. *Kidney Int.* 1997;52:1656-1662.

49. Wang E, Schneditz D, Levin NW. Predictive value of access blood flow and stenosis in detection of graft failure. *Clin Nephrol.* 2000;54:393-399.

50. Huber TS, Carter JW, Carter RL, Seeger JM. Patency of autogenous and polytetrafluoroethylene upper extremity arteriovenous hemodialysis accesses: a systematic review. *J Vasc Surg.* 2003;38:1005-1011.

51. Gibson KD, Gillen DL, Caps MT, Kohler TR, Sherrard DJ, Stehman-Breen CO. Vascular access survival and incidence of revisions: a comparison of prosthetic grafts, simple autogenous fistulas, and venous transposition fistulas from the United States Renal Data System Dialysis Morbidity and Mortality Study. *J Vasc Surg.* 2001;34:694-700.

52. Trerotola SO. Hemodialysis catheter placement and management. *Radiology.* 2000;215:651-658.

53. Centers for Medicare and Medicaid Services 2007 Annual Report. End-Stage Renal Disease Clinical Performance Measures Project. Baltimore, MD: Centers for Medicare and Medicaid Services, 2007.

54. Dawidson IJ, Ar'Rajab A, Melone LD, Poole T, Griffin D, Risser R. Early use of the Gore-Tex Stretch Graft. *Blood Purif.* 1996;14:337-344.

55. Sottiurai VS, Stephens A, Champagne L, Moradeshagi P, Frey D, Reisin E. Comparative results of early and delayed cannulation of arteriovenous graft in haemodialysis. *Eur J Vasc Endovasc Surg.* 1997;13:139-141.

56. Bartlett ST, Schweitzer EJ, Roberts JE, et al. Early experience with a new ePTFE vascular prosthesis for hemodialysis. *Am J Surg.* 1995;170:118-122.

57. Park TC (ed). The Diastat Vascular Dialysis Graft and the Stretch Graft: A 12-Month Comparative Study. Chicago: Precept Press; 1997.

58. Coyne DW, Lowell JA, Windus DW, et al. Comparison of survival of an expanded polytetrafluoroethylene graft designed for early cannulation to standard wall polytetrafluoroethylene grafts. *J Am Coll Surg.* 1996;183:401-405.

59. Lohr JM, James KV, Hearn AT, Ogden SA. Lessons learned from the DIASTAT vascular access graft. *Am J Surg.* 1996;172:205-209.

60. Kiyama H, Imazeki T, Kurihara S, Yoneshima H. Long-term follow-up of polyurethane vascular grafts for hemoaccess bridge fistulas. *Ann Vasc Surg.* 2003;17:516-521.

61. Wiese P, Blume J, Mueller HJ, Renner H, Nonnast-Daniel AB. Clinical and Doppler ultrasonography data of a polyurethane vascular access graft for haemodialysis: a prospective study. *Nephrol Dial Transplant.* 2003;18:1397-1400.

62. Kapadia MR, Popowich DA, Kibbe MR. Modified prosthetic vascular conduits. *Circulation.* 2008;117:1873-1882.

Central Venous Cannulation for Hemodialysis Access

Matthew D. Danielson, Larry-Stuart Deutsch, and Geoffrey H. White

Vascular access problems continue to be a leading cause of morbidity and hospitalization in patients with chronic kidney disease. Although surgically created arteriovenous (AV) fistulas shunt grafts are now recognized as the "gold standard" in providing vascular access for hemodialysis and offer many advantages over percutaneous catheters for long-term care (refer to www.fistulafirst.org), hemodialysis catheters still have a very important role in the treatment and longevity of hemodialysis patients. Indeed, percutaneous placement of vascular access catheters for both short- and long-term hemodialysis is still an essential tool in the care of hemodialysis patients that offers a wide range of mature catheter technologies optimized for various patient needs.

Vascular access catheters are primarily used to bridge critical time gaps in the treatment of renal failure patients, enabling rapid response to urgent dialysis needs in the case of acute renal failure or allowing uninterrupted dialysis care while patients wait for AV fistula or shunt graft placement, repair, healing at surgical sites, and maturation. Furthermore, long-tem hemodialysis catheters have also proved useful in patients in whom creation of permanent surgical vascular access is inappropriate owing to severe comorbidities including advanced peripheral vascular disease, congestive heart failure, the very elderly, patients with abnormal or inadequate vascular anatomy, or those with limited life expectancy.

Although percutaneous placement of hemodialysis access catheters is often relatively straightforward, establishing and maintaining a high-quality vascular access service capable of handling the broad range of challenges encountered in treating this patient population requires a thorough understanding of these various types of catheters, their uses, and their complications. Nothing simple is actually simple until it is finished, and the incidence of complicated vascular access situations is remarkably common, especially in chronic dialysis patients who have undergone multiple vascular access procedures and developed troublesome venous stenoses or occlusions over the course of their care.

Although initially intended as a set of evidence-based clinical practice guidelines specific to the care of dialysis patients in the United States, the Dialysis Outcomes Quality Initiative (DOQI) published by the Vascular Access Workgroup of the National Kidney Foundation (NKF) in 1997 has become widely accepted around the world as the guidelines of choice regarding vascular access in hemodialysis patients. The goal of this effort is to improve patient survival and quality of life, reduce morbidity, and increase efficiency of care. These guidelines were reissued in an updated and expanded form as the Kidney Disease Outcomes Quality Initiative (K/DOQI) in 2001 and updated again in 2006, and they have become the de facto standard of appropriateness in patient care as well as the basis for both government and private insurance payment policies (see Web site www.kidney.org/professionals/KDOQI).[1] Thus, for both technical and practical reasons, familiarity with and general adherence to those guidelines should be regarded as essential to providing quality care to patients with renal failure, and the material presented in this chapter is consistent with current NKF K/DOQI guidelines.

Equipment and Insertion Technique: Clinical Considerations

There are many commercially available hemodialysis access catheter systems designed for percutaneous placement, and the choices change as scientific advances occur and new products replace old ones. The correct selection of equipment requires a review of the available products and their differences. The list provided in Table 16-1, although certainly not exhaustive, is representative of the major types of hemodialysis access catheter systems in general use today. This discussion, however, focuses on indications for use, implantation techniques, and general considerations rather than specific products.

By convention, the blood withdrawal channel of a hemodialysis catheter is termed *arterial*, and the blood return channel is referred to as *venous*. These terms are best understood if the hemodialysis machine is thought of as an "artificial kidney," a term once in common use. The blood withdrawal channel of a catheter is the *arterial* channel because it provides the arterial inflow to the artificial kidney, and the blood return channel is the *venous* channel because it provides the venous drainage from the artificial kidney. Because these terms may be vague, we suggest referring to the channels in terms of how they relate to the

Table 16–1
Representative Hemodialysis Access Catheter Systems

Short-Term Hemodialysis Catheter Systems—Single-Lumen Nontunneled Systems

Quinton catheter (Covidien, Inc., Mansfield, Mass)
(Not the "classic" dual lumen short-term dialysis catheter originally marketed by Quinton Instrument Co., Bothell, Wash)

Short-Term Hemodialysis Catheter Systems—Dual-Lumen Nontunneled Systems

Mahurkar dual and triple-lumen noncuffed catheters (Covidien, Inc., Mansfield, Mass)
(The dual-lumen catheter is the "classic" short-term dialysis catheter originally marketed by Quinton Instrument Co., Bothell, Wash, and still generally referred to as a "Quinton Catheter")
Brevia and Niagara catheters (Bard Access Systems, Inc., Murray Hill, NJ)

Long-Term Hemodialysis Catheter Systems—Single-Lumen Tunneled Systems

Hickman central venous access catheter (Bard Access Systems, Inc., Murray Hill, NJ)
(This is the "classic" tunneled central venous access catheter generally used for nondialysis applications, not the Hickman Hemodialysis catheter discussed later)

Long-Term Hemodialysis Catheter Systems—Dual-Lumen Staggered Split End Tunneled Systems

Centros and Dynamic Flow catheters (AngioDynamics, Inc., Queensbury, NY)
HemoSplit catheter (Bard Access Systems, Inc., Murray Hill, NJ)
Split-Cath catheter (Medcomp Inc., Harleysville, Pa)

Long-Term Hemodialysis Catheter Systems—Dual-Lumen Staggered Tunneled Systems

Vaxcel catheter (Boston Scientific, Inc., Natick, Mass)
Hemo-Cath and Hemo-Flow catheters (Medcomp, Inc., Harleysville, Pa)
Quinton PermCath and Mahurkar cuffed catheters (Kendall-Covidien, Mansfield, MA)
Dura-Flow and EvenMore catheters (AngioDynamics, Inc., Queensbury, NY)
HemoStar, Hickman dual lumen, and Soft-Cell catheters (Bard Access Systems, Inc., Murray Hill, NJ)
HemoStream Concentric Lumens (Angiotech, Vancouver, British Columbia, Canada)

Long-Term Hemodialysis Catheter Systems—Dual-Lumen Spiral-Z End Tunneled System

Tal Palindrome catheter (Covidien, Inc., Mansfield, Mass)

Long-Term Hemodialysis Catheter Systems—Dual-Catheter Tunneled Systems

Bio-Flex Tesio catheter (Medcomp Inc., Harleysville, Pa)
Tandem-Cath catheter (Covidien, Inc., Mansfield, Mass)
SchonCath catheter (AngioDynamics, Inc., Queensbury, NY)

Long-Term Implantable Hemodialysis Port Systems

LifeSite system (Vasca, Inc., Tewksbury, Mass); no longer manufactured
Dialock system (Biolink, Inc., Middleboro, Mass); no longer manufactured

patient and simply calling them blood *withdrawal* and *return* channels. However, the former terms are still in common use in hemodialysis facilities, and manufacturers still label the extension tubing as either "arterial" or "venous" and often mark the channels by coloring the corresponding catheter fittings red and blue, making it important for the physician to understand these designations.

Duration of Catheterization

Hemodialysis catheters have classically been categorized into short-term and long-term systems depending on their physical and functional characteristics as well as the placement technique required for their use. Although the definitions of *short-term* and *long-term* are flexible, the use of short-term catheters should generally be limited to periods of up to 2 weeks, whereas the long-term catheters can be used reliably without replacement for periods of 1 to 2 years

and sometimes as long as 3 to 4 years with scrupulous catheter care.[2-4] Short-term catheters typically are easy to place with no subcutaneous tunneling and require little to no imaging guidance for placement. They should be used for acute dialysis and limited duration therapy in hospitalized patients. Long-term catheters, conversely, are the catheters of choice when the duration of catheter-based dialysis therapy is anticipated to be longer than 2 weeks, especially in outpatients. They are usually tunneled under the skin to emerge at a site separated from the actual point of vascular entry by a distance of several centimeters and are constructed with added barriers to reduce the risk of infection.

Catheter Design

The initial dual-lumen catheter used for short-term (acute care) hemodialysis, popularized by Uldall and associates,[5] consisted of two interlocking components: an outer cathe-

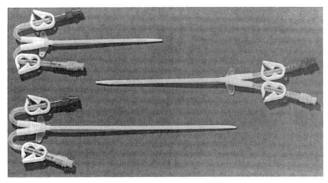

Figure 16-1.
The Quinton-Mahurkar catheter (Covidien, Inc., Mansfield, Mass), now known only as the Mahurkar catheter, is used for acute care hemodialysis with or without reverse-curved extension tubing. Although it is only one of many popular catheters used for temporary hemodialysis, it was the first catheter to be widely used for this purpose. Thus, many other temporary catheters are often referred to generically as "Quinton catheters," much as many brands of tissue paper are referred to as "Kleenex."

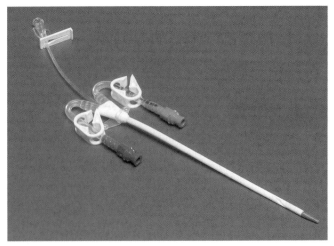

Figure 16-3.
The triple-lumen Mahurkar is identical to the classic "Quinton catheter" with the exception of an additional 19-gauge intravenous infusion port. This simple addition is very useful in patients with limited vascular access options, often saving an additional, potentially difficult venous access procedure.

ter with side holes for blood withdrawal and a thin-walled inner catheter for blood return that was introduced over an obturator through the outer catheter. Although it provided adequate access for hemodialysis, it was also plagued by frequent clotting and was soon discarded in favor of the dual-lumen Quinton-Mahurkar catheter (Quinton Instrument Co., Bothell, Wash). This is a single, round, flexible polyurethane catheter with a dividing septum that creates two back-to-back D-shaped channels connected via a molded Y-piece to separate color-coded external tubes, of which each is fitted with a flexible plastic clamp safety closure and an injectable Luer-Lok cap. The Quinton-Mahurkar is currently known and marketed as the Mahurkar catheter (Covidien, Inc., Mansfield, Mass).

Although the Quinton-Mahurkar catheter (Fig. 16-1) is certainly not the only catheter in common use for short-term hemodialysis, it is in many ways typical of the class of catheters used for this purpose. The tip of the catheter is constructed with the blood withdrawal and return ports staggered usually at 2.5 cm to minimize recirculation (Fig. 16-2) with the external blue and red catheter fittings marking the distal and proximal ends of the dual-lumen staggered tip, respectively. This relatively stiff catheter is placed via conventional Seldinger technique, and the tip is sufficiently tapered so that it can be placed over a guidewire

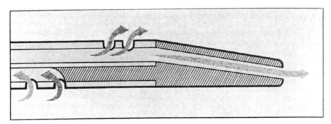

Figure 16-2.
Diagram of the Mahurkar catheter tip shows the staggered blood withdrawal and return pathways designed to minimize recirculation during hemodialysis.

without the need for ancillary vascular dilators, although they are provided in the insertion set. A recently introduced triple lumen version includes an additional 19-gauge intravenous infusion channel that eliminates the need for an additional venous access procedure in patients with limited venous access sites (Fig. 16-3).

Whereas the short straight or J-shaped guidewires supplied in most dialysis catheter insertion sets are adequate for the purpose, they are usually relatively stiff-tipped wires that can damage vessels upon insertion and tend to have relatively weak shaft strength that provides poor support during the insertion process. Using standard interventional radiologic guidewires such as the floppy-tipped, stiff-shaft Amplatz Interventional guidewire (Cook, Inc., Bloomington, Ohio) available in a convenient 80-cm length provides an extra measure of safety, maneuverability, and support, which makes it preferable to the guidewires supplied with most insertion sets.

The Brevia short-term hemodialysis catheter (Bard Access Systems, Salt Lake City, Utah) is also a tapered-tip, staggered-port device and is in most respects similar to the Mahurkar catheter. The oval Niagara catheter (Bard Access Systems), conversely, is relatively blunt tipped and requires the use of both vascular dilators and a temporary coaxial plastic stiffener for placement. The Brevia and Niagara catheters are constructed of a relatively soft and thermally sensitive Bodysoft polyurethane formulation that the manufacturer claims softens considerably when exposed to body heat, which makes the catheter more pliant and less prone to causing vascular injury. Unlike the Mahurkar and Brevia devices, which support dialysis flow rates of approximately 300 mL/min, the Niagara catheter can support flow rates of as much as 400 mL/min at normal operating pressures, thus markedly improving the efficiency and reducing the duration of dialysis sessions.

Most of the short-term hemodialysis catheters are available in a range of sizes, lengths, and configurations, with either straight or reverse-curved extension tubes designed to enhance acceptance among ambulatory patients.

Long-Term Catheters

Although some of the classic designs remain in widespread use, the range of choices in long-term hemodialysis catheter systems is considerable and frequently changing. Among these is the classic Quinton PermCath catheter (Covidien, Mansfield, MA) which is a large-caliber, soft, flexible, dual-lumen silicone rubber catheter with two side-by-side round channels in an oval catheter. The Hickman dual-lumen catheter (Bard Access Systems), which is also a long-term hemodialysis catheter, is conceptually similar to the Quinton PermCath and is constructed from a similar material; however, it is a round 13.5-Fr (4.5-mm) catheter with asymmetrical inner channels. Although the Hickman and Perm-Cath dual-lumen hemodialysis catheters are still in use, many physicians have switched to catheters such as the HemoStar catheter (Bard Access Systems), which, although it looks remarkably like the Hickman dual-lumen hemodialysis catheter, has larger lumens and is composed of the same thermally sensitive Bodysoft polyurethane material used in the Niagara catheter. Furthermore, it can accommodate flow rates up to 500 mL/min as opposed to the Quinton Perm-Cath or Hickman dual-lumen hemodialysis catheters, which generally achieve rates of approximately 350 mL/min. The distal ends of the Quinton PermCath, Hickman dual-lumen, and HemoStar catheters are not tapered like the Mahurkar catheter, but they share a similar arrangement of staggered blood withdrawal and return ports designed to minimize recirculation. These catheters have extension tubing, closures, and clamps similar to those of the Mahurkar catheter. Because these long-term catheters are all designed for tunneled implantation, they also have a polyethylene terephthalate (Dacron) cuff that provides fixation through tissue ingrowth within the subcutaneous tunnel.

Catheter Tips

A new trend in hemodialysis catheter tips has developed in which the staggered blood withdrawal and return ports that were originally fused in an asymmetrical steplike configuration are now separated from one another, commonly referred to as a *staggered split-end catheter*. Split-end catheters improve flow and eliminate positional occlusion, a phenomenon that occurs when the tip of a catheter abuts the venous wall and blocks blood return from the patient due to the relatively high negative pressure developed in the return channel. The Centros catheter (AngioDynamics, Inc., Queensbury, NY), which supports flow rates in excess of 400 mL/min, has the added benefit of permanently curving the staggered split-end tips toward midline, which automatically centers the catheter tips within the vessel, furthermore decreasing the likelihood of positional occlusion. Specially placed side holes are used in these split catheters to facilitate using a guidewire woven between the two split ends and to keep the tips together to facilitate easy insertion.

The pace of new product announcements in this field is rapid, with new advances and novel designs introduced almost daily in an effort to increase the efficacy and useful life of both short- and long-term percutaneous hemodialysis catheters. One such novel design is the Tal Palindrome catheter (Covidien). This 14.5-Fr catheter boasts a unique symmetrical Z-tip design that decreases approximation of the lumen against the vessel wall and minimizes the risk of positional occlusion. As its name suggests, it functions effectively when the withdrawal and return ports are used as labeled or reversed and it supports flow rates of up to 450 mL/min while greatly reducing recirculation.

Catheter Placement

Although relatively large, the long-term hemodialysis catheters are placed with the same technique used for many other central venous access catheters. Preplacement planning, however, is more important because the staggered ports at the catheter tip have a specialized function and this end cannot be cut to accommodate patient size, as is done with many other tunneled catheters (eg, Hickman, Leonard, and Broviac vascular access catheters) (Fig. 16-4). Thus, it is important to select an appropriate catheter length and lay the catheter out along the intended course of insertion so as to plan a subcutaneous tunnel that will yield the desired intravascular tip position. Then tunnel the catheter from its intended exit site to a small wound at the puncture site. At this point, flush the catheter with heparinized saline and close both extension tubes using the tubing clamps provided with the catheter. Because these catheters have relatively large channels, this simple maneuver is an important pre-

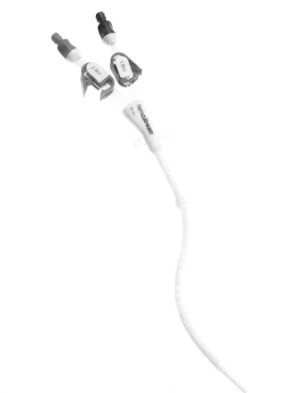

Figure 16-4.

A variety of effective catheter tip configurations (eg, staggered lumen, split end, spiral-Z) have been developed by various manufacturers in order to minimize recirculation and avoid catheter malfunction due to "side-walling" occlusion caused by vessel wall impingement on the high flow withdrawal (arterial) channel. The HemoStream (Angiotech, Vancouver, British Columbia, Canada) is a unique design that employs three radially distributed withdrawal flow channels leading to a single conventional connector. The symmetrical tapered tip configuration also permits the optional insertion over a guidewire without the use of a vascular introducer sheath.

caution against the occurrence of inadvertent and potentially serious air embolism during catheter insertion through the peel-away access sheath. Use the Seldinger technique to achieve venous access, and place the peel-away vascular access sheath supplied with the catheter into the venous system via guidewire exchange, using ancillary vascular dilators as needed. Finally, place the catheter via the peel-away sheath, and confirm appropriate position with fluoroscopy, if available. To further reduce the risk of air embolization and blood loss while transferring the catheter into the peel-away sheath, some catheter insertion sets include peel-away insertion sheaths equipped with built-in hemostatic valves (eg, EmboSafe, AngioDynamics, Inc., Queensbury, NY) that largely eliminate the risk of air embolism.[6] Other techniques such as pinching the peel-away sheath, using a hemostat to clamp the sheath, or occluding the sheath with a finger and timing the insertion to match the expiratory phase of the patient's breathing, although perhaps less convenient, have also been found to have similar results.[7] Regardless of which technique is employed to prevent air embolism, the operator must be keenly aware of the risk because a substantial portion of patients receiving these catheters are incapable of complying with breathing instructions and the onus of preventing this potentially serious complication rests with the operator. For this reason, some physicians have even chosen to eliminate the introducer sheath when using staggered-tip catheters that permit the use of a woven guidewire technique that temporarily, but very effectively, unites the separate tip lumens into a single fixed structure during the insertion process. This method allows the predilated entry tract to be occluded with simple finger pressure during the insertion process and the catheter to be advanced as a single unit over the guidewire directly through the skin entry site without the use of a sheath. No matter which technique is used for the catheter insertion, if preplacement tunnel planning has been done correctly, once the catheter has been inserted, changing the position of the catheter within the tunnel will produce small adjustments in catheter tip position. However, as with all cuffed catheters, the cuff should ideally be placed relatively close to the exit site because it is part of the infection barrier mechanism.

In addition to the fact that catheter ends cannot be shortened without impairment of their dialysis efficiency, there is an important difference between implantation of dialysis catheters and other tunneled central venous access catheters that must be noted: one has to take much greater care in preparing the puncture site to avoid kinking than one does with the smaller catheters. To avoid catheter kinking, it is essential to create a reasonably large subcutaneous pocket that extends away from the actual puncture site wound to provide sufficient room for the catheter to form a gentle curve once the peel-away sheath is removed. Many of these catheters can now be ordered with preformed curved extension tubing that serves to minimize the chance of kinking. Regardless of the catheter used, it is absolutely essential to check for kinking before conclusion of the procedure. If kinking is found, make whatever adjustments are needed to alleviate the problem. Although most cases of catheter kinking are apparent fluoroscopically, checking for adequate flow rate is still important to avoid kinking that may be more subtle. This check can be easily performed by aspirating venous blood from each lumen with a 20-cc syringe as quickly as possible. If any resistance is met or if

there is slow blood flow into the syringe, further adjustments need to be made. These are essential parts of the implantation procedure.

Dual Catheter Systems

The Bio-Flex Tesio dual-catheter (Medcomp, Inc., Harleysville, Pa) (Fig. 16-5) and other similar dual-catheter tunneled systems represent another important approach to the problem of achieving efficient hemodialysis and shortening the duration of the sessions. The Tesio system, which is capable of supporting flow rates of approximately 400 to 450 mL/min, uses two completely separate tunneled catheters placed via adjacent vascular access sites; each component is simply a large-bore tunneled catheter whose fittings are attached after tunneling. Placement of the Tesio component catheters is similar to placement of many other central venous catheters. In particular, the fact that the fittings are attached to the catheter after vascular access has been achieved allows the catheter tip to be placed at exactly the desired location using fluoroscopic guidance, with the

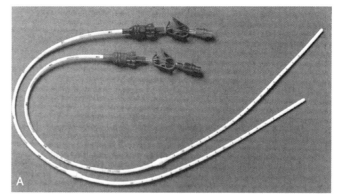

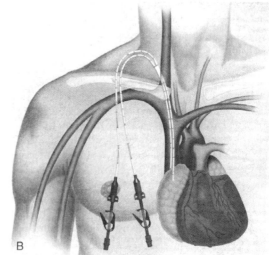

Figure 16-5.
A, The Bio-Flex Tesio system (Medcomp, Inc., Harleysville, Pa) uses two separate tunneled catheters, each capable of providing flow rates of approximately 400 to 450 mL/min. *B,* The Schon-Cath (AngioDynamics, Inc., Queensbury, NY) provides similar functionality to the Bio-Flex Tesio system but simplifies the insertion process by using a dual-catheter system in which the two catheters are joined at one point along their course to form a short anchoring hub.

length adjusted during the tunneling process as opposed to the more cumbersome and error-prone technique required when using catheters whose fittings are preattached and therefore must be tunneled before the vascular access step. The disadvantage of these dual-catheter systems is that they generally require the use of separate adjacent vascular access sites and thus incur the additional risk of a separate vessel puncture, although a single-site technique with two guidewires can sometimes be used. Furthermore, the large bullet-shaped fixation devices that secure the Tesio catheters within the subcutaneous tunnel are relatively large, making the tunneling process more difficult for this catheter than for the usual tunneled central venous catheter. Likewise, the retention bullets make removal more difficult. Nevertheless, the Bio-Flex Tesio has gained considerable popularity among nephrologists because of the high flow rates, although it should be noted that they are often not the individuals who actually place these catheters.

Conceptually similar to the Bio-Flex Tesio system, the SchonCath (AngioDynamics, Inc., Queensbury, NY) (see Fig. 16-5) simplifies the insertion process by using a dual-catheter system in which the two catheters are joined at one point along their course to form a short anchoring hub. This arrangement has the advantage of allowing the two catheters to be placed using a single-puncture access technique, whereas it has the disadvantage of requiring a relatively large vascular access sheath because the sheath must accommodate both catheters simultaneously. Once the catheters have been placed in the vessel and the peel-away sheath is removed, the two catheters are tunneled to separate exit sites, making the point at which they are bonded together a very effective anchoring hub within the tunnel.

Subcutaneous Ports

Although there are substantial advantages and disadvantages to the various short- and long-term hemodialysis catheter systems, they all share the disadvantage of being externalized devices prone to inadvertent dislodging and contamination even with meticulous care. Furthermore, patients may like their ease of use, but they also consider them to be both inconvenient and esthetically unappealing. For that reason, two companies developed subcutaneous port implants as alternatives to conventional long-term catheter systems that are capable of accommodating the high flow rates and frequent access demands of hemodialysis (Fig. 16-6). The LifeSite system (Vasca, Inc., Tewksbury, Mass) consisted of two identical subcutaneous ports that were implanted in the same manner as the usual subcutaneous ports used in cancer chemotherapy, although they had tubing and needle access valves specially designed to meet the special demands of hemodialysis. The LifeSite system was capable of supporting flow rates of 450 to 480 mL/min and could also be used as a single-port system for peritoneal dialysis. Unfortunately, although this system seemed very promising, the U.S. Food and Drug Administration (FDA) received 129 adverse incident reports and the company became the target of product liability litigation that resulted in the demise of the firm in January 2006. The Dialock System[8] (Biolink, Inc., Middleboro, Mass) was a single-body, two-access port system that used two separate catheters attached to a dual-channel access port. Flow rates in the Dialock System were reported to be around 330 mL/min on average. Unfortunately, despite promising early reports, this firm has also ceased operations and the product is no longer available.

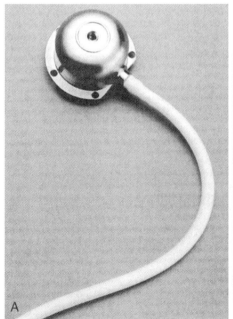
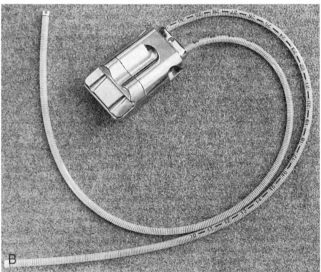

Figure 16-6.
A, The LifeSite (Vasca, Inc., Tewksbury, MA) hemodialysis system used two subcutaneous ports that are implanted like conventional subcutaneous vascular access ports, although they used valves specially designed to meet the demands of hemodialysis rather than the conventional diaphragm and reservoir (device no longer available). *B,* The Dialock System (Biolink, Inc., Middleboro, MA) uses two separate catheters attached to a single-body dual-channel access port unit equipped with special septum-less atraumatic access valves (device no longer available).

For completeness, it is important to remember that conventional small-caliber single-lumen tunneled catheters such as the Hickman, Leonard, and Quinton vascular access catheters may also be used for single-needle hemodialysis, although they are incapable of supporting high flow rates. Furthermore, the cyclic single-needle hemodialysis machines required when using these catheters are both uncommon and inefficient. Thus, this technique is now largely of historic interest and should be reserved for rare situations in which there is no feasible alternative and the need for dialysis is expected to be brief.

Antibiotic prophylaxis, using antistaphylococcal agents such as vancomycin, is still controversial despite its common use. When antibiotics are used, however, it is important to consider the route of clearance. Vancomycin clearance depends solely on renal function. In patients with anuria, a single dose will last until the next hemodialysis session and will make this the usual agent of choice despite real concern for the development of vancomycin-resistant enterococcus (VRE) either as a clinical infection or as a carrier state.

Image-Guided Placement

Some of the most important advantages of percutaneous catheter placement for short-term hemodialysis access are the speed, simplicity, and safety of the technique. When the patient's condition makes transport inconvenient or hazardous, urgent venous access can generally be accomplished with the Mahurkar catheter using a sterile bedside

approach without the use of either fluoroscopic or ultrasound guidance. Ideally, however, all central venous catheters should be placed in a sterile procedure room, operating room, or interventional suite with the aid of fluoroscopic as well as ultrasound guidance. Maintenance of strict sterile technique is simple in these areas, and the use of fluoroscopy coupled with other angiographic techniques permits the operator to deal effectively with problem catheterization situations (Fig. 16-7). Likewise, the routine use of ultrasound guidance for initial vascular access punctures has virtually eliminated complications such as pneumothorax and is by now the de facto standard of care. The large caliber of the long-term, tunneled hemodialysis catheters (eg, Quinton PermCath and Hickman dual-lumen catheters) and the potential for serious complications in the event of a failed attempt at blind placement make the use of fluoroscopic guidance and the controlled environment of an operating room or interventional suite virtually mandatory when percutaneous placement methods are used. When fluoroscopy is unavailable, however, blind placement of these catheters by surgical cutdown does, however, have the advantage that it is simpler to back out from a failed placement attempt than it is with percutaneous methods.

Blind insertion of a central venous catheter, that is, placement using anatomic landmarks rather than imaging guidance, whether performed at the bedside or in the operating room, carries with it the special obligation to desist when unexpected or unexplained difficulties are encountered because it is difficult to accurately determine

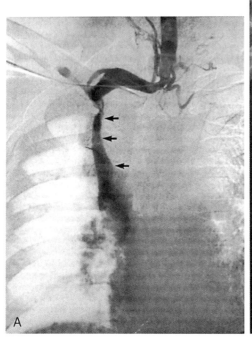 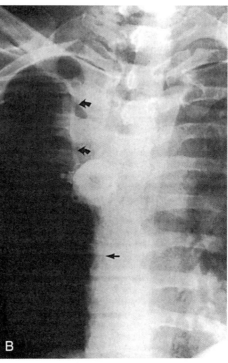

Figure 16-7.

A, A large superior mediastinal mass deviates and compresses the superior vena cava (SVC) *(arrows)* so much that blind catheterization would not have succeeded. *B,* With the use of fluoroscopy and a steerable guidewire to negotiate the distorted SVC, the catheter tip *(straight arrow)* was easily directed through the deviated SVC *(curved arrows)* toward the right atrium. (Radiation and chemotherapy reduced the size of this mass and restored normal central venous anatomy [not shown].)

the cause of the problem. The inability to freely advance a guidewire without resistance may be associated with venous occlusion, stenosis, or distortion of the regional anatomy (see Fig. 16-7). The natural tendency to avoid withdrawing the needle from a vessel once blood return has been achieved makes inexperienced operators tend to advance the needle slightly so that its tip may come to rest close to the opposite wall of the vessel, making guidewire insertion difficult. This situation can easily lead to vessel perforation because even a floppy-tipped, atraumatic guidewire can be remarkably stiff when it protrudes only a few millimeters from a needle. If resistance to guidewire passage is encountered, removal of the guidewire, readjustment of needle depth or angulation, reconfirmation of good blood return, and reintroduction of the guidewire coupled with judicious persistence may solve the problem. However, the attempt should be discontinued promptly if this maneuver is unsuccessful. Forceful attempts at blind passage of either a guidewire or a catheter can easily lead to considerable complications (Fig. 16-8).

Blind insertion of hemodialysis catheters is still routinely performed in many centers; however, it is important to recognize that most complications associated with the use of these devices are actually related to the initial placement procedure and the inability to visualize the course of the needle, guidewire, or catheter within the patient. Fluoroscopic guidance has gained widespread acceptance and is considered the standard of care in most settings because it virtually eliminates most of these hazards.

Initial Venous Access

Micropuncture technique for the initial venous access has also gained widespread, although not universal, acceptance. Rather than using conventional 18- or 19-gauge needles for the initial venipuncture, a much smaller caliber 21-gauge needle is used. On obtaining blood return from the needle, a small-caliber 0.018-inch guidewire is used in place of the usual 0.035- or 0.038-inch guidewire. A short coaxial dilator set with an inner component tapered to the 0.018-inch guidewire and an outer component that will admit a 0.035-inch guidewire is then advanced into the vessel over the 0.018-inch guidewire. Once this has been done, the inner component is removed and a conventional 0.035-inch guidewire is advanced through the outer dilator. This technique has the advantage of being far less traumatic than the standard large-bore needle technique, materially reducing the incidence of bleeding and pneumothorax. Although direct puncture of the underlying lung is certainly not an advisable maneuver, puncturing it with a 21-gauge needle will generally not produce a pneumothorax unless there is considerable underlying pulmonary pathology, a contrast to the situation encountered when this is done using the usual 18- or 19-gauge needle. In addition, the inadvertent puncture of an artery with a 21-gauge needle is far less likely to result in substantial hemorrhage than is the case with an 18- or a 19-gauge needle, a consideration of particular importance for patients with renal failure who often have platelet dysfunction and other coagulopathies.

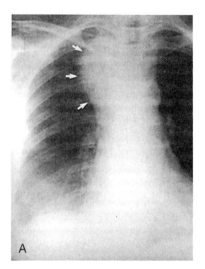

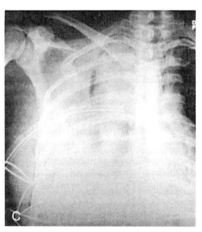

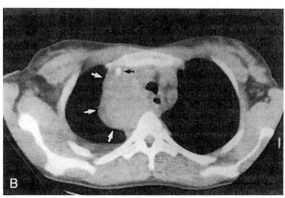

Figure 16-8.

A, Chest radiograph of patient with a new superior mediastinal mass *(arrows)* that appeared after difficult blind placement of a Quinton Perm-Cath catheter. B, Computed tomography scan shows large superior mediastinal hematoma *(white arrows)* and hemodialysis catheter *(black arrow)*. C, Portable chest radiograph just before patient's death shows severe hemothorax. (Catheter was removed by the ward team without consulting the surgery service.)

Another simple technique that is of great use in avoiding insertion complications when using either a subclavian or a jugular venous approach is visual identification of the superior vena cava by guidewire course. If the initial guidewire, whether a conventional 0.035/0.038-inch guidewire or an 0.018-inch microguidewire, is advanced through the right atrium into the inferior vena cava, one can be confident that the guidewire actually traverses the superior vena cava and has not entered either an artery or the azygos vein. Although the lack of cardiac motion should make it obvious that a guidewire has entered the azygos vein rather than the superior vena cava, the course is similar enough and the lack of cardiac motion a sufficiently subtle finding that recognition of this problem can sometimes be difficult for those not experienced in angiographic techniques. Whereas inadvertent arterial puncture or azygos vein catheterization with a guidewire (even a large-caliber 0.035/0.038-inch guidewire) may indeed cause problems, the complications that arise from the advancement of a much larger caliber hemodialysis catheter or access sheath are far more critical, making prior identification of the superior vena cava a very useful complication avoidance maneuver.

Although blind venipuncture is still an acceptable technique in placement of short-term nontunneled dialysis catheters, especially in urgent situations, the use of ultrasound guidance (gray scale with or without color-flow Doppler) is remarkably useful in determining vessel location and patency. Indeed, in difficult situations, real-time ultrasound guidance can transform a difficult puncture into a straightforward exercise, which is why ultrasound guidance is now routinely used at initial venipuncture in most facilities and its use has become the de facto standard of care at most institutions. Because most long-term tunneled dialysis catheters are placed via the internal jugular vein approach and then tunneled to emerge caudal to the clavicle, ultrasound guidance has the added benefit of allowing the operator to plan a specific vessel entry site to allow for creation of a subcutaneous pocket that will easily accommodate the catheter, providing room for a gentle catheter curve avoiding the sort of kinking than can render a newly placed catheter useless. Alternatively, in the case of subclavian catheterization, an assistant may inject radiographic contrast material via a peripheral vein in the ipsilateral arm while the operator punctures the subclavian contrast column under fluoroscopic control. If both fluoroscopy and ultrasound are unavailable, repeated unsuccessful puncture attempts should be followed by the selection of a new access site. In the case of subclavian (infraclavicular or supraclavicular) and jugular venous approaches, it is also essential to confirm the absence of pneumothorax by either fluoroscopy or chest radiography before attempting a contralateral approach.

Catheter Complications

Because dialysis flow is venovenous, the hemodialysis machine must include a blood pump. Common problems include poor flow from the catheter to the hemodialysis machine or the need to use greater-than-normal withdrawal pressures to maintain adequate flow. Often, this is a one-way obstruction of the blood withdrawal (arterial) side of the catheter resulting from positioning of the inflow holes against the vessel wall. If this is the situation, it can be

confirmed by demonstrating inability to aspirate blood despite easy flushing. Simply reversing the connections to the hemodialysis machine will often alleviate the problem, but this maneuver increases the degree of recirculation and thus decreases the efficiency of the hemodialysis process, because the arrangement of the staggered blood withdrawal and return ports at the catheter tip obviously cannot be changed. The exception to this would be the Tal Palindrome catheter (Covidien, Inc., Mansfield, Mass) with its symmetrical spiral-Z tip that specifically takes into account the occasional need for flow reversal hemodialysis. In the case of the short-term hemodialysis catheters, the problem is resolved by simply turning the catheter at the insertion or withdrawing it slightly. (Reintroduction, even for a short distance, should never be attempted without a guidewire because of the risk of vessel perforation.) These maneuvers are not applicable to long-term hemodialysis catheters, however, because they are firmly fixed within the subcutaneous tunnel within a few days.

Poor flow associated with a one-way obstruction tends to occur early in the useful life of the catheter. Later on, poor flow tends to be associated with *fibrin sheathing*, a phenomenon that occurs with virtually all indwelling catheters to some extent. This phenomenon is easily documented by injecting radiographic contrast material, using either fluoroscopy or conventional angiographic serial filming. (One-shot contrast material injections made with portable radiographic equipment can easily fail to demonstrate the finding even when a considerable obstructive fibrin sheath is present, simply as a result of timing difficulties.) Because the useful life of the Mahurkar and Niagara catheters is relatively short, the problem is best solved by exchanging the old catheter for a new one using guidewire exchange technique, preferably with disruption of the sheath using an angioplasty balloon. Conversely, the long-term hemodialysis catheters have relatively long useful lives, and both insertion and withdrawal are more complex and make catheter salvage preferable to replacement. For this reason, it is often advantageous to use a lytic infusion (eg, tissue-type plasminogen activator [t-PA]) to break up the fibrin sheath or a loop snare device to strip the fibrin sheath off the catheter.[9] Because the fibrin sheath once removed from the catheter embolizes to the lung, the technique may seem unattractive at first.[10] However, when one considers that catheters removed from a vessel will always have their fibrin sheath stripped off at the vessel entry, with some fibrin plugs adhering to the vessel at the entry site and many embolizing to the lung, it seems better to preserve catheter function than to subject the patient to the risks involved in finding a new access site; pulmonary embolization is likely in either case.[11] Fortunately, the embolic burden is sufficiently small that the occurrence of considerable cardiorespiratory symptoms on catheter removal is a rare event, even when occlusive fibrin sheathing has been angiographically documented. Although unappealing, the presence of a septic process that might involve colonization of the fibrin sheath is only a relative contraindication to lytic infusion or the loop snare technique; the prospect of causing a septic pulmonary embolus is certainly unattractive until one remembers that simply removing the catheter will likely have the same effect. In any event, instituting appropriate antibiotic therapy is essential. The availability of an appropriate venous access site for introduction of the loop snare catheter does, however, limit the applicability of the technique, sometimes making it difficult in patients with limited access.

Equipment Selection: Technical Considerations

Although it is impractical for most users to actually perform the studies involved in the technical evaluation of specific hemodialysis catheters, it is still helpful to understand the factors involved in the evaluation of catheter efficacy (Table 16-2).

Modern high-efficiency hemodialysis machines are generally operated at flow rates between 250 and 350 mL/min when using catheter access (300-400 mL/min when using prosthetic grafts or fistulas), with blood withdrawal and return pressures up to 250 mm Hg, although improvements in catheter design have made it possible to achieve rates over 400 mL/min with catheter-based hemodialysis at the same operating pressures. Thus, it is essential for a hemodialysis catheter to provide this flow without Venturi effect, wall collapse, or considerable mechanically induced hemolysis.

Ideally, the arterial inflow to the hemodialysis machine consists entirely of unprocessed blood; that is, all of the blood returned to the patient from the hemodialysis machine should mix uniformly with the patient's systemic blood pool before reentering the hemodialysis process. In practice, whether surgically created AV fistulas, shunt grafts, or percutaneous catheters are used, there is always some recirculation of the hemodialysis effluent blood with the inflow stream as a result of the proximity of the blood withdrawal and return pathways. Classically, this recirculation percentage, a measure of efficiency loss, is calculated with the following equation:

$$R (\%) = [(U_{pv} - U_a)/(U_{pv} - U_v)] \times 100$$

where U_{pv} is peripheral vein blood urea nitrogen, U_a is blood urea nitrogen for arterial inflow to dialyzer, and U_v is blood urea nitrogen for venous effluent from dialyzer. Routine assessment of recirculation is, however, generally done using noninvasive methods (eg, ultrasound dilution [Transonics, Inc., Ithaca, NY]) with the urea technique being reserved for confirmation of abnormal measurements and periodic quality control.

Recirculation associated with percutaneous dialysis catheters is primarily determined by the configuration of catheter inflow and outflow ports; however, anatomic location is also important because of the size and flow rate characteristics of each site. For example, one type of hemodialysis catheter was shown to yield recirculation rates of approximately 3% to 7% in the subclavian and jugular positions, whereas the same catheter type produced a recirculation rate of 18% in the femoral position when used in a short (15-cm) version and a rate of 10% when used in a longer (24-cm) version that actually placed the active segment of the catheter in the inferior vena cava, a larger vessel with more rapid flow than the femoral vein.[12] All other factors being equal, minimizing recirculation by either catheter design or placement enhances the efficiency of the hemodialysis process.

Most hemodialysis catheters are made of polyurethane or silicone rubber, materials that are remarkably free of adverse bioreactivity. Virtually all catheters, however, tend to become enveloped in a fibrin sheath with time. The extent to which this occurs varies with surface coating, shape, anatomic site, and anticoagulant or antiplatelet therapy, but it is still one of the major limitations of long-term catheter use. The other major factor that limits the useful life of these catheters is the occurrence of bacterial colonization. Bacterial growth, usually involving skin organisms (eg, *Staphylococcus epidermidis*) originating at the skin entry site,[13] tends to advance retrograde along the catheter, thriving in the nutrient-rich pericatheter fibrin sheath from which it disseminates in the form of microemboli. Such growth is the principal reason why the short-term catheters should be exchanged at a frequency of 1 to 2 weeks.[14] Fortunately, a guidewire exchange can be performed using the same access site, unless gross contamination of the skin entry site is present.

The Dacron fixation cuff on the long-term catheters provides an effective, but still incomplete, infection barrier. For that reason, the use of an antibacterial silver-impregnated collagen cuff (eg, VitaCuff; Bard Access Systems, Inc., Murray Hill, NJ) adjacent to the Dacron fixation cuff designed to be placed within the subcutaneous tunnel close to the skin entry site has gained some popularity. The efficacy of this device is still controversial, however, with some authors claiming a significant decrease in infection rate[15] and others reporting no significant effect.[16] Many catheters are now available constructed with various antimicrobial silver-impregnated coatings and sleeves built on to the tunnel tubing itself, but their efficacy is also still controversial.[17]

Although catheter flexibility, softness, and kink resistance are all important factors, the choice of commercially available materials and designs is limited. Nevertheless, users need to be aware of these characteristics when planning catheter insertion so as to minimize sharp bends in the intravascular and subcutaneous tunnel segments to avoid

---

Table 16-2
Technical Factors Affecting Hemodialysis Catheter Efficacy

Hemodynamic Factors

Recirculation
Maximum flow rate

Biocompatibility

Thrombogenicity
Care and duration of use
Antimicrobial cuffs and catheter coating

Mechanical Factors

Catheter tubing and tip variations
Flexibility and kink-resistance
External versus internal dimensions
Cross-sectional profile

Convenience

Radiopacity
Fixation
Availability of different sizes and lengths
Availability of access kits

obstructive kinking or exertion of undue forces on the vessel wall that may lead to erosion and perforation.

When all of the other differences in the catheter systems marketed by various firms are considered, convenience issues should also be considered. The degree of radiopacity and the presence of embedded radiopaque stripes or tip markers can have a great impact on the ease of placement when using fluoroscopic guidance. The type of external catheter fixation and the range of available sizes and lengths are also important convenience issues, as is the composition of the insertion set supplied with the catheter. The routine use of items not included with the insertion set, although perhaps necessary, adds cost and decreases efficiency.

Vascular Access Routes

Site Selection

Placement of an ipsilateral catheter at certain sites may adversely affect the long-term patency of a newly created surgical access or complicate a subsequent surgical access procedure. The selection of a specific vascular access approach for percutaneous placement of either a short- or a long-term hemodialysis catheter requires careful consideration of the relative risks and benefits of each approach and an assessment of the patient's current situation, including any prior or planned access procedures. Because these considerations are so important to patient outcome, K/DOQI, the de facto standard of care for kidney disease patients, addresses the issue of access site in detail.

Whereas the use of small-caliber vascular access catheters intended for routine nondialysis intravenous therapy (eg, fluid and medications) is beyond the range of this chapter, consideration of their impact on both current and future dialysis access is an essential part of access planning in renal failure patients whether or not these patients have reached the stage of actually requiring dialysis. For that reason, the K/DOQI guidelines are very specific in recommending against the use of peripherally inserted central catheters (PICCs) in this patient population. PICC catheter use has been associated with a vessel stenosis rate of up to 7% and a thrombosis rate variously reported as ranging from 11% to as high as 85%, a complication that continually eliminates a potential site for creation of a vascular access fistula or shunt graft and can thus materially affect patient survival. Similarly, tunneled central venous catheters should be placed in the right internal jugular vein or, if unavailable, the left internal jugular vein rather than the right or left subclavian vein in order to avoid development of flow limiting stenoses that could affect future dialysis access.

Femoral Approach

Practical percutaneous catheterization for temporary hemodialysis was first described by Shaldon and colleagues in 1961[18] using separate single-lumen catheters in the femoral artery and vein. Since that time, several venovenous hemodialysis techniques have been developed that use femoral vein catheterization. Because the Shaldon catheters and the variants that followed were relatively

large, repeated femoral vein puncture was advocated for intermittent hemodialysis[19] to avoid the risks associated with long-term femoral vein catheterization, such as thrombosis and pulmonary embolization. Use of a single-lumen device necessitated the use of two separate catheters, one for blood withdrawal and the other for blood return; these were positioned either in each femoral vein or both in the same femoral vein. Alternatively, a femoral vein was catheterized for blood withdrawal and a conventional large-bore peripheral intravenous catheter was used to accommodate the blood return from the dialyzer. When patient condition or the lack of available access sites dictated, hemodialysis could also be achieved using only one catheter, but this technique required the use of a cyclic single-needle hemodialysis machine to provide alternate blood cycling through the same channel and resulted in significant blood recirculation and inefficiency.[20] The advent of practical dual-lumen catheters such as the Mahurkar greatly simplified the process of percutaneous vascular access for hemodialysis and largely eliminated the need for cyclic single-needle hemodialysis machines.

Although occasionally indicated for short-term and long-term hemodialysis, femoral vein catheterization is far from ideal. The infection rate associated with femoral catheters is higher than that seen in other sites, especially in obese patients. In the immobilized patient, there also is a substantial risk for venous thrombosis because femoral vein flow rates are inherently lower than those seen in the subclavian and jugular veins, especially in low-output states, and continuous anticoagulation carries its own well-known risks. In an ambulatory patient, the presence of a femoral catheter markedly limits mobility. Furthermore, the forces and catheter movements associated with walking and sitting carry a risk of vein perforation when any but the most blunt-tipped soft devices are used. Although most health care workers avoid the use of femoral hemodialysis access catheters in ambulatory patients, especially the acute care catheters such as the Mahurkar and Niagara, there have been reports of small numbers of tunneled, silicone rubber catheters placed in the femoral vein for long-term hemodialysis.[21] These were generally placed via a skin puncture situated close to the groin fold with a tunnel usually directed cephalad so as to place the external segment of the catheter in a lower abdominal quadrant for patient convenience, although a tunnel that allows the catheter to take a straight line course and exit along the anterior thigh is also acceptable in most situations and flexion at the hip does not appear to be a practical problem. An ipsilateral renal transplant, or planned transplantation, is also a relative contraindication to femoral vein catheterization because of the risk of femoral vein thrombosis, which may seriously impair venous outflow from the transplant.

Subclavian Vein: Infraclavicular Approach

In 1969, Erben[22] first described infraclavicular subclavian catheterization, which is the conventional technique for subclavian catheterization. The technique has long been popular because it is convenient for both physicians and patients. Conscious patients tend to be more comfortable with a physician working on their chest wall than on their neck or groin, and the catheter can be easily hidden under clothing. Physicians also tend to prefer this approach because it eliminates concerns about risk of infection with long-term femoral catheterization or neurovascular complications with the internal jugular approach. Although hemodialysis catheters are relatively sturdy and less likely to experience catheter fracture caused by improper placement technique than the usual central venous access catheters, it is still best to place them so that the subclavian vein entry is situated lateral to the point where the vein actually passes between the clavicle and the first rib. An intravascular position at that point protects the catheter by routing it through the area of the venous groove on the anterior surface of the first rib.

Inadvertent puncture of the subclavian artery instead of the vein, although not desirable, is often relatively benign as long as it is not repeated. However, achieving hemostasis through manual compression can be rather difficult, if not impossible, in this area. The size of the puncture is very important; holes made using 21-gauge micropuncture needles or conventional 18- or 19-gauge needles will usually seal, but the hole made by placement of a larger dilator, access sheath, or catheter can lead to considerable hemorrhage, especially in an anticoagulated patient or a chronic renal failure patient, because these patients are notoriously prone to platelet dysfunction. Large false aneurysms can occur in such situations, often requiring surgical intervention. We have treated two such patients by placement of intraluminal endografts, a technique for treating a fortunately uncommon complication that avoids the morbidity of conventional surgery in an area where vessel exposure can be difficult.

Subclavian catheterization for both short- and long-term hemodialysis was once the access method of choice, but the publication of multiple reports warning that the risk of significant ($>70\%$) late stenoses associated with the use of hemodialysis catheters could be as high as 50%[23,24] led the K/DOQI consensus group to indicate that internal jugular vein (preferably the right side) is the catheter access site of choice. In addition, although the numbers are not great enough for statistical analysis, there is a possibility that African Americans who are prone to keloid formation may also be more prone to late venous stenoses than other populations.[23] The cause of late–catheter-related subclavian vein stenosis is uncertain, but some authors theorize that the pressure of the catheter on the caudal aspect of the subclavian vein as it bends to enter the superior vena cava coupled with the effect of cardiac motion causes cumulative trauma.[25] Although many of these stenoses are clinically silent, the placement of an ipsilateral prosthetic shunt graft or fistula might result in flow that exceeds the venous drainage capacity of the stenotic vein, causing swelling that is both uncomfortable and unsightly and causing hemodynamic compromise of the vascular access, leading to premature failure. For that reason, some authors advocate routine preoperative venography if the patient has ever had a percutaneous venous access catheter in the ipsilateral subclavian position.[25,26] Ultrasonography (with or without color-flow Doppler encoding) can sometimes be used instead of venography to evaluate the subclavian vein; however, a thorough ultrasound examination of this area is often very difficult. Although still not routine owing to both cost and considerations of imaging artifact, the use of CT

venography has gained some popularity. Similarly, there was a flurry of interest in the potential of using magnetic resonance (MR) venography. However, the recognition of the association between the use of gadolinium MR imaging contrast material, renal failure, and the occurrence of nephrogenic systemic fibrosis syndrome, an incurable and potentially life-threatening entity, has effectively eliminated the use of MR venography in this patient population.

Subclavian Vein: Supraclavicular Approach

The supraclavicular approach to central venous catheterization, as described by Jones and Walters,[12] Conroy and colleagues,[27] and Yoffa,[28] is accomplished by puncturing the skin approximately 1 cm medial and superior to the midpoint of the clavicle and directing the needle toward the sternoclavicular joint so as to enter the confluence of the subclavian and internal jugular veins deep to that joint. Jones and Walters[12] reported a series of 27 patients in whom the supraclavicular approach was used to place 9-, 10-, and 11-Fr dual-lumen hemodialysis catheters that were in use for 3 to 156 days (mean, 40 days). Patient acceptance of the supraclavicular catheter in their series was basically the same as for conventional infraclavicular subclavian catheters and much better than generally observed in the case of internal jugular catheter placement. Catheter position was also noted to be less affected by arm and neck movement than in the case of either the infraclavicular or the internal jugular approach. Furthermore, although the external position of the catheter is similar to that of the conventional infraclavicular subclavian catheter, the intravascular lie is closer to that seen with internal jugular catheterization. For that reason, Jones and Walters[12] also theorized that supraclavicular catheterization may not be prone to late venous stenoses, unlike conventional infraclavicular subclavian catheterization. Although Jones and Walters[12] did not encounter any clinical evidence of central venous stenoses after supraclavicular catheterization, there have not been any long-term follow-up studies involving angiographic evaluation of the regional venous anatomy in this setting.

The potential procedural complications of the supraclavicular approach are similar to those encountered with the conventional infraclavicular and internal jugular approaches, including inadvertent arterial catheterization, hemorrhage, and pneumothorax. The risk of significant damage to the large central lymphatic ducts is, however, unique to this approach because the major right and left thoracic lymph ducts join the venous system at the junction of the respective subclavian and internal jugular veins. Because the right-sided duct is generally much smaller than the left-sided duct, Jones and Walters[12] recommended limiting supraclavicular venous access to the right side to minimize the risk. Despite this precaution, they did encounter 1 case of persistent lymphorrhea that took 11 days to resolve after catheter removal.

Although enhanced patient acceptance and the probability that the supraclavicular approach, like the internal jugular approach, may be far less likely to cause late venous stenoses than the conventional infraclavicular subclavian approach are appealing, the morbidity of persistent lymphatic leakage can be substantial, and corrective therapeutic measures rarely offer definitive remedies. Thus, one should probably view the supraclavicular approach to central venous catheterization as a secondary technique to be used in situations not amenable to other approaches. Risking a chronic debilitating complication in a patient with transient renal failure should obviously be avoided, as should unnecessarily adding to the problems of a patient already burdened with chronic renal failure, hemodialysis, and the ongoing struggle to maintain effective vascular access. Thus, in practice, this approach is not commonly employed by most operators.

Internal Jugular Vein Approach

K/DOQI 2006 Vascular Access guideline 2.4.1 states that "The preferred insertion site for tunneled, cuffed venous dialysis catheters or port catheter systems is the right internal jugular vein." The choice of access site for nontunneled, temporary catheters is, however, left to the individual physician's discretion, although the most recent K/DOQI also states that "catheters should not be placed in the subclavian vessels on either side because of risk for stenosis which can permanently exclude the possibility of upper-extremity permanent fistula or graft. Catheters should not be placed on the same side as a slowly maturing permanent access." Percutaneous catheterization of the internal jugular vein using any of the conventional approaches is a straightforward technique and should be performed on the right internal jugular vein whenever possible. Catheter placement in the left internal jugular vein potentially puts the left arm vasculature in jeopardy for a permanent access on the ipsilateral side because the catheter must, by virtue of the anatomy, traverse the left brachiocephalic vein en route to the superior vena cava where it can traumatize the vessel wall, unlike the right internal jugular vein approach in which the catheter has only minimal, if any, wall contact. The left side approach may also be associated with poorer blood flow rates and greater rates of thrombosis and stenosis because it requires a longer catheter and forces the catheter to lie in a position similar to that achieved with the common infraclavicular subclavian venous approach.[29] The major drawback of the jugular approach for placement of the Mahurkar or Niagara catheters is poor patient acceptance in the ambulatory patient; the catheter tubing is uncomfortable and difficult to hide under clothing even when reverse-curved extension tubing is used. In the case of the long-term tunneled catheters, the creation of a subcutaneous pocket at the base of the neck large enough to prevent catheter kinking and tunneling the catheter caudally to exit at an acceptable site on the anterior chest wall presents some simple but very important challenges. Tunneling anterior to the clavicle to reach an acceptable exit site creates a potentially uncomfortable and unsightly bump in most patients. Tunneling under the clavicle, however, presents a greater risk and can also be both difficult and uncomfortable. These considerations certainly make the infraclavicular subclavian approach appear more attractive; however, the high incidence of significant central venous stenoses encountered when large-caliber catheters are placed via this approach is the reason for the K/DOQI recommendations. Thus, most physicians opt for the right internal jugular venous approach and a subcutaneous

catheter tunnel superficial to the clavicle whenever possible even though it is less appealing to ambulatory patients. In this patient population, preservation of the upper extremity veins for definitive surgical vascular access is a life-saving approach to the problem.

Nonstandard Approaches

The venous access approaches described here constitute the mainstay of percutaneous venous access for hemodialysis. However, improvements in hemodialysis and the overall care of the chronic renal failure patient have led to additional demands on vascular access providers. As patients survive longer, they undergo more cycles of access failure, temporary catheterization, as well as surgical revision and replacement of fistulas and grafts, progressively using up all of the standard access sites. Eventually, even the most resourceful vascular surgeon encounters situations in which no further surgery is feasible. Although these situations are equally challenging for the interventional radiologist, the nature of catheter-based access is sufficiently different that an adequate access can often be created using a dual-lumen catheter or, as a last resort, a single-lumen catheter.

Occlusion of a major vein segment such as the subclavian vein presents a significant problem while developing surgical access. However, it is often possible to traverse an occluded vein segment using interventional radiologic techniques to place the hemodialysis catheter into the patent segment beyond the occlusion without actually restoring flow in the occluded segment (Fig. 16-9). If the occlusion was asymptomatic, the presence of a catheter traversing the occlusion will not make it any more occlusive. In the case of a high-grade stenosis that precludes the creation of an ipsilateral surgical access, angioplasty, with or without adjunctive intravascular stenting, is appropriate before placing a percutaneous hemodialysis access catheter that might otherwise occlude the narrowed residual lumen, because it is impossible to make an a priori prediction of which occlusions will be symptomatic. Similarly, angioplasty, with or without stenting, is appropriate when it becomes necessary to use the affected limb for the creation of surgical access because it can also be difficult to determine whether a moderate-severity stenosis will accommodate the increased flow and pressure that result from the creation of surgical access. Both angioplasty alone and angioplasty supplemented by stent implantation have high technical success rates.[12,30,31] Unfortunately, neither technique has a high primary patency rate. Thus, once a central venous intervention has been performed, whether it is angioplasty or combined angioplasty and stenting, periodic noninvasive follow-up is essential, and secondary interventions are often required to maintain long-term patency.

When all of the usual routes (subclavian, jugular, and femoral) are occluded and the only remaining patent veins in these regions are collaterals insufficient to permit catheterization via either percutaneous or surgical techniques, hemodialysis access can still be achieved through the translumbar approach to the inferior vena cava or the transhepatic approach to the right atrium via a hepatic vein. These approaches are simply modifications of techniques

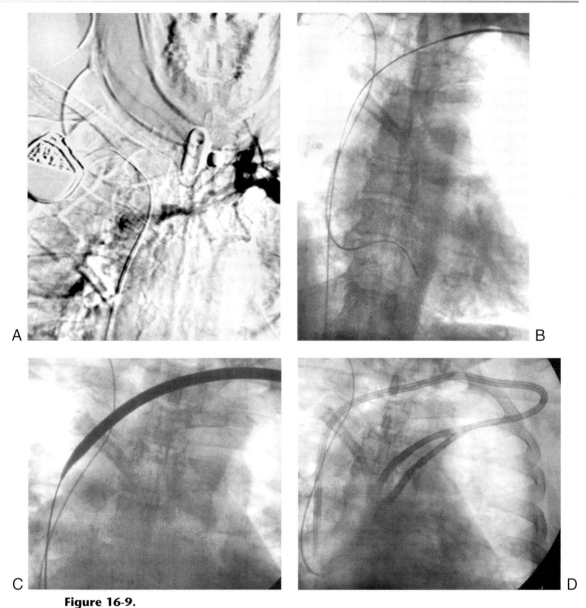

Figure 16-9.
A, A digital subtraction venogram demonstrates long, high-grade narrowing of the left bra-chiocephailic vein as well as a short segment occlusion of this vein with collateral flow beyond the occlusion. *B,* Traversal of the diseased vein segment was accomplished using standard angiographic catheter and hydrophilic guidewire technique. *C,* Serial dilation of the diseased vein segment was performed using rigid dilators and a large-bore peel-away catheter insertion sheath. *D,* A large-caliber tunneled hemodialysis catheter was placed through the diseased left brachiocephalic vein, but no attempt was made to restore venous patency. No symptoms referable to the newly placed catheter were observed.

used by interventional radiologists for other purposes. The risk of inferior vena cava thrombosis or an iatrogenic Budd-Chiari syndrome is relatively low when using conventional small-caliber venous access catheters, but the risk is unknown when using the larger-caliber catheters required for hemodialysis because there are insufficient case numbers in any one center for critical review.

Although the numbers are low and the risks are not therefore well quantified, it is also important to recognize that the placement of large-caliber catheters using nonstandard approaches also carries an increased risk of bleeding

into locations where hemostasis may be more difficult to achieve than in the case of the conventional approaches. Because the risks of a procedural mishap are of course greater with creative or nonstandard approaches, they are best left to individuals with appropriate skills and training.

Indications and Patient Selection

Prosthetic shunt grafts for hemodialysis generally require a 1- to 2-week period of healing to ensure adequate graft incorporation before use, to prevent leakage with hematoma formation along the course of the graft. In contrast, AV fistulas require a period of 3 to 5 weeks or more before the venous limb is sufficiently dilated to permit effective hemodialysis.[32] Percutaneous placement of dual-lumen hemodialysis access catheters is thus the method of choice for the institution of hemodialysis when the need for renal replacement therapy is either so acute that the patient cannot tolerate having therapy withheld during the time necessary to create and mature a definitive surgical access or so temporary that long-term access is unnecessary. The choice of which type of catheter to use depends in large part on the patient's overall condition and expected duration of catheter-based hemodialysis. Nontunneled catheters (eg, Mahurkar and Niagara) are best used in patients who require short-term hemodialysis, and the tunneled catheters are more appropriate for longer periods of need especially in patients who will be treated on an outpatient basis. Logistical factors, such as operating room constraints and the unavailability of an appropriately trained surgeon, interventional radiologist, or interventional nephrologist, may also dictate the need for percutaneous placement of a short-term catheter to ensure timely hemodialysis access. Fortunately, percutaneous placement of the Mahurkar and Niagara catheters is sufficiently straightforward and most institutions have a reasonable number of physicians in other specialties with the requisite skills and experience.

The ideal approach to a failed prosthetic shunt graft or fistula is either prompt surgical revision or endovascular treatment involving varying combinations of pharmacomechanical thrombolysis, angioplasty, and intravascular stenting.[33] Fortunately, the logistics of providing care in this situation are quite favorable because these are rarely situations requiring after-hours emergency procedures. In general, these patients can usually safely wait to receive this sort of care during normal weekday business hours. Occasionally, however, the patient's fluid or electrolyte status (ie, hyperkalemia) will mandate urgent after-hours or weekend treatment. Placement of a temporary (nontunneled) dialysis access catheter in such situations may be the most expeditious way to ensure prompt dialysis in such situations and is probably the best course of action in the face of severe cardiopulmonary decompensation or severe hyperkalemia when the patient is unlikely to tolerate a potentially more complex and prolonged intervention aimed at restoring flow in an occluded access graft or fistula. Access, however, is such a precious commodity in these patients that restoration of flow in the failed access is usually preferable to catheter placement, assuming that the patient can tolerate the procedure.

Although the endovascular approach usually renders a fistula or graft access ready for immediate use at the completion of treatment, this is not usually the situation when surgical revision is required. It is important to determine the expected recovery period, which is the period during which surgical access will be unavailable for dialysis access, and plan appropriately for catheter-based dialysis by placing either a short-term nontunneled or a long-term tunneled dialysis catheter as appropriate. Eventually, repeated cycles of surgical and/or endovascular treatments take their toll on the access, making additional surgical and endovascular treatments technically impossible and mandating the construction of a totally new vascular access fistula or shunt graft. Whereas there may be some disagreement as to the length of the interval among those charged with treating dialysis access problems, most providers agree that there eventually comes a point at which the interval between access failures becomes sufficiently short that additional salvage treatments, whether surgical or endovascular, are fruitless, subjecting the patient to more risk than benefit. An interval of less than 6 weeks between salvage treatments is a strong indication for construction of a new dialysis access or conversion to permanent long-term catheter-based hemodialysis when new surgical access is no longer technically possible or the patient is unwilling to undergo additional access surgery. If new surgical access is planned and the current access cannot be salvaged even for a short period, percutaneous placement of a long-term tunneled hemodialysis access catheter is the appropriate course of action because there is some unpredictability as to when the new access will be ready for use and most patients tolerate tunneled catheters better than notunneled catheters if they are ambulatory outpatients.

Percutaneous placement of hemodialysis access catheters is also appropriate for renal transplant patients experiencing temporary renal dysfunction associated with a rejection episode and for those who develop irreversible renal failure and no longer have a working vascular access. One should be mindful, however, that access through a femoral vein in this patient population may potentially jeopardize future transplanted kidneys in the pelvis secondary to femoral venous stenosis and clot. Hemodialysis catheter placement is also of benefit to peritoneal dialysis patients who require short-term hemodialysis during a period of peritonitis or abdominal surgery.

Patient preference can also lead to the use of long-term hemodialysis access catheters. Despite considerable technical advantages of surgically constructed long-term access over catheter-based techniques, many patients cite dissatisfaction with the cosmetics of surgically created access, repeated needle cannulation, and anxiety about undergoing surgery, especially after a number of access creation-revision cycles as reasons for depression and withdrawal from treatment. The simplicity of percutaneously placed long-term hemodialysis access catheters is often an appealing alternative for those patients. The catheters can easily be hidden under clothing and connection and disconnection from the hemodialysis machine is simple when using venous catheters and eliminates the need for repeated needle punctures and postcannulation compression of the needle access sites. The limiting factors for long-term, catheter-based hemodialysis—infection, occlusive fibrin sheathing, venous compromise (thrombosis or stenosis), longer dialysis times associated with lower blood flow rates, and the potential for limb swelling—are risks that these patients gladly accept.

Percutaneous placement of dual-lumen hemodialysis catheters is compatible with either intermittent or continuous venovenous hemodialysis techniques. Although intermittent hemodialysis is preferable for outpatients and stable inpatients, the fine control and gradual nature of continuous hemodialysis methods such as continuous AV hemofiltration with dialysis are especially important in the hemodynamically unstable, critically ill patient who cannot tolerate the cyclic swings in fluid volume and cardiac work associated with intermittent hemodialysis.[19,34] Continuous AV hemofiltration with dialysis uses the difference between arterial and venous pressure as its driving force. Although this eliminates the need for a mechanical pump, it requires the use of relatively large femoral artery and vein catheters to provide adequate flow and poses a considerable risk to the vascular supply of the lower extremity in a patient with already compromised cardiac function. Continuous venovenous hemofiltration with dialysis, conversely, does require the use of a mechanical pump, but it eliminates the risks associated with large-bore femoral artery and vein catheters. In addition, continuous venovenous hemofiltration with dialysis expands the range of vascular access alternatives because it can be carried out using a short-term dual-lumen catheter (eg, Quinton-Mahurkar or Niagara) placed in any suitable central vein.

Complications

Most of the complications of percutaneous hemodialysis catheter placement are those of conventional central venous catheterization, as discussed elsewhere in this text. Published reports cite complication rates of 4% to 6% occurring at the time of the initial venous catheterization. However, in centers in which experienced individuals frequently perform this procedure, complication rates are generally much lower. Although air embolism is a recognized risk in any central venous catheterization, especially one involving the jugular and subclavian veins, the large caliber of the dual-lumen hemodialysis catheters and vascular access sheaths used in the placement of the long-term catheters increases the risk. Accordingly, the use of slight Trendelenburg position, careful respiratory coaching of cooperative patients (exchange maneuvers should be performed during sustained maximal inspiration), access sheathes equipped with Hemostatic valves, and an appropriate measure of deliberate speed when performing critical exchange maneuvers are all important preventive measures.

Despite best efforts, catheter malfunctions do occur and steps need to be taken to correct them in a timely manner because a dysfunctional catheter is usually easier to salvage than a nonfunctional one. Signs of dysfunction during hemodialysis include decreased blood flow rates, increased arterial and venous pressures, inability to aspirate blood freely, and frequent pressure alarms not responsive to patient repositioning or catheter flushing. Catheter dysfunction should be treated when a dialyzer blood flow of 300 mL/min is not being attained in a catheter previously able to deliver greater than 350 mL/min. The catheter will need to be replaced if the actual catheter itself is dysfunctional because of a break in the tubing or a broken external fitting. Repair kits are commercially available for the external portion of some tunneled dialysis catheters that could potentially cut back on the costly nature and potential hazards of such exchanges,[35] but most catheter systems require replacement rather than repair.

The most common late complications of venous access catheters are device occlusion, usually due to thrombus or fibrin sheathing, and infection. Unfortunately, preventive measures such as the use of antiplatelet agents and anticoag-

ulation have not proved effective in preventing such events and often lead to bleeding complications.[36] Occlusive intraluminal catheter thrombus can often be removed by forceful aspiration or infusion of a thrombolytic agent (eg, t-PA, reteplase, streptokinase), and such measures are indicated before considering catheter replacement because each cycle of venous catheterization takes an inevitable toll on existing access sites, eventually leading to situations in which achieving effective access can be very difficult if not impossible.[37] Early catheter dysfunction with blood flow less than 300 mL/min for two consecutive treatments should be treated by using an intraluminal interdialytic thrombolytic lock protocol between dialysis treatments. When repeated cycles of lytic therapy are required to maintain operation of a catheter, a thorough diagnostic evaluation of the catheter itself should be made before the catheter and access site become unusable. Endoluminal catheter brushes have also been employed in declotting hemodialysis catheters.[38] These brushes were originally developed to obtain biofilm specimens from catheters in an effort to diagnose the nature of catheter-based infection, but to date, there are no convincing data regarding their efficacy in restoring catheter patency and they are expensive; consequently, they have not gained any measure of general acceptance.

Up to 10% of all dialysis access catheters are complicated by infection at a reported rate of one infection per 20 patient-weeks.[39] Infections can occur at the exit site, subcutaneous tunnel, or remotely secondary to catheter-related bacteremia. Infection continues to be the leading cause of catheter removal and morbidity in dialysis patients. Catheter exit-site infections alone, in the absence of a tunnel infection, can be treated and the catheters salvaged with topical and/or oral antibiotics, as well as appropriate local skin care. In general, it should not be necessary to remove the catheter. Conversely, obvious infection of the subcutaneous catheter tunnel or evidence of systemic sepsis usually indicates the need for prompt catheter removal. Catheter-related bacteremia in stable patients, without tunnel-tract involvement, however, has been successfully treated using two different approaches. The first is systemic antibiotics with the exchange of the catheter over a guidewire to salvage the site. This technique has been proved to save 80% to 88% of access sites without apparent negative effects.[40] The salvage of the access site is obviously beneficial because accessible venous catheterization sites significantly decrease over the life span of the hemodialysis patient. An alternative to this management allows for site and catheter salvage by combining systemic antibiotics in conjunction with interdialytic antibiotic locks. Catheter salvage without recurrence of infection has been achieved with this technique in about 65% to 70% of cases, comparing favorably with the catheter-exchange approach.[41] If a catheter-related bacteremia has occurred and the catheter is removed, typically a minimum of 5 to 10 days of systemic antibiotic therapy is needed to ensure adequate eradication of the culprit organism and prevent recolonization of the new catheter. Therefore, a nontunneled short-term catheter should be used if the patient cannot tolerate interruption of dialysis therapy and new permanent access (ie, long-term catheter, AV fistula, or shunt graft) should not be placed until culture results have been negative for at least 48 hours after cessation of antibiotic therapy. Scheduled replacement of short-term nontunneled catheters by guidewire exchange technique every 1 to 2 weeks has become widely accepted, although there is actually little evidence to support scheduled replacement except for catheters in the femoral area.

Catheter malpositioning involving inappropriate placement of the catheter in a nontarget vessel, such as retrograde catheterization of the internal jugular vein during subclavian vein catheterization, does not occur when fluoroscopic guidance is used. Before placing the catheter or vascular access sheath, simply reposition the guidewire into the target vessel using whatever angiographic tools and techniques are needed. When this occurs as a result of a blind insertion technique, it is best to perform the repositioning in the interventional suite, where these tools are available. Repositioning the short-term hemodialysis catheters, especially the relatively stiff Mahurkar catheter, involves partial withdrawal and then redirection, using either a floppy-tipped or steerable angiographic guidewire. The long-term hemodialysis catheters are sufficiently flexible that they can sometimes be displaced back to the target vessel using a guidewire alone. Because withdrawal and reintroduction of a tunneled catheter are difficult and may potentially increase the risk of infection, the tip may be snared and

pulled into the desired position using a separate catheter introduced via another venous route (eg, the femoral vein in the case of a subclavian or jugular venous catheter).

In addition to the usual complications of central venous access, contralateral hemothorax,[42] hemomediastinum, and hemopericardium[43] have been reported, associated with puncture of the superior vena cava by the tip of a temporary hemodialysis catheter (eg, Mahurkar and Niagara). These complications are often the result of an attempt at forceful passage during a blind insertion procedure or mistaken acceptance of a catheter position that causes the tip to press against the wall of the vena cava. Delayed hemothorax, a potentially life-threatening complication that can develop several weeks after placement of the catheter, is caused by caval perforation involving only the tip of the catheter, which continues to function adequately because of the remaining intravascular side holes. Hemothorax, heralded by hypotension during hemodialysis, occurs when the catheter position shifts, placing some of the blood return ports outside the vena cava or the tip, which may have been blocked by surrounding soft tissues, then becomes unblocked and flow exits the end hole (Fig. 16-10). Hemodialysis should be discontinued as soon as this

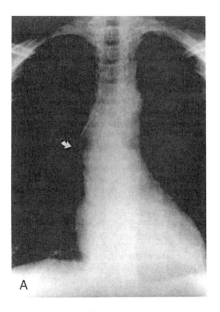

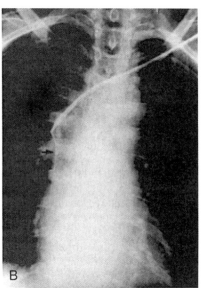

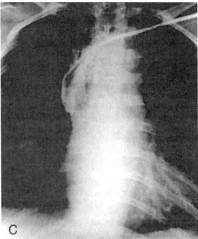

Figure 16-10.
A, Chest radiograph shows a suspect position for the Mahurkar catheter tip *(arrow).* *B,* Contrast medium injected via the red proximal (blood withdrawal) port of the Mahurkar catheter shows intravascular flow streaming along the right side of the SVC *(arrows).* *C,* Contrast medium injected via the blue distal (blood return) port of the Mahurkar catheter spreads within the soft tissues surrounding the superior vena cava, revealing its extravascular position.

complication is suspected and appropriate fluid resuscitation instituted. Simply stopping flow to the catheter will arrest the process in most cases. This complication is confirmed by obtaining a chest radiograph or injecting angiographic contrast material under fluoroscopy if the diagnosis is in doubt.[42] The complication can be avoided by scrupulous adherence to proper technique, including the use of either fluoroscopy during catheter insertion or routine chest radiography after insertion. If the orientation or position of the catheter tip is suspect, it is best to confirm acceptable placement by injecting angiographic contrast material under fluoroscopy before using the catheter.[44]

Thrombosis of the axillosubclavian or iliofemoral vein segments associated with the use of either short- or long-term hemodialysis catheters can cause edema and pain in the affected limb or it may be asymptomatic, and it can occur as early as the immediate postimplantation period or well after the offending catheter has been removed. Iliofemoral thrombosis is often symptomatic and debilitating, but axillosubclavian thrombosis is often asymptomatic until a surgical vascular access is created in the same arm.[45] For this reason, as discussed earlier, in planning a new access, consideration must be given to the patient's prior vascular access history and preoperative planning angiography considered when the situation requires use of the same arm. Catheterization of the internal jugular vein seems to be largely free of these complications, although the reason is unclear.

Obtaining hemostasis on the removal of a temporary hemodialysis catheter, especially a large-caliber catheter like the Quinton PermCath or the Niagara, can be greatly complicated by the placement of a surgical access in the ipsilateral limb. At that point, the catheterization site is no longer a low-pressure venous system because of the AV shunt, and withdrawing the catheter will not result in collapse of the tract. Prolonged manual compression is generally successful, although we have on one occasion found it necessary to place a temporary suture around the proximal end of the tract to achieve hemostasis. Good communication among the various members of the treatment team and a little forethought are usually all that is needed to avoid this problem.

Overall, the risk of catheter-related complications with the use of percutaneously placed dual-lumen hemodialysis catheters is considered to be low with strict adherence to proper insertion technique and adequate experience.

Perspective

Although AV fistula and shunt graft construction remains the gold standard for long-term hemodialysis access, the widespread use of percutaneously placed hemodialysis catheters has greatly expanded the range of treatment options for both acute and chronic renal failure patients. Institution of hemodialysis can now be accomplished without delay whenever necessary, surgical vascular access procedures can be carried out electively without compromising the patient's care, and surgical access is no longer the patient's only long-term option. However, there still is no ideal vascular access site or method. The best choice for a specific patient always involves balancing tradeoffs by assessing the overall clinical situation, prior vascular access history, planned surgical access creation, and any renal transplant history or plans, based on a thorough understanding of the available options.

REFERENCES

1. Eknoyan G, Levin NW. Impact of the new K/DOQI guidelines. *Blood Purif.* 2002;20:103-108.
2. Gibson SP, Mosquera D. Five years experience with the Quinton PermCath for vascular access. *Nephrol Dial Transplant.* 1991;6: 269-274.
3. Moss AH, Vasilakis C, Holley JL, Foulks CJ, Pillai K, McDowell DE. Use of a silicone dual-lumen catheter with a Dacron cuff as a long-term vascular access for hemodialysis patients. *Am J Kidney Dis.* 1990;16: 211-215.
4. Shusterman NH, Kloss K, Mullen JL. Successful use of double-lumen silicone rubber catheters for permanent hemodialysis access. *Kidney Int.* 1989;35:887-890.
5. Uldall PR, Woods F, Merchant N, Crichton E, Carter H. A double-lumen subclavian cannula (DLSC) for temporary hemodialysis access. *Trans Am Soc Artif Intern Organs.* 1980;26:93-98.
6. Kolbeck K, Stavropoulos SW, Trerotola SO. Over-the-wire catheter exchanges: reduction of the risk of air emboli. *J Vasc Interv Radiol.* 2008;19:1222-1226.
7. Kolbeck K, Itkin M, Stavropoulos SW, Trerotola SO. Measurement of air emboli during central venous access: do "protective" sheaths or insertion techniques matter? *J Vasc Interv Radiol.* 2005;16:1:89-99.
8. Canaud B, My H, Morena M, et al: Dialock: a new vascular access device for extracorporeal renal replacement therapy. Preliminary clinical results. *Nephrol Dial Transplant.* 1999;14:692-698.
9. Janne d'Othee B. Restoration of patency in failing tunneled hemodialysis catheters: a comparison of catheter exchange, exchange and balloon disruption of the fibrin sheath, and femoral stripping. *J Vasc Interv Radiol.* 2006;17:1011-1015.
10. Winn MP, McDermott VG, Schwab SJ, Conlon PJ. Dialysis catheter "fibrin-sheath": a cautionary tale! *Nephol Dial Transplant.* 1997; 12:1048-1050.
11. Brismar B. Diagnosis of thrombosis by catheter phlebography after prolonged central venous catheterization. *Ann Surg.* 1981;6:779-783.
12. Jones CE, Walters GK. Efficacy of the supraclavicular route for temporary hemodialysis access. *South Med J.* 1992;85:725-728.
13. Fry DE, Fry RV, Borzotta AP. Nosocomial blood-borne infection secondary to intravascular devices. *Am J Surg.* 1994;167:268-272.
14. Weijmer MC, Vervloet MG, ter Wee PM. Compared to tunneled cuffed haemodialysis catheters, temporary untunnelled catheters are associated with more complications already within 2 weeks of use. *Nephrol Dial Transplant.* 2004;19:670-677.
15. Maki DG, Cobb L, Garman JK, Shapiro JM, Ringer M, Helgerson RB. An attachable silver-impregnated cuff for prevention of infection with central venous catheters: a prospective randomized multicenter trial. *Am J Med.* 1988;85:307-314.
16. Groeger JS, Lucas AB, Coit D, et al: A prospective, randomized evaluation of the effect of silver impregnated subcutaneous cuffs for preventing tunneled chronic venous access catheter infections in cancer patients. *Ann Surg.* 1993;218:206-210.
17. Stavros K. Effectiveness of a new tunneled catheter in preventing catheter malfunction: a comparative study. *J Vasc Interv Radiol.* 2008; 19:1018-1026.
18. Shaldon S, Silva H, Pomeroy J, Rae AI, Rosen SM. Percutaneous femoral venous catheterization and reusable dialysers in the treatment of acute renal failure. *Trans Am Soc Artif Intern Organs.* 1964;10:133-135.
19. Matalon R, Nidus BD, Cantacuzino D, Eisinger RP. Intermittent hemodialysis with repeated femoral vein puncture. *JAMA.* 1970;214: 1883-1884.
20. Paganini EP, Nakamoto S. Continuous slow ultrafiltration in oliguric acute renal failure. *Trans Am Soc Artif Intern Organs.* 1980;26:201-204.
21. Weitzel WF, Boyer CJ Jr, el-Khatib MT, Swartz RD. Successful use of indwelling cuffed femoral vein catheters in ambulatory hemodialysis patients. *Am J Kidney Dis.* 1993;22:426-429.
22. Erben J. [Current possibilities of treatment of chronic renal insufficiency.] *Cas Lek Cesk.* 1968;107:1249-1253.

23. Barrett N, Spencer S, McIvor J, Brown EA. Subclavian stenosis: a major complication of subclavian dialysis catheters. *Nephrol Dial Transplant.* 1988;3:423-425.

24. Raju RM, Kramer MS, Fernandes M, Rosenbaum JL, Barber K. Subclavian vein and femoral vein catheterisation for hemodialysis: one year comparison. *Trans Am Soc Artif Organs.* 1982;28:58-60.

25. Cimochowski GE, Worley E, Rutherford WE, Sartain J, Blondin J, Harter H. Superiority of the internal jugular over the subclavian access for temporary dialysis. *Nephron.* 1990;54:154-161.

26. Surratt RS, Picus D, Hicks ME, Darcy MD, Kleinhoffer M, Jendrisak M. The importance of preoperative evaluation of the subclavian vein in dialysis access planning. *AJR Am J Roentgenol.* 1991;156:623-625.

27. Conroy JM, Rajagopalan PR, Baker JD 3rd, Bailey MK. A modification of the supraclavicular approach to the central circulation. *South Med J.* 1990;83:1178-1181.

28. Yoffa D. Supraclavicular subclavian venepuncture and catheterisation. *Lancet.* 1965;2:614-617.

29. Schillinger F, Schillinger D, Montagnac R, Milcent T. Post catheterisation vein stenosis in haemodialysis: comparative angiographic study of 50 subclavian and 50 internal jugular accesses. *Nephrol Dial Transplant.* 1991;6:722-724.

30. Farber A, Barbey MM, Grunert JH, Gmelin E. Access-related venous stenoses and occlusions: treatment with percutaneous transluminal angioplasty and Dacron-covered stents. *Cardiovasc Intervent Radiol.* 1999;22:214-218.

31. Vesely TM, Hovsepian DM, Pilgram TK, Coyne DW, Shenoy S. Upper extremity central venous obstruction in hemodialysis patients: treatment with Wallstents. *Radiology.* 1997;204:343-348.

32. Wilson SE. Autogenous arteriovenous fistulas. In Wilson SE (ed). *Vascular Surgery: Principles and Practice.* 2nd ed. St. Louis: Mosby; 1994: 82-96.

33. Kumpe DA, Cohen MA. Angioplasty/thrombolysis treatment of failing and failed hemodialysis access sites: comparison with surgical treatment. *Prog Cardiovasc Dis.* 1992;4:263-278.

34. Tominaga GT, Ingegno MD, Scannell G, Pahl MV, Waxman K. Continuous arteriovenous hemofiltration in postoperative and traumatic renal failure. *Am J Surg.* 1993;166:612-615.

35. Hwang F, Stavropoulos SW, Shlansky-Goldberg RD, et al. Tunneled infusion catheter breakage: frequency and repair kit outcomes. *J Vasc Interv Radiol.* 2008;19:2:201-206.

36. Obialo CI, Conner AC, Lebon LF. Maintaining patency of tunneled hemodialysis catheters—efficacy of aspirin compared to warfarin. *Scand J Urol Nephrol.* 2003;37:172-176.

37. Tapson JS, Hoenich NA, Wilkinson R, Ward MK. Dual lumen subclavian catheters for haemodialysis. *Int J Artif Organs.* 1985;8:195-200.

38. Tranter SA, Donoghue J. Brushing has made a sweeping change: use of the endoluminal FAS brush in haemodialysis central venous catheter management. *Aust Crit Care.* 2000;13:10-13.

39. Uldall PR, Joy C, Merchant N. Further experience with a double-lumen subclavian cannula for hemodialysis. *Trans Am Soc Artif Intern Organs.* 1982;28:71-75.

40. Shaffer D. Catheter-related sepsis complicating long-term, tunneled central venous dialysis catheters: management by guidewire exchange. *Am J Kidney Dis.* 1995;25:593-596.

41. Allon M. Saving infected catheters: why and how. *Blood Purif.* 2005;23:23-28.

42. Kozeny GA, Bansal VK, Vertuno LL, Hano JE. Contralateral hemothorax secondary to chronic subclavian dialysis catheter. *Am J Nephrol.* 1984;4:312-314.

43. Fine A, Churchill D, Gault H, Mathieson G. Fatality due to subclavian dialysis catheter. *Nephron.* 1981;29:99-100.

44. Kaupke CJ, Ahdout J, Vaziri ND, Deutsch LS. Perforation of the superior vena cava by a subclavian hemodialysis catheter: early detection by angiography. *Int J Artif Organs.* 1992;15:666-668.

45. Currier CB Jr, Widder S, Ali A, Kuusisto E, Sidawy A. Surgical management of subclavian and axillary vein thrombosis in patients with a functioning arteriovenous fistula. *Surgery.* 1986;100:25-28.

CHAPTER 17

Access in the Neonatal and Pediatric Patient

Nikunj K. Chokshi, Nam Nguyen, and Marianne Cinat

Vascular access in infants and children, especially in those who are critically ill, may be extremely challenging. Their small-caliber vessels, which are prone to collapse in states of shock, in combination with the relatively large diameter of angiocatheters have often frustrated clinicians seeking to establish reliable access. The availability of catheters with improved outer diameter–to–inner diameter ratios and improved imaging techniques for insertion has allowed for safer and more effective pediatric vascular access procedures. This chapter highlights the practical and important aspects of vascular access in children who require resuscitation, hemodynamic monitoring, total parenteral nutrition (TPN), chemotherapy, and prolonged pharmacologic therapy.

Indications

Vascular access is required both in acute settings and for the delivery of therapeutic infusions in chronic diseases (Table 17-1).

Resuscitation and Hemodynamic Monitoring

Hypovolemia is the most common cause of shock in children, followed by septic and cardiogenic shock.[1] Initially, the priority is to restore adequate volume in order to maintain vital organ perfusion. Once resuscitation is under way, a means to monitor hemodynamics might be necessary. Central venous access allows for both resuscitation and hemodynamic monitoring. With its larger diameters and central location, large volumes of fluid and vasoactive medications may be administered. Furthermore, the central venous pressure (CVP) can be measured. In the presence of a normal heart, CVP measurement provides useful clinical information. CVP measurement alone, however, may be inadequate, and placement of a Swan-Ganz catheter may be required in particular situations to further assess the patient's hemodynamics.[2,3] The Swan-Ganz catheter can be placed percutaneously or by cutdown into the subclavian, jugular, cephalic, femoral, or saphenous vein.

Therapeutic Infusions

Long-term access for continuous or recurrent infusions is necessary in many pediatric disease processes. During the 1970s, the discovery and clinical use of TPN may have

Table 17–1
Indications for Central Venous in Pediatric Patients
Hemodynamic Monitoring
Major trauma
Transplantation
Thermal injury
Sepsis
Cardiorespiratory failure
Major surgery
Alimentary Tract Disease
Intestinal perforation
Necrotizing enterocolitis
Chronic intestinal obstruction
Peritonitis
Biliary, pancreatic, enteric fistulas
Prolonged ileus
Inflammatory bowel disease
Protracted diarrhea
Pancreatitis
Short- bowel syndrome
Malabsorption
Low-Birth-Weight, Premature Infants
Metabolic Derangements
Renal failure
Reversible hepatic failure
Enzyme deficiencies
Reye's syndrome
Hypermetabolic State With Limited Oral Intake
Thermal injury
Major trauma
Adjuvant cancer therapy
Marginal cardiorespiratory reserve
Coma or neurologic alterations
Chronic Pharmacologic Therapy
Cancer chemotherapy
Cystic fibrosis
Autoimmune disease
Blood dyscrasias
Bacterial, viral, fungal infections

salvaged more infants than any other advance in pediatrics or surgery.[4,5] At birth, infants in an anabolic state have several metabolic characteristics such as limited glycogen and fat stores, immaturity of the temperature control mechanism, and a high caloric need that render them vulnerable to starvation. In general, TPN is indicated when enteral feedings are not possible or inadequate, which may occur with prematurity, alimentary tract anomalies, alimentary tract disease, or hypermetabolic states with feeding intolerance. TPN may also be given at home for chronic disease states such as short bowel syndrome and intestinal pseudo-obstruction.

The research and development of more efficacious chemotherapy agents have improved outcomes in pediatric oncology. Central venous access is required for administration of these drugs, which are often caustic in nature. Access might also be needed for blood sampling, supplemental fluid support, TPN, and the infusion of blood and blood products. This can be achieved via an external catheter or an implanted infusion port.[6] Pediatric patients with chronic medical conditions such as cystic fibrosis, sickle cell disease, and hemophilia might also require prolonged venous access for the intermittent infusion of medications, antibiotics, and blood products. In all of these patients, repeated peripheral venipuncture causes thrombosis and sclerosis of veins, and access may become progressively difficult and distressing for the patient. Long-term central venous access devices (VADs) are being used in these patients with minimal complications.[6–11] In addition, totally implantable VADs can be used successfully in hemophiliacs without serious side effects, despite their hemorrhagic diathesis.[10]

VADs

The choice of vascular access is dependent on the age, size, and condition of the patient and on the acuity of the situation. When choosing the type of VAD necessary, the clinician has to determine the purpose of the VAD and the duration of treatment. The methods used for acute or short-term vascular access (days to weeks) differ from those used for long-term access (≥1 mo).

Most of the central venous catheters are made of Teflon, polyethylene, polyurethane, or silicone elastomer (Silastic). In general, Silastic catheters are too soft for pressure monitoring. Most surgeons prefer polyurethane or polyethylene for short-term access and monitoring and Silastic catheters for long-term therapeutic needs (eg, TPN, drug infusions). Introducing cuffed polyurethane catheters for long-term use in phoresis and bone marrow transplantation has made them a preferred option. The catheter is soft enough to negotiate through the tear-away sheath, yet strong enough to withstand high-pressure infusion.

Short-Term Peripheral Venous Access

Peripheral Intravenous Catheters

Peripheral intravenous catheters are often the easiest and safest way to achieve vascular access. They are used as the first line for intravenous therapy in children of all ages and sizes. These short, flexible, plastic catheters are commonly available in sizes from 14- to 26-gauge. They are inserted into a peripheral vein of the extremities, scalp, or external jugular veins. The median antecubital vein is commonly the first choice; however, the dorsal veins on the hands and feet and the basilic, median cephalic, and cephalic veins can also be used. The greater saphenous vein is an excellent site because of its large size and consistent anatomy. It courses immediately anterior to the medial malleolus. As a result, it may be accessed even without direct visualization or palpation. Scalp veins and external jugular veins are reserved for infants whose extremity veins cannot be cannulated. Each peripheral intravenous catheter can be used for 3 to 5 days; longer use is associated with an increased incidence of infiltration or phlebitis.[12,13]

Peripheral Cutdown Venous Access

Because of its high complication rates, venous cutdown access has fallen out of favor. However, it remains a useful technique to obtain vascular access in an emergency situation when all other percutaneous access methods have been unsuccessful.[14] This is a procedure of last resort. For a pediatric surgeon, the average time to achieve access in older children (6–16 yr) was 6 minutes, and in younger children (1 mo–5 yr), 8 minutes.[15] Thus, it takes longer than percutaneous peripheral catheter placement. If it is necessary, the distal greater saphenous and antecubital veins are the best sites, but proximal saphenous, inferior epigastric, axillary, or femoral veins can also be used.

The distal greater saphenous vein can be easily accessed via a small transverse incision superior and anterior to the medial malleolus (Fig. 17-1). The vein is exposed with gentle dissection of the cutaneous tissue as it lies in the superficial cutaneous plane. Once exposed, it is secured with suture ligatures. The vein is accessed either by direct cannulation of an angiocatheter or through a venotomy.

There are four veins in the antecubital fossa: the median basilic, the basilic, the median cephalic, and the cephalic (Fig. 17-2). The median basilic vein runs obliquely across the medial aspect of the antecubital fossa, and the median cephalic runs across the lateral aspect on the superficial fascia as they enter into their respective main veins. The

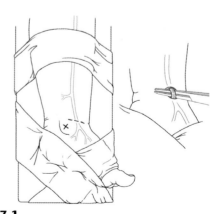

Figure 17-1.
Saphenous vein cutdown showing incision anterior to medial maleolus (x). (Adapted from Chameides L [ed]. *Textbook of Pediatric Advanced Life Support.* Dallas: American Heart Association; 1997.)

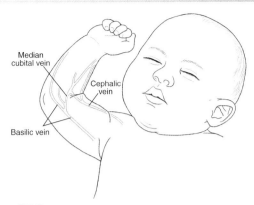

Figure 17-2.
Veins of the upper extremity. (Adapted from Chameides L [ed]. *Textbook of Pediatric Advanced Life Support.* Dallas: American Heart Association; 1997.)

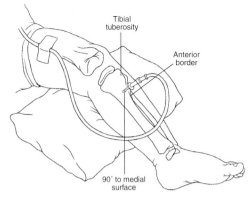

Figure 17-3.
Intraosseous cannulation technique. (Adapted from Chameides L [ed]. *Textbook of Pediatric Advanced Life Support.* Dallas: American Heart Association; 1997.)

basilic vein pierces the deep fascia to join the axillary vein. The cephalic vein runs vertically in the lateral aspect of the antecubital fossa over the long head of the biceps muscle and through the deltopectoral groove to enter the subclavian vein.

These veins may be exposed via a transverse incision in the center of the antecubital fossa. The incision may be extended medially or laterally depending on which vein is the intended target.

In comparison with percutaneous central venous access, peripheral venous cutdowns have a shorter duration of function, higher rate of infection, and more mechanical difficulties, such as line leakage, catheter slippage, and catheter occlusion. In one study, 78% of peripheral venous cutdowns had complications, whereas only 14% of the percutaneously inserted central lines had associated complications.[16]

Intraosseous Catheters

Intraosseous infusion was first introduced in the 1940s. Its use declined in the 1980s but has increased since the late 1990s with the introduction of new needles and spring-loaded devices. The procedure is taught to all trainees in Advanced Pediatric Life Support courses and is most commonly reserved for acute, life-threatening situations, when standard vascular access cannot be achieved.[14] In general, intraosseous access is indicated when two attempts at peripheral access have failed or when more than 90 seconds has elapsed in an attempt to gain access in a child who is in shock or cardiac arrest.[17] The intraosseous route is based on the presence of noncollapsible medullary sinuses in the bone marrow. This vascular network empties into the central circulation. As a result, any solution that can be infused intravenously (including resuscitative medications) can be administered intraosseously.[18]

Sites for intraosseous infusion include the tibia, iliac crest, and femur. In children younger than 5 years, insertion is performed 1 to 3 cm below the tibial tuberosity on the flat anteromedial surface of the tibia. The needle should be placed at a distal direction in a 40- to 60-degree angle away from the growth plate (Fig. 17-3). In older children, the distal femur is the preferred site, and the needle is intro-

duced in a cephalad direction, 3 cm proximal to the condyles.[18] For children younger than 18 months, an 18- to 20-gauge disposable bone marrow needle is sufficient. Children older than 18 months require a 13- to 16-gauge needle. Successful placement is confirmed through aspiration of marrow content and easy infusion of fluid.

Complications for this technique are rare but include osteomyelitis,[19] tibial fracture,[20] extravasation with tissue necrosis, and compartment syndromes.[21] Overall, intraosseous access is a rapid, safe, and simple method of obtaining vascular access in critically ill and injured children and should be an alternate route of fluid resuscitation in pediatric patients when venous access is not rapidly available.[22]

Short-Term Central Venous Access

Peripherally Inserted Central Catheters

Peripherally inserted central catheters (PICCs) are an innovation whose use has decreased the need for cutdowns and intraoperative catheter placement.[15,23–26] The PICC is a radiopaque, flexible Silastic tube that is inserted percutaneously or via a cutdown through a peripheral vein and threaded centrally. The PICC is available in a variety of sizes. The smallest PICC, for use in neonates, is 1.1 Fr and can withstand flow rates up to 125 mL/hr. These catheters have the potential to remain in place for several weeks.[25] When it is properly secured, the flexibility of the PICC allows full range of motion of an extremity. The main advantage of the PICC is the prevention of multiple intravenous sticks for venous infusion and blood sampling.

The PICC is safe to use in neonates as well as in older children. It is an excellent choice for patients in whom intermediate-term intravenous access is required. Complications associated with these catheters include catheter-related infections (4%–8%) and catheter occlusion (5%–10%).[15,31] The rate of phlebitis is significantly lower than that observed with peripheral intravenous catheters (5%–10% vs. 35%).[12,23,25,26] Catheter embolization and vessel perforations are rare complications associated with the PICC.

Percutaneous Central Venous Catheters

The placement of a central venous catheter has become the mainstay for vascular access. The percutaneous route, with the catheter placed using Seldinger's technique, is the standard. Polyethylene and polyurethane uncuffed catheters can be inserted into the subclavian, internal jugular, or femoral veins. They are intended for short-term use only (2–4 wk),[14] because these catheters have a higher rate of infection and thrombosis. The development of smaller, more flexible catheters has allowed for safe use in neonates, infants, and small children.[16,25,27–29] The multilumen plastic catheters are available in sizes ranging from 3 to 8 Fr (Table 17-2 lists age-based sizing). They can be used for hemodynamic monitoring, intravenous infusion, dialysis, and blood sampling.

Insertion can frequently be performed at bedside with the use of local anesthesia and sedation. However, general anesthesia might be necessary in neonates or children who are unable to cooperate. It is important to place the patient in a proper position to optimize the likelihood of cannulating the vein. Use a Trendelenburg position for the subclavian and internal jugular veins, ands reverse Trendelenburg position for the femoral vein. When placing a subclavian catheter, remember that the vein is more cephalad in younger children. Under aseptic conditions, insert a needle with attached small syringe (3 or 5 mL) at the medial third of the clavicle. Advance the needle toward the sternal notch, keeping the syringe and the needle parallel to the frontal plane, as in adults (Fig. 17-4). The angle of the needle with respect to the sternal notch may vary depending on the patient's age. Apply a gentle negative pressure to the syringe. It is advisable not to exert too much pressure on the syringe because it might cause the vein to collapse, giving a false impression of missing the vein.

If cannulation is not successful, slowly retract the needle, keeping constant pressure on the syringe in the event that the vein traversed completely. Remove the needle com-

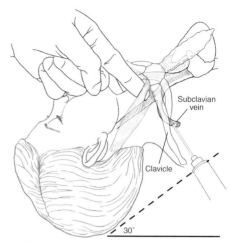

Figure 17-4.
Subclavian vein anatomy. (Adapted from Chameides L [ed]. *Textbook of Pediatric Advanced Life Support*. Dallas: American Heart Association; 1997.)

pletely before making another attempt. Negotiating the needle within the subcutaneous tissue is not advisable and might injure vital structures. Once the needle is within the vein, place the catheter using Seldinger's technique as described elsewhere in this text (see Chapter 34). If the procedure is performed in the operating room, confirm the position of the guidewire radiographically. Care should be taken during advancement of the guidewire because it might cause cardiac arrhythmia or injuries. Following placement of the catheter, also assess the location of the tip with fluoroscopy, with the ideal location at the junction of the superior vena cava and right atrium. Obtain a chest radiograph in the recovery room to confirm the position of the catheter and to evaluate for pneumothorax. If the patient is to be discharged following catheter placement, perform a chest radiograph in 2 to 4 hours to ensure that there is no development of a "late pneumothorax."

In the pediatric population, the internal jugular vein can be accessed through one of the three approaches: the middle, anterior or posterior. The middle approach is most commonly used in the pediatric population. For this approach (Fig 17-5), insert the needle at the apex of the triangle bounded by the sternal and clavicular heads of the sternocleidomastoid muscle (SCM) and the clavicle (at the level of cricoid cartilage), aiming toward the ipsilateral nipple. For the anterior approach, the initial puncture site is at a point halfway along the anterior border of the SCM. Advance the needle toward the ipsilateral nipple at a 30- to 40-degree anterior angle. Retraction of the carotid artery medially might help avoid accidental puncture of the carotid arterial (Fig 17-6). Lastly, for the posterior approach, insert the needle at the posterior border of the SCM at a point one third from the clavicle, just above the external jugular vein. Advance the needle toward the sternal notch, with the needle maintained immediately underneath the SCM (Fig 17-7).

In general, the right subclavian and right internal jugular veins are preferred sites because they are away from the thoracic duct. In addition, the dome of the pleura is higher on the left side, which makes it more susceptible to

Table 17–2

Age and Catheter Size

Catheter Type	Age	Catheter Size (Fr)
Short-term catheter (PICCs)	Premature to term infants	1.1-2
	<1 yr	3
	>1 yr	3-4
Short-term catheter (Arrow, Cook)	6 mo to 1 yr	3
	1–5 yr	4
	5–10 yr	5-6
	>10 yr	6-8\F
Long-term catheter (Broviac, Hickman)	Premature to SCA	2.7
	<6 mo	3.0-4.2
	>6 mo to 5 yr	5.0-7.0
	5–10 yr	7
	>10 yr	9

PICC, peripherally inserted central catheter; SCA, small for gestational age.

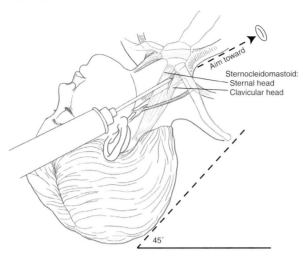

Figure 17-5.
Internal jugular vein technique, middle (central) route. (Adapted from Chameides L [ed]. *Textbook of Pediatric Advanced Life Support*. Dallas: American Heart Association; 1997.)

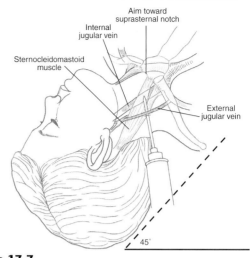

Figure 17-7.
Internal jugular vein technique, posterior route. (Adapted from Chameides L [ed]. *Textbook of Pediatric Advanced Life Support*. Dallas: American Heart Association; 1997.)

injury.[30] The right internal jugular has a straight course to the superior vena cava. Internal jugular access should not be considered in patients in whom tracheostomies or extracorporeal membrane oxygenation (ECMO) is present or contemplated.

The common femoral vein is large and superficial and has a constant relationship medial to the femoral artery. It is located at the junction of the medial and middle third of the straight line drawn between the superior iliac spine and the pubic tubercle. However, the most reliable landmark is the femoral artery pulsation (Fig 17-8). Femoral vein catheterization is safe, because it has a low complication rate and a success rate greater than 90%. Place the femoral catheter tip either below the level of the renal veins or at the level of the diaphragm to avoid visceral vessel thrombosis. Percutaneous femoral catheterization is generally discouraged in neonates because of potential injury to the femoral artery, which may lead to leg ischemia. The constant relationship of the femoral artery and vein is more pronounced with increases in muscular mass and walking,

whereas in neonates, the artery may be anterior in relation to the vein.

Acute complications generally incurred during catheter insertion may include pneumothorax, hemothorax, arrhythmia, hydrothorax, arterial puncture, hematoma, nerve injury, superior vena caval or right atrial injury, and cardiac tamponade.[31] Long-term complications include intravenous line infection, sepsis, venous thrombosis, venous embolization, vessel perforation, pericardial tamponade, hydrothorax, catheter occlusion, and mural thrombi.[32–34]

Umbilical Vein Catheters

The umbilical vein was first used in 1974 by Diamond for exchange transfusions and is still in widespread use as short-term emergency central venous access.[37] It is relatively safe, easily accessible, and cost effective during the first 2 weeks

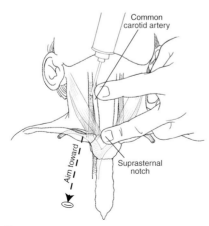

Figure 17-6.
Internal jugular vein technique, anterior route. (Adapted from Chameides L [ed]. *Textbook of Pediatric Advanced Life Support*. Dallas: American Heart Association; 1997.)

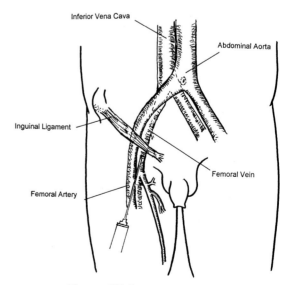

Figure 17-8.
Percutaneous femoral approach.

of life.[35] Cannulation is possible up to 7 days after birth. It has been shown that this access is more difficult after 10 days of life and associated with major infectious and thrombotic complications.[36]

Under aseptic conditions, cut the umbilical stump 1 or 2 cm above the skin. Then stabilize the stump stabilized with two hemostats places laterally. The large, thin-walled umbilical vein is located in the superior aspect of the umbilical stump (Fig. 17-9). Remove blood clots from the vein, and insert a single- or multilumen umbilical catheter (5 Fr for term infants and 3 Fr for premature infants) with an attached syringe filled with saline and advanced it centrally. The catheter should be passed easily without resistance. Overly aggressive insertion can cause the catheter to enter the portal venous system via the portal sinus or the pulmonary vein through the foramen ovale. A good blood return on aspiration of the catheter suggests that the tip is in the central venous system. If there is no blood return, withdraw the catheter is withdrawn while maintaining gentle pressure to extract possible blood clots. Then renegotiate the catheter into a proper position, and confirm its location of the catheter radiographically. The ideal location is at the junction of the inferior vena cava and the right atrium (diaphragmatic level).

Umbilical vein cannulation can be accomplished in 70% of patients with relatively low complication rates if properly placed.[35] The potential complications are sepsis, portal thrombosis, hepatic necrosis, paradoxical embolism, cardiac arrhythmias, hydrothorax, pericardial effusions with cardiac tamponade, erosion of the atrium or ventricle from the catheter tip, and phlebitis.[37–39] Several reports showed catheter-related sepsis ranging from 3% to 5% and a colonization rate of 22%.[37,38] Furthermore, there are no prospective trials suggesting increased risk of complications with multilumen umbilical vein catheters, as compared with single-lumen catheters. Although an umbilical vein catheter may remain in place for up to 14 days, it should be removed as soon as possible because of increased infection rate with a life span of the catheter beyond 10 days.[38]

Long-Term Vascular Access

Long-term VADs are necessary when venous access is required for longer than 1 month. These VADs include Dacron-cuffed Silastic catheters (Broviac[40] and Hickman[41]) and totally implantable VADs (eg, Port-a-Cath).[6,42,43]

Cuffed Silastic Catheters

These catheters are used in patients who require long-term continuous infusion of TPN (eg, patients with short gut syndrome), cancer chemotherapy, or prolonged treatment with other medications. The Broviac catheter is preferred over the totally implantable VAD when long-term access is required in patients whose catheters need to be accessed more frequently. The cuffed Silastic catheters are available with single and double lumens in sizes ranging from 2.7 to 12 Fr. They contain a polyethylene terephthalate (Dacron) cuff at the proximal end that allows ingrowth of surrounding tissue over the first 2 months after placement, serving

to anchor the catheter and possibly to prevent ascending catheter tract infections.[14] The advantage of the cuffed Silastic catheter is its easy accessibility with no discomfort to the child. Moreover, it can be removed at the bedside or in the treatment room with sedation and a local anesthetic. However, there are disadvantages. It is an external device susceptible to physical damage as well as accidental dislodgment. It requires meticulous care and carries a higher infection rate. It also costs more than the totally implantable VAD if it is used for longer than 6 months.[44–47]

Technique for Broviac-Hickman Catheter Insertion

These catheters are surgically inserted percutaneously into the subclavian, internal jugular, or femoral veins using the Seldinger technique as described in Chapter 34 or via direct vessel cutdowns.

PERCUTANEOUS TECHNIQUE. Cannulation is established with the use of the Seldinger technique as described previously. For access via the internal jugular or subclavian veins, make a small incision on the anterior chest wall, laterally near the anterior axillary line at the level of the mammary crease, or alternatively medial to the nipple at the same level. When the femoral vein is used, the exit site is on the lower abdomen or the medial aspect of the lower thigh, away from the diaper lines. Create a subcutaneous tunnel between this incision and the guidewire exit site with a tunneler. In young female patients, great care must be taken to prevent injury to the breast buds. Pass the catheter through the tunnel via the lower incision and exit next to the guidewire. Efforts should be made to place the cuff at least 2 cm from the skin incision, because it has been shown to decrease the rate of infection and dislodgment. Tailor the catheter length to place the tip into the superior vena cava, near the origin of the right atrium. Insert a peel-away sheath attached to the dilator over the guidewire. It is critical to use live fluoroscopy during this maneuver to avoid potential injury from the dilator or from the guidewire as it is being pushed. Remove the introducer and the guidewire, leaving the peel-away sheath in the vein. Thread the catheter into the sheath, and peel the sheath away from the catheter. Check the catheter for blood return, and perform fluoroscopy to confirm proper placement of the tip. Secure the catheter to the skin at the lower incision with a monofilament suture. Check the catheter again for patency because the suture may obstruct the lumen. Close the superior skin incision, and place appropriate dressings.

CUTDOWN TECHNIQUE. In small neonates, a direct cutdown of the external jugular, facial, saphenous, or internal jugular veins is preferred. This procedure may be performed at bedside with sedation and local anesthesia. It is critical to avoid hypothermia in these newborns. This technique can also be used in older children, but general anesthesia may be required.

EXTERNAL JUGULAR VEIN CUTDOWN. The external jugular vein is superficial and usually visible running across the

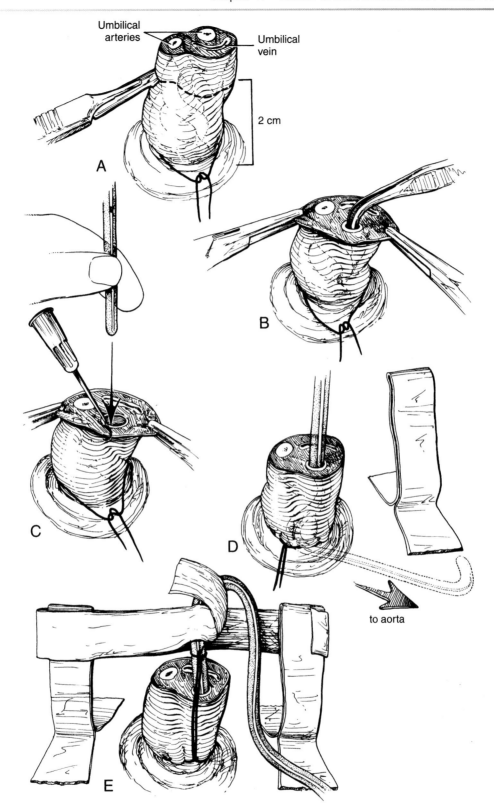

Figure 17-9.
Anatomy of the umbilicus with umbilical artery catheterization. *A,* The umbilicus, with two thick-walled arteries and one thin-walled collapsible vein. A suture is placed at the base of the stump, and the umbilicus is transected approximately 2 cm from its base. *B,* The artery should be opened, and any visible clot extracted with fine forceps. *C,* The arterial catheter is grasped 2 to 4 cm from the tip. *D,* The catheter is inserted with minimal resistance. *E,* An H-type dressing is placed to secure the catheter (*A-E,* From Fleisher GR, Ludwig S, Henretig FM [eds]. *Textbook of Pediatric Emergency Medicine.* 5th ed. Philadelphia: Lippincott Williams & Wilkins; 2005:1874-1876.)

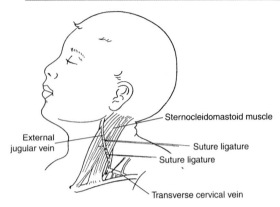

Figure 17-10.
External jugular vein cutdown technique.

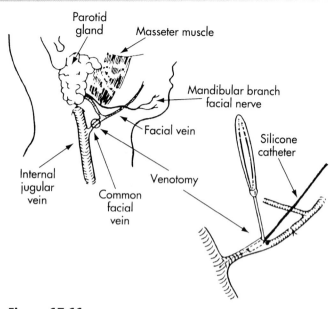

Figure 17-11.
Regional anatomy of the common facial vein and internal jugular vein. Insertion of the silicone catheter is facilitated by using a vein introducer.

sternocleidomastoid muscle (Fig 17-10). Most surgeons recommend using this vein first if it is easily visible. Unfortunately, its central placement is less reliable and is directly related to the ability to control its side branches, such as the transverse cervical vein underneath the clavicle.

Start the procedure with a small transverse incision over the inferior aspect of the vein. Carry out a gentle dissection with a fine hemostat. The external jugular vein should be easily visualized as it lies in the superficial fascia. In tracing the vein proximally, the transverse cervical vein should be encountered as it enters posteriorly. Control this vein and the external jugular vein with sutures. Tunnel the catheter in the subcuticular plane as mentioned. Cut the catheter to an appropriate length. Construct a venotomy, and insert the catheter through this venotomy and advance it centrally. Ligate the distal end of the external jugular, and tie the other suture around the catheter to prevent backbleeding. A chest radiograph confirms the position of the catheter.

FACIAL VEIN CUTDOWN.   The common facial vein is most commonly used in neonates (Fig 17-11). This vein allows direct access to the superior vena cava via the internal jugular vein. It begins at the confluence of the posterior and anterior facial veins. The anterior branch runs across the mandible with the facial artery in the mandibular notch. The pulsation of this artery provides a helpful landmark. Make an incision parallel and below the mandible. Perform the dissection bluntly to avoid injury to the mandibular branch of the facial nerve. The vein is located deep to the cervical fascia and is often located just posterior to a large lymph node or the inferior pole of the parotid gland. If the common facial vein cannot be located, ready access to the internal jugular vein can be accomplished through the same incision.

INTERNAL JUGULAR VEIN CUTDOWN.   The internal jugular vein provides reliable access when other veins cannot be used. The easiest and most direct way to approach the internal jugular vein is through an incision over the SCM in the middle of the neck. Bluntly split the muscle is bluntly split and retract it apart. The first vessel encountered is the internal jugular vein. The upper portion of the internal jugular vein may also be exposed through the incision recommended for the common facial vein. Approaching this vein along the

medial border to the sternocleidomastoid muscle, in the midportion of the neck, is considerably more difficult. Once the vessel is identified, control it controlled proximally and distally with either vessel loops or 2-0 silk sutures. Place a small pursestring suture of 5-0 or 6-0 monofilament on the anterior aspect of the vein. Cannulate the vein through a venotomy constructed in the middle of the pursestring.

GREATER SAPHENOUS VEIN CUTDOWN.   The saphenous vein at the saphenofemoral junction is a reliable and easy route to gain central access, even in premature infants. To expose the vein, make an incision inferior to the inguinal crease and medial to the femoral artery. The vein is encountered in the subcutaneous tissue. Continue the dissection to the saphenofemoral junction. Here, the saphenous vein is controlled with sutures (Fig. 17-12). Ligate the distal end of the vein with one of the sutures and retract it caudally. Pass the catheter through a saphenous venotomy and advance it centrally. The ideal location is at the diaphragm level.

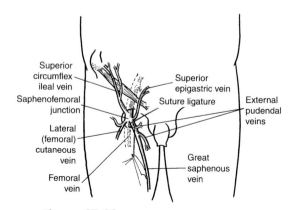

Figure 17-12.
Great saphenous vein cutdown technique.

Totally Implantable VADs

The implantable devices (eg, Port-a-Cath, Infuse-a-Port, or Mediport) provide a more permanent venous access for patients who require long-term intermittent vascular access. These devices have a single or double plastic or metal reservoir attached to a Silastic catheter. They are surgically placed in the subcutaneous tissue of the anterior chest wall, lateral chest wall, upper extremity,[48] or in rare instances, the iliac crest region. The smaller, low-profile ports are preferred in younger and smaller children, whereas bigger ports and double-reservoir ports are used in older and larger children. It is safe to use these devices in infants as young as 6 months old. Advantages of these devices include total concealment, lower infection rate, low maintenance requirements, and cosmetically acceptable. Furthermore, the patient's physical activity is not limited.[42,44]

After accessing the vein via the Seldinger technique or direct cutdown, construct a subcutaneous pocket to accommodate the port. Make a small incision on the chest wall, at the site chosen for port placement. Make a small pocket at the fascial level. Then anchor the port onto the fascia with nonabsorbable sutures in at least three different places to prevent flipping or migration. Tunnel the attached Silastic tubing subcutaneously from the port site to the puncture site or the cutdown site. Cut an appropriate length of the catheter. Central venous cannulation proceeds as described elsewhere. Confirm the position of the catheter with fluoroscopy. Access the port with a Hubber needle. Aspirate the system and flush with heparin solution. Close the incisions in layers with subcuticular absorbable sutures, and place a sterile occlusive dressing.

The peripherally inserted ports are useful in children 10 years of age and older, when they have enough subcutaneous tissue to allow placement of a low-profile port. Anesthetize the skin of the medial forearm locally. Place the port into a subcutaneous pocket through a small incision in the midforearm and secure it. Isolate the basilic or cephalic vein via cutdown at the level of the antecubital fossa. Tunnel the catheter and insert into the vein. Close the incisions with a subcuticular absorbable suture and dress appropriately.

Arterial Access

Umbilical Artery Catheterization

Many infants require direct central blood pressure monitoring, arterial blood gases, and frequent blood samplings to allow minute-to-minute management. The umbilical arteries allow easy access to the descending aorta in the first 3 to 4 days of life, and umbilical artery catheters (UACs) can also be used for exchange transfusion. Insertion of the UAC is usually done in the neonatal intensive care unit. Under aseptic conditions, encircle an umbilical tape around the base of the umbilical stump and tie it loosely (see Fig. 17-9). Cut the umbilical stump 1 to 2 cm from the base and secure with hemostats. The two thick-walled arteries that lie in the inferior aspect of the umbilicus are visible. Insert a single-lumen umbilical catheter (3.5 Fr for premature infants and 5.0 Fr for term infants) through one of these vessels and negotiate it to an appropriate location. It is recommended that the UAC tip be positioned high, at the level of the midthoracic spine (T6–T8), above the origin of all major visceral vessels, or low, below the level of the renal artery (L3 or L4). Preference for high versus low UAC tip position is controversial.[37,49–51] An increased incidence of limb ischemia and vessel perforation has been reported with low-positioned UACs.[49] High-positioned UACs last longer than low-positioned UACs, but the former have been implicated in an increased rate of intraventricular hemorrhage.[51] Although UACs remain in place for 7 to 10 days, they should be removed as soon as possible to avoid increased risks of complications.[50] Catheter-related aortic thrombosis has been reported as high as 50%[52–54] and is directly related to the duration of catheter use (5% in 3.5 days vs. 30% in 11 days). Moreover, approximately 25% of these patients have renal artery involvement. Catheter sepsis is also higher in UACs compared with peripheral arterial catheters ($<$1% vs. 5%–10%). Other complications related to UACs include vasospasm, distal embolization with extremity or visceral ischemia, necrotizing enterocolitis, bowel perforation, and vascular perforation with intraperitoneal hemorrhage. There also have been reports of arterial aneurysm[55,56] and aortic coarctation[57] as a result of umbilical catheterization. Although these complications can be catastrophic, the overall incidence of major complications is usually reported as less than 5%.

Radial Artery Cannulation

Although arterial cannulation can be done at many locations, such as the posterior tibial, dorsalis pedis, and femoral axillary arteries, the radial artery is the preferred site (Fig. 17-13). The right radial artery is an excellent source of preductal gas sampling. The radial artery is a branch of the brachial artery. At the wrist, it gives rise to a

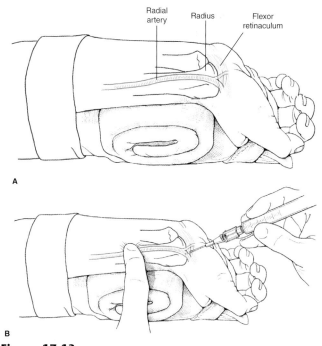

Figure 17-13.
Radial artery. *A*, Anatomy. *B*, Technique (*A* and *B*, Adapted from Chameides L [ed]. *Textbook of Pediatric Advanced Life Support.* Dallas: American Heart Association; 1997.)

Table 17–3

Indications, Advantages, and Disadvantages of Various Methods for Vascular Access in Pediatric Patients

Method	Indications	Advantages	Disadvantages
Peripheral	Short term	Easy to insert, low cost	Easily dislodged, high rate of occlusion, tissue injury with extravasation of irritants
Intraosseous	Emergency or short term	Rapid and easy to insert, relatively safe	Not suitable for long-term use, tendency to leak at site
PICC* lines	Intermediate term, patients with access problems	Excellent for neonates with access problems, low cost	Easily occluded, can be difficult to advance into central vein
Venous cutdown	Emergency or long term	Direct exposure of vein in patients with difficult access	High rate of dislodgment and infection, incision required
Polyethylene central catheter	Long term	Percutaneous insertion, safe with hypertonic solutions	Altered body image, bacterial colonization of tunnel may require surgical insertion*
Silastic central catheter	Long term	More pliable, less thrombogenic, decreased infection rate	Higher cost, requires surgical Insertion*
Central ports	Long term	Low visibility, reliable, lowest rate of infection	Higher cost, requires surgical Insertion*

*May require general anesthesia.
PICC, peripherally inserted central catheter.
From Stovroff M, Teague WG. Intravenous access in infants and children. *Pediatr Clin North Am.* 1998;45:1373-1393, viii.

deep palmar arch that joins with the superficial palmar arch (from the ulnar artery) to provide blood to the digits. In approximately 12% of patients, the radial artery contributes significant blood supply to the fingers. For this reason, it is important to perform an Allen test before inserting a radial artery catheter. Unfortunately, this test is difficult and unreliable to obtain in neonates. The use of a Doppler probe to listen for the digital arterial signals while performing an Allen test is extremely helpful. Cannulation can be done either percutaneously or via a cutdown. A 24-Fr catheter is used in newborns, and a 22-Fr catheter is used in larger children. Complications include infection, sepsis, thrombosis with distal ischemia, and catheter malfunction.

Summary

Advances have provided the clinician with a substantial armamentarium to address the problem of venous access in the pediatric patient.

The majority of short-term VADs are inserted percutaneously; these include the standard peripheral intravenous catheter, the PICC, and the Silastic, polyurethane, and polyethylene central venous catheters. The same catheters can be inserted via a cutdown, but this technique should be reserved for instances when percutaneous venous access is not available. Intraosseous access is vital in the emergency situation when immediate venous access is not possible.

Long-term VADs include the cuffed Silastic catheter and the implantable VAD. The cuffed Silastic catheter is used for prolonged, continuous infusion, and the implantable VAD is used for prolonged, intermittent infusion. Both cuffed catheter and implantable devices are available in various sizes appropriate for the pediatric patient population. Table 17-3 provides a summary of the indications, advantages, and disadvantages of the various access methods.

REFERENCES

1. Fuhrman BP, Zimmerman JJ (eds). *Pediatric Critical Care.* 3rd ed. Philadelphia: Mosby Elsevier; 2006.
2. Hunter KS, Lee PF, Lanning CJ, et al. Pulmonary vascular input impedance is a combined measure of pulmonary vascular resistance and stiffness and predicts clinical outcomes better than pulmonary vascular resistance alone in pediatric patients with pulmonary hypertension. *Am Heart J.* 2007;155:166-174.
3. Introna RPS, Martin DC, Pruett JK, Philpot TE, Johnston JF. Percutaneous pulmonary artery catheterization in pediatric cardiovascular anesthesia: insertion techniques and use. *Anesth Analg.* 1990; 70:562-566.
4. Cochran EB, Phelps SJ, Helms RA. Parenteral nutrition in pediatric patients. *Clin Pharm.* 1988;7:351-366.
5. Wessel JJ, Kocoshis SA. Nutritional management of infants with short bowel syndrome. *Semin Perinatol.* 2007;31:104-111.
6. Dillon PA, Foglia RP. Complications associated with an implantable vascular access device. *J Pediatr Surg.* 2006;41:1582-1587.
7. Ball AB, Duncan FR, Foster FJ, Davidson TI, Watkins RM, Hodson ME. Long term venous access using a totally implantable drug delivery system in patients with cystic fibrosis and bronchiectasis. *Respir Med.* 1989;83:429-431.
8. Deerojanawong J, Sawyer SM, Fink AM, Stokes KB, Robertson CF. Totally implantable venous access devices in children with cystic fibrosis: incidence and type of complications. *Thorax.* 1998;53:285-289.
9. Hockenberry MJ, Schultz WH, Bennett B, Bryant R, Falletta JM. Experience with minimal complications in implanted catheters in children. *Am J Pediatr Hematol Oncol.* 1989;11:295-299.

10. Ljung R, Petrini P, Lindgren AK, Berntorp E. Implantable central venous catheter facilitates prophylactic treatment in children with haemophilia. *Acta Paediatr.* 1992;81:918-920.

11. Sola JE, Stone MM, Wise B, Colombani PM. Atypical thrombotic and septic complications of totally implantable venous access devices in patients with cystic fibrosis. *Pediatr Pulmonol.* 1992;14:239-242.

12. Garland JS, Dunne WM Jr, Havens P, et al. Peripheral intravenous catheter complications in critically ill children: a prospective study. *Pediatrics.* 1992;89:1145-1150.

13. Maki DG, Ringer M. Risk factors for infusion-related phlebitis with small peripheral venous catheters: a randomized controlled trial. *Ann Intern Med.* 1991;114:845-854.

14. Stovroff M, Teague WG. Intravenous access in infants and children. *Pediatr Clin North Am.* 1998;45:1373-1393, viii.

15. Iserson KV, Criss EA. Pediatric venous cutdowns: utility in emergency situations. *Pediatr Emerg Care.* 1986;2:231-234.

16. Newman BM, Jewett TC Jr, Karp MP, Cooney DR. Percutaneous central venous catheterization in children: first line choice for venous access. *J Pediatr Surg.* 1986;21:685-688.

17. Cilley RE. Intraosseous infusion in infants and children. *Semin Pediatr Surg.* 1992;1:202-207.

18. de Caen AR, Reis A, Bhutta A. Vascular access and drug therapy in pediatric resuscitation. *Pediatr Clin North Am.* 2008;55:909-927, x.

19. Barron BJ, Tran HD, Lamki LM. Scintigraphic findings of osteomyelitis after intraosseous infusion in a child. *Clin Nucl Med.* 1994; 19:307-308.

20. Katz DS, Wojtowycz AR. Tibial fracture: a complication of intraosseous infusion. *Am J Emerg Med.* 1994;12:258-259.

21. Simmons CM, Johnson NE, Perkin RM, van Stralen D. Intraosseous extravasation: complication reports. *Ann Emerg Med.* 1994;23: 363-366.

22. Guy J, Haley K, Zuspan SJ. Use of intraosseous infusion in the pediatric trauma patient. *J Pediatr Surg.* 1993;28:158-161.

23. Chathas MK, Paton JB, Fisher D. Percutaneous central venous catheterization: three years' experience in a neonatal intensive care unit. *Am J Dis Child.* 1990;144:1246-1250.

24. Dolcourt JL, Bose CL. Percutaneous insertion of Silastic central venous catheters in newborn infants. *Pediatrics.* 1982;70:484-486.

25. Durand M, Ramanathan R, Martinelli B, Tolentino M. Prospective evaluation of percutaneous central venous Silastic catheters in newborn infants with birth weights of 510 to 3,920 grams. *Pediatrics.* 1986;78:245-250.

26. Loeff DS, Matlak ME, Black RE, Overall JC, Dolcourt JL, Johnson DG. Insertion of a small central venous catheter in neonates and young infants. *J Pediatr Surg.* 1982;17:944-949.

27. Eichelberger MR, Rous PG, Hoelzer DJ, Garcia VF, Koop CE. Percutaneous subclavian venous catheters in neonates and children. *J Pediatr Surg.* 1981;16(4 suppl 1):547-553.

28. Filston HC, Grant JP. A safer system for percutaneous subclavian venous catheterization in newborn infants. *J Pediatr Surg.* 1979; 14:564-570.

29. Pietsch JB, Nagaraj HS, Groff DB. Simplified insertion of central venous catheter in infants. *Surg Gynecol Obstet.* 1984;158:91-92.

30. Boon JM, van Schoor AN, Abrahams PH, Meiring JH, Welch T, Shanahan D. Central venous catheterization—an anatomical review of a clinical skill—Part 1: subclavian vein via the infraclavicular approach. *Clin Anat.* 2007;20:602-611.

31. Goutail-Flaud MF, Sfez M, Berg A, et al. Central venous catheter-related complications in newborns and infants: a 587-case survey. *J Pediatr Surg.* 1991;26:645-650.

32. Bagwell CE, Marchildon MB. Mural thrombi in children: potentially lethal complication of central venous hyperalimentation. *Crit Care Med.* 1989;17:295-296.

33. Bone DK, Maddrey WC, Eagan J, Cameron JL. Cardiac tamponade: a fatal complication of central venous catheterization. *Arch Surg* 1973; 106:868-870.

34. Farkas JC, Liu N, Bleriot JP, Chevret S, Goldstein FW, Carlet J. Single- versus triple-lumen central catheter-related sepsis: a prospective randomized study in a critically ill population. *Am J Med.* 1992;93:277-282.

35. Loisel DB, Smith MM, MacDonald MG, Martin GR. Intravenous access in newborn infants: impact of extended umbilical venous catheter use on requirement for peripheral venous lines. *J Perinatol.* 1996;16: 461-466.

36. Möller JC, Reiss I, Schaible T. Vascular access in neonates and infants—indications, routes, techniques, devices, and complications. *Intensive Care World.* 1995;12:48-53.

37. Green C, Yohannan MD. Umbilical arterial and venous catheters: placement, use, and complications. *Neonatal Netw.* 1998;17:23-28.

38. Ramachandran P, Cohen RS, Kim EH, Glasscock GF. Experience with double-lumen umbilical venous catheters in the low-birth-weight neonate. *J Perinatol.* 1994;14:280-284.

39. Morag I, Epelman M, Daneman A, et al. Portal vein thrombosis in the neonate: risk factors, course, and outcome. *J Pediatr.* 2006;148: 735-739.

40. Broviac JW, Cole JJ, Scribner BH. A silicone rubber atrial catheter for prolonged parenteral alimentation. *Surg Gynecol Obstet.* 1973; 136:602-606.

41. Hickman RO, Buckner CD, Clift RA, Sanders JE, Stewart P, Thomas ED. A modified right atrial catheter for access to the venous system in marrow transplant recipients. *Surg Gynecol Obstet.* 1979;148:871-875.

42. Hall P, Cedermark B, Swedenborg J. Implantable catheter system for long-term intravenous chemotherapy. *J Surg Oncol.* 1989;41:39-41.

43. Strum S, McDermed J, Korn A, Joseph C. Improved methods for venous access: the Port-A-Cath, a totally implanted catheter system. *J Clin Oncol.* 1986;4:596-603.

44. Ingram J, Weitzman S, Greenberg ML, Parkin P, Filler R. Complications of indwelling venous access lines in the pediatric hematology patient: a prospective comparison of external venous catheters and subcutaneous ports. *Am J Pediatr Hematol Oncol.* 1991;13:130-136.

45. La Quaglia MP, Lucas A, Thaler HT, Friedlander-Klar H, Exelby PR, Groeger JS. A prospective analysis of vascular access device-related infections in children. *J Pediatr Surg.* 1992;27:840-842.

46. Mirro J Jr, Rao BN, Kumar M, et al. A comparison of placement techniques and complications of externalized catheters and implantable port use in children with cancer. *J Pediatr Surg.* 1990;25:120-124.

47. Ross MN, Haase GM, Poole MA, Burrington JD, Odom LF. Comparison of totally implanted reservoirs with external catheters as venous access in pediatric oncologic patients. *Surg Gynecol Obstet.* 1988;167: 141-144.

48. Pearl JM, Goldstein L, Ciresi KF. Improved methods in long term venous access using the P.A.S. Port. *Surg Gynecol Obstet.* 1991;173: 313-315.

49. Kempley ST, Bennett S, Loftus BG, Cooper D, Gamsu HR. Randomized trial of umbilical arterial catheter position: clinical outcome. *Acta Paediatr.* 1993;82:173-176.

50. Kitterman JA, Phibbs RH, Tooley WH. Catheterization of umbilical vessels in newborn infants. *Pediatr Clin North Am.* 1970;17:895-912.

51. Umbilical Artery Catheter Trial Study Group. Relationship of intraventricular hemorrhage or death with the level of umbilical artery catheter placement: a multicenter randomized clinical trial. *Pediatrics.* 1992;90:881-887.

52. Hermansen MC, Hermansen MG. Intravascular catheter complications in the neonatal intensive care unit. *Clin Perinatol.* 2005;32: 141-156.

53. O'Neill JA Jr, Neblett WW 3rd, Born ML. Management of major thromboembolic complications of umbilical artery catheters. *J Pediatr Surg.* 1981;16:972-978.

54. Symansky MR, Fox HA. Umbilical vessel catheterization: indications, management, and evaluation of the technique. *J Pediatr.* 1972;80: 820-826.

55. Cribari C, Meadors FA, Crawford ES, Coselli JS, Safi HJ, Svensson LG. Thoracoabdominal aortic aneurysm associated with umbilical artery catheterization: case report and review of the literature. *J Vasc Surg.* 1992;16:75-86.

56. Kirpekar M, Augenstein H, Abiri M. Sequential development of multiple aortic aneurysms in a neonate post umbilical arterial catheter insertion. *Pediatr Radiol.* 1989;19:452-453.

57. Starc JJ, Abramson SJ, Bierman FZ, et al. Acquired coarctation of the aorta. *Pediatr Cardiol.* 1992;13:33-36.

CHAPTER 18

Surveillance, Revision, and Outcome of Vascular Access Procedures for Hemodialysis

Dmitri V. Gelfand, Apostolos K. Tassiopoulos, and Samuel Eric Wilson

The introduction of Quinton-Scribner shunt in 1960 and Brescia-Cimino radiocephalic arteriovenous fistula (AVF) in 1966 provided the conduits necessary for chronic hemodialysis in patients with end-stage renal disease (ESRD).[1,2] Today, over 300,000 ESRD patients receive hemodialysis annually in the United States.[3] Maintaining a functional hemodialysis access is crucial for optimal care of these patients. Inadequate access leads to underdialysis and repeated hospitalizations and surgical reinterventions, affects not only patients' quality of life but also their longevity, and greatly affects health care expenditures.

Maintenance of vascular access for hemodialysis remains a challenge for vascular surgeons and interventionalists. Procedures for failing or thrombosed arteriovenous grafts (AVG) occur once a year on average. Thrombosis remains the primary cause of hemodialysis access failure and is most commonly the result of compromised venous outflow.[4] A number of surveillance methods have been proposed for identifying access conduits at risk for thrombosis. Angiographic guidance has been employed more frequently for both diagnosis and treatment. Introduction of less nephrotoxic isosmolar contrast agents and the refinement of percutaneous techniques have decreased periprocedural complications in recent years. Duplex ultrasound (DU) remains the first choice for imaging of hemodialysis access conduits, providing detailed anatomic and functional information of the arterial and venous sides. Recently, DU has been used as imaging guidance during percutaneous interventions for failing AVFs and AVGs, a trend that, in these authors' opinion, is likely to expand in the future.

In 1997, the Kidney Dialysis Outcomes Quality Initiative (K/DOQI), a project initiated by the National Kidney Foundation (NKF) in order to improve the care of dialysis patients, provided evidence-based clinical practice guidelines for the management of chronic kidney disease and related complications. A significant component of the NKF K/DOQI Clinical Practice Guidelines and Clinical Practice Recommendations (updated in 2006)[5] focuses on surveillance protocols for dialysis conduits and prophylactic interventions for failing access sites in order to improve patency rates and prevent thrombosis. As of 2009, the Centers for Medicare Services (CMS) require periodic monitoring and recording to document surveillance of the vascular access.

Surveillance

The long-term success of an autogenous or nonautogenous dialysis conduit is dependent on a detailed preoperative patient evaluation for selection of the optimal vein (autogenous conduit) and arterial and venous anastomosis sites (nonautogenous grafts) and for assessing arterial inflow and venous outflow. Duplex imaging of the extremity vessels has become a routine component of the preoperative evaluation for patients with ESRD. Silva and coworkers[6] used duplex ultrasound (DU) to identify adequate vessels and found that more than 60% of the arteries and veins in the upper extremity were suitable for autogenous AVFs. These authors also reported a significant decrease in the early failure rate of fistulas from 36% to 8.3% when preoperative duplex scanning was employed. Duplex imaging may not be necessary for the preoperative assessment of all ESRD patients, but it is particularly valuable for assessing veins that are not visible on physical examination. Given the usual history of previous hospitalizations with multiple peripheral and central venous catheterizations in ESRD patients, duplex is a sensitive test for detecting stenosis or thrombosis of both the superficial and the deep proximal veins. It also provides detailed information about arterial occlusive disease in diabetic or elderly patients, thus limiting the potential for early failures and/or hemodynamic complications (arm edema, steal).

Physical Examination

Once the patient has acquired a functional arteriovenous (AV) conduit, prevention of AVF or AVG thrombosis is of paramount importance. The hemodialysis center serves as a convenient and cost-effective site for routine surveillance of functioning access conduits, and hemodialysis access evaluation should start there. On routine physical examination prior to each dialysis session, palpation of the graft should reveal a continuous thrill and a low-frequency bruit throughout its length. A strong pulsatile flow pattern or a high-pitch bruit should raise suspicion of stenosis, and further evaluation is indicated. Additional findings on examination that raise suspicion of graft or fistula dysfunction include development of collateral veins, worsening arm edema, hand pain that worsens during dialysis, and prolonged bleeding postdialysis from the needle puncture sites. Current recommendations call for at least monthly physical examination of the fistula or graft by trained professionals to allow for early detection of a stenosis. Early detection is critical in preventing development of "functionally significant stenosis," defined by K/DOQI as a greater than 50% reduction of normal vessel diameter, together with hemodynamic or clinical signs of stenosis, such as increased recirculation, decreased flow, elevated venous pressures, or increased swelling of the extremity.[5]

Pressure Measurements

Pressure measurements from the dialyser circuit were originally designed to assess the mean transmembrane pressure to establish optimal ultrafiltration rate. This was later replaced by volumetric control systems. When employed in surveillance of hemodialysis access, venous pressure monitoring is based on the premise that resistance to flow is the result of venous outflow stenosis. Static venous pressure monitoring has replaced dynamic pressure monitoring and is currently endorsed by NKF K/DOQI work force as one of various methods for surveying hemodialysis access.[5] Static venous pressure monitoring corrects for resistance in dialysis tubing and needles that affect the venous pressure measured during hemodialysis.[7] The role of venous pressure measurements is less valuable in surveying forearm fistulas because of the significant collateralization seen with these conduits. Direct venous pressures are measured by cannulation of the arterial and venous segments of the access conduit, using an appropriate pressure-measuring device.[8] When the measured pressure is elevated by more than 25% compared with the baseline measurements, a hemodynamically significant stenosis should be suspected.

Access Flow

Decreasing flow is a sign of stenosis in the arterial inflow, conduit, or venous outflow. Sveral direct and indirect methods are available for measuring flow in a dialysis access conduit. DU[9,10] and magnetic resonance angiography (MRA)[11,12] are the most commonly described direct methods. In addition to flow measurements, DU and MRA allow for anatomic visualization and assessment of the severity of stenosis. MRA is rarely used for AV access conduit surveillance because of the very high cost. Indirect methods employ various indicator dilution techniques during hemodialysis sessions. The most commonly used indirect methods are ionic dialysance, ultrasound dilution, glucose infusion, timed ultrafiltration, and differential conductivity. Results are comparable with those of DU flow assessment. Depner and colleagues[13] reported a 77% rate of failure in AVGs with baseline flow of less than 600 mL/min over 6 months. Sands and associates[14] found that patients who had monthly access flow monitoring had decreased thrombosis rates for both AVFs and AVGs compared with those of

patients who had static venous pressure monitoring. A 5-year prospective study by Tessitore and coworkers[15] showed that using access blood flow (Qa) for monitoring mature AVFs increases the short term (3-year) cumulative patency of AVFs by better detection and early treatment of subclinical stenoses, which they found to contribute to lower AVF thrombosis rates.

Imaging

DU combines anatomic visualization of an AVF or AVG with measurement of blood flow through the conduit. Direct measurement of diameter reduction by B-mode and color-flow imaging combined with Doppler criteria (peak systolic velocities >400 cm/sec and peak systolic velocity ratio >3) can accurately diagnose conduit and anastomotic stenoses. Advantages of DU include patient comfort, reproducibility, and the ability to fully study the arterial inflow, conduit and venous outflow anatomy, and hemodynamics while avoiding radiation exposure and the complications of invasive diagnostic tests. In recent years, DU has become the preferred imaging modality for surveillance of AV access sites. Despite its proven accuracy for detecting stenoses, however, whether DU can predict conduit thrombosis or whether intense surveillance is associated with prolonged overall hemodialysis access survival are questions that remain unanswered.

Early Intervention

Correction of subclinical AV access conduit stenosis detected during surveillance is an attractive preventative measure. Strauch and colleagues[16] found that 57% of patients with functioning AVGs and DU evidence of venous stenosis greater than 50% progressed to thrombosis within 6 months as compared with 9.5% of the patients with 30% to 50% stenosis. In a prospective, randomized trial Lumsden and associates[17] used DU to discover greater than 50% stenosis in functioning polytetrafluorethylene (PTFE) grafts and then confirmed the findings with angiography. Patients were randomized to duplex surveillance and prophylactic angioplasty of all stenoses greater than 50% versus ongoing surveillance but no intervention. No improvement was found in the patency of PTFE grafts at 12 months. A more recent randomized trial by Tessitore and colleagues[18] compared two groups of ESRD patients with hemodynamically significant (>50%) stenosis in AVFs with regards to preemptive percutaneous intervention. This study showed reduced thrombosis rates and improved access survival in patients with prophylactic angioplasties. Whether this reflects an improvement of diagnostic and interventional techniques over the intervening decade or a difference in angioplasty results between AVFs and AVGs is uncertain. The most recent K/DOQI update recommends access surveillance and preemptive interventions because it allows for advanced planning and team coordination toward elective interventions as opposed to urgent or emergent hemodialysis access salvage procedures.

K/DOQI recommends monitoring at monthly intervals that should include physical examination, static venous pressures, and flow measurements, followed by DU or fistulogram when a significant stenosis is suspected (Table 18-1). In general, it is not advised to respond to an isolated abnormal value. Instead, one should follow the trend in the

Table 18–1

Clinical Recommendations of the Society for Vascular Surgery

The Role of Monitoring and Surveillance in Arteriovenous Access Management

Regular clinical monitoring (inspection, palpation, auscultation, and monitoring for prolonged bleeding after needle withdrawal).

Flow monitoring or static dialysis venous pressures for routine surveillance.

Duplex ultrasound study or contrast imaging study in accesses that display clinical signs of dysfunction or abnormal routine surveillance.

From Sidawy AN, Spergel LM, Besarb A, et al. The Society for Vascular Surgery: clinical practice guidelines for the surgical placement and maintenance of arteriovenous hemodialysis access. *J Vasc Surg.* 2008;48:2S-25S.

observed values. Access imaging is indicated when flow rates persistently decrease (<400 mL/min in fistulas and 600 mL/min in grafts) or elevate in venous (>0.5) or arterial (>0.75) static pressure ratio.[5]

Revision

Patients with clinical signs of a malfunctioning AV conduit should be considered for elective intervention to repair the underlying abnormality and prevent thrombosis. Autogenous fistula maturation during the first 6 months after creation is critical for its long-term function. A weak thrill, persistent arm swelling, and/or failure to mature should trigger initiation of a diagnostic workup (DU or fistulogram) in order to identify and correct the underlying cause, as early as 6 weeks after the initial procedure.[19] Patients with AVGs who have arm swelling beyond 2 weeks should undergo a DU study to evaluate patency of the central veins.[20] Recently, in an attempt to improve utilization and shorten maturation time of primary AVFs, Miller and coworkers[21] suggested a "balloon angioplasty maturation" (BAM) technique. This technique is based on "staged sequential dilation" of the AVF conduit. With an initial technical success rate of 98.6%, patients with AVFs who underwent BAM had primary patency over 90% in 1 year.

Patients with functional access should be referred for further evaluation with DU or fistulogram if they cannot complete hemodialysis owing to poor flow or high static pressures. Development of aneurysmal dilation of the fistula or persistent bleeding after decannulation should raise suspicion of venous outflow obstruction or stenosis and requires further evaluation as well. Ischemic changes due to steal syndrome require immediate referral to a vascular surgeon for an appropriate evaluation and intervention to restore adequate perfusion of the affected limb.[22] The current K/DOQI recommendation for patients with the previously discussed clinical signs who are diagnosed with an AV conduit stenosis of greater than 50% by DU or fistulogram is to proceed with percutaneous transluminal angioplasty (PTA) of the stenosis.[18] Successful PTA is defined as that resulting in a residual stenosis less than 30% and in normalization of all hemodynamic and clinical parameters.[23] Ac-

cording to K/DOQI guidelines, when elastic recoil after PTA results in more then 50% residual stenosis, stent placement may be considered. In addition, restenosis within 3 months after a successful PTA may be regarded as an indication for stenting. If, however, a percutaneous intervention for the same lesion is required more than twice within a 3-month period, open surgical revision should be considered.[5] Tessitore and associates[24] prospectively compared surgical versus endovascular repair for patients with failing forearm AVFs. The study showed significantly higher restenosis rates after PTA, but there was no difference in overall hemodialysis access survival, procedural success rate, or cost. The current trend is to employ endovascular techniques as the initial approach for identified hemodynamically significant stenoses and reserve open techniques for persistent or recurrent lesions and for the management of aneurysms, pseudoaneurysms, or steal complications.

Salvage of a thrombosed fistula or graft should be performed as soon as possible in order to avoid temporary hemodialysis access.[25] It can be performed via either surgical or endovascular approaches. The most common lesion responsible for AVG failure and thrombosis is development of a stenosis at the venous anastomosis as a result of intimal hyperplasia. Surgical thrombectomy is followed by a revision at the venous anastomosis aimed at improving outflow stenosis. This can be accomplished by a patch angioplasty or an extension graft targeting a more suitable proximal outflow segment.[24] Initially described by Rodkin and coworkers in 1983,[26] endovascular treatment techniques with fluoroscopic or ultrasound guidance have become much more common over time. Mechanical thrombectomy techniques combined with conventional PTA, cutting balloon PTA, and/or use of bare or covered stents have increased the AVG salvage rate while minimizing patient discomfort, surgical trauma, and the need for hospitalization. The following chapters provide a detailed description of various techniques employed in the management of hemodialysis access complications.

Outcome

In the past, the higher use of nonautogenous hemodialysis access conduits in the United States as compared with Europe was possibly a reflection of delays in referring ESRD patients to vascular surgeons and of a preference by patients, vascular surgeons, and dialysis personnel for AVGs versus AVFs. It is generally believed that the patency rates for AVFs are superior to those of AVGs. Therefore, NKF K/DOQI Clinical Practice Guidelines 2006[5] recommend AVF (radiocephalic, brachiocephalic, and brachiobasilic transposition) as *preferred* permanent hemodialysis access. Synthetic or biologic AVGs are considered *acceptable*, whereas long-term central venous tunneled catheters should be avoided if possible. Although there are no level-one data available comparing autologous to nonautologous hemodialysis access options, AVFs are favored because of lower incidence of infection, thrombosis, and secondary interventions.[27] Data from experienced vascular surgeons and established dialysis centers show primary patency rates for AVG to be just under 50% in the first year. In an analysis of 632 patients with PTFE grafts, Schuman and colleagues[28] reported a primary patency rate of 44% at 1 year. In a prospective study by Cinat and associates,[29] the primary patency was 43% at 1 year. Kennedy and coworkers[30] calculated a 37% overall graft survival rate at 2 years in a review of Medicare records for 1477 northern New England hemodialysis patients. Secondary patency rates for PTFE grafts are considerably higher, ranging between 85%[28] and 64%[29] in the first year. A study by Huber and colleagues[31] reviewed studies comparing patency of AVGs and AVFs and performed a meta-analysis of all available data. According to these authors, autogenous AVFs had significantly higher primary patency rates (72% and 51% vs. 58% and 33% at 6- and 18-mo intervals) and secondary patency rates (86% and 77% vs. 76% and 55% at 6 and 18 mo) when compared with AVGs. Although based on case series and nonrandomized studies, these results support the "fistula first" initiative recommending that AVF should be the primary choice for hemodialysis access.

It is critical to remember, however, that the decision on the type of access should not be based on a single factor. A multivariate regression analysis by Gibson and associates[32] evaluated 2247 patients undergoing new hemodialysis access procedures to determine differences in access performance by type of access among patient subgroups. The study examined the performance of 1574 prosthetic grafts, 492 simple autogenous fistulas, and 181 venous transposi-

tions, with a mean follow-up time of 340 days. Prosthetic grafts were shown to have a 32% greater risk of failure compared with simple fistulas and a 78% higher incidence of revision procedures. At 2 years, autogenous fistulas demonstrated superior primary patency (42.9% vs. 31.0%) and equivalent secondary patency (64.2% vs. 59.5%) rates compared with prosthetic grafts. Vein transpositions showed inferior primary patency rates but equivalent secondary patency rates at 2 years, validating the increased efforts to use transposition fistulas when regional vein targets are suboptimal. Not all patient subgroups, however, demonstrated similar results in this study. *AVGs had primary patency similar to that of AVFs in women, African Americans, diabetic patients, and patients older than 66 years.* Furthermore, the data showed that diabetic patients had a higher risk of primary access failure and demonstrated no benefit from autogenous access compared with prosthetic grafts. This report suggests that selection of the most appropriate hemodialysis access procedure may need to be subgroup-specific in order to balance patency and function limitations with the need for a reliable and easily accessible site while minimizing the use of central venous catheters. Other factors that need to be considered include time available until the projected onset of hemodialysis, patient comor-

---

Table 18–2

National Kidney Foundation Dialysis Outcomes Quality Initiative Clinical Practice Guidelines for Vascular Access[5]

Clinical Outcome Goals

Goals of access placement
- Each center should establish a database and quality assurance process to track the types of accesses created and complication rates for these accesses.
- The goals for permanent hemodialysis access placement should include:
- Prevalent functional AVF placement rate of greater than 65%.
- Cuffed catheter for permanent dialysis access in less than 10%.

The *primary* access failure rates of hemodialysis accesses in the following locations and configurations should not be more than the following:
- Forearm straight grafts: 15%
- Forearm loop grafts: 10%
- Upper arm grafts: 5%

Access complications and performance
- Fistula thrombosis: fewer than 0.25 episodes/patient-year at risk.
- Fistula infection: less than 1% during the use-life of the access.
- Fistula patency greater than 3.0 years (by life-table analysis).
- Graft thrombosis: fewer than 0.5 thrombotic episodes/patient-year at risk.
- Graft infection: less than 10% during the use-life of the access.
- Graft patency greater than 2 years (by life-table analysis).
- Graft patency after PTA: longer than 4 months.

Efficacy of corrective intervention
- AVF patency after PTA: greater than 50% unassisted patency at 6 months (and <30% residual stenosis);
  AVF patency following surgery: greater than 50% unassisted patency at 1 year.
- AVG after either PTA or surgery: greater than 90% with postprocedure restoration of blood flow and greater than 85% postprocedure ability to complete one dialysis treatment.

Adapted from The National Kidney Foundation Kidney Disease Outcomes Quality Initiative (NKF K/DOQI). *Clinical Practice Guidelines and Clinical Practice Recommendations 2006 Updates.* Available at www.kidney.org (accessed September 10, 2008).

bidities, and estimated life expectancy. Taking all these parameters into consideration, NKF K/DOQI set the expected target for AVF prevalence within a hemodialysis center patient population to 65% by year 2009, with cuffed catheters representing less than 10% of all access sites. The rate of thrombosis for AVGs should approach 0.5 events per patient-year and for AVFs 0.25.[5] The clinical outcome goals for hemodialysis access in the next several years as set by NKF K/DOQI are listed in Table 18-2.

In conclusion, collaboration between vascular specialists and nephrologists aimed at standardizing graft surveillance, optimizing function, and prevention of complications is essential. ESRD patients should be referred to the vascular surgeon as early as possible to provide ample time for the creation and maturation of an autogenous AVF. Dialysis staff must be proficient in proper aseptic cannulation techniques to minimize mechanical and infectious complications. Static conduit pressure and flow assessment via a standardized method should be done on a monthly basis. If a trend of increasing pressures is seen or if there is abnormal blood flow, a DU scan of the graft should be obtained early to detect a subclinical stenosis. When a significant stenosis is detected, correction should proceed promptly. The intervention (surgical revision vs. PTA with or without stenting) should be planned for a day between dialysis sessions. Accurate records of outcome data should be maintained by vascular surgeons and nephrologists in order to assess the accuracy of surveillance methods and the effectiveness of prophylactic interventions in prolonging the life of hemodialysis access conduits in the specific institution.

REFERENCES

1. Quinton W, Dillard D, Scribner BH. Cannulation of blood vessels for prolonged hemodialysis. Trans Am Soc Artif Intern Organs. 1960;6:104-113.
2. Brescia MJ, Cimino JE, Appel K, Hurwich BJ. Chronic hemodialysis using venipuncture and a surgically created arteriovenous fistula. N Engl J Med. 1966;275:1089-1092.
3. United States Renal Data System. USRDS 2007 Annual Data Report. Bethesda, Md: National Institute of Diabetes and Digestive and Kidney Diseases (NIDDK), National Institutes of Health (NIH), U.S. Department of Health and Human Services (DHHS); 2007. Available at www.usrds.org (accessed September 10, 2008).
4. Schwab SJ, Raymond JR, Saeed M, Newman GE, Dennis PA, Bollinger RR. Prevention of hemodialysis fistula thrombosis. Early detection of venous stenoses. Kidney Int. 1989;36:707-711.
5. The National Kidney Foundation Kidney Disease Outcomes Quality Initiative (NKF K/DOQI). Clinical Practice Guidelines and Clinical Practice Recommendations 2006 Updates. Available at www.kidney.org (accessed September 10, 2008).
6. Silva MB Jr, Hobson RW 2nd, Pappas PJ, et al. A strategy for increasing use of autogenous hemodialysis access procedures: impact of preoperative noninvasive evaluation. J Vasc Surg. 1997;27:302-307.
7. Besarab A, Sullivan KL, Ross RP, Moritz MJ. Utility of intra-access pressure monitoring in detecting and correcting venous outlet stenoses prior to thrombosis. Kidney Int. 1995;47:1364-1373.
8. Besarab A, Frinak S, Aslam M. Pressure measurements in the surveillance of vascular accesses. In Gray RJ, Sands JJ (eds). Dialysis Access: A Multidisciplinary Approach. Philadelphia: Lippincott Williams & Wilkins; 2002:137-150.
9. Basseau F, Grenier N, Trillaud H, et al. Volume flow measurement in hemodialysis shunts using time-domain correlation. J Ultrasound Med. 1999;18:177-183.
10. Bay WH, Henry ML, Lazarus JM, Lew NL, Ling J, Lowrie EG. Predicting hemodialysis access failure with color flow Doppler ultrasound. Am J Nephrol. 1998;18:296-304.
11. Laissy JP, Menegazzo D, Debray MP, et al. Failing arteriovenous hemodialysis fistulas: assessment with magnetic resonance angiography. Invest Radiol. 1999;34:218-224.
12. Oudenhoven LF, Pattynama PM, de Roos A, Seeverens HJ, Rebergen SA, Chang PC. Magnetic resonance, a new method for measuring blood flow in hemodialysis fistulae. Kidney Int. 1994;45:884-889.
13. Depner TA, Rizwan S, Cheer AY, Wagner JM, Eder LA. High venous urea concentrations in the opposite arm. A consequence of hemodialysis-induced compartment dysequilibrium. ASAIO Trans. 1991;37:M141-M143.
14. Sands J, Young S, Miranda C. The effect of Doppler flow screening studies and elective revisions on dialysis access failure. ASAIO J. 1992;38:M524-M527.
15. Tessitore N, Bedogna V, Poli A, et al. Adding access blood flow surveillance to clinical monitoring reduces thrombosis rates and costs, and improves fistula patency in the short term: a controlled cohort study. Nephrol Dial Transplant. 2008;23:3578-3584. Epub 2008;May 29.
16. Strauch BS, O'Connell RS, Geoly KL, Grundlehner M, Yakub YN, Tietjen DP. Forecasting thrombosis of vascular access with Doppler color flow imaging. Am J Kidney Dis. 1992;19:554-557.
17. Lumsden AB, MacDonald MJ, Kikeri D, Cotsonis GA, Harker LA, Martin LG. Cost efficacy of duplex surveillance and prophylactic angioplasty of arteriovenous ePTFE grafts. Ann Vasc Surg. 1998;12:138-142.
18. Tessitore N, Lipari G, Poli A, et al, Can blood flow surveillance and pre-emptive repair of subclinical stenosis prolong the useful life of arteriovenous fistulae? A randomized controlled study. Nephrol Dial Transplant. 2004;19:2325-2333.
19. Malik J, Slavikova M, Malikova H, Maskova J. Many clinically silent access stenoses can be identified by ultrasonography. J Nephrol. 2002;15:661-665.
20. Schwab SJ, Quarles LD, Middleton JP, Cohan RH, Saeed M, Dennis VW. Hemodialysis-associated subclavian vein stenosis. Kidney Int. 1988;33:1156-1159.
21. Miller GA, Schur I, Song M, et al. Balloon angioplasty maturation of arteriovenous fistulae: a new technique to facilitate placement and utilization of primary arteriovenous fistulae. Vascular. 2005;13(suppl 1):S80-S81.
22. Thermann F, Wollert U, Dralle H, Brauckhoff M. Dialysis shunt-associated steal syndrome with autogenous hemodialyis accesses: proposal for a new classification based on clinical results. World J Surg. 2008;32:2309-2315.
23. Tessitore N, Mansueto G, Bedogna V, et al. A prospective controlled trial on effect of percutaneous transluminal angioplasty on functioning arteriovenous fistulae survival. J Am Soc Nephrol. 2003;14:1623-1627.
24. Tessitore N, Mansueto G, Lipari G, et al. Endovascular versus surgical preemptive repair of forearm arteriovenous fistula juxta-anastomotic stenosis: analysis of data collected prospectively from 1999 to 2004. Clin J Am Soc Nephrol. 2006;1:448-454. Epub 2006;March 1.
25. Turmel-Rodrigues L. Application of percutaneous mechanical thrombectomy in autogenous fistulae. Tech Vasc Interv Radiol. 2003;6:42-48.
26. Rodkin RS, Bookstein JJ, Heeney DJ, Davis GB. Streptokinase and transluminal angioplasty in the treatment of acutely thrombosed hemodialysis access fistulas. Radiology. 1983;149:425-428.
27. Perera GB, Mueller MP, Kubaska SM, Wilson SE, Lawrence PF, Fujitani RM. Superiority of autogenous arteriovenous hemodialysis access: maintenance of function with fewer secondary interventions. Ann Vasc Surg. 2004;18:66-73. Epub 2004;January 20.
28. Schuman E, Standage BA, Ragsdale JW, Gross GF. Reinforced versus nonreinforced PTFE grafts for hemodialysis access. Am J Surg. 1997;173:407-410.
29. Cinat ME, Hopkins J, Wilson SE. A prospective evaluation of PTFE graft patency and surveillance techniques in hemodialysis access. Ann Vasc Surg. 1999;13:191-198.
30. Kennedy MT, Quinton H, Bubolz TA, Wennberg JE, Wilson SE. An analysis of the patency of vascular access grafts for hemodialysis using the Medicare Part B claims database. Semin Vasc Surg. 1996;9:262-265.
31. Huber TS, Carter JW, Carter RL, Seeger JM. Patency of autogenous and polytetrafluoroethylene upper extremity arteriovenous hemodialysis accesses: a systematic review. J Vasc Surg. 2003;38:1005-1011.
32. Gibson KD, Gillen DL, Caps MT, Kohler TR, Sherrard DJ, Stehman-Breen CO. Vascular access survival and incidence of revisions: a comparison of prosthetic grafts, simple autogenous and venous transposition fistulas from the United States Renal Data System Dialysis Morbidity and Mortality Study. J Vasc Surg. 2001;34:694-700.

CHAPTER 19

Endovascular Management of Dialysis Graft Stenosis

Russell A. Williams and Kimberly S. Stone

Currently, there are three options for provision of chronic vascular access in patients requiring hemodialysis, native or autogenous arteriovenous (AV) fistulas, synthetic grafts, and tunneled double-lumen catheters. Native fistulas are the preferred access, given that they have the best long-term patency rates, require the fewest interventions, and have the lowest associated morbidity and mortality. Long-term studies have demonstrated that with aggressive re-intervention, mature fistulas can have cumulative patency rates at 5 and 10 years of 53% and 45%, respectively.[1,2] However, they are more likely to have primary failure (i.e., to never provide reliable hemodialysis access) and are not available to be cannulated for a minimum of 1 month, and at times upward of 6 months.

Therefore, synthetic grafts made of polytetrafluoroethylene (PTFE) are commonly constructed because they can be used for hemodialysis within days of construction. Grafts are more likely than native fistulas to develop certain complications including outflow stenosis, which leads to thrombosis, infection, and seromas, particularly at the time of placement. The cumulative patency for PTFE grafts at 1, 2, and 4 years is 67%, 50%, and 43%, respectively.[3]

Double-lumen tunneled catheters are typically used temporarily as an intermediate site for dialysis while a fistula or graft is maturing or if dialysis is needed for lesser time up to 1 year. This is due to the high risk of infection and malfunction and consequently high associated morbidity and mortality with these catheters. These large-diameter catheters have been shown to also have the delayed consequence of central venous stenosis and occlusion.

The inciting events for pathogenesis of these stenotic lesions caused by percutaneous central venous catheters include initial trauma at the time the device is placed as well as continued alteration in flow dynamics and endoluminal contact. Later, the increased flow and turbulence from an AV fistula or graft, or chronic dialysis, contributes to activation of factors in the vessel wall and eventually the formation of central venous stenosis.[4] The duration for use of percutaneously placed tunneled catheters should be kept to a minimum to decrease the incidence of central stenosis, which may ultimately preclude construction of access sites in that arm because of severe venous outflow obstruction, in effect losing a limb for construction of access sites in patients who require chronic hemodialysis.

The use of each of the means for dialysis varies between clinical sites, but the 2006 National Kidney Foundation

Kidney Disease Outcomes Quality Initiative (NKF K/DOQI) guidelines[5] recommend that autogenous AV fistulas be used for 65% of patients undergoing dialysis. However, in the United States, only 28% of patients are dialyzed via fistula, whereas 49% of patients are dialyzed via synthetic grafts and 23% via catheter.[6]

Access Patency Rates, Complications, and Treatments

The seemingly inevitable failure and secondary complications with hemodialysis access continue to be a challenge with few successful solutions. Despite the relatively long cumulative patency of fistulas mentioned previously, the primary patency of grafts is expected to be only 10% to 40% at 1 year.[7] Aggressive re-intervention with numerous procedures is necessary to maintain vascular access once the patency has been compromised. The most common complication of vascular access is venous thrombosis, which leads to loss of the access if the thrombosis is unable to be corrected. AV fistulas and grafts are predisposed to thrombose when there is anatomic stenosis in the inflow (arterial) or outflow (venous) anastomotic sites or bridge material itself in the case of a synthetic graft. *Stenosis* is typically defined as a narrowing of equal to or greater than 50% of the adjacent vessel. The majority of efforts are aimed at identifying and treating venous stenosis because these account for the majority of complications.

Late stenosis at the venous outflow of a graft is caused by neointimal hyperplasia, which is initiated by endothelial cell injury, leading to the up-regulation of adhesion molecules on the endothelial cell surface and adherence of leukocytes. The activated endothelium releases various factors that are chemotactic and mitogenic to vascular smooth muscle cells, resulting in migration and proliferation. In addition, the neointimal hyperplasia is triggered by shear stress from turbulent blood flow and excessive mechanical stretch due to unequal elasticity on either side of an anastomosis. It has been proposed that the previously mentioned pathogenesis is responsible for stenosis at the AV anastomotic site, whereas stenosis in autogenous AV fistulas is due to a different mechanism. Beathard[8] suggested that venous lesions are likely due to phlebosclerosis and perivenous fibrosis, resulting in the constriction of the outflow tract and, therefore, may be more amenable to intervention such as stenting.[8] There are a number of other potential complications of fistulas and grafts that are not discussed here but include infection, ischemia distal to the fistula, aneurysm formation, injury or ischemia of the median nerve, venous hypertension, and high-output heart failure.

Thrombotic complications with vascular access sites are a major cause of morbidity and are responsible for 16% to 23% of all hospitalizations of dialysis patients. Also, maintaining patency of vascular access is costly and accounts for about 15% of total annual spending on hemodialysis.[9] Therefore, much research has gone into developing effective ways to prevent and treat thrombosis of AV fistulas and grafts. There are currently two basic options available for treating stenosis: percutaneous transluminal angioplasty (PTA) with or without insertion of endovascular stents (PTA plus stent) and surgical revision.

PTA

PTA is currently used to treat stenosis in both AV fistulas and grafts and can be used for lesions on the arterial and venous sides as well as at the anastomosis. The basic technique involves inserting a large-diameter, high-pressure balloon catheter into the access graft and venous outflow tract and inflating the balloon to disrupt the lesion (Figs. 19-1 and 19-2). The balloon should be 20% to 30% larger in diameter than the vein and should be inflated to a pressure of at least 10 atmospheres in order to dilate the lesion. It is common to perform multiple dilations and inflate the balloons to pressures of 15 to 20 atm in order to disrupt lesions. There are also ultrahigh-pressure balloons available that inflate to pressures as high as 30 to 40 atm, and use of these devices has decreased the incidence of PTA-resistant lesions.[10] Another option for the treatment of resistant lesions is to use a cutting balloon, which has been shown to be an effective alternative; however, it has not been shown to result in improved patency when compared with standard PTA.

The advantages of PTA are that it preserves other potential access sites; all venous sites are accessible including central lesions; it is minimally invasive; the graft can continue to be used, immediately if necessary; and the procedure can be performed on an outpatient basis. The primary shortcoming of PTA is that it is not a permanent solution and there is a high rate of recurrent stenosis, often requir-

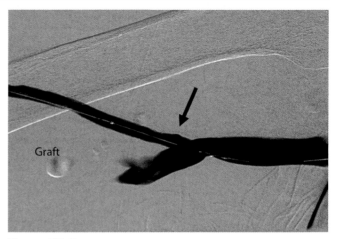

Figure 19-2.
Venous outflow stenosis shown in diagram 4 treated with percutaneous transluminal angioplasty (PTA).

ing early re-interventions. If repeat angioplasty is required more frequently than twice in 3 months, the NKF-K/DOQI guidelines[5] recommend surgical intervention or the placement of a stent. Recurrent stenosis may be due to elastic recoil even after successful balloon dilatation. The most common complication of AV fistula and graft PTA is venous rupture, with an incidence of at least 1% to 2%; however, some reports cite a significantly higher rate of rupture of 10% to 20%.[11–13] The clinical significance of these tears also varies, and the majority are small tears of no clinical significance besides a small ecchymosis over the site. Larger ruptures result in the significant extravasation of contrast and blood and can form large unstable hematomas that disrupt flow and even cause dehiscence of the vein and complete loss of the access site. Therefore, all ruptures must be evaluated and treated appropriately to ensure access integrity. Many tears can be successfully treated by inflating the balloon and leaving it in place for a few minutes; however, if this is not successful, the deployment of an endovascular stent can help salvage the access and stabilize the hematoma.

If the AV fistula is complicated by a stenotic lesion that cannot be dilated, it can be surgically revised with a patch angioplasty of the stenosed segment or jump graft, bypassing the stenosis, moving the venous outflow of the graft further up the arm. Surgical thrombectomy with a Fogarty embolectomy catheter can be accomplished through a small incision into the midregion of the graft. This incision is then used to obtain an angiogram and treat any identified underlying stricture with PTA and possibly stenting. Alternatively, the clot may be macerated and aspirated with a mechanical device placed into the clot in the graft lumen, using an endovascular sheath for access.

Lesions that are not suitable for or do not resolve with PTA can be revised surgically. However, the same problem of recurrence still holds, with the additional problem that surgical revision results in loss of potential access sites as the fistula or graft is moved farther up the arm. Other disadvantages include the possible need for hospitalization and, other than strictly local anesthesia to perform the procedure, more postoperative pain than after PTA. Occasionally, a tunneled catheter is temporarily needed after surgery.

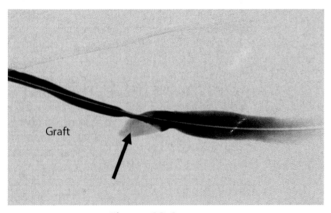

Figure 19-1.
Venous outflow stenosis.

Endoluminal Stents in Hemodialysis Access

Since the introduction of endoluminal stents for the treatment of vascular access complications in 1988, there has been much debate over their utility.[14] The U.S. Food and Drug Administration (FDA) has not specifically approved the use of stents in dialysis applications; however, numerous available stents are used for vascular applications and have been studied in both grafts and AV fistulas. Originally, it was hoped that stents could both treat and prevent access stenosis, and although they are effective at treating even difficult stenoses, it is clear that they do not prevent restenosis. Theoretically, stents might prevent restenosis based on the process of re-endothelialization that has been studied in animal and human models. After a graft has been surgically implanted, a fibrin layer forms on the inner surface that is in contact with bloodstream, then fibrous encapsulation occurs, followed by organization of the fibrin lining. It has been shown that in humans, PTFE fails to completely re-endothelialize, a process that is closely related to the porosity of the material. It has been theorized that a very low porosity stent material would lead to failure of complete endothelialization and consequently less intimal hyperplasia; however, it is now clear that stents do not prevent restenosis.[14]

Although stents are not a permanent solution for vascular access thrombosis or stenosis, when appropriately used, they can help extend the life of an access, salvage a failed access, and sometimes help avoid surgery in a high-risk patient. Because stents are expensive, particularly those that are covered, averaging $1,000 to $2000 per device, PTA is often considered a primary intervention for stenosis or thrombosis of hemodialysis access sites, with surgical intervention as a second alternative.

The three generally accepted indications for using a stent in hemodialysis vascular access sites are (1) a peripheral lesion that has failed PTA when surgery is contraindicated or there are limited remaining access sites; (2) an elastic central lesion that has failed balloon angioplasty or recurred twice within 3 months after PTA; and (3) to control an unstable hematoma after venous rupture, if it cannot be managed by inflating a balloon across the lesion under low pressure for 3 to 5 minutes. There is continued debate about the use of stents for other indications such as in rapidly recurrent and elastic lesions; however, there has not been enough conclusive evidence to date to justify their routine use in these applications. A rapidly recurrent lesion is one that recurs more than twice in less than 3 months after what seemed to be a successful dilatation with PTA. Some of these lesions may be due to residual stenosis that was not adequately treated with the PTA, and therefore, the use of ultrahigh-pressure balloons should help decrease the incidence of these lesions and provide a better solution than stents. Another reason that stenoses recur soon after a seemingly successful intervention is elastic recoil. In the case of elastic recoil, surgical intervention should be considered; however, if the lesion is not easily accessible, as in the case of central lesions, then stents are preferred to PTA alone.

A variety of different stents are available, each with unique benefits and drawbacks. In order to be used for hemodialysis access, Beathard[12] proposed that the ideal material would include the following properties: high radiopacity, high hoop strength to resist recoil, longitudinal flexibility to avoid kinking, radial elasticity to resist external compression, ability to be cannulated, minimal inducer of intimal hyperplasia (perhaps via low porosity, given the foregoing proposed theory), and also resistance to thrombosis. Furthermore, the delivery system of this ideal stent should be simple to use with a high expansion ratio and low profile so that it can be passed through a small-diameter sheath. It should also undergo minimal shortening upon deployment, be retrievable in the case of faulty deployment, be potentially removable if surgery is needed at that vascular site, and affordable. No currently available stent, whether balloon expandable, self-expanding, covered, and drug-eluting, comes close to meeting these expectations.

Balloon expandable stents including the Palmaz (Cordis) and Strecker (Boston Scientific) are less suitable for hemodialysis access because they are rigid and will collapse if an external force is applied. Further, they may migrate if placed in a central vein because these large veins change diameter with respiration. The Wallstent (Boston Scientific) is made of woven stainless steel alloy and is highly flexible along the longitudinal axis, thereby resisting kinks when used in curved vessels. It is a commonly used stents for hemodialysis applications. The Gianturco Z-stent (Cook, Inc.) has a zig-zag configuration that results in the lowest metallic surface area of all the stainless steel stents and might offer increased patency when used at the venous anastomosis. A few available models are made of titanium and nickel alloy called nitinol, including Symphony Stent (Boston Scientific), SMART stent (Cordis), Zilver stent (Cook), Bard Luminex Stent, and Memotherm (both Bard Peripheral Technologies). Nitinol has extremely high elasticity and thermal shape memory so that upon deployment, it expands to its predetermined configuration without shortening. Each nitinol stent has its own unique properties, for example, the SMART stent is very flexible and can be used in regions with sharp angles whereas other nitinol stents would break if used in the same situation. Covered stents are also available that are a combination of a stent sheath and PTFE or Dacron graft material; these include the Cragg and Wallgraft (both by Boston Scientific), Viabahn (WL Gore), and Fluency (CR Bard, Inc.). Early research indicates that covered stents (also known as stent grafts) have comparable and possibly superior patency rates when compared with standard PTA. Lastly, drug-eluting stents have not been studied for dialysis vascular access, but have been shown to have short-term effectiveness in animal studies. At this point in stent development, nitinol stents are most commonly used.

The primary patency rate of vascular access sites after stent placement is unfortunately low, but multiple re-interventions extend the cumulative patency rate. A number of observational studies have evaluated the primary and secondary patency rates after stent placement in AV fistulas and grafts. Overall, the primary patency is about 20% at 1 year, which is in comparison to the primary patency after PTA alone of 31% to 45% at 1 year. The secondary patency rate for grafts and AV fistulas treated with stents is approximately 70% at 1 year, in comparison with the 60% to 70% patency at 1 year for PTFE grafts (Table 19-1).

Table 19–1
Primary and Secondary Patency Rates of Grafts and Fistulas

Author, Year	Type of Access	Primary Patency	Secondary Patency
Vesely et al, 2008[24]	Grafts	47% at 1 yr	74% at 1 yr
Sapoval et al, 1996[14]	Grafts and AV fistulas combined	28.5% at 6 mo	67.8% at 6 mo
Pan et al, 2005[13]	AV fistulas	31% at 1 yr	82% at 1 yr
Turmel-Rodrigues et al, 1997[7]	Grafts	10% at 1 yr	88% at 1 yr
	AV fistulas	20% at 1 yr	79% at 1 yr

AV, arteriovenous.

PTA and Stent Versus PTA Alone

Studies directly comparing treatment with stents with either PTA alone or surgical intervention often reach different conclusions, still leaving this subject up to considerable debate. A prospective trial compared mechanical thrombectomy with angioplasty alone to thrombectomy followed by stent placement and found that stenting resulted in significantly longer primary and secondary patency.[15] This study compared 14 patients with thrombosed arteriovenous grafts who received stents at the venous anastomosis with 34 patients matched for age, sex, and date (controls) who underwent angioplasty alone. The indications for stenting included severe elastic recoil or significant residual stenosis. A variety of devices were used including the SMART (nitinol), Wallstent (metallic), Protégé (metallic), and Fluency (covered) stents. During the stent procedure, 3000 to 4000 Units of heparin was administered, and no patients received antiplatelet agents after the intervention. The stent group had a somewhat disappointing primary patency of 85 days as compared with 27 days for the angioplasty alone ($P = .02$). The secondary patency was also longer with a survival of 1215 days for the stent group and only 46 days for the angioplasty group ($P = .049$). This small study using a variety of metal, nitinol, and covered stents makes it unclear which type provided the most benefit over angioplasty alone.[15]

Another prospective, nonrandomized trial compared the use of SMART stents versus PTA alone in PTFE grafts and found that stents significantly improved the primary patency rate of the grafts.[16] This study had 60 patients, 35 in the PTA alone group and 25 in the stent group. Most of the treated stenoses (58/60) were at the graft-to-vein anastomosis, and the indications for stent placement were acute PTA failure, rapid restenosis, and vessel perforation. The mean primary patency for the PTA group was 5.6 months and for the stent group was 8.2 months ($P = .050$), with primary patency rates of 22% at 12 months for the PTA group and 41% for the stent group. The secondary patency rates were 41% and 81%; however, this was not statistically significant. Some have indicated that the location of a graft influences the patency rate, but this study separately evaluated lower and upper arm grafts and found that the patency was not significantly influenced by the graft location. This study was not randomized, but it demonstrates results that

are comparable with those of Wallstents and surgical graft revision. The authors pointed out the importance of balancing the added cost of placing a stent with the potential savings of improving the primary patency, concluding that the short-term benefit would not offset the additional cost of routinely placing stents. More detailed financial analysis is warranted to further evaluate this issue.[16]

In 1993, Beathard[8] published a randomized trial of 58 patients with greater than 50% stenosis of the graft-vein anastomosis who received either PTA alone ($N = 30$) or PTA followed by placement of the Gianturco self-expanding stent ($N = 28$). The treatment group failed to show any significant difference at any time period between 30 to 360 days in the duration of efficacy, which was defined as the period of time from intervention to an end-point event. End-point events included graft thrombosis, need for surgical intervention, or the need for repeat PTA. The primary patency rate was 17% at 12 months for the stent group and 28% for the PTA only group, which were not significantly different. Importantly, the study included only stenotic lesions that could be dilated to 100% normal vessel size, thereby excluding any resistant lesions, which has been one of the indications for stent placement in other studies that have shown benefit to stents. In the study design, similar lesions were randomized to receive the different interventions, which is in contrast to most other studies that use particularly challenging lesions or PTA failure as an indication for stenting. The authors pointed out that the lesions included in this study were only graft-vein anastamoses; venous lesions were excluded even though they are very common and often concurrent. They also explained that there might be different pathophysiologic mechanisms behind the various types of lesions, and if venous lesions are due to sclerosis leading to constriction, then stents might be particularly useful for treating venous lesions. In conclusion, this study failed to show any short- or long-term benefit with the use of stents over PTA in stenotic graft-vein anastomoses.

Hoffer and coworkers[17] published a similar prospective, randomized trial comparing PTA alone with PTA and the Wallstent self-expandable stents in recurrent graft stenoses. In this study, the lesions were located both at the graft-vein junction and in the draining veins. The only notable difference in their methods was that after deployment of the self-expandable stent, the stent was balloon dilated if there was any significant residual stenosis. They also found similar primary and secondary patencies (128 and 431 days, respectively) for both groups, despite a 90%t increase in cost. The primary and secondary patency rates at 360 days for the PTA group were 7% and 47%, respectively. In comparison, the primary and secondary patency rates for the stent group at 360 days were 0% and 60% (no differences in these comparisons). Therefore, they also concluded that stents did not provide an advantage for recurrent graft stenosis. One problem with this study is that the two comparison groups had significant differences at the start that could have confounded the data. The stent group had more previous interventions, perhaps indicating deterioration of the grafts at the onset of the study. However, there were also more nontarget lesions and a greater number of previous accesses in the PTA group (although similar duration of dialysis), which could have indicated worse underlying vascular disease in this group. Regardless of these differences, the authors concluded that stents should not be used as a primary treatment of peripheral venous stenosis in grafts.[17]

Lombardi and colleagues[18] published a case-control study that compared angioplasty with stent placement and surgical intervention with patch angioplasty in patients with thrombosed and stenotic PTFE grafts. Both groups consisted of patients with either brachial or axillary grafts who had multiple graft revisions. The indication for stent placement was residual stenosis of greater than 30% diameter after balloon angioplasty. They found that primary patency for stent placement compared with patch angioplasty was not statistically different at any time up to 1 year after the intervention. The secondary patency rates were slightly better for the patch angioplasty group at all time points; however, the differences were not statistically significant. There was also no difference in complication rates, so it was concluded that the stents could be a reasonable alternative when surgery is particularly high-risk or surgical access is difficult, such as in the case of high-axillary grafts.[18]

Stents for Central Venous Stenosis or Occlusion

One consequence of percutaneous centrally placed tunneled catheters is the development of central stenosis. This is particularly troublesome for patients with AV fistulas and grafts because central stenosis can cause loss of the existing vascular access as well as compromise of the entire ipsilateral side for placement of future access. Central vein stenosis usually manifests as edema of the extremity and pain, AV access failure, and inadequate hemodialysis. The prevalence of this complication ranges from about 16% to 29% of dialysis patients with access failure depending on the study; however, it is clearly a common cause of vascular access malfunction. Central stenoses have historically been successfully treated with PTA, similar to the way peripheral stenoses are treated (Figs. 19-3 and 19-4). Despite good initial success, it has been documented that there is a much higher rate of recurrence of central lesions than peripheral lesions after PTA.[19] The availability of intravascular ultrasound has shown that a significant number of these central lesions have dramatic elastic recoil after angioplasty despite

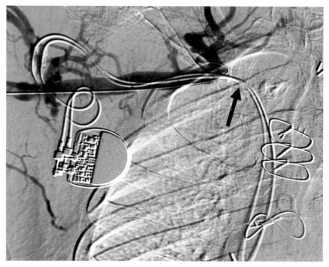

Figure 19-3.
Central vein stenosis *(arrow)* caused by pacemaker wires. The patient had marked swelling of the right arm, and high pressures were noted during dialysis using his right brachioaxillary shunt.

early normal morphologic appearance. Therefore, Kovalik and associates[19] proposed that stents might be superior to angioplasty in the treatment of central stenosis.

In their study, standard angiographic imaging was used to determine the percent of diameter stenosis before and after PTA, as well as intravascular ultrasound to evaluate elasticity. In the first phase of the study, patients received PTA alone (7% failed), although 23% of these had elastic lesions that did not improve at all after angioplasty.[19] The other 70% had greater than 50% improvement in the lumen diameter and were deemed successful. During the second phase, Wallstents were placed in the central lesions of 5 patients with elastic lesions that demonstrated greater than 50% elastic recoil after angioplasty, and in 5 patients who had recurrence of the same central lesion within 6 months of PTA. In the angioplasty alone group, 100% of the elastic

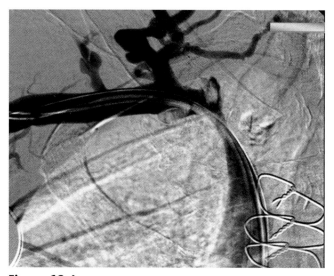

Figure 19-4.
Following percutaneous transluminal angioplasty of the central stenosis shown in Figure 19-3.

lesions occluded after an average of 2.9 months, and 81% of the successful PTAs restenosed at an average of 7.6 months. In the patients who received stents for recurrent lesions, there was a significantly worse patency rate, with restenosis occurring at an average of 4.2 months compared with 7.6 months for the group that had PTA alone. The patients who had stents placed for elastic lesions had significantly better patency, with recurrence at an average of 8.9 months after the stent was placed. Therefore, it was concluded that central stenoses include two distinct types of lesions—nonelastic caused by intimal hyperplasia or fibrosis similar to peripheral lesions, which should be treated with standard PTA, and elastic lesions that recur rapidly if treated with PTA alone but respond relatively well to stent placement.

Stents for Venous Rupture

As described earlier, one of the most common complications during angioplasty is vessel injury resulting in extravasation of contrast and blood. Most cases of venous rupture are minor and require little or no intervention; however, when the vessel injury is substantial, the rupture can lead to loss of the access via intravascular thrombosis as well as stenosis from external compression by the large hematoma that results from the expelled material. There are three treatment options for these venous ruptures including stent placement, protamine sulfate administration to reverse the effects of heparin (used during the PTA thrombolysis procedure), and intentional graft thrombosis. If the patient is taking protamine insulin then administering protamine sulfate, caution is advised because there are reports of increased incidence of anaphylactic reactions. If the graft is intentionally thrombosed, a temporary catheter is placed so that the injured vein can have time to heal and then PTA is repeated to attempt to salvage the thrombosed access. This process is time-consuming and expensive and has added risk to the patient because of the multiple interventions necessary. Further, there are the complications associated with the tunneled central venous catheter for temporary access.

Several mechanisms have been proposed to successfully treat venous rupture with stenting. First, if there is an intimal flap in the lumen of the access, it will be compressed against the lumen wall upon deployment of the stent, thereby closing off the leak.[20] Deployment of a stent creates less forward resistance to blood flow in the vessel and therefore promotes blood flow along the vascular access as opposed to out into the surrounding tissues. This might explain why bare stents that are a lattice of material are still effective at stopping bleeding even though they do not completely occlude the leak.[21] Also, metallic stents are somewhat thrombogenic and promote thrombosis of the rupture. Lastly, stents help to decrease the external pressure applied by the surrounding hematoma and therefore lower the intraluminal pressure and decrease the amount of leak.

Raynaud and coworkers[20] published one of the largest studies of venous rupture treated with endoluminal stents in 1998. During a 5-year period, the authors performed 2414 PTAs and there were 37 severe ruptures treated with Wallstent placement. All but 1 of the ruptures were located on the vein or the venous anastomosis to the graft; the other 1 was of the graft itself. Of the 37 ruptures, 4 were isolated pseudoaneurysms without bleeding, and these were also treated with stents to avoid further enlargement of the pseudoaneurysm. Stents with balloon inflation were effective at stopping the bleeding in all the remaining 33 cases, although 1 required the implantation of a covered stent within the metal stent. The primary and secondary patency rates for the stented vascular accesses were 48% and 86$ at 1 year, which is comparable with the expected patency after PTA alone without complications. In their study, the stents controlled bleeding after a rupture, treated residual stenosis caused by the surrounding hematoma, and prevented or treated the pseudoaneurysms. Therefore, the authors concluded that stents should always be available when performing PTA because, if severe rupture occurs, they are usually successful at saving the access.

Another smaller study reports the use of Wallstents for venous rupture during PTA procedures.[21] These authors had 23 cases of venous rupture and placed 27 stents, with 4 patients receiving more than one stent. They had 100% technical success, 96% successfully underwent dialysis after the procedure, and 78% had no sequelae at all of the hemorrhage. The 5 complications included 4 moderate-sized hematomas and 1 delayed pseudoaneurysm. The primary and secondary patency rates of the stents at 1 year were 11% and 56%. These patency rates are similar to those of stents placed for other reasons, and the authors concluded that stents are effective and safe for treating venous rupture and were able to salvage grafts that otherwise would have thrombosed.

Both of these studies, as well as several smaller ones that specifically studied stents in venous rupture,[22,23] indicate that the deployment of metallic stents is the best option for the treatment of severe ruptures that do not respond to prolonged balloon dilatation alone. Venous rupture is a sound indication for stent placement and clinical reports confirm the safety and utility of stents in this application.[7,13,14,24]

Additional Considerations

Access cannulation through a stent could possibly result in damage to the stent material by the needle. An animal study demonstrated that puncturing either metallic or nitinol stents was technically feasible, did not result in deformation of the stents, and did not have any major short-term complications.[25] However, it did demonstrate that the nitinol stents had more pronounced intimal thickness when punctured. Turmel-Rodrigues and colleagues[7] reported that they had four patients with metallic self-expandable Craggstents that were routinely punctured for hemodialysis without any consequences. There have also been reports of cannulating through covered stents without problem; however, this topic needs more careful studies in order to determine safety.

Of all the reviewed studies, only one reported use of an antiplatelet agent after stent placement for vascular stenosis.[26] In this study, patients who had a stent placed received 300 mg of clopidogrel immediately after stent placement and 75 mg daily for at least 4 weeks after the procedure. They found a relatively high primary patency rate at 6 months of 63%; however, at 1 year, it was similar to other studies at 36%. Their overall graft patency of 86% at 1 year was again similar to other studies.

Antiplatelet agents have been studied in the prevention of thrombosis of vascular accesses, and it has been found that neither dipyridamole nor aspirin is effective in patients who have had a previous thrombus, but these agents reduce the rate of thrombus formation in patients with a new graft. It is not clear what role antiplatelet agents have in the setting of endoluminal stents used for hemodialysis access, and most centers do not routinely use antiplatelet agents or systemic anticoagulation. Whereas clopidogrel reduced early AV fistula thrombosis, it failed to improve AV fistula dialysis function.[27]

Conclusion

Endovascular techniques are a valuable method for prolonging the life of an AV fistula that has developed segmental stenosis and also for some patients whose autogenous vein has failed to mature. For correction of prosthetic graft-to-vein outflow stenosis, stents placed by endovascular methods provide a useful extension in patency but are not as durable as surgical repair (eg, patch angioplasty).

REFERENCES

1. Rodriguez JA, Armadans L, Ferrer E, et al. The function of permanent vascular access. *Nephrol Dialysis Transplant*. 2000;15:402-408.
2. Bonalumi U, Civalleri D, Rovida S, Adami GF, Gianetta E, Griffanti-Bartoli F. Nine years' experience with end-to-end arteriovenous fistula at the "anatomical snuffbox" for maintenance haemodialysis. *Br J Surg*. 1982;69:486-488.
3. Munda R, First MR, Alexander JW, Linnemann CC Jr, Fidler JP, Kittur D. Polytetrafluoroethylene graft survival in hemodialysis. *JAMA*. 1983; 249:219-222.
4. Agarwal AK, Patel BM Haddad NJ. Central vein stenosis: a nephrologist's perspective. *Semin Dial*. 2007;20:53-62.
5. National Kidney Foundation/Kidney Disease Outcomes Quality Initiative. Clinical Practice Guidelines for vascular access: update 2006. *Am J Kidney Dis*. 2006;48(suppl):S248-S273.
6. Reddan D, Klassen P, Frankenfield DL, et al. National profile of practice patterns for hemodialysis vascular access in the United States. *J Am Soc Nephrol*. 2002;13:2117-2124.
7. Turmel-Rodrigues LA, Blanchard D, Pengloan J, et al. Wallstents and Craggstents in hemodialysis grafts and fistulas: results for selected indications. *J Vasc Interv Radiol*. 1997;8:975-982.
8. Beathard GA. Gianturco self-expanding stent in the treatment of stenosis in dialysis access grafts. *Kidney Int*. 1993;43:872-877.
9. Feldman HI, Held PJ, Hutchinson JT, Stoiber E, Hartigan MF, Berlin JA. Hemodialysis vascular access morbidity in the United States. *Kidney Int*. 1993;43:1091-1096.
10. Trerotola SO, Stavropoulos SW, Shlansky-Goldberg R, Tuite CM, Kobrin S, Rudnick MR. Hemodialysis-related venous stenosis: treatment with ultrahigh-pressure angioplasty balloons. *Radiology*. 2004;231:259-262.
11. Pappas JN, Vesely TM. Vascular rupture during angioplasty of hemodialysis graft-related stenoses. *J Vasc Access*. 2002;3:120-126.
12. Beathard, GA. Use of stents for venous stenosis associated with dialysis vascular access. In: Basow DS (ed). *UpToDate*. Waltham, MA: UpToDate, 2009.
13. Pan HB, Liang HL, Lin YH, et al. Metallic stent placement for treating peripheral outflow lesions in native arteriovenous fistula hemodialysis patients after insufficient balloon dilation. *AJR Am J Roentgenol*. 2005; 184:403-409.
14. Sapoval MR, Turmel-Rodrigues LA, Raynaud AC, Bourquelot P, Rodrigue H, Gaux JC. Cragg covered stents in hemodialysis access: initial and midterm results. *J Vasc Interv Radiol*. 1996;7:335-342.
15. Maya ID, Allon M. Outcomes of thrombosed arteriovenous grafts: comparison of stents vs angioplasty. *Kidney Int*. 2006;69:934-937.
16. Vogel PM, Parise C. Comparison of SMART stent placement for arteriovenous graft salvage versus successful graft PTA. *J Vasc Interv Radiol*. 2005;16:1619-1626.
17. Hoffer EK, Sultan S, Herskowitz MM, Daniels ID, Sclafani SJ. Prospective randomized trial of metallic intervascular stent in hemodialsis graft maintenance. *J Vasc Interv Radiol*. 1997;8:965-973.
18. Lombardi JV, Dougherty MJ, Veitia N, Somal J, Calligaro KD. A comparison of patch angioplasty and stenting for axillary venous stenosis of thrombosed hemodialysis grafts. *Vasc Endovascular Surg*. 2002;36:223-229.
19. Kovalik EC, Newman GE, Suhocki P, Knelson M, Schwab SJ. Correction of central venous stenoses: use of angioplasty and vascular Wallstents. *Kidney Int*. 1994;45:1177-1181.
20. Raynaud AC, Angel CY, Sapoval MR, Beyssen B, Pagny JY, Auguste M. Treatment of hemodialysis access rupture during PTA with Wallstent implantation. *J Vasc Interv Radiol*. 1998;9:437-442.
21. Funaki B, Szymski GX, Leef JA, Rosenblum JD, Burke R, Hackworth CA. Wallstent deployment to salvage dialysis graft thrombolysis complicated by venous rupture: early and intermediate results. *AJR Am J Roentgenol*. 1997;169:1435-1437.
22. Rundback JH, Leonardo RF, Poplausky MR, Rozenblit G. Venous rupture complicating hemodialysis access angioplasty: percutaneous treatment and outcomes in seven patients. *AJR Am J Roentgenol*. 1981; 171:1081-1084.
23. Welber A, Schur I, Sofocleous CT, Cooper SG, Patel RI, Peck SH. Endovascular stent placement for angioplasty-induced venous rupture related to the treatment of hemodialysis grafts. *J Vasc Interv Radiol*. 1999;10:547-551.
24. Vesely TM, Amin MZ, Pilgram T. Use of stents and stent grafts to salvage angioplasty failures in patients with hemodialysis grafts. *Semin Dial*. 2008;21:100-104.
25. Schürmann K, Vorwerk D, Kulisch A, Rosenbaum C, Biesterfeld S, Günther RW. Puncture of stents implanted into veins and arteriovenous fistulas: an experimental study. *Cardiovasc Interv Radiol*. 1995;18:383-390.
26. Sreenarasimhaiah VP, Margassery SK, Martin KJ, Bander SJ. Salvage of thrombosed dialysis access grafts with venous anastomosis stents. *Kidney Int*. 2005;67:678-684.
27. Dember LM, Beck GJ, Allon M, et al. Effect of clopidogrel on early failure of arteriovenous fistulas for hemodialysis: a randomized controlled trial. *JAMA*. 2008;299:2164-2171.

CHAPTER 20

Axillosubclavian Vein Thrombosis

Sukgu Han, Vincent L. Rowe, and Fred A. Weaver

Thrombosis of the axillary and subclavian veins accounts for less than 5% of all cases of deep venous thrombosis. The most common cause is catheter-induced thrombosis of the axillary and subclavian veins, which comprises approximately one third of all cases of upper extremity deep venous thrombosis. Other causes include effort thrombosis, thoracic outlet syndrome, thoracic tumors, congestive heart failure, and trauma.

Overall incidence of axillosubclavian vein thrombosis (ASVT) is estimated to be 6 out of 10,000 hospital admissions.[1] It has been observed that this overall incidence is increasing.[2,3] Although this increase may not be universally noted,[4] it is certain that the proportion of ASVT resulting from iatrogenic causes is increasing. There has been an explosive increase in the use of the subclavian vein for a variety of purposes: hemodynamic monitoring, short- and long-term provision of parenteral nutrition and other intravenous agents, placement of pacemaker wires, and acute hemodialysis. Along with this increased use of central venous access, the prevalence of related complications remains substantial, with the incidence of catheter-associated ASVT reported to be up to 32% in patients with cancer.[5]

Pathogenesis

A number of factors has been reported to increase the risk of catheter-induced ASVT,[6] including the number of attempts at catheter placement, the duration of catheterization, the composition and stiffness of the catheter, catheter diameter and length, the composition of the infusate, and the indication for placement of the catheter. The relationship of these factors in the pathogenesis of ASVT may be better understood on the basis of Virchow's triad: intimal injury, stasis, and hypercoagulability.

Placement of a catheter into the subclavian vein produces the initial intimal injury. In fact, in a prospective review of registry of 592 patients, Joffe and associates[7] found that an indwelling catheter was the strongest predictor of upper extremity deep vein thrombosis (DVT) with the odds ratio of 7.3; 95% confidence interval of 5.8 to 9.2, compared with the patients with lower extremity DVT. This is also consistent with the experience at our institution. Our retrospective cohort study of 189 patients who underwent upper extremity vein duplex scanning showed that the presence of a central venous catheter was the only significant risk factor ($P = .03$) for upper limb DVT among numerous variables including renal failure, diabetes, malignancy, and intensive care unit status.[8] Repeated, unsuccessful attempts at placement compound this injury. The most common method of placement is via the Seldinger technique, in which the vein is punctured with a needle, a wire is passed through the needle, a large dilator is inserted over the wire, and finally, a catheter is threaded into the vein. Any or all of these steps will cause varying degrees of intimal injury, which may promote platelet deposition and thrombus formation. Notably, the use of a dilator that is larger than the catheter itself produces a hole in the vein wall that is not sealed by the catheter but must be sealed by newly formed thrombi. This initial thrombus may propagate and occlude the vein. Sustained contact between the catheter and the vein wall leads to further intimal ulceration with exposure of subendothelial collagen, a procoagulant. The longer the catheter, the greater the amount of intimal damage incurred. Catheter movement that occurs with exercise of the upper extremity or with respiration will cause additional trauma to the endothelial surface. Catheter materials also have an impact on intimal injury. Catheters made of polyvinyl chloride or other stiff materials have the potential to cause more intimal damage and are associated with a greater likelihood of thrombosis than are catheters made of more-pliable silicone elastomer (Silastic). This finding was confirmed in a report by Monreal and colleagues,[9] who found a greater than threefold increase in catheter-induced ASVT with polyethylene and polyvinyl chloride catheters compared with polyurethane or silicone catheters. Other potential causes of intimal injury include hypertonic or irritating infusates and mechanical disruption of the intima by balloon thrombectomy catheters used to salvage ipsilateral upper extremity hemodialysis access sites.

A catheter placed into the lumen of the subclavian vein alters the normal pattern of blood flow through the vein. This disruption of normal flow is another important mechanism in the development of thrombosis, particularly when combined with endothelial injury. Flow may become sluggish or turbulent and produce eddy currents. The magnitude of flow disruption varies according to the size of the catheter relative to the size of the vein. When the cross-sectional diameter of the catheter approaches that of the vein, flow becomes increasingly sluggish. Also, as the length of the catheter increases, the more sluggish venous blood flow becomes in a longer segment of vein. In patients with congestive heart failure and sluggish central venous flow, these indwelling catheter effects are further magnified.

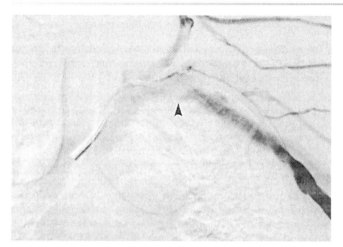

Figure 20-1.
Short-segment occlusion of subclavian vein *(arrow)* with central venous catheter still in place. Note the presence of collaterals around the site of occlusion.

Frequently, subclavian vein catheters are placed into patients being treated for malignancy, many of whom have cancer-induced hypercoagulable states. Spontaneous episodes of ASVT are well recognized in these patients, even without a history of prior subclavian vein catheterization. Other forms of hypercoagulable states that increase the risk of catheter-induced ASVT include prolonged parenteral nutrition and inherited thrombophilia. Inherited hypercoagulable states are found up to 30% of patients with upper extremity DVTs. Among these cases, lupus anticoagulant or anticardiolipin antibodies are the most common, followed by factor V Leiden. Other types of inherited hypercoagulable states include protein C or S deficiencies, antithrombin III deficiency, and altered prothrombin G20210A gene.[10,11]

When ASVT does occur, it most commonly results in a short-segment occlusion of the subclavian vein that may extend to its junction with the internal jugular vein (Figs. 20-1 and 20-2). The thrombus, however, can extend centrally into the innominate vein and even into the superior vena cava (SVC). Peripheral extension of thrombus past the level of the axillary vein is uncommon. Important collateral

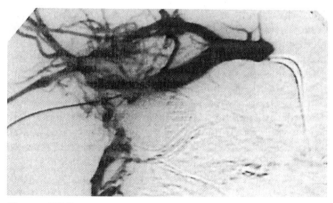

Figure 20-2.
Complete occlusion of subclavian vein with transvenous pacemaker wires in place.

pathways around the site of venous obstruction include those to the chest wall, to the vertebral vein in the posterior neck, to the internal jugular vein in the anterior neck, and to the contralateral neck through the jugular venous arch.

Clinical Presentation

Although prospective studies that use venography to detect thrombosis have shown that approximately 30% of patients with a history of subclavian vein catheterization develop ASVT, fewer than 5% of such patients develop clinical symptoms.[12] To a large degree, the proximal and distal propagation of thrombus determines whether clinical symptoms are produced. Many, if not most, short-segment occlusions remain asymptomatic because blood is shunted through venous collaterals around the site of occlusion. Thrombosis that extends peripherally into the arm or centrally to involve the innominate vein or SVC is more likely to cause symptoms because more collaterals become occluded.

Most episodes of catheter-induced ASVT are insidious in onset, but are more likely to become symptomatic when thrombosis occurs abruptly. The most common symptom of ASVT is edema of the ipsilateral arm, which extends to the forearm and hand. In the dialysis patient with an ipsilateral arteriovenous fistula, this edema can be dramatic. Pain in the arm and shoulder, especially with physical activity or exercise, is also common in symptomatic patients.

Physical signs of ASVT include the presence of dilated superficial veins on the ipsilateral upper extremity and across the shoulder. There will be increased circumference of the arm and forearm. Occasionally, the axillary vein will be palpable and present as a tender cord that is suggestive of thrombophlebitis. Occasionally, the thrombus may extend centrally and involve the SVC, in which case edema is usually present in both upper extremities as well as the head and neck regions. Constans and coworkers[13] developed a clinical score to predict likelihood of developing upper extremity DVT by evaluating the presence of a catheter, unilateral pitting edema, localized upper extremity pain, and absence of another diagnosis.

Diagnosis

When signs and symptoms of ASVT occur in a patient with a recent history of subclavian vein catheterization or in a patient with an indwelling catheter, the diagnosis is almost certain. Confirmation may be obtained with the noninvasive methods of duplex scanning, computed tomography (CT), or magnetic resonance imaging, or with venography.

Thrombus can frequently be visualized on the ultrasound image as a nonechogenic density in the lumen of the vein (Fig. 20-3). With the addition of color-flow technology to the duplex scanner, thrombus appears as a color void. When using the duplex scanner, the distal subclavian and proximal axillary veins are imaged below the clavicle and the proximal subclavian and innominate veins are imaged from the supraclavicular fossa. A thrombus-filled vein will not be compressible, although this maneuver is not always possible, particularly when the thrombosis is located beneath the clavicle or within the tight confines of supraclavicular fossa.

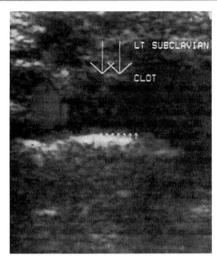

Figure 20-3.
Duplex image of subclavian vein with intraluminal thrombus.

Normal respiratory variation of the venous diameter or collapse of the vein on deep inspiration will be absent in the thrombosed vein. Doppler examination of the thrombosed or obstructed segment will reveal either the absence of flow or nonphasic flow. When compared with venography, the sensitivity and specificity of duplex scanning for correctly identifying ASVT approach 100%.[14,15] False-negative results do occur. The proximal subclavian and innominate veins are often difficult to image, and the SVC cannot be imaged in the chest. However, obstruction of these central veins may be inferred by an abnormality or absence of the normal respiratory variation of the Doppler examination. The subclavian vein is also difficult to image because it passes under the clavicle; therefore, a short-segment occlusion in this area may be obscured. Another potential source of error might be a large collateral vein that is mistaken for the subclavian vein. Nevertheless, the duplex scan is a very useful noninvasive screening test that, if abnormal, is sufficient to confirm the diagnosis of ASVT.

Further diagnostic testing may be necessary when faced with a patient who has a high clinical likelihood of ASVT on the basis of history and symptoms but has normal results from a duplex study. CT and magnetic resonance imaging are other noninvasive methods used to visualize central venous thrombi, and they are particularly appropriate to evaluate the mediastinum in the patient with a suspected SVC thrombosis. These tests are most helpful in patients in whom a mediastinal tumor may be the cause of SVC compression or thrombosis. There has been more interest in and experience with the use of magnetic resonance venography; Thornton and associates[16] demonstrated 100% sensitivity, specificity, and accuracy in the diagnosis of central vein thrombosis and anomalies. In the setting of limited ultrasound study, successful diagnosis of upper extremity deep venous thrombosis can be achieved with spiral CT venography.[17] Contrast venography is still considered the "gold standard" by most clinicians for the diagnosis of ASVT. Compared with duplex scanning, venography better defines the extent of thrombosis or stenosis and the location of collateral veins.[18] However, venography performed through a peripheral arm vein can be painful and carries the small risk of contrast toxicity.

Treatment

The goals of therapy for catheter-induced ASVT are to alleviate the acute symptoms when present, to prevent complications caused by the thrombus, and to minimize late sequelae. The asymptomatic patient without complications requires no therapy. When symptoms such as edema develop, conservative therapy consisting of catheter removal followed by extremity elevation and systemic anticoagulation is adequate treatment for the majority of patients. Anticoagulation is initiated with intravenous heparin or low-molecular-weight heparin to immediately arrest the propagation of thrombus and to prevent the obstruction of collateral venous pathways. Collateral veins usually enlarge and cause rapid resolution of symptoms. Oral anticoagulation with warfarin should then be continued for 3 months, by which time the intimal injury should have healed and the thrombus organized.

Patients who develop more serious complications may require more aggressive therapy. Pulmonary embolism should be treated initially with full heparin anticoagulation, followed by warfarin. If embolization recurs while the patient is therapeutically anticoagulated or the patient has a contraindication to anticoagulation, a filter device may be placed in the SVC.[19]

Septic thrombophlebitis is best treated with systemic antibiotics directed at the causative organism plus anticoagulation. Unlike septic thrombophlebitis in peripheral veins, excision of the involved segments of vein is surgically difficult with unrewarding results. There is some evidence that dissolution of the infected thrombus with thrombolytic agents provides more rapid resolution and fewer treatment failures than anticoagulation alone.[20,21] The lytic agent is best administered via catheters placed directly into the thrombus to optimize drug delivery, limit the necessary dose, and minimize hemorrhagic complications. Surgical or endovascular thrombectomy may be considered if thrombolytic therapy is contraindicated. Krauthamer and colleagues[22] report such a case successfully managed with a combination of balloon angioplasty, thrombectomy devices, and local intraluminal antibiotics infusion in a patient with contraindication to thrombolysis. The reported case was a 26-year-old woman with history of pure red cell aplasia and idiopathic thrombocytopenic purpura, who presented with septic thrombophlebitis of basilic, axillary, and subclavian veins ipsilateral to the indwelling peripherally inserted central venous catheter. Thrombolysis was considered to be contraindicated based on her thrombocytopenia, anemia, and extensive thrombosis. Following the removal of the central line and initiation of enoxaparin, her upper extremity septic thrombophlebitis was treated with the rheolytic thrombectomy AngioJet catheter, followed by Arrow-Trerotola thrombolytic device and balloon angioplasty. Within 48 hours from treatment, the patient's sepsis as well as arm swelling resolved. The follow-up venogram revealed patent axillary and subclavian veins without lesions.[22]

Proximal extension of thrombus producing an SVC syndrome and the rare case of venous gangrene are best treated by immediate systemic anticoagulation followed by thrombolytic therapy. Residual high-grade stenosis in the SVC should be corrected to prevent recurrence. Management options include balloon angioplasty with or without stent placement and surgical reconstruction.[23,24]

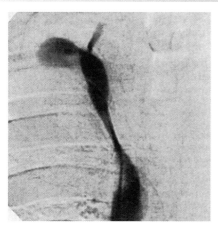

Figure 20-4.
Stenosis of innominate vein in patient with ipsilateral upper extremity hemodialysis access fistula.

Subclavian vein stenosis is rarely a clinical problem except in the dialysis patient who requires an ipsilateral arteriovenous fistula. All patients being considered for the placement of such a fistula who have a prior history of subclavian vein catheterization for any reason should be evaluated for the presence of central venous stenosis[25] (Fig. 20-4). Venography is often required because duplex scanning is limited in precise definition of the location of axillosubclavian vein stenosis. These lesions should be treated if no other site is available for placement of the fistula or if a threatened, but still functional, fistula is to be salvaged. Surgical repair of subclavian vein stenosis may be quite challenging. In the absence of extrinsic compression, balloon angioplasty alone is initially successful in most cases. Stent placement can be readily accomplished by an interventional radiologist or surgeon. In these cases, a guidewire may be advanced up the arm and across the area of stenosis. Alternatively, access may be obtained via the femoral vein. Balloon angioplasty is performed with the appropriately sized balloons (usually 8-12 mm) at a maximum inflation pressure of 12 to 15 atm. A metallic stent, along with its delivery system, is advanced over the guide and deployed. Completion venography is then performed to document stent function and position (Fig. 20-5).

Early studies with endovascular management of subclavian vein stenosis demonstrated excellent patency rates. However, these studies had short-term follow-up, and studies with longer follow-up times have not been as successful.[26–28] Many central venous stenoses are resistant to successful dilation because of the fibrotic nature and elastic recoil properties of these lesions, producing an initial failure rate of 30%.[23,28] Primary use of expandable metallic stents across lesions with elastic recoil and a significant residual stenosis after dilation improves the initial success rate of balloon angioplasty, but long-term success is questionable. For example, Vesely and coworkers[29] reported patency rates of 90% at 1 month for stenting of central venous stenoses in dialysis patients. However, at 1-year follow-up, patency rates declined to 25%. Lumsden and associates[30] reported similar results: a 1-year patency rate of 17% for endovascular management of central venous stenosis in dialysis patients. Interestingly, Quinn and colleagues[31] found no statistical difference in 1-year patency rates for angioplasty of central vein stenosis with or without stent placement in dialysis patients. In a recent study, Bakken andcoworkers[32] also found that primary and assisted 1-year patency rates were equivalent between angioplasty and stenting. When recurrent stenosis does occur, the lesions are at the ends of the stent and usually amenable to repeat dilation. When endovascular methods are judged against surgical revision, early trials show comparable outcome results, but later studies report an advantage with surgical intervention.[8,33–35]

Complications

In the past, ASVT was thought to be a relatively innocuous, self-limited entity with few sequelae. However, it is apparent that the complications of catheter-induced ASVT are frequent and may be severe or even fatal (Table 20-1). The loss of central venous access may be critical to patients with few or no other options for access who are receiving life-sustaining therapy via these catheters. Although pulmonary embolization from upper extremity venous thrombosis was formerly thought to be a rare event, this is not the case. Becker and associates[2] reported that 7.4% of patients with catheter-induced ASVT had this complication, with half of the cases documented by lung scan or autopsy studies. Hingorani and colleagues[36] reported a 7% incidence of pulmonary embolism and a 3-month mortality rate of 34% in patients with ASVT. However, no deaths were directly attributable to pulmonary embolism. Recently, Muñoz and coworkers[37] reported similar findings: 9% of the patients

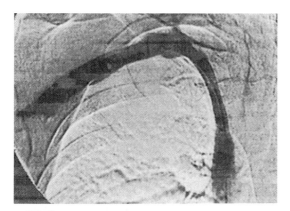

Figure 20-5.
Same patient as in Figure 20-3 after stent placement to relieve innominate vein stenosis.

Table 20–1
Complications of Catheter-Induced Axillosubclavian Vein Thrombosis
Loss of central venous access
Pulmonary embolism
Septic thrombophlebitis
Chronic venous insufficiency
Venous gangrene
Loss of ipsilateral upper extremity dialysis access

with symptomatic upper extremity DVT developed clinically overt pulmonary embolism, and 3-month outcome was significantly worse for cancer patients with upper extremity DVT. Using CT angiography to document pulmonary embolism, Major and associates[8] showed a similar rate of pulmonary embolism (7.9%) in patients with upper extremity DVT.

Infection of the thrombus, producing a septic thrombophlebitis, is another potential complication that can be difficult to control and is frequently fatal.[20] The most common responsible organisms are staphylococcal species, but Gram-negative and *Candida* organisms are also important pathogens. Venous gangrene has been reported to occur below catheter-induced ASVT, although this is extremely rare.

Although it is often stated that most of these occlusive lesions will spontaneously recanalize, the natural history of catheter-induced ASVT is not well defined. Reports on ASVT frequently contain a large number of patients with thrombosis from other causes, such as effort thrombosis. The reported incidence of chronic venous insufficiency in these instances may be as high as 75%.[2,3,38] Donayre and colleagues[39] analyzed 41 patients with ASVT according to cause (extrinsic or intrinsic) and correlated long-term sequelae with cause. Although 46% of patients with an extrinsic cause of ASVT (e.g., effort thrombosis, malignant compression, or trauma) developed long-term symptoms, none of the 10 patients with catheter-induced ASVT acquired such symptoms. Although arm swelling is the most common complaint of ASVT, Hingorani and colleagues[36] reported only a 4% incidence of significant arm edema at 1-year follow-up. These data suggest that catheter-induced ASVT is usually an acute condition and that once the inciting cause is removed, symptoms will resolve without long-term problems.

Up to 50% of patients with a prior subclavian vein catheterization for temporary hemodialysis access can be shown on venography to have a stenosis within the subclavian vein.[15] It is possible that some of these stenoses represent previous, unrecognized episodes of ASVT that have spontaneously recanalized and healed, leaving a residual stenosis. Alternatively, these stenoses may result from intimal hyperplasia at the site of venipuncture without an episode of thrombosis. Subclavian vein stenosis or occlusion is usually without consequence but may become hemodynamically important if an arteriovenous fistula is placed in the ipsilateral upper extremity for permanent dialysis access. The resulting increased flow into the venous system of the extremity may overwhelm the capacity of the compromised outflow system, producing early and massive edema in the arm and thrombosis of the access graft.

Prevention

Attention to technical factors during catheter insertion can reduce the risk of thrombosis. Meticulous catheter insertion technique will reduce the number of placement attempts, minimize endothelial injury, and decrease the contamination risk. We have found that insertion of the needle into the deltopectoral groove, aiming 1 to 2 cm above the sternal notch and just below the clavicle, with the patient laying flat on the bed and in slight Trendelenburg position,

provides a high initial puncture success rate. Strict asepsis, both at the time of initial insertion and with chronic use, is essential to reduce infection rates. The tip of the catheter should be placed into the SVC, preferably at its junction with the right atrium, where high flow rates will rapidly dilute potentially damaging infusates. This procedure can be facilitated by the use of intraoperative fluoroscopic guidance, which is especially important with dialysis catheters. Catheters of different lengths are available to ensure proper placement depending on whether an approach from the right or the left side is used. The catheter diameter should be as small as clinical circumstances permit and should be removed as soon as no longer necessary.

Prophylactic low-level anticoagulation has been shown to diminish the incidence of catheter-induced ASVT. Heparin may be added to and administered concurrently with the solution to be infused; the usual dose is 1000 units/L infusate.[6] Low-dose warfarin (1 mg/day) has previously been shown to reduce the risk of thrombosis without causing a significant prolongation of the prothrombin time.[40] However, a recent multicenter, randomized, controlled trial showed that incidence of catheter-related thrombosis was not reduced with low-dose warfarin prophylaxis in cancer patients.[41]

Catheter-related factors that can decrease the risk of thrombosis include the pliability of the catheter, the softness of the tip, and the smoothness of the surface both in overall design and microscopically. Heparin-bonded central venous catheters have been shown to reduce the risk of catheter-related thrombosis as well. In a prospective cohort study, Krafts-Jacobs and coworkers[42] compared incidence of venous thrombosis after placement of heparin-bonded and standard venous catheters in pediatric intensive care unit patients. The incidence of DVT was significantly lower with heparin-bonded catheter group; 2 (8%) of the 25 patients in the heparin-bonded catheter group versus 11 (44%) of the 25 patients in the standard-catheter group (*P* = .004).

The best therapy for catheter-induced ASVT is prevention. Although the risk of developing this complication of central venous cannulation cannot be eliminated, its likelihood can be reduced.

REFERENCES

1. Otten TR, Stein PD, Patel KC, Mustafa S, Silbergleit A. Thromboembolic disease involving the superior vena cava and brachiocephalic veins. *Chest.* 2003;123:809-812.
2. Becker DM, Philbrick JT, Walker FB 4th. Axillary and subclavian venous thrombosis. Prognosis and treatment. *Arch Intern Med.* 1991; 151:1934-1943.
3. Horattas MC, Wright DJ, Fenton AH, et al. Changing concepts of deep venous thrombosis of the upper extremity—report of a series and review of the literature. *Surgery.* 1988;104:561-567.
4. Hill SL, Berry RE. Subclavian vein thrombosis: A continuing challenge. *Surgery.* 1990;108:1-9.
5. Bona RD. Central line thrombosis in patients with cancer. *Curr Opin Pulm Med.* 2003;9:362-366.
6. Clagett GP, Eberhart RL. Artificial devices in clinical practice. In Colman RW, et al (eds). *Hemostasis and Thrombosis: Basic Principles and Clinical Practice.* 3rd ed. Philadelphia: JB Lippincott; 1994.
7. Joffe HV, Kucher N, Tapson VF, Goldhaber SZ, and the Deep Vein Thrombosis (DVT) FREE Steering Committee. Upper-extremity deep vein thrombosis: a prospective registry of 592 patients. *Circulation.* 2004;110:1605-1611.

8. Major KM, Bulic S, Rowe VL, Patel K, Weaver FA. Internal jugular, subclavian, and axillary deep venous thrombosis and the risk of pulmonary embolism. *Vascular.* 2008;16:73-79.

9. Monreal M, Raventos A, Lerma R, et al. Pulmonary embolism in patients with upper extremity DVT associated to venous central lines—a prospective study. *Thromb Haemost.* 1994;72:548-550.

10. Hendler MF, Meschengieser SS, Blanco AN, et al. Primary upper-extremity deep vein thrombosis: high prevalence of thrombophilic defects. *Am J Hematol.* 2004;76:330-337.

11. Leebeek FW, Stadhouders NA, van Stein D, Gómez-García EB, Kappers-Klunne MC. Hypercoagulability states in upper-extremity deep venous thrombosis. *Am J Hematol.* 2001;67:15-19.

12. Bozzetti F, Scarpa D, Terno G, et al. Subclavian venous thrombosis due to indwelling catheters: a prospective study on 52 patients. *JPEN J Parenter Enteral Nutr.* 1983;7:560-562.

13. Constans J, Salmi LR, Sevestre-Pietri MA, et al. A clinical prediction score for upper extremity deep venous thrombosis. *Thromb Haemost.* 2008;99:202-207.

14. Baarslag, HJ, van Beek EJ, Koopman MM, Reekers JA. Prospective study of color duplex ultrasonography compared with contrast venography in patients suspected of having deep venous thrombosis of the upper extremities. *Ann Intern Med.* 2002;136: 865-872.

15. Barrett N, Spencer S, McIvor J, Brown EA. Subclavian stenosis: a major complication of subclavian dialysis catheters. *Nephrol Dial Transplant.* 1988;3:423-425.

16. Thornton MJ, Ryan R, Varghese JC, Farrell MA, Lucey B, Lee MJ. A three-dimensional gadolinium-enhanced MR venography technique for imaging central veins. *AJR Am J Roentgenol.* 1999;173:999-1003.

17. Sabharwal, R, Boshell D, Vladica P. Multidetector spiral CT venography in the diagnosis of upper extremity deep venous thrombosis. *Australas Radiol.* 2007;51(suppl):B253-B256.

18. Richard HM 3rd, Selby JB Jr, Gay SB, Tegtmeyer CJ. Normal venous anatomy and collateral pathways in upper extremity venous thrombosis. *Radiographics.* 1992;12:527-534.

19. Spence LD, Gironta MG, Malde HM, Mickolick CT, Geisinger MA, Dolmatch BL. Acute upper extremity deep venous thrombosis: safety and effectiveness of superior vena cava filters. *Radiology.* 1999; 210:53-58.

20. Kelly RF, Yellin AE, Weaver FA. Candida thrombosis of the innominate vein with septic pulmonary emboli. *Ann Vasc Surg.* 1993;7:343-346.

21. Seigel EL, et al. Thrombolytic therapy for catheter-related thrombosis. *Am J Surg.* 1993;166:716.

22. Krauthamer R, Milefchik E. Endovascular treatment of upper extremity septic thrombophlebitis without thrombolysis. *AJR Am J Roentgenol.* 2004;182:471-472.

23. Gloviczki P, Pairolero PC, Toomey BJ, et al. Reconstruction of large veins for nonmalignant venous occlusive disease. *J Vasc Surg.* 1992; 16:750-761.

24. Khanna S, Sniderman K, Simons M, Besley M, Uldall R. Superior vena cava stenosis associated with hemodialysis catheters. *Am J Kidney Dis.* 1993;21:278-281.

25. Surratt RS, Picus D, Hicks ME, Darcy MD, Kleinhoffer M, Jendrisak M. The importance of preoperative evaluation of the subclavian vein in dialysis access planning. *AJR Am J Roentgenol.* 1991;156:623-625.

26. Glanz S, Gordon DH, Lipkowitz GS, Butt KM, Hong J, Sclafani SJ. Axillary and subclavian vein stenosis: percutaneous angioplasty. *Radiology.* 1988;168:371-373.

27. Hood DB, Yellin AE, Richman MF, Weaver FA, Katz MD. Hemodialysis graft salvage with endoluminal stents. *Am Surg.* 1994; 60:733-737.

28. Kovalik EC, Newman GE, Suhocki P, Knelson M, Schwab SJ. Correction of central venous stenoses: use of angioplasty and vascular Wallstents. *Kidney Int.* 1994;45:1177-1181.

29. Vesely TM, Hovsepian DM, Pilgram TK, Coyne DW, Shenoy S. Upper extremity central venous obstruction in hemodialysis patients: treatment with Wallstents. *Radiology.* 1997;204:343-348.

30. Lumsden AB, MacDonald MJ, Isiklar H, et al: Central venous stenosis in the hemodialysis patient: incidence and efficacy of endovascular treatment. *Cardiovasc Surg.* 1997;5:504-509.

31. Quinn SF, Schuman ES, Demlow TA, et al. Percutaneous transluminal angioplasty versus endovascular stent placement in the treatment of venous stenosis in patients undergoing hemodialysis: intermediate results. *J Vasc Interv Radiol.* 1995;6:851-855.

32. Bakken AM, Protack CD, Saad WE, Lee DE, Waldman DL, Davies MG. Long-term outcomes of primary angioplasty and primary stenting of central venous stenosis in hemodialysis patients. *J Vasc Surg.* 2007;45: 776-783.

33. El-Sabrout RA, Duncan JM. Right atrial bypass grafting for central venous obstruction associated with dialysis access: Another treatment option. *J Vasc Surg.* 1999;29:472-478.

34. Schuman E, Quinn S, Standage B, Gross G. Thrombolysis versus thrombectomy for occluded hemodialysis grafts. *Am J Surg.* 1994;167: 473-476.

35. Wisselink W, Money SR, Becker MO, et al. Comparison of operative reconstruction and percutaneous balloon dilatation for central venous obstruction. *Am J Surg.* 1993;166:200-204.

36. Hingorani A, Ascher E, Lorenson E, et al. Upper extremity deep venous thrombosis and its impact on morbidity and mortality rates in a hospital-based population. *J Vasc Surg.* 1997;26:853-860.

37. Muñoz FJ, Mismetti P, Poggio R, et al. Clinical outcome of patients with upper-extremity deep vein thrombosis: results from the RIETE registry. *Chest.* 2008;133:143-148.

38. Elman EE, Khan SR. The post-thrombotic syndrome after upper extremity deep vein thrombosis in adults: a systematic review. *Thromb Res.* 2006;117:609-614.

39. Donayre CE, White GH, Mehringer SM, Wilson SE. Pathogenesis determines late morbidity of axillosubclavian vein thrombosis. *Am J Surg.* 1986;152:179-184.

40. Bern MM, Lokich JJ, Wallach SR, et al. Very low doses of warfarin can prevent thrombosis in central venous catheters. *Ann Intern Med.* 1990; 112:423-428.

41. Couban, S, Goodyear M, Burnell M, et al. Randomized placebo-controlled study of low-dose warfarin for the prevention of central venous catheter-associated thrombosis in patients with cancer. *J Clin Oncol.* 2005;23:4063-4069.

42. Krafte-Jacobs, B, Sivit CJ, Mejia R, Pollack MM. Catheter-related thrombosis in critically ill children: comparison of catheters with and without heparin bonding. *J Pediatr.* 1995;126:50-54.

CHAPTER 21

Complications of Vascular Access: Thrombosis, Venous Hypertension, Congestive Heart Failure, Neuropathy, and Aneurysm

Samuel Eric Wilson

In North America, the typical patient who begins hemodialysis today has diabetes mellitus as the cause of renal disease and is older than 65 years. These risk factors, taken together with the propensity of access routes to clot, tax the ingenuity of the surgeon in maintaining a means for long-term hemodialysis. The most common treatment for chronic renal failure, hemodialysis is used for the majority of patients with end-stage renal disease (Fig. 21-1). Since the 1970s, the number of renal transplants has been limited by a lack of available donors (Fig. 21-2); thus, it is likely that hemodialysis will remain the mainstay for the treatment of chronic renal failure in the foreseeable future.

Complications associated with established vascular access sites or the inability to obtain suitable vascular access are important causes of morbidity and mortality in patients with end-stage renal disease. The most frequent complication leading to failure of the vascular access site is thrombosis. Infection is second but may be more acutely life-threatening. Hemodynamic and neurologic complications do not jeopardize the access site but result in considerable patient discomfort and morbidity and may be a reason for revision or removal. This chapter reviews clinical complications other than infection, which is discussed in Chapter 24, and considers methods for prevention and treatment.

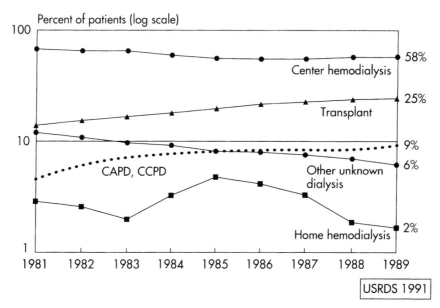

Figure 21-1.
Percent of patients alive on December 31 by treatment modality. All patients by year 1981 to 1989. *CAPD,* Continuous ambulatory peritoneal dialysis; *CCPD,* continuous cycling peritoneal dialysis. (From US Renal Data System. 1991 annual report. *Am J Kidney Dis.* 1991;18[suppl 2]:9.)

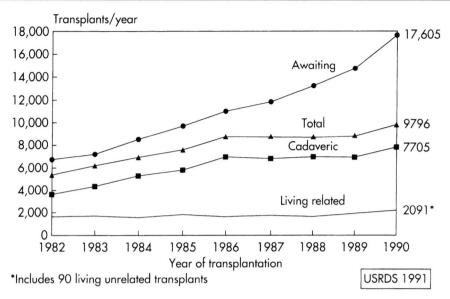

Figure 21-2.
Kidney transplants by donor types and patients awaiting transplants, 1982 to 1990. (From US Renal Data System: 1991 Annual Report. *Am J Kidney Dis.* 1991;18[suppl 2]:1-16.)

The complications of vascular access surgery occurring at one institution during a 4-year period were retrospectively reviewed by Ballard and coworkers.[1] Of the total 435 access procedures performed, which included 81 autogenous fistulas and 166 polytetrafluoroethylene (PTFE) grafts, just over 25% (111) were for thrombectomy and for revisions. In fact, Ballard and coworkers[1] concluded that 18% of total vascular access procedures involve the correction of major complications. It is no surprise, then, that almost 20% of all dialysis patient admissions are related to vascular access problems and that the most frequent cause of access failure is thrombosis.

Thrombosis

Certainly the foremost complication to be anticipated in the construction of vascular access procedures is clotting of the fistula or graft.

Patency rates are often considered as primary and secondary. *Primary functional patency* refers to the useful duration of fistula or graft function from initiation of successful dialysis at that site until the first intervention designed to maintain patency occurs.[2] Note that it is presumed that the access construction is satisfactory for hemodialysis. *Assisted primary patency* is the functional interval to thrombosis including use of percutaneous and surgical methods to correct a nonoccluding stenosis. *Secondary patency* refers to the total period of time until the access site is abandoned. Usually, several thrombectomies, revisions, and/or angioplasties have been performed within the time defined as secondary patency. In vascular access sites using prosthetic materials, secondary patency rates may be twice those of primary patency.

The likelihood of thrombosis depends on multiple factors, including the development of myointimal hyperplasia, anatomic configuration of the fistula or graft constructed,

site of arteriovenous (AV) anastomosis, selection of prosthetic material, and intrinsic clotting ability, but adequacy of the patient's veins and arteries is probably most important. The autogenous radiocephalic AV fistula is associated with fairly high early failure rates that have increased in recent years. The cumulative patency of autologous AV fistulas was 63% at 1 year in 2005.[3,4] Failure may be caused by small vessels, excessive dehydration in a debilitated patient, or venous outflow obstruction. Once successfully constructed, however, the autogenous radiocephalic AV fistula with adequate flow for dialysis has the most satisfactory long-term functional patency rate. Long-term patency rates of 60% to 70% at 1 to 2 years for radiocephalic AV fistulas have been reported by Biuckians and colleagues[4] and Mandel and associates.[5] Perhaps the most realistic data to date on patency rates are those from the U.S. Renal Data System Dialysis Morbidity and Mortality Study by Gibson and coworkers.[6] At 2 years, autogenous fistulas had a primary patency rate of 43% versus 31% for prosthetic grafts, and secondary patency rates were 64% and 60%, respectively. Vein transpositions in this analysis demonstrated a primary patency rate of 31% and a secondary patency rate of 64.2% at 2 years.

The patency rate of bridge fistulas are higher postoperatively, but the primary patency rates at 1 and 3 years drop below those of the autogenous AV fistula. For example, graft patency calculated by the life table method for the bovine heterograft was 92% at 3 months but 75% at 1 year.[7] Two-year secondary patency rates for prosthetic PTFE bridge grafts approach those of autogenous fistulas but usually at the cost of one or more revisions.

Patency rates vary according to dialysis centers in part because of both surgical skill and care in management of the functioning AV fistula or graft. For example, life table analysis of patency for 75 bovine heterografts at one center showed that at 1 year, only 45% of the grafts were still patent.[8] In another experience that compared the bovine heterograft and PTFE graft, primary patency rates have been higher and similar at 66% at 1 year.[9] Furthermore, in a review of Medicare data from a northeastern U.S. region, Kennedy and associates[10] demonstrated differences in outcome data between the dialysis centers.

Another consideration is the durability of prosthetic materials. More revisions were required for PTFE grafts, but in our experience, complications that occur in bovine heterografts often required excision of the graft. Cumulative patency rates for the polyethylene terephthalate (Dacron) velour graft of 80% at 24 months were reported by Jamil and colleagues.[11] Even so, Dacron grafts are not commonly used for dialysis access, because of greater resistance to needle penetration.

The anatomic site chosen for placement of the AV fistula also has important bearing on the duration of function before a complicating thrombosis. A graft with a diameter of 8 mm that connects a large artery and vein (e.g., the femorosaphenous AV shunt in the thigh) often has flow rates that exceed 1000 mL/min. Consequently, this graft is more likely to remain patent for a long period but has a greater likelihood of hemodynamic complications. Conversely, a smaller-diameter 6-mm graft placed between the radial artery and the cephalic vein in the forearm has a lower flow rate and lower patency rate at 1 year but usually is hemodynamically safe. At present, a 6-mm-diameter conduit is selected for most sites.

Thrombosis of shunts may occur soon after surgery or in the follow-up period. *Early thrombosis*, defined here as occurring within the first month after placement, is often caused by technical factors, whereas *late thrombosis*, which occurs from 1 month on, is generally caused by venous run-off stenosis (neointimal hyperplasia), continued trauma to the access site by needle puncture for hemodialysis, external pressure on the graft, hypotension, or central venous thrombosis.

Early Thrombosis

Clotting of a vascular access construction may be noted in the operating room soon after completion of the last anastomosis by the absence of a pulse and no palpable thrill. Thrombosis of the radiocephalic (Brescia-Cimino-Appel) fistula is most frequently caused by selection of an inadequate vein. Rohr and coworkers[12] recommended that the vein be at least 3 mm in diameter and open beyond the antecubital fossa. Preoperative ultrasound mapping will provide this information. Gentle dilation of the cephalic vein immediately proximal to the site of anastomosis with coronary dilators overcomes spasm and ensures a wide AV communication. Topical papaverine is also useful.

In some elderly patients and diabetics, the radial artery is involved with atherosclerotic disease and may not have sufficient pressure to sustain a fistula. Ideally, the patient with a poor radial pulse should have a Doppler systolic pressure measurement of at least 100 mm Hg confirmed in the radial artery before coming to surgery. Compression of the radial artery at the wrist should not result in blanching of the hand, and the collateral capability of the ulnar artery should be confirmed before surgery (Allen test). Plethysmographic recording of finger pulse volume or digital Doppler pressure and the response to compression of the

radial and ulnar arteries provide an objective evaluation if there is any doubt as to the adequacy of collateral circulation.[13] The characteristic eggshell calcification of the arterial wall is not a contraindication for fistula construction or conduit anastomosis, providing the artery is open, but requires careful suturing to avoid tears.

Early thrombosis of the bovine or prosthetic graft placed in the femorosaphenous position originating from the distal superficial femoral artery may be due to atherosclerosis of the superficial femoral artery as it traverses the distal thigh. Again, this condition is best evaluated preoperatively with Doppler measurement of the dorsalis pedis systolic pressure and duplex imaging. If the ankle-to-wrist ratio is less than 0.80, arterial imaging studies should be performed before selection of the superficial femoral artery for the site of origin of a graft.

Thrombosis of the fistula or graft during surgery may be caused by inadequate anticoagulation. Remember that patency of all vascular access sites depends to some extent on the coagulopathy of end-stage renal disease. In most patients, a Brescia-Cimino radiocephalic fistula can be easily accomplished without heparinization, taking advantage of the already diminished platelet function of the patient with chronic renal failure and the short occlusion time necessary for the procedure. However, when the brachial, femoral, or other major artery is occluded for insertion of a prosthetic shunt, systemic heparinization is warranted in the order of 40 to 50 units heparin/kg body weight intravenously. Heparinization also retards clotting of blood within the prosthetic graft during completion of the second anastomosis. The lower dose of heparin is selected, taking into account the relatively brief procedure.

Technical factors are often responsible for thrombosis of the newly placed fistula or graft. In particular, one must be careful not to narrow the lumen of the artery or vein during suturing and not to incorporate the back wall of the artery or vein in the vascular suture. When suturing a prosthesis to the artery, it is especially important to include all layers of the arterial wall to prevent subintimal dissection and subsequent thrombosis.

In the early postoperative period, thrombosis may be caused by external compression of the graft by a tight extremity bandage. Inadequate hemostasis during the procedure or early puncture of the graft for hemodialysis may result in extravasation of blood into the graft tunnel, requiring prolonged pressure for control. In such cases, reexploration with evacuation of the hematoma and declotting of the graft will usually result in salvage of the graft.

When placing a loop graft in the brachiocephalic or axilloaxillary position, take care to avoid a kink or twist in the distal portion of the loop. Inspection of the distal curve through a counterincision during placement of the graft and a recheck of the position when flow is established ensure proper alignment. I prefer to complete the arterial anastomosis first and then allow pressurization of the graft to check its conformation within the subcutaneous tunnel before completing the venous anastomosis. Suction blood from the graft before beginning the venous anastomosis.

Thrombosis of fistulas or grafts may occur after a hemodialysis run. Undue pressure over the needle puncture site for hemostasis or application of a tight compression dressing may result in graft thrombosis. Occasionally, a needle-induced flap or tear of the prosthetic wall, as can occur in PTFE grafts, is responsible for clotting. The diagnosis is often not apparent until the patient returns for the next dialysis run.

Late Thrombosis

Clotting of the autogenous radiocephalic fistula after the first months of successful use is caused by repeated trauma from needle punctures, with subsequent fibrosis and narrowing of the arterialized vein. Repetitive puncture of the fistula in the same area, extravasation of blood with local fibrosis, and cellulitis of the fistula all lead to fibrosis and stenosis. Correction may be accomplished by a more proximal direct anastomosis. In the worst of these situations, it may be necessary to convert the fistula to a bridge fistula using a prosthetic graft.[14] Percutaneous transluminal angioplasty with or without a stent has been used successfully to salvage failed or thrombosed AV fistulas.

Late thrombosis of a prosthetic graft is usually due to obstruction at the site of venous outflow secondary to myointimal hyperplasia. Development of stenosis at the venous end may be recognized by a gradual increase in pressure within the graft (venous return pressure) or by dialysis personnel reporting "recirculation" caused by sluggish flow. The combination of forceful pulsation throughout the graft and a loud bruit at the venous end may suggest progressive stenosis. Duplex ultrasound will confirm this diagnosis (Figs. 21-3 and 21-4). Correction of outflow

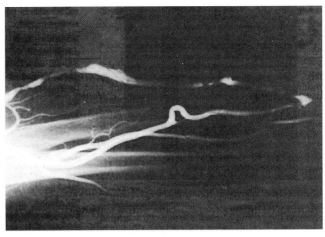

Figure 21-4.
A PTFE radiocephalic graft filled with laminated fibrin and clot after 5 years' use. Note hypertrophy and elongation of the feeding radial artery. Repair was successfully accomplished by interposing a new segment of PTFE, retaining the venous and arterial ends of the old graft.

stenosis is always easier for the patient and the surgeon if it is recognized before graft thrombosis occurs.

Anastomotic intimal hyperplasia that causes venous stenosis in AV fistulas has been attributed to mechanical endothelial damage; the shearing effect of blood flow; and the high-pressure, pulsatile nature of arterial flow in the venous system. Venous stenosis also may be caused by mechanical factors, such as angulation and stretching of the vein, or by compliance mismatch between prosthesis and vein. Currently, no methods clinically approved to reduce the myointimal hyperplasia that causes venous run-off stenosis, although research on irradiation, photodynamic therapy, immunosuppression- and biochemical growth factors is ongoing.

The placement of a graft across a flexion crease may give rise to obstruction due to kinking when the extremity is flexed. This situation may be avoided by preoperative planning of the site in conjunction with correct intraoperative positioning of the prosthesis. Having warned about kinking of graft material crossing a joint, most (but not all) PTFE grafts are flexible enough to extend across the elbow and shoulder during revision and to provide an adequate result without kinking. I do not find it necessary to use externally supported grafts when adding an extension across the elbow or shoulder joints, although this is an option. In PTFE grafts that have lasted for years, buildup of laminated fibrin and cellular elements of the blood leads to gradual occlusion or wearing out of the graft through the creation of multiple tiny "trapdoor" defects in PTFE caused by repeated needle punctures (see Fig. 21-4). These grafts may be replaced using the same vessels.

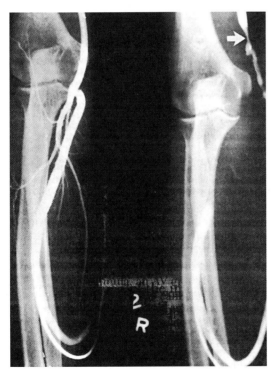

Figure 21-3.
Arterial anastomosis of this brachiobasilic polytetrafluoroethylene (PTFE) loop graft *(left)* is normal, but typical venous run-off stenosis *(arrow)* will cause thrombosis unless repaired. Graft was extended to a more superior venous anastomosis using an interposition of PTFE.

Thrombectomy

The role of thrombolysis for the clotted graft is discussed in Chapter 19. Thrombosis of a prosthetic graft may be treated successfully by thrombectomy, usually with local revision of the graft to vein anastomosis. Unfortunately, in some cases, salvage will not be possible, and a new access site will have to be constructed. When a strong pulse is palpated at the site of the arterial anastomosis, the surgical approach for thrombectomy of the occluded graft should be directed first to the venous anastomosis, because complications of venous outflow are usually responsible for late failure. The PTFE prosthesis with an external wrap will be surrounded by a fibrous capsule. Mobilization of graft material within this capsule is generally readily performed. The PTFE prosthesis without an external wrap is more tightly incorporated into the subcutaneous tissue, and it may be torn if dissection from the surrounding tissue is rough. Alternatively, one may decide not to mobilize the entire circumference but rather to control venous and arterial bleeding by manual compression or the insertion of Fogarty catheters to occlude the lumen. This procedure is not as safe as gaining complete circumferential control but requires less dissection. Adequate, although temporary, hemostasis can be achieved through manual compression of the graft by the assistant.

The following technique is most useful. After exposure, open the graft-to-vein anastomosis by a 3- to 4-cm longitudinal incision beginning just proximal to the venous anastomosis and carry it through the neointimal hyperplasia to the dilated, normal vein. Systemic heparinization may be given. Use a Fogarty embolectomy catheter (No. 4) to remove thrombus from the venous outflow tract, although this is often free of clot. Advance the catheter into the major vein and withdraw gently until all clot is removed. During venous thrombectomy, clot may be dislodged into the central venous system, but this is rarely evident clinically. On one occasion, I observed an episode of hemoptysis while declotting a femorosaphenous shunt; the procedure was terminated immediately, and the patient recovered uneventfully. Asymptomatic minor pulmonary emboli undoubtedly complicate some thrombectomies. After satisfactory venous runoff is ascertained, suture an oval patch of PTFE in place, beginning at the venous end and sewing toward the prosthesis; 5-0 Prolene serves the purpose well. Before placement of the last few sutures, the graft is thrombectomized. Recovery of the "bullet"—the pale, compressed portion of the clot most proximal in the graft—as recognized by an arterial indentation is the best signal for a complete thrombectomy. After clot removal from the graft, brisk arterial bleeding should be apparent. In some patients, it will be necessary to explore the graft at the arterial anastomosis to remove clot from the artery itself. If an excellent pulsatile flow or thrill is not obtained in the graft after thrombectomy, perform intraoperative arteriography to determine the status of arterial inflow and venous outflow. The advantages of this method, which leaves the graft thrombectomy until the last, are that heparinization is not required and that graft rethrombosis does not occur while the patch is being sutured in place. Furthermore, minimal dissection is needed for control of bleeding from the graft because hemostasis can be obtained by an assistant with finger pressure while the last few sutures are placed and tied.

Intimal hyperplasia at the venous anastomosis is best managed through one of three surgical methods, depending on the extent of disease and adjacent venous anatomy: (1) widening of the lumen with a patch angioplasty (as described earlier), (2) interposition of a short segment of new graft material and construction of a more proximal venous anastomosis, or (3) transfer of the venous end of the graft to an adjacent vein, such as from an antecubital vein to the cephalic vein. Endovascular methods are reviewed in Chapter 19.

Reasonable, but not spectacular, results can be obtained with thrombectomy; about 15% of grafts fail immediately after thrombectomy, and an additional 15% reocclude within 3 months. Implantation of a new graft or fistula will have a greater likelihood of success than will a declotted graft. Because the number of vascular access sites is limited, however, every effort should be made to obtain maximum duration of an established access. The secret to successful thrombectomy and graft salvage lies in reconstruction of the venous outflow tract. A successful graft revision has the advantage of allowing dialysis to continue with central venous catheterization using the undissected graft.

An episode of hypotension secondary to an unrelated surgical procedure or a medical complication (e.g., sepsis, congestive heart failure, or any cause of low cardiac output) may cause early or late thrombosis. When the complication is detected, successful thrombectomy and preservation of the graft or fistula usually are possible. This is also a clinical situation in which thrombolysis should be considered. Thrombosis may also occur secondary to efforts to obtain hemostasis after routine dialysis. Personnel and patients should be encouraged to report this finding rather than wait for its discovery just before the next dialysis session, thereby losing a 2- or 3-day window for thrombectomy.

Silent proximal venous thrombosis is indicated by venous distention and swelling of the entire extremity after construction of a distal AV fistula. In an excellent description, Mindich and colleagues reported two patients,[15] in whom the cephalic vein was occluded proximal to the fistula, and diversion of the fistula flow was recognized on the basis of dilated, tortuous veins. These venous collaterals involved the hand and thumb, resulting in progressive swelling of the hand, impaired function of the thumb and fingers, and extreme pain. In addition, ulceration of the digits occurred, which did not respond to intensive local measures. In both patients, interruption of the fistula entirely relieved the symptoms. The swelling, pain, and ulceration developed as a characteristic manifestation of chronic venous obstruction with venous stasis. Axillosubclavian thrombosis and its treatment are considered in Chapter 20. Although endovascular methods are the standard first-line treatment for the occluded subclavian vein, when they fail, anastomosis of the internal jugular vein to the axillary vein, "jugular turndown procedure," can be performed to maintain a distal arm fistula.[16]

Treatment of the thrombosed access site has been emphasized here, but the recognition of decreased flow in a graft or fistula, increased pressure in the venous return line, recirculation, or decreased dialysis efficiency (often reported by the dialysis nurse or technician) should prompt the nephrologist and surgeon to investigate and correct the stenosis before clotting. Color-flow Doppler imaging is a useful noninvasive technique for the detection of graft stenosis. So far, identification of graft stenosis without accompanying hemodynamic abnormalities by routine surveillance has not led to an overall increase in graft longevity.[17] Arteriography via the graft will show significant stenosis, and when associated with hemodynamic abnormalities, these stenoses can be treated successfully with fistula revision before the development of thrombosis.

Balloon catheter dilation of stenotic areas in patients with failing AV fistulas may be successful in carefully selected cases.[18] In general, the application of this technique results in shorter patency than does surgical revision. Dilation of autogenous veins may result in rupture of the vein, and stenosis of a prosthetic graft may not respond to dilation. Although thrombolysis and percutaneous transluminal angioplasty may successfully extend the patency of vascular access sites by several months, the procedure time, inconvenience to the patient, and cost are not better than those for surgical correction. The interventional radiologist and surgeon should work together to select the best approach for the individual patient rather than to apply one method to all.

Hemodynamic Complications

When Emil Holman conducted his classic experiments on abnormal AV communications, his observations were clinically applicable only to congenital or traumatic fistulas. He could not have anticipated how his findings would apply to the far greater number of fistulas constructed today by surgeons for hemodialysis.

The three principal hemodynamic complications of the AV fistula are congestive heart failure, peripheral vascular insufficiency (steal phenomenon), and venous hypertension. As discussed in Chapter 5, the following are physiologic responses to an AV fistula: (1) decrease in total systemic vascular resistance, (2) increase in cardiac output, with a rise in heart rate and stroke volume, (3) increase in venous pressure, and (4) reversal of flow in the artery distal to the site of the fistula when the diameter of the fistula opening exceeds the diameter of the feeding artery. In the first years of vascular access surgery, most surgeons shared the opinion of Hunter, who wrote in 1757 with regard to an AV shunt, "If not disturbed, such a shunt produces no mischief. I presume it will be best to do nothing." Nevertheless, detailed studies as early as 1970 by Johnson and Blythe[19] showed that each of eight patients with autogenous AV fistulas constructed for hemodialysis had a slight increase in cardiac output and pulse rate, with a decrease in total peripheral resistance. Although these alterations in hemodynamics did not produce overt congestive heart failure or cardiomegaly, the authors were wise enough to predict the occurrence of these complications in patients on hemodialysis.

High-Output Heart Failure

Depending on the diameter of the AV communication and the size of the feeding artery, an AV fistula increases venous return to the heart. Thus, the cardiac output and work of the heart increase, eventually leading to cardiomegaly and congestive heart failure. It is estimated that heart failure occurs only when 20% to 50% of the cardiac output is shunted through a fistula.[19] Because most of the fistula flow rates from radiocephalic forearm (Brescia-Cimino-Appel) fistulas are in the range of 400 mL/min, high-output failure

is unusual. Flow rates, however, may vary considerably, depending on whether the fistula is based on a distal (small) artery or on a proximal (large) artery and on the diameter of the fistula opening or bridge graft. For example, Anderson and associates[20] measured blood flow in AV dialysis fistulas shortly after construction in the operating room. In the distal radial artery–to–cephalic vein autogenous fistula, the mean blood flow was 242 ± 89 mL/min; however, in fistulas arising from the brachial artery, the flow rates were twice as great, averaging 599 ± 126 mL/min. Similarly, grafts placed in the thigh originating from the femoral artery had flow rates of 592 ± 134 mL/min.

Ahearn and Maher[21] reported two patients with Brescia-Cimino AV fistulas who had developed congestive heart failure. In one of these patients, the Nicoladoni-Branham sign was elicited; temporary occlusion of the AV fistula resulted in slowing of the heart rate. Measurements showed flow rates through the fistula of 2700 to 3800 mL/min. With occlusion of the fistula, cardiac output decreased from 11.2 to 8.4 L/min. This fistula was diverting as much as 25% of the resting cardiac output.

Anderson and associates[20] described six patients with cardiac failure and summarized nine other cases collected from the literature. Decreases in cardiac output with temporary fistula occlusion ranged from 0.3 to 11 L/min and averaged 2.9 L/min. The fistula flow rates in these patients varied from 0.6 to 2.9 L/min, with an average of 1.5 L/min. The earliest cardiac failure occurred 3 months after fistula construction, with the latest at 48 months. In all cases, the artery that contributed to fistula formation was either the radial or the brachial. Although the mean flow in the newly constructed radiocephalic fistula is approximately 300 mL/min, with dilation of the venous outflow tract, the shunted blood flow may greatly increase.

The effect of the standard distal forearm hemodialysis fistula on cardiac function was investigated in seven patients who had average flow rates of 0.71 L/min.[7] The cardiac index was raised significantly to 4.31 $L/min/m^2$ and fell into the normal range after occlusion of the fistula. The heart rate fell from 82 to 76 beats/min with closure of the fistula. Although none of the patients had congestive heart failure, those with poor left ventricular function and septal hypertrophy showed improved cardiac performance after occlusion of the AV fistula. Echocardiographic studies may be useful preoperatively in the selection of candidates with poor contractility, manifested by changes in the mean velocity of fiber shortening and ejection fraction and by left ventricular or septal hypertrophy. Abnormal results may warn the clinician of future development of cardiac failure and lead to construction of the smallest AV fistula compatible with adequate access.

When cardiac failure complicates high-flow AV fistulas, surgical correction is, fortunately, simple. In the patient with a successful renal transplant, closure of the fistula with repair of the artery by lateral suture may be carried out. In most patients in whom dialysis is still necessary, revision with narrowing of the anastomosis or construction of a completely new fistula may be used to correct the problem. One simple procedure to reduce flow is to narrow the graft close to its arterial origin with several interrupted sutures or clips. For investigational purposes, the flowmeter may be placed on the vein distal to the banding (not on the PTFE) and continuous flow recorded to document the excess flow and to monitor the fistula flow until it is within the desired range of 400 to 600 mL/min. In clinical practice, this is not feasible, and Doppler can substitute. We have noted that reduction in flow to values lower than 300 mL/min results in thrombosis of the graft. The step graft or tapered graft with a 4-mm arterial end was designed to avoid later development of this complication.

Venous Hypertension

Arterialization of the venous system results in venous hypertension and, if the valves are incompetent, in retrograde venous flow. Venous hypertension is marked by distention of the veins, swelling, and bluish discoloration and pigmentation of the skin (Fig. 21-5). Ulceration and pain occur in long-standing cases (Fig. 21-6). Surgical correction is obtained with ligation of the vein or veins immediately distal to the fistula or, in the case of a side-to-side anastomosis converting to a functional end of vein–to–side of artery radiocephalic fistula.

Persistent swelling of the entire extremity after the construction of an AV fistula may indicate a previously unrecognized major central venous thrombosis. This serious complication can be corrected by dismantling the fistula or, in certain patients, by reimplanting the venous end of the graft proximal to a limited thrombosis. Some clinicians are cautiously optimistic about the results of percutaneous transluminal dilation of the occluded subclavian vein followed by stenting;[16] a review of the results of this procedure is included in Chapter 20.

The ideal autogenous fistula in the forearm or wrist, avoiding both arterial and venous complications, would have an end-to-end anastomosis. This technique has not been generally accepted because it is technically more

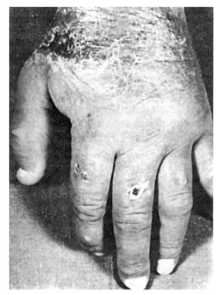

Figure 21-6.
Advanced stasis ulceration of the hand secondary to venous hypertension caused by a side-to-side fistula. (Courtesy of Dr. O. N. Fernando.)

difficult to construct an end-to-end anastomosis without stenosis or rotation. Complications that follow fistula construction are more often caused by thrombosis than by excessive flow. Consequently, most surgeons proceed with an end of vein–to–side of artery anastomosis, realizing that should a hemodynamic complication develop, it may be corrected by the local procedures that have been outlined. Subclavian venous occlusion can on occasion be bypassed by the internal jugular vein turndown procedure. The most distal portion of the internal jugular vein is divided, and the vein is mobilized in the neck and then anastomosed to the subclavian vein just distal to the occlusion.

Increased local hemodynamic stresses in the cephalic vein associated with construction of an AV fistula have been described as causing venous atherosclerosis in patients with long-standing access sites.[22] Clubbing of the fingertips may occur secondary to an AV fistula used for hemodialysis.[23] Anoxia is postulated as the mechanism responsible.

Vascular Access Neuropathy

Peripheral neuropathies, especially uremic polyneuropathy, have long been recognized in patients receiving chronic hemodialysis. Peripheral nerve symptoms resembling carpal tunnel syndrome have also been described. Although uncommon, this latter complication produces painful and sometimes disabling symptoms, which may be difficult to diagnose. Compression of the median nerve within the carpal tunnel of the wrist may occur either from a decrease in capacity of the canal or from an increase in the volume of its contents. Few dialysis patients with carpal tunnel syndrome–like symptoms have readily identifiable anatomic causes. Osteophytes, rheumatoid granulation tissue, and benign tumors have all been responsible for carpal tunnel syndrome in nonuremic patients but not usually in dialysis patients.

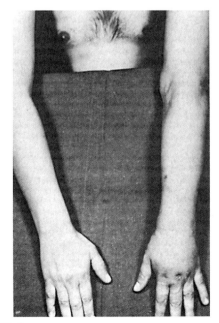

Figure 21-5.
Moderate chronic edema of the left arm secondary to venous hypertension in a patient with a side-to-side radiocephalic fistula. (Courtesy of Dr. O. N. Fernando.)

When first reported by Mancusi Ungaro and coworkers in 1976,[24] compression of the median nerve was thought to be caused by increased venous hypertension and by the secondary development of congestion within the carpal tunnel. In support of this causative factor was a study of 36 dialysis patients, of whom 23 reported symptoms of carpal tunnel syndrome in the hand containing the vascular access fistula.[25] Warren and Otieno[26] measured the volumes of both hands and found that the expected difference in volume between the dominant and the nondominant hands was reversed. The volume of the nondominant hand or hand with the fistula was largest due to its significantly elevated venous pressure. The authors related the development of symptoms in the fistula side during dialysis to a greater increase in hand volume than in the contralateral hand (the one without a fistula). Increased venous pressure in the hand may follow construction of an AV fistula, and it causes edema, resulting in greater hand volume. The resultant venous hypertension was considered to be the primary physiologic abnormality leading to edema and to symptoms of median nerve compression in the carpal tunnel of dialysis patients.

If venous hypertension and edema are the cause of carpal tunnel syndrome, why, then, do we not see symptomatic carpal tunnel syndrome with such conditions as axillary vein thrombosis or lymphedema of the arm, which give rise to edema and venous distention?[26] Furthermore, other studies have shown that venous occlusion produced by a pressure cuff around the arm has no influence on nerve conduction. This observation led Harding and Le Fanu[27] to propose that the symptoms are really provoked by ischemia caused by a vascular steal phenomenon resulting from the AV fistula. With the establishment of a successful radiocephalic fistula, it is likely that there will be reversal of blood flow through the distal artery, as documented by decreased blood flow to the first and second digits. The pain of the carpal tunnel syndrome may then be a manifestation of a relative ischemia of the median nerve during hemodialysis. Partial relief of symptoms has been obtained by ligation of the radial artery distal to the AV fistula in the forearm, lending further support to the ischemic etiology.[25,27]

Taking a strictly anatomic view, one may postulate that compression of the median nerve is most likely caused by an increase in the volume of the contents of the carpal tunnel. Indeed, a definite thickening of the flexor synovium within the carpal tunnel is occasionally observed either in patients with a functioning shunt or as a late complication after removal of an external shunt.

Ischemic monomelic neuropathy is defined as dysfunction of several peripheral nerve trunks in one extremity with the apparent absence of arterial insufficiency.[28] At its worst, weakness or paralysis of muscles innervated by the radial, ulnar, and median nerves results in a claw-hand deformity with substantially decreased function and severe neuropathic pain.[29] This condition is detailed in Chapter 23.

In summary, the pathophysiology of the development of carpal tunnel syndrome in dialysis patients remains controversial and has been variously ascribed to edema of the hand during dialysis, compression of the nerve, or thickening of the carpal ligaments and flexor retinaculum, but most likely represents ischemia secondary to a vascular steal phenomenon.[30]

The most prominent symptom of carpal tunnel syndrome in dialysis patients is painful, nocturnal acroparesthesia of the affected limb. The pain and numbness are in the distribution of the median nerve. Wasting of the muscles of the thenar eminence is a relatively late sign found in only a few patients. Abnormal motor signs and persistent sensory loss are usually not detected on examination. A diminished tactile sensation over the distribution of the median nerve may be present immediately after dialysis but usually resolves within 24 hours.

In differentiation of the carpal tunnel syndrome from uremic peripheral neuropathy, one should consider that the symptoms of uremic neuropathy are symmetrical, often beginning as a burning sensation in the soles of the feet, with progressive involvement in the legs. The upper extremities are involved only after the presence of severe lower extremity disease. Physical examination should also rule out severe ischemic changes. Absent or markedly decreased flow on Doppler examination of the digital arteries to the index finger and thumb confirms severe ischemia.

Suspicion of carpal tunnel syndrome in uremic patients should be confirmed by measurement of nerve conduction impairment. In patients with generalized uremic nephropathy, peripheral nerve conduction slows. In carpal tunnel syndrome, decrease in nerve conduction velocity is limited to slowing across the wrist. Typically, the distal motor latent period at the wrist for the median nerve is increased in carpal tunnel syndrome. Early diagnosis of carpal tunnel syndrome is important to prevent loss of reversible sensory and motor function.

The excellent results obtained with surgical release of the transverse carpal ligament for correction of median nerve compression in nondialysis patients has been found to be equally true for a few patients with end-stage renal disease treated surgically. The neurilemmal sheath is opened microsurgically, with care taken not to damage either the nerve fascicles or the intraneural vessels.[31] The sheath is then divided for a distance of about 2 cm above the carpal ligament to the distal bifurcation in the palm where the vessels leave the neural sheath. Surgical decompression has resulted in prompt relief of carpal tunnel syndrome symptoms in a few very carefully selected patients with marked fibrosis.

Some patients may achieve relief from symptoms through conservative measures such as simply moving the hand during dialysis. The use of digital compression of the needle puncture site rather than a compression bandage avoids increased venous pressure. Pain that limits the patient's competence for self-dialysis or makes dialysis at a center intolerable is an indication to search for an ischemic or other cause of the carpal tunnel syndrome.

Aneurysms

Vascular access bridge grafts may develop pseudoaneurysms secondary to trauma or true aneurysmal dilatation due to degeneration of the graft material.[32] We have observed pseudoaneurysms most commonly at needle puncture sites in biologic materials (Fig. 21-7) and less frequently at puncture sites in PTFE grafts. If there is no infection, treatment is simply local suture repair of the small

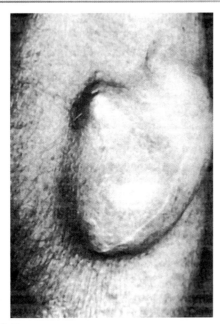

Figure 21-7.
Aneurysmal dilatation of a brachiocephalic fistula at the elbow. (Courtesy of Dr. O. N. Fernando.)

defect in the graft or, in some cases, interposition of a small segment of new graft.[33]

Formerly, prostheses constructed of expanded PTFE with a wall thickness of less than 0.5 mm were subject to aneurysmal degeneration. In an experience between 1975 and 1977, Owens and colleagues[34] noted aneurysmal changes in five PTFE grafts. None ruptured; some dilated up to a diameter of 7 to 8 cm, and excision was necessary (Fig. 21-8). In the 1980s and 1990s, dilation of aneurysms

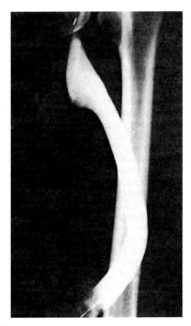

Figure 21-8.
Angiogram of a PTFE graft (implanted in 1975) that has undergone gradual dilatation after 8 months in situ. This does not occur with currently available PTFE grafts.

has not been reported in PTFE grafts with a wall thickness of 0.75 mm or with a reinforced wall structure. True aneurysms and false aneurysms that develop in biologic grafts may be treated with ligation or excision and graft revision using a new interposition segment.[32] Remember that infection, which accounts for about 25% of these aneurysms, renders treatment much more difficult, as discussed in Chapter 24. Large aneurysmal dilations frequently occur in the run-off veins of an AV fistula after some years of use. If the overlying skin is thinning or eroding, these should be repaired with local measures such as excision or interposition of prosthetic material.

REFERENCES

1. Ballard JL, Bunt TJ, Malone JM. Major complications of angioaccess surgery. *Am J Surg.* 1992;164:229-232.
2. Sidawy AN, Gray R, Besarab A, et al. Recommended standards for reports dealing with arteriovenous hemodialysis accesses. *J Vasc Surg.* 2002;35:603-610.
3. Ehrenfeld W, Grausz H, Wylie E. Subcutaneous arteriovenous fistulas for hemodialysis. *Am J Surg.* 1972;124:200-206.
4. Biuckians A, Scott EC, Mier GH, Panneton JM, Glickman MH. The natural history of autologous fistulas as first-time dialysis access in the KDOQI era. *J Vasc Surg.* 2008;47:415-421.
5. Mandel S, Martin PL, Blumoff RL, Mattern WD. Vascular access in a University transplant and dialysis program. *Arch Surg.* 1977;112:1375-1380.
6. Gibson KD, Gillen DL, Caps MT, Kohler TR, Sherrard DJ, Stehman-Breen CO. Vascular access survival and incidence of revisions: A comparison of prosthetic grafts, simple autogenous and venous transposition fistulas from the United States Renal Data Systems Dialysis Morbidity and Mortality Study. *J Vasc Surg.* 2001;34:694-700.
7. Oakes D, Spees EK Jr, Light JA, Flye MW. A three year experience using modified bovine arterial heterografts for vascular access in patients requiring hemodialysis. *Ann Surg.* 1978;187:423-429.
8. Hertzer N, Beven E. Venous access using the bovine carotid heterograft: techniques, results, and complications in 75 patients. *Arch Surg.* 1978;113:696-700.
9. Anderson CB, Sicard GA, Etheredge EE. Bovine carotid artery and expanded polytetrafluoroethylene grafts for hemodialysis vascular access. *J Surg Res.* 1980;29:184-188.
10. Kennedy MT, Quinton H, Bubolz TA, Wennberg JE, Wilson SE. An analysis of the patency of vascular access grafts for hemodialysis using the Medicare Part B Claims database. *Semin Vasc Surg.* 1996;9:262-265.
11. Jamil Z, O'Donnell JA, Merk EA, Hobson RW 2nd. A comparison of knitted Dacron velour and bovine heterograft for hemodialysis access. *J Surg Res.* 1979;26:423-429.
12. Rohr M, Browder W, Frentz GD, McDonald JC. Arteriovenous fistulas for long-term dialysis. Factors that influence fistula survival. *Arch Surg.* 1978;113:153-155.
13. Fronek A, King D. An objective sequential compression test to evaluate the patency of the radial and ulnar arteries. *J Vasc Surg.* 1985;2:450-452.
14. Mennes P, Gilula LA, Anderson CB, Etheredge EE, Weerts C, Harter HR. Complications associated with arteriovenous fistulas in patients undergoing chronic hemodialysis. *Arch Intern Med.* 1978;138:1117-1121.
15. Mindich B, Dunn I, Frumkin E, Levowitz BS. Proximal venous thrombosis after side-to-side arteriovenous fistula. *Arch Surg.* 1974;108:227-229.
16. Schoenfeld R, Hermans H, Novick A, et al. Stenting of proximal venous obstructions to maintain hemodialysis access. *J Vasc Surg.* 1994;19:532-538.
17. Bay WH. Correlation of color flow Doppler and angiography. In Henry ML, Ferguson RM (eds). *Vascular Access for Hemodialysis.* Vol 3. Hong Kong: WL Gore & Associates and Precept Press; 1993.
18. Lawrence PF, Miller FJ Jr, Mineau DE. Balloon catheter dilatation in patients with failing arteriovenous fistulas. *Surgery.* 1981;89:439-442.

19. Johnson G Jr, Blythe WB. Hemodynamic effects of arteriovenous shunts used for hemodialysis. *Ann Surg.* 1970;17:715-723.

20. Anderson CB, Etheredge EE, Harter HR, Codd JE, Graff RJ, Newton WT. Blood flow measurements in arteriovenous dialysis fistulas. *Surgery.* 1977;81:459-461.

21. Ahearn D, Maher J. Heart failure as a complication of hemodialysis arteriovenous fistula. *Ann Intern Med.* 1972;77:201-204.

22. Stehbens W, Karmody A. Venous atherosclerosis associated with arteriovenous fistulas for hemodialysis. *Arch Surg.* 1975;110:176-180.

23. Leb DE Sharma JK. Clubbing secondary to an arteriovenous fistula used for hemodialysis. *JAMA.* 1978;240:142-143.

24. Mancusi Ungaro A, Corres JJ, Di Spaltro F. Median carpal tunnel syndrome following a vascular shunt procedure in the forearm. Case report. *Plast Reconstr Surg.* 1976;57:96-97.

25. Lindstedt E, Westling H. Effects of an antebrachial Cimino-Brescia arteriovenous fistula on the local circulation in the hand. *Scand J Urol Nephrol.* 1975;9:119-124.

26. Warren DJ, Otieno LS. Carpal tunnel syndrome in patients on intermittent haemodialysis. *Postgrad Med J.* 1975;51:450-452.

27. Harding AE, Le Fanu J. Carpal tunnel syndrome related to antebrachial Cimino-Brescia fistula. *J Neurol Neurosurg Psychiatry.* 1977;40:511-513.

28. Padberg FT, Calligaro KD, Sidawy AN. Complications of arteriovenous hemodialysis access: recognition and management. *J Vasc Surg.* 2008; 48(5 suppl):55S-80S.

29. Miles AM. Upper limb ischemia after vascular access surgery: differential diagnosis and management. *Semin Dial.* 2000;13:312-315.

30. Fullerton PM. The effect of ischaemia on nerve conduction in the carpal tunnel syndrome. *J Neurol Neurosurg Psychiatry.* 1963;26:385-397.

31. Bosanac P, Bilder B, Grunberg RW, Banach SF, Kintzel JE, Stephens HW. Post-permanent access neuropathy. *Trans Am Soc Artif Intern Organs.* 1977;23:162-167.

32. Garvin PJ, Castaneda MA, Codd JE. Etiology and management of bovine graft aneurysms. *Arch Surg.* 1982;117:281-284.

33. Owens ML, Stabile BE, Gahr JA, Wilson SE. Vascular grafts for hemodialysis: An evaluation of sites and materials. *Dial Transplant.* 1979;8:521-530.

34. Owens ML, Wilson SE. Aneurysmal enlargement of e-PTFE A-V fistulas. *Dial Transplant.* 1978;7:692-694.

CHAPTER 22

Dialysis Access–Associated Ischemic Steal Syndrome

Al Hassanein and Samuel Eric Wilson

Vascular steal syndrome, also known as ischemic steal syndrome, refers to the process by which the arterial inflow to a vascular bed is diverted to another vascular network, thus reducing inflow to the point at which it cannot meet the demands of the tissue of the primary vascular network. This may result in ischemic symptoms such as pain, weakness, pallor, distal tissue loss, and ulceration. Ischemic steal syndrome is a known complication of vascular access. Constructing vascular access for hemodialysis alters blood flow to the extremity and might potentially trigger ischemic steal.

This chapter reviews the pathophysiology of ischemic steal syndrome, methods of preoperative recognition, and techniques and results of correction of steal syndrome.

Pathophysiology

The surgical construction of an arteriovenous (AV) fistula leads to predictable physiologic changes in blood flow such as decreased resistance through the network and a subsequent increase in cardiac output. In 80% to 90% of AV fistulas, there is a reversal of blood flow in the distal vascular bed, leading to a retrograde flow in the artery distal to the graft. Despite these frequent and expected physiologic changes from an AV fistula, pathologic clinical symptoms of ischemic steal occur only 10% to 20% of the time and severe symptoms requiring re-intervention occur only 4% of the time.

Predicting which patients will experience symptomatic ischemic steal syndrome is a challenging but critical question. Three major factors that can create symptomatic ischemic steal are inadequate collateral arterial networks to refill the vascular network distal to the AV fistula, a very high flow fistula, or arterial stenosis. Hemodialysis patients, particularly diabetics, may have preexisting vascular occlusive disease that contributes to ischemia regardless of access construction techniques. In female patients with small arteries, a high-flow fistula or graft (>750 mL/min) may exceed the capacity of the feeding arterial system even in the absence of arterial inflow disease. The combination of an inadequate collateral network, high-flow fistula, and arterial stenosis leads to hypoperfusion of the extremity. A more accurate descriptive term in place of "steal syndrome" would be "distal hypoperfusion ischemic syndrome."[1]

Prevalence

Steal syndrome will develop in 2% to 20% of patients with AV fistulas or grafts (Table 22-1).[2-8] Most recent retrospective studies show operative intervention for steal in about 4% of patients after vascular access surgery. Prospective studies typically diagnose symptomatic steal in 15% to 20% of patients. The difference likely represents bias from the study design because follow-up interviews with patients are more likely to elicit ischemic symptoms. Despite advances in preoperative evaluation and surgical techniques, this incidence has been largely unchanged since the 1980s. Chronic hemodialysis patients remain at risk for ischemic complications in the absence of an AV fistula (see Table 22-1).

Diagnosis

The diagnosis of ischemic steal syndrome is clinically based off the history and physical examination with symptoms of parasthesias, pain, and ulceration and tissue loss. A history of an AV graft versus an autologous fistula is critical in the expected time of presentation of steal syndrome after surgery. Steal syndrome typically presents immediately or shortly after surgery following an AV graft. Conversely, ischemic steal following autologous fistulas presents later as the vein matures and dilates, which allows for increased blood flow. The median time to recognize symptoms is 2 days for the AV graft group compared with 165 days for the autologous graft group.[3]

Patients often complain of the usual array of symptoms associated with arterial insufficiency including ischemic neuropathy, hand stiffness, tissue loss, ulceration, and gangrene. Physical examination will show pallor, diminished sensation, and ultimately, ulceration and gangrene. The radial pulse is usually absent, although ischemia of the fingers may be present with a palpable radial pulse in some patients. Compression of the shunt often relieves symptoms temporarily and augments the distal pulse. Increased heart rate and blood volume or symptoms of congestive heart failure usually are not caused by the AV fistula in hemodialysis patients, probably because of the blood volume adjustment that occurs during each dialysis.

Dialysis access associated steal syndrome is classified into four categories (Table 22-2).[9] Grade 0 exhibits no

Table 22–1

Incidence of Ischemic Steal Syndrome

Study	Study Design	Number of Patients/ Procedures	Ischemia Symptoms Not Requiring Operation	Ischemia Requiring Operative Intervention
Knox et al, 2002[8]	Retrospective review	1138 patients over 6 yr	Not described	55 (4.8%)
Valentine et al, 2002[5]	Prospective review	72 patients over 3 yr	Not described	14 (19%)
Papasavas et al, 2003[6]	Prospective review	35 patients	6 (17%)	3 (9%)
Lazarides et al, 2003[3]	Retrospective review of *proximal procedures*	569 procedures	Not described	24 (4.2%)*
Davidson et al, 2003[4]	Prospective review	325 procedures on 217 patients	4 (1.2%)	16 (4.9%)
Meyer et al, 2002[7]	Retrospective review	1253 patients over 5 yr	Not described	21 (1.7)%
Morsy et al, 1998[2]	Retrospective review	409 procedures on 352 patients over 5 yr	Not described	13/299 (4.3%) of AV grafts, 2/110 (1.8%) AV fistulas

AV, arteriovenous.

symptoms of steal. Grade I is mild steal and exhibits mild extremity coolness with few symptoms but shows improvement of symptoms and flow augmentation with graft occlusion. No treatment is needed for Grade I steal syndrome because symptoms are usually tolerable and do not interfere with function. Grade II is moderate steal syndrome in which there are symptoms of ischemia during dialysis or extremity claudication. Treatment may occasionally depend on tolerance of the symptoms and limitations of function. Finally, grade III is severe steal and includes ischemia and pain at rest with or without tissue loss. Intervention in grade III steal syndrome is mandatory. Table 22-2 shows a classification of steal syndrome with the subsequent need for treatment based on the grade.

Predicting Steal

Although a history of diabetes and previous vascular access operations are established risk factors, it remains difficult to predict who will get steal syndrome. Arterial occlusive disease in critical areas such as the palmar vessels or collateral vessels leads to steal as retrograde flow diverts blood away from the hand and collateral filling is inadequate. Multiple previous vascular operations are also risk factors because each shunt progressively becomes more proximal and decreases the inflow. In one series, all patients who required the distal revascularization interval ligation (DRIL) procedure for ischemic steal had brachial artery vascular access.[10]

Although there is no practical routine screening test for steal syndrome, several predictive measurements exist. The digital brachial index (DBI) is useful; it is the ratio of digital artery–to–brachial artery blood pressure as measured by Doppler technique. There is no single value that is indicative of steal syndrome. However, preoperative DBI at less than 0.8 provides a sensitivity of 29% and a specificity of 93%[5] at predicting ischemic steal. Another retrospective review revealed that a postoperative DBI of less than 0.6 was selected to predict steal and had a sensitivity of 100% and a specificity of 76%. The purpose of using DBI as a pre-

Table 22–2

Classification of Steal Symptoms in Patients with Arteriovenous Shunts

Grade	Symptoms	Treatment
Grade 0	No steal	None
Grade I—Mild	Cool extremity with few symptoms but demonstrable by flow augmentation with access occlusion	None
Grade II—Moderate	Intermittent ischemia only during dialysis/claudication	Intervention sometimes needed
Grade III—Severe	Ischemic pain at rest/tissue loss	Intervention mandatory

From Sidawy AN, Gray R, Besarab A, et al. Recommended standards for reports dealing with arteriovenous hemodialysis accesses. *J Vasc Surg.* 2002;35:603-610.

operative tool to detect ischemic steal syndrome is limited because steal syndrome is relatively unusual. However, ultrasound is useful to study the graft in addition to helping determine the etiology of steal syndrome and for operative planning if the patient is symptomatic. If revision for steal syndrome is indicated, the postoperative DBI should be over 0.6 or the patient will be at risk for continued steal syndrome.[11]

Operative Treatment

When the diagnosis of ischemic steal syndrome after dialysis access is established, there are several possible interventions that aim to heal ulcerations and resolve steal symptoms. These possibilities include ligation of the fistula or graft, percutaneous transluminal angioplasty (PTA), banding or restrictive procedures, and DRIL. Generally, operative interventions are successful in resolving ischemic steal in 80% to 95% of patients. Pain may sometimes persist despite the healing of ulceration.

One method to correct ischemic steal is ligation of the AV fistula or graft in order to restore the preoperative inflow. This can be done by simple ligation of the fistula or division and oversewing of the graft and leaving a small polytetrafluoroethylene (PTFE) cuff. This technique is useful for patients such as diabetics with severe atherosclerotic changes because other interventions may not be as effective in restoring adequate inflow. One major drawback to access ligation is that the access is rendered useless and an entirely new access site must be established. Any attempts or interventions aimed at addressing ischemic steal while maintaining the access site might not entirely resolve symptoms. Most series report complete resolution of pain in 70% to 80% and partial resolution in 80% to 95%.

Angiography is an extremely valuable preoperative or perioperative tool in the treatment of ischemic steal syndrome. Proximal stenosis of the inflow artery can cause ischemic steal.[12] If the etiology is proximal stenosis of the inflow artery, PTA may be employed to correct ischemic steal and save the need for intervention within the actual AV fistula or graft. If greater than 30% stenosis remains after dilation angioplasty, a stent could be deployed in the area of stenosis in the inflow artery proximal to vascular access. However, high flow through the fistula along with inadequate collateral circulation is the most frequent cause of ischemic steal and would not be corrected by PTA.

Reducing the velocity of flow through the fistula or graft is another technique aimed at treating ischemic steal. This can be accomplished through numerous approaches including banding, partial suturing, application of a hemoclip, or endovascular means, all which are intended to restrict shunt diameter. Thrombosis of the shunt is a major complication with these techniques. Partial suturing or application of a hemoclip at the vein adjacent to the arterial anastomosis can be a successful strategy in shunt-diameter restriction and subsequent high-flow reduction. This can be done while monitoring the digital or radial artery Doppler signals. Test narrowing can help determine where to place the clip or suture. The loss of anastomotic thrill indicates too much restriction with subsequent likely thrombosis. Other restrictive techniques described include the use of PTFE bands circumferentially adjacent to the arterial anas-

Table 22–3
Results of Distal Revascularization Interval Ligation Procedure

Study	Number of Patients	Patency
Knox et al, 2002[8]	55	83% at 12 mo, and 71% at 48 mo
Korzets et al, 2003[†]	11	90% and 80% at 12 and 24 mo
Sessa et al, 2004[‡]	18	94% at 12 mo
Walz et al, 2007[§]	36	
Yu et al, 2008[10]	24	96% postoperative

*Korzets A, Kantarovsky A, Lehmann J, et al. The "DRIL" procedure—a neglected way to treat the "steal" syndrome of the hemodialysed patient. *Isr Med Assoc J.* 2003;5(11):782-785.
†Sessa C, Riehl G, Porcu P, et al. Treatment of hand ischemia following angioaccess surgery using the distal revascularization interval-ligation technique with preservation of vascular access: description of an 18-case series. *Ann Vasc Surg.* 2004;18(6):685-694.
‡Walz P, Ladowski JS, Hines A. Distal revascularization and interval ligation (DRIL) procedure for the treatment of ischemic steal syndrome after arm arteriovenous fistula. *Ann Vasc Surg.* 2007;21(4):468-473.

tomosis.[13] Another method involves placing a ligature adjacent to the anastomosis after inserting an angioplasty balloon to maintain a standard 4- or 5-mm diameter.[14]

Reconstruction with distal bypass with ligation is another proven technique particularly useful in patients whose access site is the last available or critical to maintain dialysis. DRIL is a well-described technique. The operation consists of two fundamental phases. The first is a bypass from a proximal portion of the inflow artery to a site distal to the fistula opening. A reverse saphenous vein graft can be employed for the bypass. The second phase of the DRIL procedure is ligation of the artery just distal to the access site. This subsequently results in halting retrograde flow in the artery and reperfusion of the extremity with the bypass. An autogenous vein of suitable length and diameter is necessary because prosthetic conduits are more prone to late thrombosis. Thrombosis is particularly an undesirable outcome in this case because occlusion of the graft with the inflow artery ligated can be limb-threatening. The results of DRIL show 78% to 94% patency at 12 months and 71% to 80% at 24 months (Table 22-3).

Although the DRIL procedure remains the most likely intervention to correct steal syndrome and alleviate symptoms, some fistulas are not amendable by the DRIL procedure. Distal fistulas, in particular distal radiocephalic AV fistulas, are too distal to allow for distal revascular->tion. Fortunately, these types of fistulas very rarely cause steal syndrome. However, an endovascular approach using coil embolization of the distal radial artery and collaterals is one method of successfully treating this rare cause of steal syndrome.[15]

Summary

Ischemic steal syndrome is a rare complication of vascular access. Diabetes, previous multiple access surgeries, and brachial artery site for inflow are risk factors for the development of steal syndrome. The mechanism of steal syndrome involves high-flow fistulas, poor collaterals, and proximal inflow stenosis. There is no screening tool or test to predict or help prevent steal syndrome, but a decreased DBI less than 0.8 is a potential red flag. Ultrasound is useful in determining the cause of steal syndrome. Angiography can be used to define the anatomy and potentially intervene if proximal stenosis is the etiology of steal syndrome. Endovascular methods are increasingly being explored to expand the treatment of steal syndrome, but the method with consistently successful results continues to be the DRIL procedure.

REFERENCES

1. Leon C, Asif A. Arteriovenous access and hand pain: the distal hypoperfusion ischemic syndrome. *Clin J Am Soc Nephrol.* 2007;21:175-183.
2. Morsy AH, Kulbaski M, Chen C, Isiklar H, Lumsden AB. Incidence and characteristics of patients with hand ischemia after a hemodialysis access procedure. *J Surg Res.* 1998;74:8-10.
3. Lazarides MK, Staramos DN, Kopadis G, Maltezos C, Tzilalis VD, Georgiadis GS. Onset of arterial "steal" following proximal angioaccess: immediate and delayed types. *Nephrol Dial Transplant.* 2003;18:2387-2390.
4. Davidson D, Louridas G, Guzman R, et al. Steal syndrome complicating upper extremity hemoaccess procedures: incidence and risk factors. *Can J Surg.* 2003;46:408-412.
5. Valentine RJ, Bouch CW, Scott DJ, et al. Do preoperative finger pressures predict early arterial steal in hemodialysis access patients? A prospective analysis. *J Vasc Surg.* 2002;36:351-356.
6. Papasavas PK, Reifsnyder T, Birdas TJ, Caushaj PF, Leers S. Prediction of arteriovenous access steal syndrome utilizing digital pressure measurements. *Vasc Endovascular Surg.* 2003;37:179-184.
7. Meyer F, Muller JS, Grote R, Halloul Z, Lippert H, Burger T. Fistula banding—uccess-promoting approach in peripheral steal syndrome. *Zentralbl Chir.* 2002;127:685-688.
8. Knox RC, Berman SS, Hughes JD, Gentile AT, Mills JL. Distal revascularization-interval ligation: a durable and effective treatment for ischemic steal syndrome after hemodialysis access. *J Vasc Surg.* 2002;36:250-255.
9. Sidawy AN, Gray R, Besarab A, et al. Recommended standards for reports dealing with arteriovenous hemodialysis accesses. *J Vasc Surg.* 2002;35:603-610.
10. Yu SH, Cook PR, Canty TG, McGinn RF, Taft PM, Hye RJ. Hemodialysis-related steal syndrome: predictive factors and response to treatment with distal revascularization-interval ligation procedure. *Ann Vasc Surg.* 2008;22:210-214.
11. Goff CD, Sato DT, Bloch PH, et al. Steal syndrome complicating hemodialysis access procedures: can it be predicted? *Ann Vasc Surg.* 2000;14:138-144.
12. Malik J, Slavikova M, Maskova J. Dialysis access-associated steal syndrome: the role of ultrasonography. *J Nephrol.* 2003;16:903-907.
13. Papalois VE, Haritopoulos KN, Farrington K, Hakim NS. Successful reversal of steal syndrome following creation of arteriovenous fistula by banding with a ringed Gore-Tex cuff: a new technique. *Int Surg.* 2003;88:52-54.
14. Goel N, Miller GA, Jotwani MC, Licht J, Schur I, Arnold WP. Minimally Invasive Limited Ligation Endoluminal-assisted Revision (MILLER) for treatment of dialysis access-associated steal syndrome. *Kidney Int.* 2006;70:765-770.
15. Plumb TJ, Lynch TG, Adelson AB. Treatment of steal syndrome in a distal radiocephalic arteriovenous fistula using intravascular coil embolization. *J Vasc Surg.* 2008;47:457-459.

CHAPTER 23

Vascular Access Neuropathic Syndrome: Ischemic Monomelic Neuropathy

Larry A. Scher and Amit R. Shah

Distal ischemia is a known complication of vascular access placement in patients with end-stage renal disease. The incidence varies based on the location and type of access and patient demographics and ranges from less than 1% for radiocephalic arteriovenous fistulas (AVFs) to 1% to 5% for brachiocephalic and brachiobasilic AVFs and 2% to 6% for arteriovenous grafts (AVGs).[1-3] Symptoms can vary from mild pain or paresthesias to devastating arterial insufficiency with limb-threatening ischemia. Two distinct variants of upper extremity ischemia can be seen following the placement of AVFs or AVGs.[4,5] In the typical vascular steal syndrome, distal ischemia is invariably present and manifested by symptoms such as numbness, pain, and paresthesias and clinical findings including diminished or absent pulses, delayed capillary refill, and in severe cases, impending or frank tissue necrosis in the involved extremity. Symptoms may begin immediately after access placement but may also be delayed for days, weeks, or months.

Ischemic monomelic neuropathy (IMN) is a distinct clinical entity involving dysfunction of multiple upper extremity peripheral nerves either predominantly or exclusively. Symptom onset is usually immediate and neurologic symptoms are dominant, often in the absence of significant clinical ischemia of the hand. Typically, the hand is warm, capillary refill is preserved, and a palpable radial or ulnar pulse or audible Doppler signal is present. Diagnosis and treatment are often delayed, and even with early intervention, neurologic dysfunction may be irreversible. Because IMN can lead to significant long-term disability, potential medicolegal issues exist as well. The proposed etiology, clinical presentation, and management strategies for IMN are reviewed.

Background

In 1971, Matolo and coworkers[6] reported two patients with neurovascular complications of brachial AVFs. Although one patient had only a median neuropathy, the other had involvement of both the median and the ulnar nerves. This patient presented with pain, tingling, and progressive forearm and hand weakness. Although no additional details are available, this may be the first reported case of IMN. Despite this report, the initial description of ischemic neuropathy related to hemodialysis access is generally attributed to a report by Bolton and colleagues published in 1979[7] in which two patients presented with complications of bovine arteriovenous (AV) shunts. They described findings consistent with axonal degeneration of motor and sensory nerve fibers in two patients who developed hand and forearm weakness, numbness, and burning after bovine AV graft placement. The term *ischemic monomelic neuropathy* was first used by Wilbourn and associates[8] in 1983. Their initial report described a clinical entity with arterial insufficiency (*ischemic*) involving a single extremity (*monomelic*) and causing selective dysfunction (*neuropathy*) of multiple peripheral nerves. In their report, Wilbourn and associates[8] described three patients, two with acute arterial occlusions and one with placement of an AVF for hemodialysis access. The common etiologic factor was a sudden decrease in arterial blood flow caused by an acute noncompressive major arterial occlusion or shunting of arterial blood away from the distal extremity such as occurs after placement of an AVF. This resulted in damage to distal nerve fibers with acute neurologic symptoms but insufficient ischemia to cause muscle or skin ischemia or necrosis. Since these initial descriptions of this entity, numerous additional reports have appeared describing patients with IMN and attempting to provide additional insight into this condition.[9-14] Several reports have highlighted the differences between IMN and vascular steal syndrome (see Chapter 22), identifying IMN as a distinct clinical entity that occurs in patients after hemodialysis access surgery.[4,5]

Incidence

Although numerous reports document the frequency of vascular steal syndromes, the true incidence of IMN after hemodialysis access surgery is not known. Zanow and coworkers[1] reviewed a personal experience of more than 5000 procedures and found the incidence of access related ischemia to be 0.3% for wrist fistulas, 1.8% for elbow fistulas, and 2.2% for upper extremity polytetrafluoroethylene (PTFE) grafts. Unfortunately, similar data are not available to determine the true incidence of IMN. Almost all cases of IMN occur with brachial artery–based access procedures and the vast majority of patients are diabetic. Recognition of IMN may be delayed because the condition occurs infrequently and there is a high incidence of diabetic neuropathy in this population.[9,10,13] IMN also appears to develop more frequently in women than in men.[5,14] Raheb and colleagues[14] reviewed 12 cases of IMN that occurred in 273 patients (4.4%) all of whom underwent placement of a forearm PTFE brachial artery–based loop graft and found that all patients who developed IMN were diabetic and female.

Clinical Features

The pathognomic feature of IMN is the presence of diffuse neurologic dysfunction, usually in the absence of significant clinical ischemia. Table 23-1 reviews the clinical features of IMN and contrasts this condition with typical vascular steal syndrome. Symptoms of IMN include pain, paresthesias, and numbness in the distribution of all three forearm nerves and diffuse motor weakness or paralysis. Poor wrist extension, poor function of the intrinsic hand musculature, and poor thumb opposition are frequently present, suggesting radial, ulnar, and median nerve dysfunction, respectively. These deficits often are less severe proximally and more severe distally. Often, the sensory deficits are more prominent than the motor deficits. Because the forearm muscles may be relatively spared when compared with the intrinsic hand musculature, complete paralysis of the intrinsic hand muscles may be present with less severe weakness of wrist flexion and extension. This polyneuropathy may result in a profound functional deficit and claw hand deformity with persistent neuropathic burning pain (Fig. 23-1). Onset of symptoms is often acute and may occur within minutes to hours after placement of an

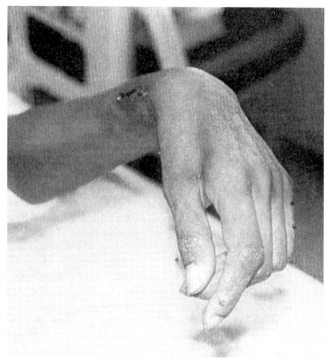

Figure 23-1.
Typical appearance of ischemic monomelic neuropathy with wrist drop and claw hand. The patient had a failed radiocephalic arteriovenous (AV) fistula and developed symptoms after placement of a brachial-based AV graft.

Table 23–1

Comparison Between Vascular Steal Syndrome and Ischemic Monomelic Neuropathy

	Vascular Steal Syndrome	Ischemic Monomelic Neuropathy
Onset	Insidious	Immediate
Diabetes	++	++++
Sex	Variable	Female >> Male
Access location	Wrist, forearm, upper arm	Forearm, brachial artery based
Affected tissue	Skin > muscle > nerve	Nerve (multiple)
Clinical ischemia	Severe	Mild
Radial pulse	Absent	+/−
Digital pressure	Markedly decreased	Normal or slightly decreased
Reversibility	Variable	Poor
Treatment options	Access revision (DRIL, banding) Ligation	?Access closure

DRIL, distal revascularization interval ligation.
　Adapted with permission from Miles AM. Vascular steal syndrome and ischaemic monomelic neuropathy: two variants of upper limb ischaemia after haemodialysis vascular access surgery. *Nephrol Dial Transplant.* 1999;14: 297-300.

AV access. The condition results from sudden diversion of the blood supply away from the nerves of the forearm and hand. This typically occurs in the absence of significant ischemia to other tissues in the extremity, thereby producing a neurologic deficit in the absence of significant clinical ischemia or necrosis of non-neurologic tissues. The hand is usually warm and often a palpable radial pulse or audible Doppler signal is present. As previously mentioned, the condition occurs typically with brachial artery–based access procedures and occurs almost exclusively in female patients with diabetes.

Pathophysiology and Electrodiagnostic Studies

Nerve conduction studies in patients with IMN show axonal loss and reduced motor and sensory nerve conduction velocities in the radial, ulnar, and median nerves.[8] These findings develop acutely and simultaneously in multiple forearm nerves as a result of sudden ischemia of the nerve trunks. Although ischemia is acute, it may be transient. Despite this, global sensorimotor dysfunction may result in prolonged or permanent injury owing to the increased sensitivity of nerve tissue to interruption in arterial blood flow. The ischemic event is often too brief or insufficient to cause detectable skin or muscle ischemia.

　Several experimental studies have attempted to clarify the mechanism for developing selective ischemia in the microcirculation of peripheral nerves. Kelly and associates[15]

experimentally assessed changes in the microvasculature of peripheral nerves after acute large vessel ligation. The vasa nervorum or nerve microcirculation was examined with scanning electron microscopy and demonstrated underfilling of the microcirculation with good filling of vessels proximal and distal to this area. This suggests that in generalized hypoperfusion states, the area of poorest perfusion and maximal damage is not the distal vascular bed but a "watershed zone" between two adjacent nutrient vessels to the nerve.

Sladky and coworkers[16] developed an experimental method for producing chronic regional endoneural ischemia in rats by creating proximal limb AV shunts. They concluded that reduced endoneural blood flow, insufficient to cause infarction, may result in measurable functional and morphologic abnormalities in peripheral nerves.

Electromyography in patients with IMN generally reveals acute denervation of all forearm motor and sensory nerves supplying the limb.[5,8] In attempting to correlate the results of electrophysiologic studies with the development of clinical symptoms, Kaku and colleagues[17] documented partial motor conduction block in the forearm in two patients with IMN following brachial artery–to–cephalic vein fistulas. Conduction block was observed shortly after the onset of symptoms of burning, paresthesias, and pain. Improvement in electrophysiologic studies correlated with clinical improvement after ligation of the AVF.

Recommendations/Management

Recognition of IMN may be problematic because of its infrequent occurrence and absence of significant clinical ischemic findings in the involved extremity. The importance of careful neurologic assessment of the operated extremity in the immediate postoperative period cannot be overemphasized. The differential diagnosis of IMN includes vascular steal, neurologic complications of axillary block anesthesia or patient positioning, carpal tunnel syndrome[18] or other peripheral nerve compression,[19] and postoperative pain and functional deficit secondary to surgical trauma or venous hypertension and postoperative swelling. Patients with only single nerve involvement likely do not have IMN.[19,20] Reinstein and associates[19] described three cases of direct peripheral nerve compression as a result of complications (hematoma, abscess, aneurysm) of brachial artery–to–basilic vein vascular access. As mentioned earlier, patients may have diabetic neuropathy, further complicating the clinical assessment. Although prompt recognition is important, diagnosis is often delayed and re-intervention has unpredictable results. If the diagnosis of IMN is in question, electrophysiologic studies may be helpful.[10,17]

Raheb and colleagues[14] described 12 patients with IMN. These patients were part of a larger series of 273 patients with forearm brachial artery–based loop AVGs, giving the authors an opportunity to evaluate clinical characteristics of IMN, estimate the frequency of the condition (4.4% in this series), and evaluate outcomes. The diagnosis was established more than 24 hours after development of symptoms in all patients. Treatment included banding only (5 patients), banding followed by access occlusion (2 patients), or observation only (5 patients). Patients who underwent

observation without intervention had limited sites for future vascular access, an often challenging problem in this patient population. All patients underwent aggressive physical therapy. One patient, who underwent banding 111 days after AVG placement followed by intensive physical therapy, had complete recovery. One patient had no recovery despite surgical occlusion of the AVG. The remaining 10 patients demonstrated only partial recovery.

Redfern and coworkers[5] reported 22 patients with neuropathic or ischemic problems following placement of AV access for hemodialysis. They divided the patients into two groups. Ten patients had nonhealing wounds or significant tissue loss. In this group, 5 were women and 9 were diabetic. The remaining 12 patients developed neuropathic or ischemic complications immediately following AVF creation at the brachial or antecubital level. Ten patients in this group were women and 8 were diabetic. Eleven of the 12 patients had involvement of more than one forearm nerve, suggesting a diagnosis of IMN. Nerve conduction studies, noninvasive vascular studies, and arteriography were used to confirm the diagnosis. The authors recommended early intervention and suggested that optimal recovery occurred in patients who underwent fistula ligation as soon as possible after the diagnosis of IMN was made. They also recommend that if there are no other options for vascular access, or if peritoneal dialysis is not possible, an attempt may be made to preserve the fistula. Flow-limiting procedures such as banding were utilized, but the authors reported that their experience with these procedures in this setting was both limited and disappointing.

Miles[21] presented a review comparing the clinical presentation of IMN and vascular steal syndromes. She also recommended immediate access closure upon diagnosing IMN to prevent severe and irreversible neurologic injury. Even so, paralysis and pain may be permanent or only partially reversible. A delay in diagnosis may reduce the likelihood of improvement, mandating the early recognition of this uncommon complication by surgeons, nephrologists, and dialysis personnel.

A literature review by Greason and colleagues[11] of 17 patients with IMN suggested that the level of improvement after treatment is related to the duration of ischemia. They reported significant improvement in patients treated within 21 days of onset of symptoms. Unfortunately, these results have not been universally reproducible.

Table 23-2 is a summary of clinical features, treatment, and outcome for cases of IMN reported in the English literature.[5–11,13,14,17,22] These data are again notable for the predominance of diabetes, female gender, and brachial-based access in patients with IMN. Most patients reported in the literature were treated with access ligation, and the results of treatment were variable, with the majority of patients demonstrating only partial clinical recovery.

The National Kidney Foundation Kidney Disease Outcomes Quality Initiative (NKF K/DOQI) has provided evidence-based clinical practice guidelines for all stages of chronic kidney disease and related complications since 1997. The most recent (2006) update of these guidelines[23] includes recommendations for the management of access-related ischemia. K/DOQI Clinical Guideline 5.6.1 identifies "older patient with diabetes with an elbow/upper arm AVF who may be at risk for monomelic ischemic neuropathy."

Table 23–2

Reported Cases of Ischemic Monomelic Neuropathy After Vascular Access Surgery

Study	Patients	Female	Diabetic	Type of Access	Treatment	Recovery
Matolo et al, 1971[6]	1	0/1	1/1	Brachial AVF	Ligation	Partial
Bolton et al, 1979[7]	2	2/2	Unknown	Bovine graft upper arm	Banding 1	Partial 2
					Observation 1	
Wilbourn et al, 1983[8]	1	1/1	Unknown	Brachiocephalic fistula	Ligation	Partial
Wytrezes et al, 1987[9]	3	2/3	3/3	Brachial-antecubital vein fistula	Banding 2	Partial 3
					Ligation 1	
Riggs et al, 1989[13]	4	2/4	4/4	Brachial-based AVG	Ligation 3	None 4
Kaku et al, 1993[17]	2	1/2	1/2	Brachial-antecubital vein fistula	Ligation 2	Partial 1
						Complete 1
Hye and Wolf, 1994[10]	5 (6 cases)	2/5	5/5	Brachial-based AVG	Ligation 2	Partial 2
					Other 2	None 4
					Observation 2	
Redfern and Zimmerman, 1995[5]	12	10/12	8/12	Brachial-based fistula	Ligation 5	Partial 8
					Banding 1	Complete 2
					Other 2	None 2
					Observation 4	
Greason et al, 1998[11]	1	1/1	1/1	Brachial-based AVG	Banding	Partial
Raheb et al, 2001[14]	12	12/12	12/12	Brachial-based forearm PTFE loop graft	Banding 5	Partial 10
					Ligation 2	Complete 1
					Observation 5	None 1
Brennan et al, 2005[22]	1	1/1	1	Brachial-based fistula	Ligation	Partial
Total	*44*	*34/44*	*36/44*	*All brachial based*	*Ligation 18*	*Partial 30*
					Banding 10	*Complete 4*
					Observation 12	*None 11*

AVF, arteriovenous fistula; AVG, arteriovenous graft; PTFE, polytetrafluoroethylene.

They describe the presentation as "an acute neuropathy with global muscle pain, weakness, and a warm hand with palpable pulses starting within the first hours after creation of the AVF." No mention is made of IMN related to AVGs. With only a single paper referenced,[4] K/DOQI guidelines suggest that "a diagnosis of monomelic ischemic neuropathy is a clinical diagnosis, and immediate closure of the AVF is mandatory." Miles[4] appropriately stated that even with early access closure, paralysis and pain may be permanent or only partially reversible. She also stated that delay in diagnosis will reduce the likelihood of improvement; hence, recognition of this uncommon complication of vascular access surgery by surgeons and nephrologists is crucial. Although this may seem logical in concept, significant data to support this statement are lacking. Closure of a functioning access is always problematic, with the need to consider alternative sites for access placement and the potential for similar complications to occur at these alternative sites. In patients with extremely limited access sites, given the lack of data and variability of clinical improvement following access closure, it seems appropriate to allow the clinician to exercise some clinical judgment in the management of these challenging patients. Nevertheless, the K/DOQI guidelines present very specific recommendations regarding the management of IMN. In addition, a recent document published by the Society for Vascular Surgery attempts to establish Clinical Practice Guidelines for the Surgical Placement and Maintenance of Arteriovenous Hemodialysis Access. Padberg and associ-

ates[24] addressed similar issues regarding the diagnosis and treatment of IMN, suggesting that recognition of IMN is an indication for deconstruction or revision of the AV access. Although these guidelines may not legally define the standard of care for managing patients with end-stage renal disease, treating physicians must carefully consider the medicolegal consequences of decisions made in treating these potentially devastating complications. If and until more effective strategies can be developed to prevent or manage IMN, it seems reasonable to recommend early diagnosis and intervention with access closure in patients with available alternative access sites. In addition, occupational or physical therapy may be important adjuncts in the long-term management of these patients. Despite these recommendations, recovery from this condition is at best unpredictable. Even with appropriate management strategies and early intervention, patients may be left with a significant clinical deficit.

REFERENCES

1. Zanow J, Petzold M, Petzold K, Kruger U, Scholz H. Diagnosis and differentiated treatment of ischemia in patients with arteriovenous vascular access. In Henry ML (ed): *Vascular Access for Hemodialysis.* VII. Chicago: Gore; 2001:201-208.
2. Morsy AH, Kulbaski M, Chen C, Isiklar H, Lumsden AB. Incidence and characteristics of patients with hand ischemia after a hemodialysis access procedure. *J Surg Res.* 1998;74:8-10.

3. Odland MD, Kelly PH, Ney AL, Anderson RC, Bubrick MP. Management of dialysis-associated steal syndrome complicating upper extremity arteriovenous fistulas: use of intraoperative digital photoplethysmography. *Surgery.* 1991;110:664-669.

4. Miles AM. Vascular steal syndrome and ischaemic monomelic neuropathy: two variants of upper limb ischaemia after haemodialysis vascular access surgery. *Nephrol Dial Transplant.* 1999;14:297-300.

5. Redfern AB, Zimmerman NB. Neurologic and ischemic complications of upper extremity vascular access for dialysis. *J Hand Surg [Am].* 1995;20:199-204.

6. Matolo N, Kastagir B, Stevens LE Chrysanthakopoulos S, Weaver DH, Klinkman H. Neurovascular complications of brachial arteriovenous fistula. *Am J Surg.* 1971;121:716-719.

7. Bolton CF, Driedger AA, Lindsay RM. Ischaemic neuropathy in uraemic patients caused by bovine arteriovenous shunt. *J Neurol Neurosurg Psychiatry.* 1979;42:810-814.

8. Wilbourn AJ, Furlan AJ, Hulley W, Ruschhaupt W. Ischemic monomelic neuropathy. *Neurology.* 1983;3:447-451.

9. Wytrzes L, Markley HG, Fisher M, Alfred HJ. Brachial neuropathy after brachial artery-antecubial vein shunts for chronic hemodialysis. *Neurology.* 1987;37:1398-1400.

10. Hye RJ, Wolf YG. Ischemic monomelic neuropathy: an underrecognized complication of hemodialysis access. *Ann Vasc Surg.* 1994;8:578-582.

11. Greason KL, Murray JD, Hemp JR, Hatter DG, Riffenburgh RH. Ischemic monomelic neuropathy: a case report and literature review. *Vasc Endovascular Surg.* 1998;32:385-390.

12. Ballard JL, Bunt TJ, Malone JM. Major complications of angioaccess surgery. *Am J Surg.* 1992;164:229-232.

13. Riggs JE, Moss AH, Labosky DA, Liput JH, Morgan JJ, Gutmann L. Upper extremity ischemic monomelic neuropathy: a complication of vascular access procedures in uremic diabetic patients. *Neurology.* 1989;39:997-998.

14. Raheb J, Esterl R, Reuter R, et al. Ischemic monomelic neuropathy as a complication of forearm PTFE loop grafts in uremic diabetic patients. In Henry ML (ed). *Vascular Access for Hemodialysis.* VII. Chicago: Gore; 2001:193-199.

15. Kelly CJ, Augustino C, Rooney BP, Bouchier-Hayes DJ. An investigation of the pathophysiology of ischaemic neuropathy. *Eur J Vasc Surg.* 1991;5:535-539.

16. Sladky JT, Tschoepe RL, Greenberg JH, Brown MJ. Peripheral neuropathy after chronic endoneurial ischemia. *Ann Neurol.* 1991;29:272-278.

17. Kaku DA, Malamut RI, Frey DJ, Parry GJ. Conduction block as an early sign of reversible injury in ischaemic monomelic neuropathy. *Neurology.* 1993;43:1126-1130.

18. Holtmann B, Anderson CB. Carpal tunnel syndrome following vascular shunts for hemodialysis. *Arch Surg.* 1977;112:65-66.

19. Reinstein L, Reed WP, Sadler JH, Baugher WH. Peripheral nerve compression by brachial artery-basilic vein vascular access in long-term hemodialysis. *Arch Phys Med Rehabil.* 1984;65:142-144.

20. Thermann F, Brauckhoff M, Kornhuber M. Dialysis shunt-associated ischaemic monomelic neuropathy: neurological recovery preserving the dialysis access. *Nephrol Dial Transplant.* 2006;22:3334-3336.

21. Miles AM. Upper limb ischemia after vascular access surgery: differential diagnosis and management. *Semin Dial.* 2000;13:312-315.

22. Brennan AM, McNamara B, Plant WD, O'Halloran DJ. An atypical case of acute ischaemic monomelic neuropathy post vascular access surgery in a patient with type I diabetes mellitus. *Diabet Med.* 2005; 22:813-4.

23. NKF—K/DOQI Clinical practice guidelines for vascular access: update 2006. *Am J Kidney Dis.* 2006;48 (suppl):S176-S247.

24. Padberg FT, Calligaro KD, Sidawy AN. Complications of arteriovenous hemodialysis access: recognition and management. *J Vasc Surg.* 2008; 48:55S-80S.

CHAPTER 24

Infection in Vascular Access Procedures

Andrew R. Ready, Al Hassanein, John A. C. Buckels, and Samuel E. Wilson

Vascular access is the Achilles heel of the dialysis patient[1] partly because of the consequences of access site infection, which remains a major source of complications and even death. Infection is the most common complication of vascular access surgery after thrombosis and a frequent cause of hospitalization of hemodialysis patients. Infection of surgical sites or graft material may prematurely end the function of autogenous or prosthetic fistulas and threatens life, through hemorrhage or systemic sepsis, and jeopardizes limb, through disruption of arterial supply.[2]

The European Dialysis and Transplant Registry has ranked infection second to cardiovascular disease as the major cause of morbidity and mortality in chronic hemodialysis patients. The management of hypertension and hypercholesterolemia, however, has improved to the extent that infection, in which access sites predominate, has become an important limitation on the life and well-being of the hemodialysis patient.[3]

The indications for hemodialysis have been progressively broadened, so that access procedures are now increasingly performed in elderly, diabetic, or medically compromised patients. Thus, complications, such as infection, are frequently encountered in patients with multisystem disease and little reserve to counter infection or endure surgical treatment. These patients constitute a major challenge to the vascular access surgeon, who must recognize and treat infection expeditiously and effectively if morbidity and mortality risks are to be minimized.

This chapter reviews the pathogenesis of vascular access infection in the hemodialysis patient and discusses its presentation, prevention, and management.

Pathogenesis

The overall risk of infection is increased in chronic renal failure. Uremia has a suppressive effect on many elements of immunity. Localization of infection to hemodialysis sites is enhanced by increased bacterial access to tissues and grafts through multiple diagnostic and therapeutic procedures, chronic indwelling cannulas, and repeated needle punctures. The altered bacterial flora of uremic patients also predisposes to infection.

Altered Immune Response

Uremia has been called "nature's immunosuppressant" because of its modulating effects on immune responses, which results in an increased incidence of infection and neoplasia. Indeed, infection is one of the most common causes of death in uremic patients and remains the principal reason for hospital admission.[4] Pulmonary, urinary, gastrointestinal, and wound infections are all more common in these patients, as are episodes of peritonitis and septicemia.

The function of many elements of immunity is impaired in uremia, although the underlying mechanisms are often obscure. Most aspects of polymorphonuclear granulocyte (PMG) function, including chemotaxis, phagocytosis, and adherence, are impaired, and evidence exists for both metabolic disturbances and circulating plasma factors as causative agents.

Deficient chemotaxis has been attributed to an intrinsic cellular deficit[5] but increasingly appears related to circulating chemotactic inhibitory factors,[6] whose effects are proportional to the level of uremia.[7] Circulating neutrophils and monocytes displayed reduced expression of chemokine receptors in patients with end-stage renal disease on dialysis.[8] These factors are ameliorated by hemodialysis, and after each treatment, chemotaxis returns toward normal.

Phagocytosis by polymorphonuclear neutrophil (PMN) leukocytes is also impaired in dialysis patients,[9] but Fc receptor function appears normal,[10] and the mechanism is unclear. Uncharacterized circulating factors may be responsible for both impaired phagocytosis and bactericidal activity. Granulocyte-inhibiting protein (molecular weight 28 kDa), a serum protein isolated from hemodialysis patients, inhibits chemotaxis and intracellular killing of bacteria. The factors, degranulation-inhibiting protein and β_2-microglobulin fragment GIPII, present in uremic serum, inhibit PMG function in vitro. Their physiologic importance remains obscure.[11,12]

Neutrophil function is also impaired by metabolic abnormalities that occur in uremia. The maintenance of correct intracellular calcium concentrations is critical both for PMG function and when abnormal chemotaxis, adherence, phagocytosis, generation of toxic oxidative species, and intracellular killing of bacteria become impaired.[13] In uremia, PMG calcium levels rise[14] after secondary increases in parathyroid hormone. Via an associated reduction in cell membrane Ca^{2+},Mg^{2+}-ATPase pump activity, increased levels of calcium are sustained and PMG function is impaired.[9] Normalization of intracellular calcium can be achieved in uremia using calcium channel blockers, but their effect on PMG function remains unclear.

Polymorphonuclear cells demonstrate increased rates of apoptosis in patients with chronic kidney disease. Dialysis normalizes this increased level of apoptosis in uremic patients. The exact mechanism remains unknown but Fas Ligand appears to play a significant role. Fas protein is expressed on PMN plasma membrane and the binding of the Fas ligand induces apoptosis of the PMN. PMN releases the Fas ligand to induce apotosis and is expressed at increased levels in patients with chronic renal failure.[15]

PMG motility correlates with granulocyte zinc levels and the moderate zinc deficiency encountered in hemodialysis impairs motility.[16] Zinc-treated patients show improved granulocyte responsiveness to zymosan-activated serum and greater chemokinetic activity.[16] Iron overload also impairs PMG function, notably phagocytosis, possibly because of effects on the cell membrane.[17] As a result, the risk of infection, particularly bacteremia, increases in hemodialysis patients who risk hemosiderosis if anemia is treated with iron or repeat transfusions. Treatment with human recombinant erythropoietin reduces iron overload and improves phagocytic function.[18] The association of iron overload with *Yersinia* and *Listeria* infections[19] probably does not reflect these impaired defenses but rather the lack of iron chelates in these organisms and their enhanced ability to obtain iron from overloaded tissues.

Uremic patients have depressed natural killer cell and monocyte[7,20] activity, and acquired immunity is also impaired, with cell-mediated rather than humoral responses being most affected. Clinically, deficient cell-mediated immunity (CMI) is exposed as impaired cutaneous hypersensitivity and enhanced skin allograft survival. Uremic patients have correspondingly impaired T-cell responses when tested in vitro and a worsening of CMI, as demonstrated by a progressive reduction in skin reactivity, which frequently occurs with increasing duration of hemodialysis.[21]

Many aberrations in CMI have been described in uremia, but the etiology and clinical relevance of most remain enigmatic. Lymphopenia is a frequent occurrence in chronically uremic patients, with a reduction in T-cell numbers becoming more pronounced with increasing duration of hemodialysis.[21,22] A reduction in the T-helper and T-inducer subset appears to be a specific finding with normal accompanying levels of T-suppressor and T-cytotoxic cells. Paradoxically, suppressor activity appears to increase.[21] In vivo, cytokine production appears deranged, whereas in vitro, both suppression of the mixed lymphocyte reaction and a decrease in antibody-dependent cytotoxicity are observed. The ability of lymphocytes to undergo blast transformation in response to mitogens or antigens is also frequently depressed, and lymphocyte survival is reduced. Structural and functional abnormalities of the thymus have been linked with uremia, and impaired thymocyte function has been associated with parathyroid hormone–induced increases in cytosolic calcium levels. The zinc deficiency of uremia also impairs CMI, and although the mechanism remains uncertain, improvements with zinc therapy have been reported.[23]

Humoral immunity appears less affected by uremia, and immunoglobulin levels tend to be normal or increased. Responses to most antigens are normal, but depressed responses have been reported to *Salmonella typhi* O and H antigens, bovine serum albumin, and rabbit antihuman

β_2-microglobulin.[24,25] The clinical implications of these findings are unknown.

Hemodialysis itself can impair host defenses through the physical contact of cells with dialysis membranes. Granulocyte adherence is aggravated during hemodialysis,[26] which can either activate or inhibit PMGs, depending on the membrane material. Dialysis-generated neutropenia is possibly due to cell sequestration in the lungs,[27] which, although usually corrected within 1 to 2 hours of dialysis, may be significant because it coincides with a period of increased risk of bacterial invasion.

Altered Natural Barriers

The integument and mucosal defenses are arguably the most important components of innate immunity, and when altered or deficient, infection becomes likely. The medical management of patients with renal failure is characterized by multiple invasive procedures that breach the integument, and the greatest risk of infection, apart from intraoperative contamination, is through direct bacterial inoculation occurring at any of many needle punctures. Cannulation sepsis is the most frequent cause of late arteriovenous (AV) graft infection and may be twice as common as sepsis originating from the surgical procedure. Its incidence increases dramatically when the sterile techniques of fistula puncture are relaxed. The appearance of any infection should provoke a review of skin preparation and puncture technique. Manipulations required for shunt connection and surgical procedures to form and salvage fistulas (eg, after clotting, stenosis, or pseudoaneurysm formation) also predispose to infection, providing an easy portal of entry for pathogens. Procedures to repair pseudoaneurysms may be particularly prone to infection as late sequelae.

Alterations in mucosal barrier function occur in uremia, and enhanced intestinal permeability and transmural bacterial migration provide the most common source of bacteremia when access sites are excluded. Bacteremia causes vascular access infection less frequently than direct inoculation, but is worrisome because systemic septic episodes can occur very frequently in dialysis patients. In animal studies, intravenous inocula of *Staphylococcus aureus* administered immediately after graft implantation often precipitate graft infection, but the infection risk is reduced if the challenge is delayed for 3 to 4 weeks until the graft neointima and pseudointima are developed.[28] Delaying dialysis for several weeks after graft implantation would seem appropriate in the elective circumstance in view of the frequent systemic sepsis that occurs in uremic patients. Nevertheless, the risk of secondary prosthetic infection from early graft cannulation is sufficiently low that on balance, early graft use may be safer than the considerable risks of percutaneous central line placement. The hematogenous seeding of access grafts can probably occur, but its importance has been questioned.[29]

Altered Bacterial Flora

In virtually all reported series of vascular access sepsis, *S. aureus* is the predominant organism, and because phage typing reveals autocolonization, most infections result from staphylococci already carried by the patient. This situation is compounded by the unusually high rate of *S. aureus* carriage found in hemodialysis patients, of whom 60% to 70% have the organism in their nose, throat, and skin, compared with 10% to 14% of control populations.[30] Dialysis unit employees have an intermediate carrier incidence of 30%, but most phage-typing studies do not indicate staff-patient cross-colonization. Colonization with *S. aureus* occurs progressively, so that after 6 months of hemodialysis, more than 50% of patients have already become carriers. This finding has considerable clinical importance because access-related infections occur most frequently in patients who become persistent staphylococcal carriers. The etiology of the staphylococcal colonization in dialysis patients is not fully understood, but it has been linked to needle puncture of fistulas, which allows *S. aureus* to colonize breaks in the skin. Multidrug-resistant gram-negative bacteria are rising in prevalence among patients requiring chronic hemodialysis.

Increased colonization by pathogenic bacteria, the breakdown of innate immunity, and aberrant acquired immunity increase the threat of bacterial infection in uremic patients, and regular needling makes access sites particularly vulnerable to infection. The type of vascular access used and its location are, however, the most important factors influencing the development and outcome of infection.

Access Type and Site

External shunts of the Quinton-Scribner type traverse the skin and are particularly prone to infection. Infection may occur any time after insertion. Although percutaneous catheters are a satisfactory, alternative means of short-term access, long-term use should be avoided if possible. External shunts have in large part been abandoned in favor of central venous catheters, which afford convenient temporary access. Nevertheless, these catheters also traverse the skin and are responsible for the majority of contemporary dialysis-related infection.

An immediate reduction in access-site infections occurred after the development of the Brescia-Cimino fistula in 1965, which superseded external shunts for long-term access. Infection rates for autologous fistulas continue to be low, and because of this low potential for infection, their superior patency, and their prolonged functional life, they remain the long-term access of choice. Vascular access constructed using prosthetic materials is required in many patients in whom autologous fistulas have been consumed by complications or have simply failed to mature.

Reinforced, expanded polytetrafluoroethylene (PTFE) grafts are the preferred alternative to autologous fistulas, but the complication rate for every 100 graft-month follow-up is three to four times greater. The percentage of patients who require prosthetic grafts continues to grow, as does the age of the patients and the severity of the coexisting vascular disease, factors that all reduce the functional life of the access site. Prosthetic graft sepsis is likely to constitute the majority of access-related infections that require surgery by the vascular access surgeon.

Infection rates for prosthetics, such as PTFE, can be daunting, with overall rates of approximately 10% during the lifetime of the graft. Furthermore, infection rates associated with graft insertion may be as high as 15%, and those for secondary procedures may be as high as 10%.[2] The present postoperative infection rates are perceived to be lower, perhaps as a consequence of outpatient surgery.

The site of graft implantation influences the risk of infection developing in prosthetic fistulas. The most common sites used are the forearm and the groin, with the latter generally having a higher infection rate and significant incidence of life- and limb-threatening sepsis.[30] This finding is probably associated with intraoperative contamination by skin bacteria that is more frequent in the groin, where, particularly around the medial thigh and inguinal skin fold, greater difficulty is encountered in preparing a sterile surgical field. We consider it prudent to reserve the groin for patients in whom forearm sites are unavailable.

A new risk for hemodialysis graft infection is the use of percutaneous methods to dissolve the clot in the thrombosed graft or to dilate the narrowed run-off site. Strict aseptic technique, equivalent to that of the operating room, must be followed in the interventional suite to prevent infection at the site of needle or instrument penetration of prosthetic material. Other risk factors that may increase the incidence of infection in prosthetic grafts include diabetes mellitus and poor nutrition.

Bacteriology

S. aureus (methicillin-susceptible and -resistant) predominates as the causative organism in vascular access infection and is responsible for about 70% to 90% of shunt infections and more than 90% of fistula infections.[30] The organism is resistant to methicillin in the majority of patients from whom *S. aureus* is isolated. A surveillance study conducted by the Centers for Disease Control and Prevention (CDC) in 2005 found that 15.4% of all reported cases of invasive MRSA were in dialysis patients, indicating that dialysis patients had a 100-fold higher risk of MRSA than the general population.[30] *S. aureus*, however, is not unique in causing access sepsis, and. in one series, 54% of infections were due to organisms other than *S. aureus*: 29% of organisms were streptococci (*Streptococcus viridans, Enterococcus faecalis*) and 25% were gram-negative bacilli, including two cases of *Pseudomonas aeruginosa*. Other reports[31-33] describe a similar array of organisms and in particular implicate *Staphylococcus epidermidis* and *S. aureus* as frequent pathogens. The reported increase in *S. epidermidis* infection rates in reconstructive arterial surgery has not occurred with vascular access.[33] *S. epidermidis* causes somewhat indolent infections. Gram-negative infections and *S. aureus* are more aggressive and frequently result in anastomotic rupture. *S. epidermidis* can also produce problematic infections of central venous cannulas, as characterized by low-grade fever and positive blood cultures. The organism produces a mucoid substance that facilitates adhesion to silicone rubber,[34] making eradication by antibiotic therapy unlikely. Cannula replacement at an alternative site is usually required.

S. viridans, a ubiquitous organism in saliva and on tooth surfaces, has been reported to infect vascular access sites after dental procedures that are not covered by antibiotics. Patients with intravascular prostheses should therefore receive antibiotic prophylaxis for dental and surgical procedures in accordance with the regimens proposed for bacterial endocarditis.

Resistant gram-positive organisms are more prevalent in dialysis access site infections. The National Nosocomial Infection Surveillance System collected data showing the rates of resistance of *S. aureus* to semisynthetic penicillins to have increased from approximately 28% in 1994 to 55% in 1999.[30] Accordingly, vancomycin has become a widely used antimicrobial in the treatment of gram-positive infections in dialysis patients. New agents are necessary for patients who are intolerant or allergic to vancomycin or in whom vancomycin has not been effective. The first of the new agents to be effective against *S. aureus* (and vancomycin-resistant *Enterococcus faecium*) is dalfopristin/quinupristin, a combination of two streptogramin antibiotics. It is administered in 5% dextrose and water over a 60-minute period via a central venous line to avoid thrombophlebitis. Approximately 10% of patients who receive dalfopristin/quinupristin will develop arthralgias or myalgias. This agent is bactericidal against most *S. aureus* strains, including vancomycin-resistant strains.

An important new antimicrobial, linezolid, the first of a new class of oxazolidinones, is effective against methicillin-susceptible and -resistant *S. aureus* as well as *E. faecalis* and *E. faecium*. This bacteriostatic agent has bioequivalence whether administered intravenously or orally. Reversible bone marrow suppression occurs with linezolid therapy, so the agent is not recommended for more than 28 days of therapy, and a white blood cell count should be obtained every week while the patient is receiving the antimicrobial either intravenously or orally. Antimicrobials alone are rarely the sole treatment for an established graft infection, but they provide essential coverage for bacteremia and resolution of the infection upon removal of the foreign material.

Two new antibiotics that have demonstrated efficacious against bloodstream MRSA are daptomycin and tigecycline.[35,36] Daptomycin is a cyclic lipopeptide with bactericidal activity against MRSA as well as VRE. It has a distinct mechanism of action that involves binding the bacterial cell membrane and causing rapid depolarization of the cell. It has been shown to not be inferior to vancomycin in the treatment of MRSA. The antimicrobial drug is tigecycline, which belongs to a new class of antibiotics called glycycylines. It inhibits the bacterial 30S ribosome.

Vancomycin–intermediate resistant and resistant *Staphylococcus aureus* (VISA, VIRSA) is so far not a major clinical problem, although emergence of this resistant organism is expected to spread worldwide. Typically, patients have undergone long-term vancomycin therapy for infection related to chronic ambulatory peritoneal dialysis. Organisms show alterations in their cell shape and wall thickness that confer resistance.

Central venous catheters impregnated with minocycline and rifampin are associated with a lower rate of infection than those associated with the use of catheters impregnated with chlorhexidine and silver sulfadiazine. The data from the clinical trial reported by Darouiche and associates[37] were obtained from a cooperative study carried out in 12 university-affiliated hospitals. This observation is of most use for patients who require vascular access for a relatively short period, 1 to 3 weeks, while awaiting maturation of a permanent access site. The benefit is achieved by enhanced resistance to colonization with coagulase-negative *S. aureus*.

Single organisms are responsible for more than 80% of vascular access infection, with two organisms being isolated in fewer than 15%. Under certain circumstances, multiple organisms may be cultured, but evidence exists that mixed growths may be increasing in frequency.[38]

In approximately one third of cases, no bacteriologic growth is obtained despite clinical evidence of infection. This finding usually relates to prior antibiotic treatment. Conversely, patients with positive blood cultures and no local signs of sepsis can pose management problems. In shunt and cannula infections, up to one third of infections have bacteremia without any obvious local signs. If *S. aureus* or *S. epidermidis* is cultured from the blood of access patients in whom other sources of infection (eg, endocarditis) have been excluded, the access site should be suspected. Under such circumstances, improvement invariably follows removal or excision of the access.

Clinical Features

The classic signs of inflammation accompany most vascular access infections. Localized warmth in the overlying tissues with erythema, swelling, pain, and tenderness is usually apparent from the early stages of infection. The severity of each sign may be modified by the type of access, its position, the duration of the infection, and previous antibiotic therapy. In the later stages of infection, abscess formation with eventual skin breakdown and chronic discharge of pus may occur.

Early shunt and cannula infections usually have local erythema and seepage of purulent material around the tubing. Peritubular bleeding, with or without disruption of the vessel, and false aneurysm formation are late signs (Fig. 24-1) associated with neglected shunt infections.

Autologous fistula infections are rare, but superficial cellulitic wound infections after fistula formation are common. Repeated needle puncture may cause hematoma formation, with subsequent infection and the typical signs of inflammation, which may proceed to abscess formation if neglected. If anastomotic infection develops, disruption of the anastomosis and pseudoaneurysm formation may occur.

A prosthetic graft infection may also be either a postoperative wound infection or related to needle puncture. The former occurs early after implantation and may range from cellulitis to complete wound breakdown and the formation of an infected cavity containing the exposed graft in its base. Needle puncture and other late causes of infection usually show erythema over the prosthesis, with local tenderness and occasional skin breakdown exposing the graft. Even with initial antibiotic treatment, aggressive infections can result in an abscess, cumulating in a purulent discharge that is likely to become chronic. In severe graft tunnel infections, the cellulitic signs can extend along the length of the graft, with the development of multiple abscesses. If the anastomoses become involved, destruction of the arterial wall may lead to anastomotic disruption,

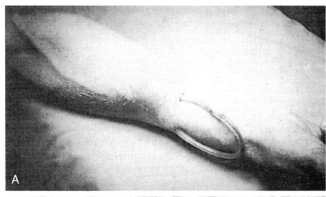

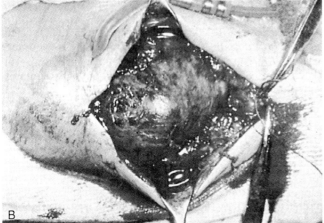

Figure 24-1.
A, False aneurysm secondary to infection of external arteriovenous shunt. *B,* Surgical exposure of aneurysm just before excision of shunt.

pseudoaneurysm formation, and eventually life-threatening hemorrhage. Graft infection is occasionally heralded by bleeding or enlargement of a pseudoaneurysm, as indicated by a pulsatile mass over the graft, which may also exhibit local tenderness, warmth, and erythema.

Most acute access infections are indicated as described earlier, but more indolent forms of infection may be encountered in which chronic infection produces walled-off sinuses that contain exposed graft. If such infections remain distant from the anastomosis, few immediate problems arise. The graft is exposed but infection is limited, and time is available to tailor the solution to the individual patient's needs.

In addition to local signs, many patients have evidence of systemic infection with bacteremia, usually caused by *S. aureus,* accompanying about 50% of autogenous fistulas and prosthetic graft infections.

Systemic effects may be severe, and some series report a 10% mortality rate due to the effects of overwhelming sepsis, including metastatic abscesses and endocarditis.

Management

Vascular access infection may have catastrophic effects on dialysis patients, and the management of established infection must be secondary to measures aimed at preventing bacteremia and secondary metastatic infections.

Prevention

The mainstay of prevention in vascular access surgery is strict adherence to aseptic technique. This is good surgical practice during any operation, but it is mandatory for vascular procedures, especially those involving prosthetics. Techniques should be no less rigorous in hemodialysis units where correct preparation of the skin before needle puncture must become an obsessional requirement. Staff and patients alike must understand the importance of such care. Patients should also be fully trained in such techniques before commencing home hemodialysis.

Other preventive measures must be considered as additions to, not substitutes for, aseptic techniques. These measures include perioperative antibiotics, although evidence for whether they reduce access infection rates remains contradictory, with some prospective studies suggesting infection rates can be decreased.[39] Even when reduced infection rates have been observed, resistant bacterial strains have resulted. There is substantial agreement, however, that perioperative antibiotics are effective in elective vascular reconstruction,[39] and we continue to administer a single dose of perioperative antibiotic, covering *S. aureus* and gram-negative organisms. Because of the prevalence of MRSE, vancomycin is often administered for one dose perioperatively.

Active infection from other sources should ideally be resolved before the implantation of vascular prostheses, and treatment to eliminate *S. aureus* carriage may be considered. Nasal staphylococcal carriage can be reduced either with oral rifampin and topical bacitracin or with topical mupirocin calcium ointment. Both regimens reduce the incidence of intravascular hemodialysis catheter sepsis, but evidence is lacking for a reduction in PTFE graft infection. This type of treatment is best reserved for patients in whom recurrent staphylococcal infection is associated with well-documented nasal staphylococcal carriage.

The site of implantation of a prosthetic graft should also be included when preventive measures are considered because infection rates and the sequelae of infection are minimized if forearm vessels, particularly the radial and ulnar, are preferred over those in the thigh.

Finally, the high incidence of infection of vascular access sites and the morbidity and mortality rates associated with access infection mandate that dialysis personnel remain constantly alert for either local or general signs of bacterial infection so that treatment may be commenced promptly.

Treatment

Established sepsis in hemodialysis access presents a major problem. Prompt treatment can both salvage access and prevent the tragedies of advanced infection, such as anastomotic disruption, hemorrhage, septic venous thrombosis, and potentially fatal blood-borne dissemination of infection. For each individual infection, achieving the appropriate balance between medical and surgical management is critical, and decisions must be made based on the type of access involved and the severity of infection.

In most access infections, antibiotic therapy plays an important role that complements rather than replaces surgical treatment. Antibiotic selection is based on the bacterial growths and sensitivities obtained from wound and blood cultures, but while sensitivities are awaited, therapy should commence with an antistaphylococcal agent appropriate to the sensitivity patterns seen in individual units. Vancomycin is usually the drug of choice for patients requiring parenteral therapy. It is normally excreted by the kidneys, with about 80% to 90% of the dose eliminated in 24 hours. In anuric patients, elimination is much delayed and drug levels should be measured because it does not dialyze. Our policy is to commence antibiotic treatment with vancomycin alone in mild to moderate infections and to add a gram-negative agent such as a third-generation cephalosporin, aminoglycoside, or carbapenem when there are severe local signs or evidence of systemic infection. These initial regimens are adjusted once cultures and sensitivity results are available. Antibiotics, if successful in reducing infection, may be required for several weeks, depending on individual circumstances, during which time, a conversion to oral preparations should occur. Surgical treatment must be considered whenever a poor response to antibiotics is observed. If the patient is intolerant or resistant to vancomycin or if response is poor, daptomycin may be used for gram-positive cocci.

Early infection of external shunts and cannulas indicated only as erythema or purulent discharge along the tubing may respond to systemic antibiotic therapy and scrupulous local care. More severe cases usually require drainage of collections and removal of the shunt or cannula. If this action is required, all ligature material should be removed because it may become chronically infected and lead to sinus formation.

Minor puncture infections and early postoperative cellulitic infections involving Brescia-Cimino fistulas may also respond to antibiotic therapy. Infected perifistula hematomas require incision and drainage, which may allow preservation of fistula function. Postoperative wound infections with deep collections, larger puncture infections in which skin cover has been lost, and rarer anastomotic infections of autologous fistulas are usually intractable problems that require ligation of the fistula and removal of anastomotic suture material.

Formation of a more proximal fistula, through a clean surgical field and using the same vessels, can often provide an early return of fistula function. The appearance of infective complications, such as false aneurysm formation, also requires urgent fistula ligation.

One of the more trying surgical challenges in vascular access surgery is the treatment of established sepsis in prosthetic grafts. Patients who have these grafts often have a limited potential for further access; therefore, each graft attains enormous importance. The loss of a graft constitutes a major setback for the patient whose life may be put at risk. Graft excision is always a safe and effective option, but graft salvage is ideal. Salvage can be achieved if management is based on assessment of the severity of infection and its location in relation to the anastomosis.

Early and superficial cellulitic infections may respond to aggressive antibiotic therapy, but deeper infections with evidence of suppuration invariably require surgical treatment and, if localized away from the anastomosis, can be managed by either graft excision or segmental bypass. Excision need not be complete because it is possible to leave a cuff of

graft adjoining the arterial anastomosis in situ after having oversewn it through a clean incision. This technique reduces risks to the artery and is associated with few complications related to the graft stump. A high rate of healing can be anticipated, and the technique provides a definitive treatment, but graft loss occurs in patients for whom access is at a premium. By contrast, segmental bypass preserves access and should be considered whenever infection is adequately localized away from the anastomoses.

To perform segmental bypass, the graft is exposed through clean wounds proximal and distal to the infected area and is divided at both sites (Fig. 24-2). A new subcutaneous tunnel is created away from the infected area, and a fresh segment of graft is interposed between the divided ends of the original graft. After the clean incisions are closed and covered, the area of infection is exposed and the infected segment is excised. The infected wound is left open and packed with gauze. The patient may continue undergoing dialysis through a segment of the original graft that remains undisturbed until the fresh segment has matured in about 3 weeks.

This procedure may be performed in one or two stages, depending on the degree of sepsis. Single-stage bypass procedures are acceptable when sepsis is well localized and particularly so if a single, chronically infected sinus is present (Fig. 24-3). Double-stage bypass is best used when the graft is involved in more widespread sepsis or when there is evidence of bacteremia. In the presence of abscesses or tis-

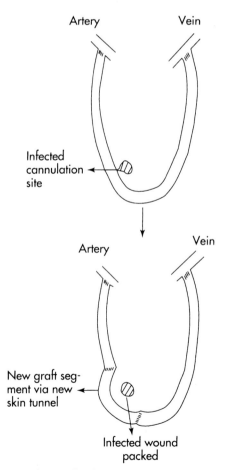

Figure 24-2.
Technique of local graft revision.

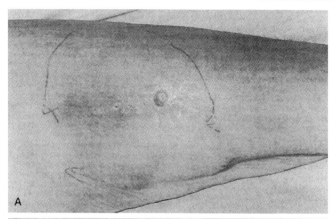

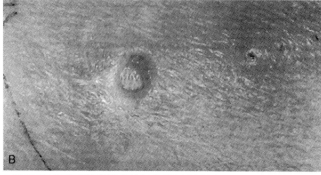

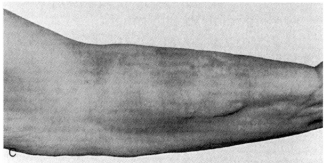

Figure 24-3.
Example of a single-stage segmental bypass to salvage an infected polytetrafluoroethylene (PTFE) arm fistula. After an infected puncture site broke down, exposing the prosthesis (A, B), a new segment of PTFE (placed approximating to the *upper arrow* in A) was used to bypass the infected area, and the infected segment was removed. C, Healing occurred, leaving the graft available for dialysis.

sue necrosis, incision and drainage should be performed as a first stage along with débridement of all inviable tissue. After 3 to 4 days, during which the wound is dressed and systemic antibiotics are administered, the bypass procedure itself is performed.

An approach to graft sepsis in which segmental bypass is used wherever possible has been reported to yield overall graft salvage rates of 50% to 60%.[40] For grafts that actually receive segmental bypass, salvage rates as high as 90% have been attained, with rates generally higher for puncture infections (77%) and erosions (90%) than for abscesses (40%). Reduced salvage rates are associated with positive blood cultures and gram-negative infections, but these effects may be reduced if double-stage procedures are used.

Graft salvage has also been reported using skin flap coverage of exposed grafts,[41] but the benefit of this technique over segmental bypass remains to be proved.

We advocate double-stage procedures. Schwab and associates detailed a series of 17 patients in whom partial infected graft excision and segmental bypass with PTFE have been successful.[42]

Segmental bypass is not without risk, and subsequent reexploration for further sepsis may be required. Some have recorded instances of severe morbidity caused by recurrent sepsis; therefore, careful follow-up of patients after these reconstructions should be standard practice. Segmental bypass can be repeated, and in this way, we maintained a number of patients with limited scope for other access.

When infection involves most of the subcutaneous graft tunnel or the anastomosis or when complications such as local hemorrhage, false aneurysm, systemic sepsis, or metastatic abscesses develop, the surgeon must be resigned to total graft excision because antibiotics and local therapy will not eradicate infection. Similarly, although most surgeons have observed healing of a superficial postoperative wound infection overlying an exposed graft (Fig. 24-4),

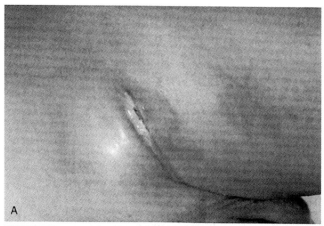

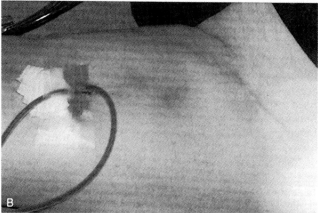

Figure 24-4.
A, A wound in the left groin became grossly infected after the insertion of a femorosaphenous PTFE arteriovenous fistula. On débridement, the prosthesis, distal to the anastomosis, became exposed in the base of the wound. The prosthesis was covered with subcutaneous tissue, the skin was loosely closed, and the patient was treated with parenteral antibiotics. B, Healing occurred, allowing the fistula to be used.

such healing is by no means common, and when major sepsis or anastomotic infection supervenes, graft excision will again be required. A delay of several days is recommended after graft excision to eliminate any associated bacteremia before implantation of a new prosthesis at a different site. Under such circumstances, either a central venous cannula or temporary peritoneal dialysis will be required.

Closing an arteriotomy after total graft excision can be problematic. Simple arteriotomy closure risks a further suture line infection, increasing the possibility of anastomotic disruption and life-threatening hemorrhage. Arterial ligation is the most secure way of addressing the problem but may cause severe ischemia. Limb ischemia is a serious problem, but this may not occur if the brachial artery is occluded distal to the profunda brachii. Mild arm claudication may result, but this can be minimized if grafts are based on the forearm vessels rather than on the brachial artery itself. This artery is then lost for future procedures. In the leg, grafts arise from the superficial femoral artery; the profunda femoris is spared, and at the time of arterial ligation, ischemia is usually limited to an acceptable degree of intermittent claudication. Nevertheless, the outcome of arterial ligation cannot always be predicted and may result in a loss of the extremity. If a small rim of prosthetic graft is left at the arteriotomy site and closed if not grossly infected, the arterial inflow is occasionally preserved and often resolves the acute process safely.

Ligation is an effective option in preventing late hemorrhage in patients requiring complete graft excision, but one may use an individualized approach to the artery after graft excision with cautious use of primary closure and vein patch repair. This approach maintains arterial continuity, but hemorrhage from disrupted suture lines is possible. Arterial continuity can also be maintained if an infected graft is replaced with the arterialized vein onto which it was anastomosed. The vein is mobilized and swung over for end-to-side anastomosis, with the arteriotomy of the excised graft allowing immediate use of the fistula. Encouraging results for this technique have been reported, and along with other closure methods, it may be useful in selected patients with recognized vascular insufficiency for whom ligation may carry high risks of ischemia. During graft excision and arterial ligation, care should be taken to avoid damage to nearby neurologic structures that may be hidden in infected debris. These structures are particularly vulnerable during emergency procedures to control hemorrhage from pseudoaneurysms. The use of a pneumatic tourniquet to reduce bleeding can be beneficial during these procedures.

An integrated protocol of segmental bypass and graft excision may minimize complications associated with prosthetic access infection. Rates for both limb loss and death are higher in patients with femoral triangle sepsis, emphasizing the importance of using the arm vessels whenever possible. Morbidity and mortality rates are also lower for grafts based on the radial and ulnar arteries than for brachial artery grafts.

Effect of Human Immunodeficiency Virus

Metropolitan health care centers have experienced an increase in patients infected with the human immunodeficiency virus (HIV) and with nephropathies related to intravenous drug abuse, either singly or in combination. Such patients are at an increased risk for all complications of vascular access surgery, including infection. Data are limited, but PTFE appears to be a principal risk factor for sepsis in these groups,[43] with significantly higher PTFE infection rates occurring in HIV-infected patients and in intravenous drug abusers than in other groups. Rates for patients with fully developed acquired immunodeficiency syndrome (AIDS) are even greater. Vancomycin prophylaxis appears to have little effect in either group. In view of these findings, PTFE grafts should be avoided in patients with AIDS and in intravenous drug abusers, and autologous vein fistulas should be constructed if at all possible. PTFE grafts may be acceptable in HIV-positive and otherwise asymptomatic individuals, but more data are required for this to be confirmed. Curi and associates[44] concluded that prosthetic graft infections were increased and patency rates are decreased in HIV-positive patients and strongly recommended autologous AV fistulas.

The overall survival of patients in these groups and particularly of those with AIDS may be limited, but most of these patients have intact fistulas at the time of death from which they have derived benefit, and these patients should not be denied access to procedures.

Hemodialysis Equipment

Microbial overgrowth in a dialysis machine has been linked to an outbreak of bloodstream infection. Multiple pathogens were associated with the removal of 23 dialysis catheters in 25 patients, and on the basis of this experience, Arnow and colleagues[45] emphasized the need for better education regarding asepsis for dialysis personnel. They concluded that percutaneous catheters amplified the risk of bloodstream infection when small numbers of bacteria were introduced during hemodialysis.

REFERENCES

1. Kjellstrand CM. The Achilles' heel of the hemodialysis patient [editorial]. *Arch Intern Med.* 1978;138:1063.
2. Nghiem DD, Schulak JA, Corry RJ. Management of the infected hemodialysis access grafts. *Trans Am Soc Artif Intern Organs.* 1983;29:360-362.
3. Lowrie EG, Lazarus JM, Mocelin AJ, et al. Survival of patients undergoing chronic hemodialysis and renal transplantation. *N Engl J Med.* 1973;288:863-867.
4. Levi J, Robson M, Rosenfeld JB. Septicaemia and pulmonary embolism complicating the use of arteriovenous fistula in maintenance haemodialysis. *Lancet.* 1970;2:288-290.
5. Raskova J, Morrison AB. A decrease in cell-mediated immunity in uremia associated with an increase in activity of suppressor cells. *Am J Pathol.* 1976;84:1-10.
6. McIntosh J, Hansen P, Ziegler J, Penny R. Defective immune and phagocytic functions in uremia and transplantation. *Int Arch Allergy Appl Immunol.* 1976;51:544-559.
7. Gowland G, Smiddy FG: The effect of acute experimental uraemia on the immunological responses of the rabbit to bovine serum albumin. *Br J Urol.* 1962;34:274-279.
8. Sengar DPS, Rashid A, Harris JE. In vitro cellular immunity and in vivo delayed hypersensitivity in uremic patients maintained on hemodialysis. *Int Arch Allergy Appl Immunol.* 1974;47:829-838.
9. Alexiewicz JM, Smogorzewski M, Fadda GZ, Massry SG. Impaired phagocytosis in dialysis patients: studies on mechanisms. *Am J Nephrol.* 1991;11:102-111.

10. Hallgren R, Fjellström KE, Håkansson L, Venge P. Kinetic studies of phagocytosis. II. The serum-independent uptake of IgG-coated particles by polymorphonuclear leucocytes from uremic patients on regular dialysis treatment. *J Lab Clin Med.* 1979;94:277-284.

11. Haag-Weber M, Hörl WH. Uremia and infection: mechanisms of impaired cellular host defense. *Nephron.* 1993;63:125-131.

12. Raskova J, Ghobrial I, Shea SM, Eisinger RP, Raska K Jr. Suppressor cells in end-stage renal disease. *Am J Med.* 1984;76:847-853.

13. Meshulam T, Diamond RD, Lyman CA, Wysong DR, Melnick DA. Temporal association of calcium mobilization, inositol triphosphate generation, and superoxide anion release by human neutrophils activated by serum opsonized and nonopsonized particulate stimuli. *Biochem Biophys Res Commun.* 1988;150:532-539.

14. Haag-Weber M, Mai B, Hörl WH. Effect of hemodialysis on intracellular calcium in human polymorphonuclear neutrophils. *Miner Electrolyte Metab.* 1992;18:151-155.

15. van Asbeck BS, Marx JJ, Struyvenberg A, van Kats JH, Verhoef J. Effect of iron (III) in the presence of various ligands on the phagocytic and metabolic activity of human polymorphonuclear leukocytes. *J Immunol.* 1984;132:851-856.

16. Briggs WA, Pedersen MM, Mahajan SK, Sillix DH, Prasad AS, McDonald FD. Lymphocyte and granulocyte function in zinc-treated and zinc-deficient haemodialysis patients. *Kidney Int.* 1982;21:827-832.

17. Bell JD, Kincaid WR, Morgan RG, et al. Serum ferritin assay and bone marrow iron stores in patients on maintenance dialysis. *Kidney Int.* 1980;17:237-241.

18. Boelaert JR, Cantinieaux BF, Hariga CF, Fondu PG. Recombinant erythropoietin reverses polymorphonuclear granulocyte dysfunction in iron-overloaded dialysis patients. *Nephrol Dial Transplant.* 1990; 5:504-517.

19. Boelaert JR, van Landuyt HW, Valcke YL, et al. The role of iron overload in *Yersinia enterocolitica* and *Yersinia pseudotuberculosis* bacteremia in hemodialysis patients. *J Infect Dis.* 1987;156:384-387.

20. Bender BS, Curtis JL, Nagel JE, et al. Analysis of immune status of hemodialyzed adults: association with prior transfusions. *Kidney Int.* 1984;26:436-443.

21. Raska K, Raskova J, Shea SM, et al. T cell subsets and cellular immunity in end-stage renal disease. *Am J Med.* 1983;75:734-740.

22. Holdsworth SR, Fitzgerald MG, Hosking CS, Atkins RC. The effect of maintenance dialysis on lymphocyte function. I. Haemodialysis. *Clin Exp Immunol.* 1978;33:95-101.

23. Antoniou LD, Shalhoub RJ. Zinc-induced enhancement of lymphocyte function and viability in chronic uremia. *Nephron.* 1985;40:14-21.

24. Goldblum SE, Van Epps DE, Reed WP. Serum inhibitor of CF fragment-mediated polymorphonuclear leucocyte chemotaxis associated with chronic hemodialysis. *J Clin Invest.* 1979;64:255-264.

25. Cosio FG, Giebink GS, Le CT, Schiffman G. Pneumococcal vaccination in patients with chronic renal disease and renal allograft recipients. *Kidney Int.* 1981;20:254-258.

26. Clark RA, Hamory BH, Ford GH, Kimball HR. Chemotaxis in acute renal failure. *J Infect Dis.* 1972;126:460-463.

27. Toren M, Goffinet JA, Kaplow LS. Pulmonary bed sequestration of neutrophils during hemodialysis. *Blood.* 1970;36:337-340.

28. Akhondzadeh L, Wilson SE, William A, Owens ML. Infection of materials used in vascular access surgery: an evaluation of Dacron, bovine heterograft, Teflon, and human umbilical vein grafts. *Dial Transplant.* 1980;9:697-701.

29. Buckels JAC, Noardestgaard AG, Wilson SE. Microporous vascular grafts do not require neointima for resistance to bacteremic infection. *J Vasc Surg.* 1987;5:198-202.

30. Morgan AP, Knight DC, Tilney NL, Lazarus JM. Femoral triangle sepsis in dialysis patients: Frequency, management and outcome. *Ann Surg.* 1980;191:460-464.

31. Centers for Disease Control and Prevention (CDC). Invasive methicillin-resistant *Staphylococcus aureus* infections among dialysis patients—United States, 2005. *MMWR Morb Mortal Wkly Rep.* 2007; 56:197-199.

32. Lowy FD, Hammer SM. *Staphylococcal epidermidis* infections. *Ann Intern Med.* 1983;99:834-839.

33. Pop-Vicas A, Strom J, Stanley K, D'Agata EM. Multidrug-resistant gram-negative bacteria among patients who require chronic hemodialysis. *Clin J Am Soc Nephrol.* 2008;3:752-758.

34. Bayston R, Penny SR. Excessive production of mucoid substance in staphylococcal SIIA: a possible factor in the colonisation of Holter shunts. *Dev Med Child Neurol Suppl.* 1972;27:25-28.

35. Steenbergen JN, Alder J, Thorne GM, Tally FP. Daptomycin: a lipopeptide antibiotic for the treatment of serious Gram-positive infections. *J Antimicrob Chemother.* 2005;55:283-288.

36. Rose W, Rybeck M. Tigecycline: first of a new class of antimicrobial agents. *Pharmacotherapy.* 2006;26:1099-1110.

37. Darouiche RO, Raad II, Heard SO, et al: A comparison of two antimicrobial-impregnated central venous catheters. Catheter Study Group. *N Engl J Med.* 1999;340:1-8.

38. Bunt TJ. Synthetic vascular graft infections. I. Graft infections. *Surgery.* 1983;93:933-746.

39. Bennion RS, Hiatt JR, Williams RA, Wilson SE. A randomized, prospective study of perioperative antimicrobial prophylaxis for vascular access surgery. *J Cardiovasc Surg.* 1985;26:270-274.

40. Bhat DJI, Tellis VA, Kohlberg WI, Driscoll B, Veith FJ. Management of sepsis involving expanded polytetrafluoroethylene grafts for hemodialysis. *Surgery.* 1980;87:445-450.

41. Tellis VA, Weiss P, Matas AJ, Veith FJ. Skin-flap coverage of polytetrafluoroethylene vascular access graft exposed by previous infection. *Surgery.* 1988;103:118-121.

42. Schwab DP, Taylor SM, Cull DL, et al. Isolated arteriovenous dialysis access graft segment infection: the results of segmental bypass and partial graft excision. *Ann Vasc Surg.* 2000;14:63-66.

43. Brock JS, Sussman M, Wamsley M, Mintzer R, Baumann FG, Riles TS. The influence of human immunodeficiency virus infection and intravenous drug abuse on complications of hemodialysis access surgery. *J Vasc Surg.* 1992;16:904-910.

44. Curi MA, Pappas PJ, Silva MB Jr, et al. Hemodialysis access: influence of the human immunodeficiency virus on patency and infection rates. *J Vasc Surg.* 1999;29:608-616.

45. Arnow PM, Garcia-Houchins S, Neagle MB, Bova JL, Dillon JJ, Chou T. An outbreak of bloodstream infections arising from hemodialysis equipment. *J Infect Dis.* 1998;178:783-791.

Assessment and Intervention for Arteriovenous Fistula Maturation

Ankit Bharat and Surendra Shenoy

The mortality rate for hemodialysis (HD) patients has fallen by 21% since 1986 due to an overall improvement in the management of patients with end-stage renal disease (ESRD).[1] Because patients with ESRD are living longer, the need for reliable, long-term HD vascular access remains critical.

Arteriovenous fistulas (AVFs) have been shown to be superior to arteriovenous grafts (AVGs) for HD but both are superior to central venous catheters (CVCs). The National Kidney Foundation Kidney Disease Outcome Quality Initiative (NKF-K/DOQI) guidelines recommend the use of AVFs, AVGs, and CVCs, in 50%, 40%, and 10% of patients, respectively, for HD.[2] Further, the Fistula First campaign has stipulated that patients be referred to surgery for "fistula-only" evaluations.

The push for the fistula-first approach has been associated with an increase in CVC dependency, possibly due to prolonged fistula maturation times and poorly functioning fistulas. Although AVFs have been shown to be superior to AVGs and CVCs have lower thrombotic complications with decreased morbidity and mortality in certain HD populations, they continue to have a higher primary failure rate.[3-6] However, there is very little literature that directly addresses the problem of nonmature fistulas, fistula maturation evaluation, and secondary procedures to promote fistula maturation. This chapter discusses approaches to promoting early fistula maturation and methods of evaluating AVF maturation as well as secondary interventions for AVF.

Definition and Characteristics of a Well-Functioning Fistula

A well-functioning (mature) fistula can be defined as "a subcutaneous conduit that is capable of delivering flows necessary for adequate dialysis."[7] Depending on the type of HD prescribed (ie, intermittent three times a week or intermittent daily), flow rates for dialysis vary between 100 to 500mL/min. In the United States, a majority of patients undergo intermittent HD performed three times a week with average flow rates of 350 to 500 mL/min. A mature fistula should be capable of providing these flows. Thus, intra-access blood flow becomes the most important determinant of AVF maturation. The other determinant includes the quality of the cannulation segment, which determines the ease of cannulation.

Blood Flow

When the flow in the fistula is low, the supple vein wall tends to collapse as the dialysis pump flow approaches intra-access flow. For this reason, to deliver a flow of 350 to 500mL/min required for dialysis, the AVF flow should be at least 250 to 300 mL more than the dialysis flow rate. The additional baseline fistula blood flow is necessary to prevent collapsing of the cannulation segment during dialysis. Thus, it is reasonable to expect a minimum flow of 600 mL/min in an AVF. Most well-functioning AVFs have flow ranging between 800 and 1000 mL/min.

The normal blood flow to the upper extremity, as determined by blood flow measurements in the brachial artery in an ESRD patient, without an arteriovenous (AV) access ranges between 6 and 78 mL/min (mean, 31 mL/min). With the creation of an AVF, there is a 10- to 40-fold increase in the flow to the limb and this is determined by the capacity of the heart to generate an increased cardiac output to overcome the loss of resistance resulting from creation of the AV anastomosis and to provide adequate circulation to the extremity beyond the anastomotic site.[8] The quality of the arterial wall and its capability to distend play an important role in providing the flow increase because the rate of flow is determined the diameter, the length of the artery, and the viscosity of the blood at any given blood pressure. Therefore, in medium-sized artery such as the radial artery, the quality of the vessel wall and its capability to dilate and accommodate the increased flow play a critical role in the maturation of the AVF.

Cannulation Segment

The diameter and depth of the cannulation segment also is an equally important maturation characteristic for an AVF. This becomes even more important because the current practice of dialysis access does not mandate any image guidance. Dialysis personnel carry out access cannulation through palpation of the cannulation segment for a pulse after applying a proximal tourniquet. This makes the technique more subjective because it depends on the size and depth of the fistula and the experience of the person cannulating and can pose an even greater problem when veins are narrow and deep. This is often responsible for infiltration and cannulation complications that result in mistrust between patients and caregivers. It also results in abandonment of AVF use as an

Table 25–1

Objective fistula maturation criteria

Flow	>600 mL/min
Cannulation segment	>10 cm long or two 4-cm segments >6 mm in diameter <5 mm deep from skin surface

access that is difficult to cannulate. Optimizing the length, diameter, and depth of the cannulation segment can make this process less subjective and more optimal.

When a cannulation segment is straight, it should be a minimum of 10 cm long. If the outflow vein is tortuous, there should be two straight segments that are at least 4 cm in length. These criteria allow placement of two needles with their tips far enough apart to prevent recirculation with standard pump flows. A cannulation segment diameter greater than 6 mm should provide for better accessibility because most AVGs are conventionally 6 mm in diameter. Lastly, from measuring these parameters in a large cohort of patients, we have learned that cannulation becomes increasingly difficult as the depth of the vein exceeds 5 mm from the skin surface. Hence, a cannulation segment less than 5 mm deep from the skin is more optimal. Table 25-1 outlines the objective maturation characteristics set for the evaluation of an AVF. Although none of these is absolute, these parameters provide an objective guideline to assess AVF maturation.

The 2005 NKF-K/DOQI Guidelines for Vascular Access[9] refer to these attributes as "The Rule of 6s," that is, 600 mL/min blood flow, 6 mm diameter, and 6 mm depth.

Determinants of Fistula Maturation

The maturation and function of a fistula depends on several factors. These can be classified as anatomic, surgical, and circulatory.[7] The anatomic factor includes the inflow artery, the cannulation segment of the vein (or conduit), and the outflow vein (vein between needle stick segment and central vein). Although all three have a distinct bearing on fistula maturation, the contribution of an individual component is not predictable because they are influenced by factors such as surgical technique, blood pressure, quality of the vessel wall, presence of collaterals, and rheology of the blood. Maturation of AVFs has been referred to as *arterialization* of the vein wall following surgical anastomosis to the artery.[10] Although conventionally arterialization has been described as thickening of the vein wall making it more robust to withstand cannulation, in practicality, the success of a fistula depends more on the blood flow, diameter, length, and depth of the cannulation segment. Therefore, the quality (size and distensibility) of the inflow artery and quality (size, distensibility, and length) of the outflow vein become most important determinants of AVF maturation.

Large-caliber arteries (brachial or larger) are usually capable of accommodating the increased blood flow resulting from AV anastomosis because their diameter is capable of accommodating the increased flow. But a medium-sized artery with significant calcification, as in the case of a calcified radial artery that is only 2 to 2.5 mm in diameter, is unlikely to handle the increased flow required for a well-functioning fistula. For this reason, it is not unusual in clinical practice to encounter fistulas that are patent but are not suitable for dialysis and collapse despite having adequate-sized outflow veins. This is often a result of low blood flow in the fistula. Using preoperative ultrasound vessel mapping provides the surgeon an opportunity to evaluate not only the outflow veins but also the size and quality of the inflow artery that needs to provide the flow necessary for the maturation of AVF. Thus, using ultrasound to complement clinical examination during preoperative patient assessment plays a crucial role in evaluating this determinant of fistula maturation.[11] The role of provocative testing to objectively evaluate the inflow artery is not yet an established approach.[12,13]

Similar to the inflow artery, intrinsically diseased veins (chronic thrombosis and recanalization from old needle sticks) with short- or long-segment stenosis intervene with fistula flow owing to an inability to distend in response to the increased flow. A comprehensive preoperative patient evaluation including ultrasound mapping sometimes helps to identify such situations, thereby reducing the incidence of AVF maturation failure due to anatomic flow restrictions caused by preexisting disease in the vessels.

Surgical technique plays an important role in fistula maturation. A fistula created with proper preoperative evaluation and with good surgical technique should mature in 4 to 6 weeks.[8,14] There is also emerging evidence to suggest that recognition of outflow vein problems, and early intervention may increase rates of fistula maturation. Rheologic factors such as increased viscosity and thrombophilic states do influence access maturation. In a recent study, clopidogrel, an antiplatelet agent, showed efficacy in increasing AVF patency but did not have any effect on maturation.[15] The role of uremia and associated platelet dysfunction is well exemplified by the fact that fistulas and grafts fail over a period of time after the patient's renal function is normalized as seen in patients who receive renal transplants. However, the exact impact of these factors on fistula maturation cannot be objectively quantified.

Fistula Failure

As previously discussed, NKF-K/DOQI vascular access guidelines propose that AVF is the best access for providing HD.[2] However, published literature has demonstrated a high fistula failure rate ranging from 28% to 53%.[16-20] An AVF that fails early can be defined as an AVF that has thrombosed after creation or has never matured to support successful dialysis.[21] Several mechanisms contribute to fistula failure (Fig. 25-1) Starting with the capability of the heart to increase the output, quality of inflow artery, surgical anastomotic technique, configuration, development of juxta-anastomotic stenosis (JAS), outflow vein stenosis, and circulatory factors contribute to maturation failure.

Failure of Arterial Dilatation

AVF creation results in an increase in shear stress that leads to vascular dilatation in order to bring the wall stress back to normal. However, when the vessel wall is diseased, for example, in a calcified vessel of an elderly uremic patient

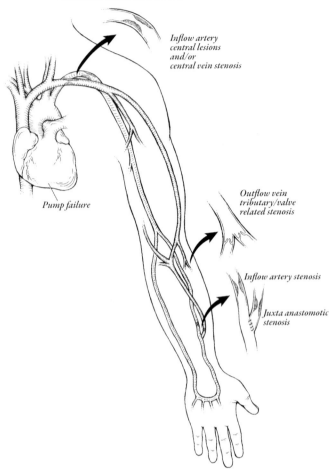

*Inflow artery
central lesions
and/or
central vein stenosis*

Pump failure

*Outflow vein
tributary/valve
related stenosis*

Inflow artery stenosis

*Juxta anastomotic
stenosis*

Figure 25-1.
Factors leading to maturation failure.

with diabetes, the ability to secrete mediators required for vasodilatation is diminished. Moreover, circumferential calcification acts as a fixed stenotic segment preventing any diltation of the vessel at this point. This results in inability of the artery to dilate to provide increased flow necessary for the outflow vein dilatation. Low flows in a fistula are most often the result of inability of the artery to dilate due to diffuse disease or occasionally due to a critical flow-limiting stenosis situated more centrally in the arterial circulation. A preoperative ultrasound evaluation is very useful to assess the quality of the artery in the periphery. Comparing the blood pressure in the extremity helps to determine a flow-limiting central stenosis.

Failure of Venous Dilatation

Factors that lead to failure of arterial dilatation can also apply to the veins. Furthermore, selection of an improper venous segment that has lost its ability to vasodilate, such as recanalized veins with wall thickening from previous chronic thrombosis or veins with scarred valve leaflets from old needle stick injuries, can also lead to fistula failure. In addition, genetic polymorphisms for mediators involved in vasodilatation could play a role in problems with arterial and venous dilation.

Accelerated Venous Neointimal Hyperplasia

Different configurations of AVF creation result in differing levels of shear stress in the venous segment. For example, there may be low shear stress at the AV anastomosis because of differences in compliance between the artery and the vein. The response of the vessel wall to the increased flow and shear stress could vary based on the configuration of the outflow vein. Thus, JAS has a tendency to develop in the area of torsion in radiocephalic fistula.[22,23] JAS is currently the single most important reason for an AVF to fail to mature. Furthermore, the impact of vascular injury resulting from trauma of skeletonization and use of vascular clamps, impact of vessel and tissue edema from inflammation, hematoma, and seroma formation are some of the many surgical variables that could affect access maturation.

Dilatation of the outflow veins results in alteration in the configuration of the venous valves, resulting in altered valve dynamics. An unfavorable alteration resulting in flow restriction could precipitate vessel wall injury due to flow jets. It is not unusual to encounter midfistula stenosis in otherwise normally developing outflow veins; these are almost always seen in the vicinity of a valve or near the entry point of a tributary.

Maturation of the AVF starts almost immediately following creation. It has been demonstrated that soon after fistula creation, there is significant increase in the blood flow. Won and coworkers[20] investigated radiocephalic fistulas and showed an increase in flow from 20.9 ± 1.1 mL/min in the radial artery to 174 ± 13.2 mL/min only 10 minutes after completion of the anastomosis. Similarly, Yerdel and colleagues[24] demonstrated that blood flow increased to 539 ± 276 and 848 ± 565 mL/min at postoperative day 1 and week 1, respectively. Other data also support changes in the diameter of an AVF postoperatively. Lin and associates[25] published a prospective analysis of 152 successful radiocephalic fistulas that found augmentation of AVF blood flow and cross-sectional area as early as 2 weeks. Robbin and coworkers[26] determined the minimum venous diameter and blood flow for predicting AVF outcomes. They showed that a venous diameter of 0.4 cm correlated with a 67% adequacy of fistulas for dialysis and a blood flow rate of at least 500 mL/min was associated with an adequate AVF in 70% of cases. Furthermore, when both variables were met, 95% of fistulas were adequate for dialysis.

AVF that are going to mature will do so within the first 3 to 6 weeks. Therefore, all AVF should be evaluated within this timeframe after creation. The majority of fistulas with early failure demonstrate stenotic lesions within the access circuit.[14] It is important to emphasize that vascular stenosis can be progressive. Therefore, a low-grade stenosis can eventually culminate into complete occlusion. Failure to recognize problems early may result in lost opportunities to salvage fistulas. Both identification of early failure and corrective measures are important. Hence, postoperative follow-up and evaluation of fistula maturation should be an integral part of AVF creation. Fistula procedures should not be considered complete until the fistula has been successfully used for dialysis.

Fistula Maturation Evaluation

Following fistula creation, the patient should be evaluated approximately 10 to 14 days after surgery. A thorough clinical evaluation during this visit helps to identify problems such as infection and vascular or neurologic complications that can occasionally develop after an access surgery. It also gives the surgeon an opportunity to identify any stenotic problems in the outflow vein from old needle trauma or valve inflammation that is unmasked by the increasing flow. When identified, these are easily fixable with early surgical or radiologic intervention, thereby helping early fistula maturation.

The second postoperative evaluation of the fistula should be performed at 4 weeks. This is true maturation evaluation in which the clinician utilizes duplex ultrasound for objective evaluation to assess the fistula maturation pattern in conjunction with a thorough clinical examination. During this examination, a decision is made whether the fistula is ready for use or will need a secondary procedure to make it suitable for dialysis use.

Clinical Examination

Clinical examinations provide reliable information on fistulas that are constructed in patients who are ideal candidates and have well-developing fistula. A normal mature AVF has a thrill that may be felt 6 to 8 cm beyond the anastomosis during both phases of the cardiac cycle and a complete absence of pulse. A normal-functioning fistula is easily compressible, and elevation of the limb above the level of the heart makes the bulge of the outflow vein disappear. The thrill completely disappears and is replaced by a strong pulse when the outflow vein is occluded more centrally beyond the cannulation segment.

Careful clinical examination can easily identify subtle problems such as intra-access stenosis in the cannulation segment. This manifests as a pulsatile flow that changes to a thrill just beyond the point of stenosis, with the pulse being strongest just proximal to the stenosis. Often, this finding is subtle and can be easily missed.

Conversely, a JAS usually presents as a bounding pulse felt at the anastomosis. As one moves distally, the pulse disappears at the site of maximum stenosis and a thrill is felt beyond. Depending on the rapidity and degree of stenosis, outflow vein development is varied. When the arm is elevated, one sees a pulse at and beyond the anastomosis with complete collapse of the rest of the cannulation segment.

The strength of the pulse in a fistula when the outflow is occluded is directly proportional to the arterial inflow pressure. The pulse augmentation test[14] can be used to evaluate the stenosis. It is performed by completely occluding the access several centimeters downstream from the arterial anastomosis and assessing the increment in the volume of the pulse by palpation. A normal AVF augments well, or in other words, has a strong pulse that indicates good arterial inflow. In contrast, the AVF that has a poor arterial inflow will be found to augment poorly.

Accessory veins also can be identified at times by visual inspection. Palpation can provide further sensitivity to detect their presence. Occlusion of the main outflow of an AVF should result in disappearance of the thrill. Failure of such an occurrence suggests the presence of an accessory outflow vein between the point of digital occlusion and the fistula anastomosis. With downstream stenosis (central stenosis), AVFs become more forcefully pulsatile (hyperpulsatile) with a discontinuous and predominantly systolic thrill. When the extremity is elevated, the portion of the AVF distal to the stenosis remains distended while the proximal portion collapses in the normal manner. Flow in the fistula with the main outflow stenosis depends on presence of collaterals. For this reason, fistulas with stenosis beyond the cannulation segments (stenosis farther away from the anastomosis) tend to have better preserved flows but higher intra-access pressure. Swelling of the extremity is also an important physical finding. Persistent swelling of the upper extremity after AVF creation is suggestive of central vein stenosis and deserves evaluation. Swelling of the distal extremity is the result of venous hypertension that is entirely dependent on the fistula blood flow, degree of stenosis in the main outflow vein, and status of collaterals. It is also not unusual to encounter an occasional patient with a functioning fistula in the arm without any swelling despite having a complete occlusion of the central vein.

Thus, a carefully performed clinical examination provides significant information that often may be sufficient in planning necessary intervention. This information can also lead the examiner toward the area of that problem that may require further evaluation. Studies have reported overall accuracy of physical examination to be about 80%. This compared favorably with the 67% and 70% adequacy when only AVF diameter ($\geq$0.4 cm) or blood flow ($\geq$500 mL/min) on ultrasound is met.[19]

Clinical examination, however, has several limitations. Whereas it is a very useful tool in identifying subtle obstructive outflow problems, it is a very poor tool to evaluate the anatomic reason for the problem as well as the actual physiologic compensatory mechanisms (ie, collateral circulatory pattern). Often, one or both of these parameters play an important role in determining the interventions necessary to help fistula maturation. Clinical examinaiton is also not reliable in situations in which the outflow veins are deeply situated. Further, clinical examinations are often subjective and depend on the experience of the examiner. Hence, a fistula maturation evaluation clinical examination should always be followed by duplex ultrasound for maturation evaluation.

Duplex Ultrasound Examination

Ultrasonography adds an entirely new dimension to fistula maturation evaluation. This not only helps to further evaluate the problems identified on physical examination but also provides objective information on the length, depth, and diameter of the cannulation segment. When combined with duplex, Doppler ultrasound provides an excellent estimate of the intra-access flow (see Chapter 30). Whereas measuring the flow in the cannulation segment (vein) is not reliable, measuring the flow in the inflow artery to the extremity (brachial or axillary) is very reliable and reproducible. For this reason, we prefer measurement of brachial artery flow, which provides an indirect estimate of the AVF flow. Hence, a duplex ultrasound evaluation should follow clinical evaluation as part of the fistula maturation evaluation.

Interpretation of Maturation Evaluation

Depending on the maturation evaluations, at week 4, fistulas can be categorized as one of the following (Fig. 25-2):

Group I—Fistulas that meet all the objective maturation criteria (see Table 25-1). These fistulas are ready for use without any further evaluation.

Group II—Fistulas that are maturing well (ie, close to but not meeting all maturation criteria). These fistulas need to be carefully evaluated with clinical and ultrasound evaluation to make sure that subtle problems are not missed. In the absence of any detectable problems, they should be followed for a further period of 4 weeks and reassessed. A small percentage of patients belong to this category. During the repeated evaluation, they usually shift to group I, remain unchanged, or deteriorate. The latter two events would require *further evaluation*.

Group III—This is the most common group with the fistula meeting flow criteria with excellent brachial artery (feeding artery to the limb) flows but the outflow veins do not meet the maturation criteria. Most of the outflow veins are of adequate diameter but situated deep from the skin surface. A few have branched outflow veins or outflow veins collateralizing owing to a stenosis/blockage in the main outflow vein. These fistulas may need *further evaluation* but certainly need *secondary intervention* to make them suitable for use.

Group IV—Fistulas that have flows greater than 400mL/min. This happens in fistulas that have obvious clinically identifiable problems in the cannulation segment (such as JAS or outflow vein occlusion with inadequate collateralization). This can also happen when a poor-quality small-caliber artery (calcified radial) was used to provide inflow or the artery has previously unrecognized proximal stenotic problem. In either case, these fistulas need immediate *further evaluation*.

Some of the problems identified during maturation evaluation using clinical examination and duplex ultrasound evaluation need surgical intervention without further evaluation. Many of them, however, need *further evaluation* with fistulogram. For fistulas with low flow, a fistulogram should

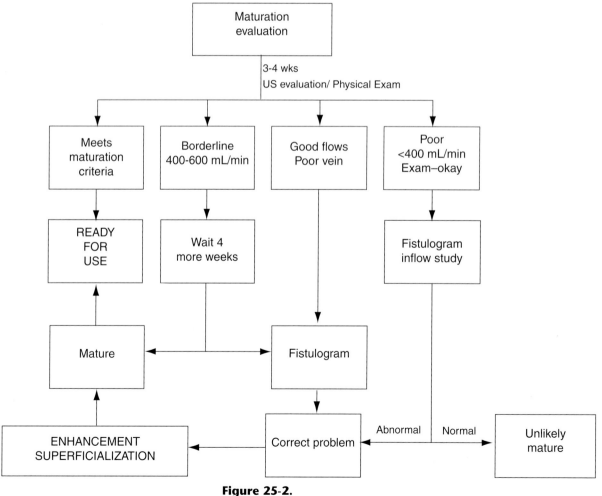

Figure 25-2.
Fistula maturation evaluation.

always pay special attention to complete evaluation of the inflow artery. Most often this can be achieved by negotiating the angiographic catheter through the AVF anastomosis in a retrograde fashion all the way up to the aortic arch and performing an adequate evaluation of the arterial tree. Decisions for secondary intervention should be based on the findings of this evaluation. Certain secondary interventions may be performed during the fistulogram.

Secondary Interventions for AVF Maturation

Secondary interventions that help fistulas meet maturation criteria can be either interventional or surgical. Whereas for some maturation problems, the decision of modality is clear, in other situations, the decision may depend upon expertise and experience available. In the following paragraphs, we attempt to address some of these scenarios and describe some useful procedures and guidelines that may be used to increase fistula maturation based on problems identified at maturation evaluation.

Low Flows Secondary to Inflow Artery Stenosis

Well-defined stenosis in the central artery is considered a favorable lesion for angioplasty or stenting and can be managed with radiologic intervention alone. As a general rule, angioplasty should be offered as the first intervention unless there is clear evidence that a stent is necessary and beneficial. Whereas stents have some proven benefit in large arteries, there is not much literature on successful long-term outcome using stents. Stenotic segments in smaller arteries have been successfully dilated with balloon angioplasty. Some of these lesions are surgically correctable with patch angioplasty.

JAS and Cannulation Segment Stenosis

In the setting of radiocephalic fistulas, JAS is the single most common cause of fistula failure.[19,21,27] This stenosis typically occurs in the outflow vein within 1 to 4 cm of the anastomosis. Although not very well documented, many stenoses develop early after fistula creation. There is also some suggestion that many go unnoticed and eventually lead to aggressively early fistula thrombosis. Successful interventional and radiologic approaches have been described to manage JAS. Early intervention is the most important part of their management. When recognized early, these lesions have been treated with balloon angioplasty.[14,21] However, when recognized early, balloon angioplasty often may not be very attractive because the veins are not well dilated and interventions are more difficult. Whereas surgical repair usually involves using autologous vein patch to widen this narrowed segment, attempting a balloon angioplasty may avert an early surgical intervention and help dilatation of outflow vein. Angioplasty also provides the surgeon a good road map of the entire fistula cir-

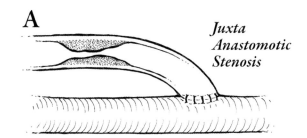

Juxta Anastomotic Stenosis

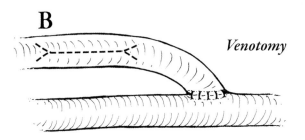

Venotomy

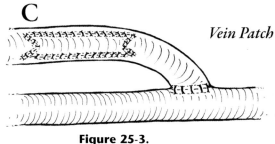

Vein Patch

Figure 25-3.
Vein patch venoplasty.

cuit, which is often useful to plan surgical interventions. A surgical approach can be contemplated in patients who fail to respond to angioplasty but otherwise have a healthy outflow vein (Fig. 25-3).

Cannulation Segment Stenosis

Cannulation segment stenoses are often short-segment stenosis. More frequently, they start as point stenosis at the site of venous valves. When left untreated, they tend to progress into longer-segmental stenosis. Some emergent data suggest that early intervention for these stenoses provides for fistula maturation. However, long-term observational follow-up data are not available. The anatomic structure of the vein wall is different at valve base and valve pillars. As a result, the rate of dilatation of a normal vein wall and that of vein walls in the region of the valve are different. This alters the function of the valve. An unfavorable functional alteration could result in alteration of blood flow resulting in valve and vein wall injury and lead to development of a stenosis. It is not uncommon to encounter such stenosis in a developing AVF often in the close vicinity of a valve near the entry of a vein tributary. With the use of ultrasound for postoperative evaluation, one can easily identify these problems.

In the presence of good access flow, early lesions can be easily missed. However, when identified with careful angiographic evaluation, they respond well to balloon angioplasty. Longer segmental stenoses tend to recur. There are no good long-term data on interventional management of these problems. For such stenosis, it is a good clinical strategy to use radiologically guided venoplasty as the first-line management. This would provide the fistula an opportunity to successfully mature. Decisions regarding further management of the problem depend on the response to angioplasty and time of recurrence (early-poor result vs. late-good result), state of maturation of AVF (maturing well vs. not maturing AVF despite first successful intervention), and the collateral autologous materials available to plan a repair.

If the angioplasty fails early (within 3 mo) in an otherwise well-maturing fistula, it is reasonable to offer surgical venoplasty, especially when there are collateral veins available for reconstruction of the stenotic segment. Peripheral vein stents should be avoided under all circumstances because they eliminate the option of surgical repair. Whereas recurrent stenosis in a surgically performed venoplasty still keeps the option of balloon venoplasty open, some data suggest better results for angioplasty after a surgical repair.[28,29] Stents should be reserved only for peripheral vein lesions with failed surgical repairs. This approach provides the patient with the best opportunity to maximize the utility of an AVF.

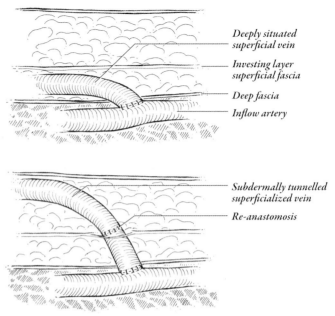

Figure 25-4.
Vein superficialization by retunneling.

Secondary Surgical Procedures

Group II is the largest group in our patient population with nonmature fistulas. These are patients with good flows with cannulation segments that do not meet maturation criteria. In addition, these patients have the best chance of fistula maturation with a secondary surgical procedure. We describe two techniques that have been successfully used for this purpose.

Vein Superficialization

Anatomically, the superficial veins are situated at an investing layer of superficial fascia in the subcutaneous tissue. However, this depth could be variable in a given individual depending on the subcutaneous fat. Use of these deeply situated superficial veins has increased owing to the ability of the ultrasound to visualize them during preoperative vein mapping. However, many patients have deeply situated enlarged outflow veins with excellent blood flow that is difficult to cannulate. Owing to the lack of defined maturation evaluation criteria, fistulas with such outflow veins are often the cause of frustration to the patient and dialysis personnel. Vein superficialization is a very useful technique to overcome these cannulation problems and increase the success of AVF maturation.

The technique involves use of intraoperative ultrasound to mark the path of the outflow vein. The surgeon then marks the proposed site for vein superficialization. Based on these plans, the surgeon places the incision required to mobilize the outflow vein and the technique used for superficialization. For an outflow vein that meets the diameter criteria (>6 mm) with very few tributaries, mobilization

may be achieved with two well-placed, small incisions that allow complete mobilization. Once mobilized, the vein is divided at one of the two incisions, released out from underneath the skin flap between the two incisions, retunneled in a subdermal plain, and reanastomosed to maintain venous continuity (Fig. 25-4). The outflow vein may require enhancement if it has many tributaries or is of marginal size. If it has a stenotic area, it will require reconstruction of the mobilization. Reconstruction may be performed using a single incision to raise a skin flap and dissect out the vein. Once the vein is reconstructed, a subdermal groove is created, and the reconstructed vein is placed in this groove and supported in place using fat pads from either side (Fig. 25-5).

Vein Enhancement

This procedure is useful for fistulas that have good blood flow. As determined by brachial artery flow measurements, outflow veins can be branched or have outflow vein stenosis with collateralization. The goal of the enhancement procedure is to construct a tubular segment of vein that is approximately 10 cm long. This tubular segment is constructed using tributaries and collateral veins that are available, which helps channelize inflow into one segment. The segment is placed in the subdermal groove as in a superficialization procedure; this procedure requires complete evaluation of the outflow venous anatomy using ultrasound mapping and venograms when necessary for the operating surgeon to plan an often extensive reconstruction. Patients are reevaluated for assessment of maturation 5 to 6 weeks after the procedure to allow the flap to heal and the vein to establish a new domicile. Figure 25-6 demonstrates one such procedure performed in a patient with anatomic snuffbox fistula. The 4-week follow-up clinical evaluation failed to identify the second tributary and revealed a poorly maturing fistula. An ultrasound performed as a complement to the

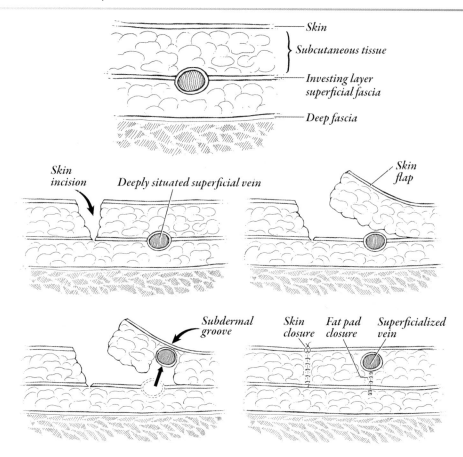

Figure 25-5.
Vein elevation under skin flap.

clinical examination revealed that the outflow vein dividing into two tributaries each measuring 3 and 4 mm, respectively. Evaluation with Doppler duplex ultrasound demonstrated a blood flow of 1100 mL/min in the brachial artery. The fistula was revised at a second stage procedure in which a long-segment vein enhancement procedure was performed by splaying open both the tributaries. The outflow vein now measured 8 to 9 mm with all the flow channeled into one single tube. This was placed underneath the skin flap. The fistula was accessed 5 weeks after the second procedure, and this fistula has required no further interventions in the past 2 years.

Tributary/Collateral Ligation

In a prospective study, percutaneous balloon angioplasty and accessory vein obliteration using one of three techniques (percutaneous ligation using 3-0 nylon, venous cutdown, or coil insertion) were used to salvage the failed AVF. The success after angioplasty was 98% and after vein obliteration about 100%. After intervention, it was possible to initiate dialysis using the AVF in 92% of the cases. Further follow-up revealed that 84% were functional at 3 months, 72% at 6 months, and 68% at 12 months. All adverse events were associated with angioplasty procedures.[21] Percutaneous ligation techniques have been described for accessory

veins.[27] In another study, Turmel-Rodrigues and colleagues[30] demonstrated the successful application of endovascular techniques to salvage AVFs that failed to mature.

Currently, collateral ligation is a commonly utilized procedure, the utility of which is least understood. Anatomic tributaries are smaller veins that drain into the major vein. Blood in the venous system always flows from the periphery to the center and from superficial to deeper veins. The venous values maintain directional flow, and it is quite common to see valves in the superficial veins proximal to the site of tributary drainage and in the tributary close to the site of drainage, both to prevent reverse flow. In the setting of AVF, tributaries tend to develop only in the presence of main outflow vein obstruction. Obliteration of the flow-diverting tributary in such situations results in exacerbation of the existing outflow problem rather than enlargement of the outflow vein. Conversely, collateral veins are flow-diverting tributaries that have developed to support the flow. Obliterating such veins leaving the major outflow does not always enlarge the remaining vein. The venous anatomy may rarely be a variant of normal anatomy with main outflow veins branching into two equally sized small veins. Once again, in such situations, ligation or obliteration of the lesser of the two tributaries does not guarantee the development of the remaining tributary. Perforating veins are veins that communicate between the superficial and the deep venous system. Occasionally, one may encounter perforat-

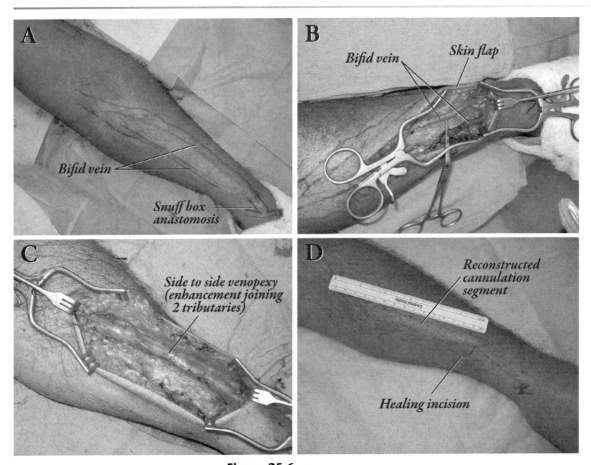

Figure 25-6.
Anatomic snuff box fistula.

ing veins that may be the flow-diverting vein and requires ligation or obliteration. However, it is very unusual to encounter perforating veins in the cephalic system. Hence, it is very important to understand the anatomy and the implication of the tributary or collateral or the perforator vein prior to obliteration or ligation. Any vein that develops after an AVF creation may act as a significant source of autologous material for secondary surgical procedures that could be used to help fistula maturation. In our experience, vein obliteration/ligation is necessary and beneficial in a significantly small proportion (5%-7%) of patients.

Recent reports have highlighted a newer technique of sequential dilation to salvage an AVF that fails to develop because of diffuse stenosis.[19,31,32] In this technique, the AVF is gradually dilated with a progressively increasing size of angioplasty balloon at 2- to 4-week intervals until a size optimal for dialysis cannulation is achieved. There are no good long-term follow up data yet for this procedure.

Conclusions

A mature AVF is an autologous vein conduit that can be accessed for HD. The most important contributors to the success of AVF are the flows in the fistula, diameter, length, and depth of needle stick segment. It is the surgeon's responsibility to identify the veins that can be used as good cannulation segments. Adequate planning and utilization of

pre- and intraoperative ultrasound imaging help surgeons plan the creation of successful AVF. Maturation evaluation using clinical examination complemented by an objective duplex ultrasound evaluation helps surgeons determine whether AVF can be successfully cannulated or whether secondary interventions could be offered for AVF maturation. A structured approach should increase AVF maturation and decrease cannulation problems at dialysis units. Ultimately, a well-functioning fistula is the greatest boon for an ESRD patient on HD.

REFERENCES

1. Annual Data Report. Atlas of End-Stage Renal Diseases in the United States. In U.S. Renal Data System. Bethesda, MD: National Institute of Health, National Institute of Diabetes and Digestive and Kidney Diseases, 2006.
2. III. NKF-K/DOQI Clinical Practice Guidelines for Vascular Access: update 2000. *Am J Kidney Dis.* 2001;37(1 suppl 1):S137-S181.
3. Allon M, Robbin ML. Increasing arteriovenous fistulas in hemodialysis patients: problems and solutions. *Kidney Int.* 2002;62:1109-1124.
4. Feldman HI, Kobrin S, Wasserstein A. Hemodialysis vascular access morbidity. *J Am Soc Nephrol.* 1996;7:523-535.
5. Schwab SJ, Harrington JT, Singh A, et al. Vascular access for hemodialysis. *Kidney Int.* 1999;55:2078-2090.
6. Dhingra RK, Young EW, Hulbert-Shearon TE, Leavey SF, Port FK. Type of vascular access and mortality in U.S. hemodialysis patients. *Kidney Int.* 2001;60:1443-1451.
7. Shenoy S. Innovative surgical approaches to maximize arteriovenous fistula creation. *Semin Vasc Surg.* 2007;20:141-147.

8. Shenoy S, Middleton WD, Windus D, et al. Brachial artery flow measurement as an indicator of forearm native fistula maturation. In Henry ML, Ferguson RM (eds). *Vascular Access for Hemodialysis*. Chicago: WL Gore and Associates, Precept Press;2001:223-239.

9. Clincal Practice Guidelines and Clinical Practice Recommendations for Vascular Access, Update 2006. Guideline 1. Initiation of dialysis. Available at www.kidney.org/professionals/KDOQI/guideline.cfm.

10. Konner K, Nonnast-Daniel B, Ritz E. The arteriovenous fistula. *J Am Soc Nephrol*. 2003;14:1669-1680.

11. Silva MB Jr., Hobson RW 2nd, Pappas PJ, et al. A strategy for increasing use of autogenous hemodialysis access procedures: impact of preoperative noninvasive evaluation. *J Vasc Surg*. 1998;27:302-307; discussion 307-308.

12. Lockhart ME, Robbin ML, Allon M. Preoperative sonographic radial artery evaluation and correlation with subsequent radiocephalic fistula outcome. *J Ultrasound Med*. 2004;23:161-168; quiz 169-171.

13. Malovrh M. Non-invasive evaluation of vessels by duplex sonography prior to construction of arteriovenous fistulas for haemodialysis. *Nephrol Dial Transplant*. 1998;13:125-129.

14. Asif A, Roy-Chaudhury P, Beathard GA. Early arteriovenous fistula failure: a logical proposal for when and how to intervene. *Clin J Am Soc Nephrol*. 2006;1:332-339.

15. Dember LM, Beck GJ, Allon M, et al. Effect of clopidogrel on early failure of arteriovenous fistulas for hemodialysis: a randomized controlled trial. *JAMA*. 2008;299:2164-2171.

16. Palder SB, Kirkman RL, Whittemore AD, Hakim RM, Lazarus JM, Tilney NL. Vascular access for hemodialysis. Patency rates and results of revision. *Ann Surg*. 1985;202:235-239.

17. Miller PE, Tolwani A, Luscy CP, et al. Predictors of adequacy of arteriovenous fistulas in hemodialysis patients. *Kidney Int*. 1999;56:75-280.

18. Allon M, Lockhart ME, Lilly RZ, et al. Effect of preoperative sonographic mapping on vascular access outcomes in hemodialysis patients. *Kidney Int*. 2001;60:2013-2020.

19. Asif A, Cherla G, Merrill D, Cipleu CD, Briones P, Pennell P. Conversion of tunneled hemodialysis catheter-consigned patients to arteriovenous fistula. *Kidney Int*. 2005;67:2399-2406.

20. Won T, Jang JW, Lee S, Han JJ, Park YS, Ahn JH. Effects of intraoperative blood flow on the early patency of radiocephalic fistulas. **Ann Vasc Surg**. 2000;14:468-472.

21. Beathard GA, Arnold P, Jackson J, Litchfield T. Aggressive treatment of early fistula failure. *Kidney Int*. 2003;64:1487-1494.

22. Corpataux JM, Haesler E, Silacci P, Ris HB, Hayoz D. Low-pressure environment and remodelling of the forearm vein in Brescia-Cimino haemodialysis access. *Nephrol Dial Transplant*. 2002;17:1057-1062.

23. Ballermann BJ, Dardik A, Eng E, Liu A. Shear stress and the endothelium. *Kidney Int Suppl*. 1998;67:S100-S108.

24. Yerdel MA, Kesenci M, Yazicioglu KM, Doseyen Z, Turkcapar AG, Anadol E. Effect of haemodynamic variables on surgically created arteriovenous fistula flow. *Nephrol Dial Transplant*. 1997;12:1684-1688.

25. Lin SL, Huang CH, Chen HS, Hsu WA, Yen CJ, Yen TS. Effects of age and diabetes on blood flow rate and primary outcome of newly created hemodialysis arteriovenous fistulas. *Am J Nephrol*. 1998;18:96-100.

26. Robbin ML, Chamberlain NE, Lockhart ME, et al. Hemodialysis arteriovenous fistula maturity: US evaluation. *Radiology*. 2002;225:59-64.

27. Faiyaz R, Abreo K, Zaman F, Pervez A, Zibari G, Work J. Salvage of poorly developed arteriovenous fistulae with percutaneous ligation of accessory veins. *Am J Kidney Dis*. 2002;39:824-827.

28. Kian K, Asif A. Cephalic arch stenosis. *Semin Dial*. 2008;21:78-82.

29. Kian K, Unger SW, Mishler R, Schon D, Lenz O, Asif A. Role of surgical intervention for cephalic arch stenosis in the "Fistula First" era. *Semin Dial*. 2008;21:93-96.

30. Turmel-Rodrigues L, Mouton A, Birmele B, et al. Salvage of immature forearm fistulas for haemodialysis by interventional radiology. *Nephrol Dial Transplant*. 2001;16:2365-2371.

31. Beathard GA. Angioplasty for arteriovenous grafts and fistulae. *Semin Nephrol*. 2002;22:202-210.

32. Achkar K, Nassar GM. Salvage of a severely dysfunctional arteriovenous fistula with a strictured and occluded outflow tract. *Semin Dial*. 2005;18:336-342.

CHAPTER 26

Coordination and Patient Care in Vascular Access

Victoria Holmes

Effective dialysis requires a reliable and functioning access. Since the early days of dialysis therapy, maintaining vascular access has been problematic. By definition, an arteriovenous fistula (AV fistula) is the connection of a vein and an artery, usually in the forearm, which allows access to the vascular system for hemodialysis. This chapter will provide a review of the dialysis population, a discussion of arteriovenous fistula, and an explanation of the importance of coordination of vascular access care.

Background of End-Stage Renal Disease Population

In the book *Epidemic of Care*, George Isham illustrates that the distribution of healthcare resources is disproportionate to the payers' contribution in a health plan. The least expensive 70% of patients account for 10% of the expenditures. The most expensive 1% of patients account for 30% of the expenditures. Patients with end stage renal disease (ESRD) constitute a major portion of the most expensive 1% of health care patients.[1]

Increasing numbers of patients require some form of renal replacement therapy. Reviewing US Renal Data System (USRDS) statistics reveals that chronic kidney disease (CKD), congestive heart failure (CHF), diabetes, and ESRD are consuming more and more of the general Medicare dollar (Fig. 26-1).[2]

Gilbertson and Collins (2007) examined USRDS statistics using a Markov model and projected the prevalence of ESRD in the United States to the year 2020.[3] Using this model, the prevalence of patients with ESRD will be 784,613, with 533,800 on dialysis. Why so many new patients? USRDS statistics indicate that these numbers are increasing due to aging "baby boomers," declining death rates as a result of improved care of patients on dialysis, higher diabetic prevalence rates, and improved treatment of persons with chronic kidney disease prior to dialysis.

The cost of vascular access is also rising (Fig. 26-2). According to USRDS statistics, the average cost of vascular access per year for placement and complications is $64,155 per patient. The most costly access is a catheter, and the least costly access is a fistula. In addition, fistulas generally have fewer complications. If medically possible, placing a fistula is the fiscally responsible access to place.

Since the late 1990s, significant strides have been made to promote the arteriovenous fistula as the access of choice for hemodialysis patients. Beginning in 1997, the National Kidney Foundation set forth Clinical Practice Guidelines, also known as the Kidney Disease Outcome Quality Initiative (KDOQI), for placement of vascular access by physicians and clinicians.[4] The KDOQI guidelines were followed by AV Fistula First. AV Fistula First was created by a coalition of groups including the Centers for Medicare and Medicaid Services (CMS), the ESRD Networks, and the renal community. This group works together to ensure that patients will receive the optimal form of vascular access, preferably an arteriovenous fistula. Another focus of this group is to work towards reducing catheter usage and vascular access complications.[5]

The success or failure of placing an arteriovenous fistula as the primary vascular access depends on when the patient is identified. KDOQI guidelines encourage the referral of patients to a nephrologist once they have reached Stage 4 CKD (eGFR 15-29 min/1.73 m²).[4] Educating patients about their disease process allows early decision-making related to treatment modality and early referral for placement of an access. It is known that unplanned or urgent initiation of dialysis is associated with less favorable outcomes than planned initiation.[6,7]

For those patients who are referred late for dialysis access placement or who are started emergently on dialysis, the tunnel or temporary catheter will be the most likely access. It is important to get this group of patients assessed for placement of other vascular access. The goal is for a patient to have minimum time with a catheter unless the patient has extremely limited vasculature for access, is so physically debilitated that they cannot have access placed, or has a very limited life expectancy.

For patients already on dialysis who do not have a functioning fistula, it is important to educate the patient about the available access options. For the patient with a catheter, it is important to stress the possible long-term problems associated with catheters, such as central venous stenosis and infection. In the patient with a graft, it is crucial to assess the patient for the possibility of secondary fistula placement.

Not only is it important to place a vascular access early in the patient with CKD, but it is also important to look at vascular access in the peritoneal dialysis population and the

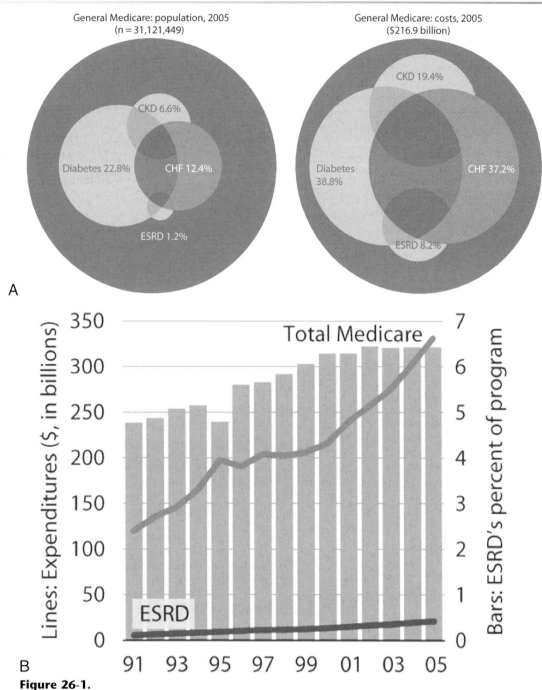

Figure 26-1.

A, Distribution of Medicare patients and costs for CKD, CHF, diabetes, and ESRD: Populations were estimated from the 5% Medicare sample and include patients surviving the entire cohort year (2004) with Medicare as primary payer, plus period prevalent ESRD patients, 2005, with Medicare as primary payer. Diabetes, CKD, and CHF costs were determined from claims (2004 and 2005). *B,* Costs of the Medicare and ESRD programs: Total ESRD expenditures were from paid claims as well as estimated costs for HMO and organ acquisitions. ESRD costs in 2005 were inflated by 2% to account for costs incurred, but not reported. Total Medicare expenditures were obtained from the CMS Office of Financial Management, Division of Budget. *CKD,* Chronic kidney disease; *CHF,* congestive heart failure; *ESRD,* end-stage renal disease. (From US Renal Data System. 2007 Annual Report).

renal transplant population. Patients on peritoneal dialysis often require frequent blood draws and are often admitted to the hospital for care related to complications of peritoneal dialysis, such as infection or for other medical conditions. Multiple insults to the vessels of these patients in the form of venous sticks or intravenous catheters will possibly yield few vessels viable for fistula placement. In the early days of dialysis, it was not uncommon for a patient to have both a peritoneal catheter for dialysis as well as a developing fistula.

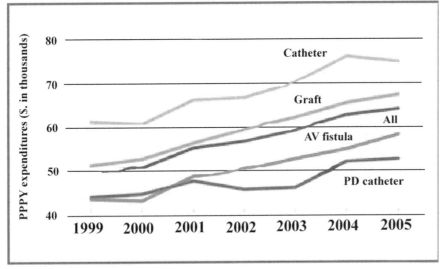

Figure 26-2.
Cost of Vascular access placement and complications per year. (From US Renal Data System. 2007 Annual Report.)

- Total Access $64,155
- AVF $58,294
- AVG $67,479
- Catheter $74,963

For the transplant patient who is gradually losing the function of his or her transplanted organ, it is also necessary to address vascular access placement early. These are difficult conversations to have with patients who may be in denial or are fearful of losing the graft and returning to dialysis therapy. It is still important to educate the patient about their dialysis treatment choices and ensure early referral for access placement.

Arteriovenous Fistula

Vascular Access Assessment

The goal for all patients is a functioning access, preferably a fistula. Prior to the placement of the access, a detailed history should be done to include the following information:

- Dominant arm—it is preferable to place the access in the non-dominant arm so that the patient maintains function and mobility.
- Previous central venous catheters—intravenous lines, Swans, pacemakers—the presence or history of these types of devices is associated with central venous stenosis, which may limit the access placement site and long-term success of the access.
- Previous chest, arm, or neck surgery—types of surgery that may involved damage to the central vessels.
- Anticoagulant therapy or coagulation disorders—may cause clotting or problems with hemostasis.
- History of diabetes—associated with damage to the vasculature necessary for internal access.
- History of severe CHF—access may alter hemodynamics and cardiac output.
- Previous vascular access—may limit options for access placement.

- Co-morbid conditions with limited life expectancy.
- Anticipated transplant from living donor.[4,8]

Physical examination

Physical examination of the patient prior to vascular access should include the following:

Arterial system

- Character of pulses
- Allen test
- Bilateral upper extremity blood pressures
- Doppler evaluation

Venous system

- Evaluation of edema
- Examination of collateral veins
- Vein mapping
- Examination for evidence of previous central or peripheral catheterization
- Examination for evidence of arm, chest, or neck surgery/trauma[4,8]

Venous and arteriography studies should be used only as a last resort on patients who are pre-renal, because the dye used in the studies may destroy the remaining renal function and hasten the need for dialysis.

Management of the New Fistula

To ensure a successful outcome with a fistula, it is important to frequently monitor and evaluate the new vessel. Once the fistula is surgically created, the patient is taught to check the incision site for warmth, redness, bleeding, and the presence of a "buzzing" over the vessel. The patient should have a return visit to the surgeon within 2–3 weeks of access placement. It is important for the patient to understand that creation of a fistula may not consist of a single surgery, but may require several procedures to optimize the vessel for long-term use.

Assessing the Fistula

A fistula should mature in 6 to 8 weeks, and should not be cannulated during the first month after construction. When evaluating the fistula it is helpful to use the Rule of 6s[5]:

- Fistula blood flow greater than an 600 ml/min
- Diameter greater than 0.6 cm with discernible margins with a tourniquet in place
- Depth approximately 0.6 cm from the skin surface

If the fistula does not meet the above criteria at 4 to 6 weeks after surgical creation, the patient is referred to the surgeon for further evaluation.

When performing the physical examination (Fig. 26-3), it is important to look for:

- Well-developed main venous outflow
- Collateral venous effluent vessels
- Vessel collapses or softens when arm is raised

Listen for:

- Low-pitched continuous systolic-diastolic bruit

Palpate for:

- Gentle thrill at the arterial anastomosis. It should not be hyperpulsatile.[8]

Cannulation of Fistulas

It is important to have an established protocol for fistula cannulation. Initially the vessel is cannulated with 17-gauge needles with a blood flow that does not exceed 250 mL/min. The size of the needle and the blood flow rate increase as the vessel matures. Experienced staff should be the initial can-

nulators of a new fistula.[5] Each dialysis unit should have a training program for instructing staff in cannulation techniques.[5]

Methods of Cannulation

Rope Ladder Technique

The most frequently used method of fistula cannulation is the rope ladder technique. This technique rotates the needle placement sites each time the fistula is cannulated. A site for cannulation is chosen about 1.5 to 2 inches from the last puncture site. The goal of this technique is to prevent excessive use of one area and creating problems such as aneurysms.[9]

Buttonhole Technique

The buttonhole cannulation technique was first used in Europe approximately 25 years ago for patients with limited sites for cannulation. It was discovered that cannulating the fistula repeatedly in the same spot had benefits. With repeated cannulation into the same puncture site, a scar tissue tunnel tract develops. The scar tissue tunnel tract allows the needle to pass through to the vessel of the fistula and follow the same path each time. Fewer incidents of infiltration and pain have been associated with this cannulation method.

When choosing the sites, select straight, relatively unused sections of the fistula. It takes 6 cannulations with a standard sharp fistula needle to establish a buttonhole site.[10] Once a buttonhole site is established, a dull needle may be used (Buttonhole Needle Sets; Medisystems Corporation, Seattle, WA). Using the dull needle minimizes tissue damage and eliminates bleeding from the site.[10]

Monitoring Fistulas

Once a fistula is placed and is successfully cannulated, ongoing evaluation should occur to identify and correct problems. A gross measure of access function can be obtained by

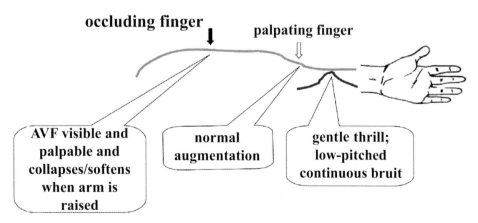

Figure 26-3.
Examination of fistula—normal physical findings. (From Urbanes AQ, RMS Lifeline 2007. Diagnosis and Timing of Intervention in Early Failure, with permission).

monitoring dialysis adequacy or Kt/V. If the access blood flow, dialysis time, and dialyzer have all been maximized and the Kt/V value is still below the target, the access should be evaluated for problems. The KDOQI Guidelines recommend that access flow be measured on a monthly basis by ultrasound dilution, conductance dilution, thermal dilution, Doppler, or other techniques.[4] Two commonly used tools are the CritLine (Hemametrics Inc., Salt Lake City, UT) and the Transonics (Transonics Systems Inc., Ithaca, NY). The CritLine uses photo-optical technology to non-invasively measure access blood flow.[11] Transonic Flow QC uses ultrasound velocity dilution to measure access flow and is recognized as the gold standard for flow measurement.[12,13]

Vascular Access Coordination

The coordination of vascular access for pre-ESRD patients as well as patients on dialysis is critical to overall care and long-term survival.[6,7] The earlier a patient is identified and referred for early access care, the better the outcome. Even with the KDOQI initiatives for early identification of patients at risk, about 50% of all known cases of Stage 4 and 5 CKD are late referrals. Navaneethan and associates did a meta-analysis of the abstracts of 256 articles and 18 observational studies about late referral in CKD and concluded that "a combination of patient and health system characteristics are associated with late referral of patients with CKD. Overall, being older, belonging to a minority group, being less educated, being uninsured, suffering from multiple co morbidities, and the lack of communication between primary care physicians and nephrologist contribute to late referral of patients with chronic kidney disease."[14]

The goal of vascular access coordination in chronic kidney disease is early fistula creation.

To achieve this goal, patients must be educated about their disease process and treatment options. There must be collaboration between nephrologist and surgeon to facilitate early fistula placement and patient follow-up after AV fistula placement. It is very important that primary care physicians are educated on early referral of patients to nephrologists.

Role of the Vascular Access Coordinator

According to Dinwiddie, the primary role of a vascular access coordinator should be quality management of access-related issues, tracking of access once placed, noting complications and interventions, making recommendations for referrals and treatment, following up after interventions, and analyzing outcomes.[15] The vascular access coordinator is the point person for not only the patient and family, but also for the dialysis unit, surgeon, nephrologists, and interventional radiologist. This person is charged with coordinating care for the patient among all of the above noted professionals, and getting the coordination done in a timely manner. The benefits of a vascular access coordinator include better access performance, reduced hospitalizations, and fewer emergency situations.

Gable et al. demonstrated the cost effectiveness of a vascular access coordinator. A vascular access coordinator was hired to manage the access issues at a large tertiary care medical center. Management of the care was evaluated over an 18-month period. The presence of the coordinator improved patient care by decreasing the need for urgent thrombectomy, temporary line placement, and emergency department visits related to vascular access. The calculated cost savings using a vascular access coordinator was calculated to be $381,000.[16]

Teamwork is required to provide access coordination. Open and fluid communication with the patient, family/partner, nephrologists, and dialysis staff is critical. The patient suffers when the team does not function well. Skill sets necessary for a vascular access coordinator are communication, collaboration, and flexibility. It is important to have an organized system in which to collect and maintain data sets for the purpose of patient care, research, and quality management.

Reviewing the literature reveals that insufficient management of access in the predialysis or CKD period directly impacts access management once a patient is on dialysis. The value of access coordination in both pre CKD and ESRD is important for improved patient outcomes, forwarding the Fistula First Initiative, and providing cost-effective care.

REFERENCES

1. Halvorson G, Isham G. *Epidemic of Care: A Call for Safer, Better, and More Accountable Health Care*. San Francisco: Jossey-Bass, 2003.
2. US Renal Data System. 2007 Annual Report. Available at http://www.usrds.org/slides_2007.htm.
3. Gilbertson DT, Collins AJ. Projecting the ESRD population to 2020. Presented at American Society of Nephrology Renal Week; October 31-November 5, 2007; San Francisco, CA. Abstract FC046.
4. National Kidney Foundation. NKF-KDOQI Guidelines. Available at http://www.kidney.org/PROFESSIONALS/kdoqi/guidelines.cfm.
5. AV Fistula First Web site. Available at http://www.fistulafirst.org. Accessed: May 13, 2009.
6. Lorenzo V, Martin M, Rufino M, Hernandez D, Torres A, Ayus JC. Predialysis nephrology care and a functioning arteriovenous fistula at the entry are associated with better survival in incident hemodialysis patients: an observational cohort study. *Am J Kidney Dis*. 2004;43: 999-1007.
7. Stack AG. Impact of timing of nephrology referral and pre-ESRD care on mortality risk among new ESRD patients in the United States. *Am J Kidney Dis*. 2003;41:310-318.
8. Urbanes AQ, RMS Lifeline 2007. Diagnosis and Timing of Intervention in Early Failure. Presented at 3rd Annual Meeting. American Society of Diagnostic and Interventional Nephrology. April, 2007
9. Ball LK. Improving arteriovenous fistula cannulation skills. *Nephrol Nursing J*. 2005;32(6):611-617.
10. Ball LK. The buttonhole technique for arteriovenous fistula cannulation. *Nephrol Nursing J*. 2006;33(3):299-304.
11. Hema Metrics Inc Web site. The CRIT-LINE IIITQA System. Available at http://www.hemametrics.com/Usersmanual/Section1.pdf.
12. Besarab A. Preventing vascular access dysfunction: which policy to follow. *Blood Purif*. 2002;20(1):26-35.
13. Transonic Systems Inc Web site. Available at http://www.transonic.com/PDF/DL-20.pdf.
14. Navaneethan SD, Aloudat S, Singh S. A systematic review of patient and health system characteristics associated with late referral in chronic kidney disease. *BMC Nephrol*. 2008;9:3.
15. Dinwiddie LC. Investing in the lifeline: The value of a vascular access coordinator. *Nephrol News Issues*. 2003;17(6):49, 52-53.
16. Gable DR, Munschauer CE, Garrett WV, et al. Vascular access coordination at a large tertiary care hospital. Presented at Texas Transplantation Society, June 24, 2004; Austin, TX.

CHAPTER 27

Cardiovascular Consequences of Rapid Hemodialysis

Orly F. Kohn, Todd S. Ing, Subhash Popli, and Nosratola D. Vaziri

End-stage renal disease (ESRD) patients have a high mortality rate that is largely attributable to cardiovascular disease. Increased cardiovascular mortality is seen in chronic kidney disease patients long before they reach end-stage organ failure. Most patients suffer from left ventricular hypertrophy by the time of their first dialysis. Conventional hemodialysis is intermittent and of relatively short duration, resulting in incomplete removal of many uremic toxins, wide fluctuations in intravascular volume, and solutes such as electrolytes. The past couple of decades have seen shortening of dialysis treatment time, with most patients receiving only 9 to 12 hours of dialysis per week. This approach is particularly true for US dialysis units and is referred to as *rapid hemodialysis* in this chapter. The impact of rapid hemodialysis on the heart, intravascular volume, and sudden death, as well as on the vascular access, will be reviewed and contrasted, where available, with slower, longer, and/or more frequent forms of hemodialysis.

Achieving Urea Kt/V Targets With Short Weekly Dialysis Time

Delivery of adequate urea clearance with a weekly dialysis time of approximately 9 to 12 hours (ie, 3- to 4-hour sessions three times a week) necessitates a high dialyzer blood flow rate, a high dialysate flow rate, a dialyzer with a high mass transfer area coefficient (KoA) value for urea,[1] and a bicarbonate-based dialysate. In the 1990s, two forms of rapid dialysis therapy evolved[2,3]:

- **High-efficiency dialysis** utilizes a dialyzer with a high KoA for urea that is greater than 700 mL/min. Such dialyzers typically have a large surface area and/or a thin membrane, facilitating substantial removal of low–molecular weight waste products such as urea and creatinine.
- **High-flux dialysis** utilizes dialyzers with highly permeable membranes with large pores that readily allow the passage of bigger molecules, such as β_2-microglobulin (β_2-microglobulin clearance greater than 20 mL/min),[4] and also of water (hence the term *high-flux*). Permeability to water is defined by ultrafiltration coefficient (Kuf). For a high-flux dialyzer, Kuf must exceed 10 to 14 mL/hr/mmHg of transmembrane pressure.[4,5] High-flux dialyzers currently used by most centers are also characterized by their high efficiency.

Both dialysis techniques require a high dialyzer blood flow rate (usually 400 mL/min or higher) and a dialysate flow rate of 500 to 800 mL/min to maximize small solute removal in the shortest time. This magnitude of blood flow places considerable demands on the cardiovascular system, including the vascular access, and presents a major challenge for the growing ESRD population of the elderly and the seriously ill.

Effect of Rapid Dialysis on Access Recirculation

Access recirculation results from the routing of just-dialyzed blood returning from the dialyzer back into the afferent limb of the vascular access (either arteriovenous [AV] access or central venous catheter) and then into the dialyzer to be dialyzed again (Fig. 27-1). Because this recirculated, just-dialyzed blood contains lower levels of uremic toxins, the efficiency of the dialysis procedure is compromised. As a result, patients are often underdialyzed, as evidenced by (1) a reduction in urea and other solute clearance measurements obtained during dialysis, and (2) an elevation in pre-dialysis blood waste-product levels.

Traditionally, the magnitude of access recirculation has been gauged by the degree of mixing of incoming systemic blood with recirculated, just-dialyzed blood. This mixing has been reflected by differences in blood urea nitrogen (BUN) levels measured at various sites. The previous standard method for evaluation of access recirculation is the "three-needle" technique using (1) undialyzed systemic arterial blood obtained from the arterial blood line after the blood pump rate has been reduced to 120 mL/min for 10 seconds, (2) blood obtained from the arterial blood line during dialysis, and (3) blood from the venous blood line during dialysis.[6-8] More sophisticated methods have emerged to replace this classic approach. Access flow measurement techniques that are commonly used include (1) sonography dilution method,[9] (2) differential conductivity method,[10] and (3) blood concentration–altering methods utilizing changes in levels of temperature, hematocrit, impedance, glucose, and potassium.[11-13] Although results obtained from some of these innovative methods have been satisfactory, the most popular technique has been the sonography dilution approach. It should be noted that measuring recirculation is ideally carried out at the begin-

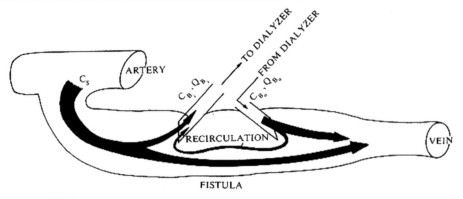

Figure 27-1.
Access recirculation in an arteriovenous fistula. (Reproduced with permission from Gotch FA. Hemodialysis: technical and kinetic considerations. In: Brenner BM, Rector FC Jr (eds). *The Kidney*. Philadelphia, PA: WB Saunders, 1976:1672-1704)

ning of a dialysis session (e.g., during the first 90 min).[14] The beginning of dialysis is preferred, because increasing cumulative fluid loss during dialysis leads to hypotension-induced reduction in arterial access flow and hence recirculation.

Recirculation was found to increase after dialyzer blood flow rate had been raised from 300 to 400 mL /min.[15] Arterial (inflow) stenosis may lead to recirculation from a reduction in the inflow of fresh systemic arterial blood. In the case of venous (outflow) stenosis, recirculation can occur because of the failure of just-dialyzed blood to return freely to the general venous circulation, an impediment that is caused by the stenotic lesion. Both of these stenosis-induced recirculation mechanisms are the consequence of the high blood-pump rate required for the performance of a rapid dialysis treatment.[15] Access recirculation has also been found in patients whose brachial artery flow rate was less than 350 mL /min, which exceeds the dialyzer blood flow rate by less than 60 mL /min.[16]

The 2006 National Kidney Foundation KDOQI (Kidney Disease Outcomes Quality Initiative) Clinical Practice Guidelines for vascular access suggest further evaluation for the following abnormalities: (1) Fistulas with an access flow rate of less than 400 to 500 mL/min and (2) grafts with (a) an access blood flow of less than 600 mL/min or (b) an access with a blood flow of 1,000 mL/min where the flow has fallen by more than 25% over 4 months.[14] Current literature provides no conclusive evidence that screening and surveillance of access blood flow can prolong vascular access survival.[17]

Effect of Dialysis Access on Cardiovascular Function

The blood flow through a newly created AV fistula increases rapidly through arterial and venous dilatation and remodeling, and the process of fistula maturation is usually achieved by 4 to 8 weeks after surgery. Blood flow rates through mature fistulas are ordinarily in the range of 500 to 3000 mL /min, with the higher values being seen in more proximal mature fistulas (upper arm or thigh). A

large AV access can place considerable stress on the cardiovascular system through the induction of a hyperdynamic state.[18] Pulse rate and cardiac output rise, whereas peripheral vascular resistance and blood pressure fall. In patients with very large fistulas that bypass 20% to 50% of the cardiac output, the result can be cardiovascular decompensation in the form of significant hypotension, cardiomegaly, and high-output congestive heart failure.[19] In asymptomatic patients with underlying cardiomyopathy or other cardiac ailments, cardiac decompensation may occur even if the fistula is smaller and the consequent shunting of cardiac output is less marked. In these patients, after occlusion of the AV fistula, improvement in cardiac function has been demonstrated by echocardiography.[20]

Because most properly functioning fistulas provide a blood flow rate of approximately 800 mL /min[21] such a flow rate can readily handle the dialyzer blood flow demands of 400 to 500 mL /min that are required for rapid dialysis. Indeed, with the use of Doppler ultrasonography, it has been shown that rapid dialysis does not bring about changes in fistula blood flow.[22] The volume of blood present in a hollow-fiber dialyzer and its accompanying blood tubing is constant and independent of dialyzer blood flow rates.[22] The constancy of the blood volume of a hollow-fiber dialyzer is related to the noncompliance of its fibers.

When access flow is excessive, interventions in the form of graft banding, plication, or placement of an interposition graft may be tried, but are often either ineffective or conducive to access thrombosis. In refractory cases, surgical ligation may be necessary.[23]

High dialyzer blood flow may have a negative impact on fistula survival. Of the countries participating in the Dialysis Outcomes and Practice Patterns Study (DOPPS), the United States has the highest prescribed blood flow rates (averaging 400 mL/min).[24] Twardowski raised the concern that the inferior survival of AV fistula in the United States might be a consequence of these excessive flow demands.[25] The poor fistula survival may be related to (1) premature abandonment of the fistula because of its inability to support the required dialyzer blood flow, (2) damage to the intima of the fistula caused by the suction force applied through the inflow needle, or (3) frequent intradialytic and early postdialytic hypotensive episodes (secondary to rapid ultrafiltration) fostering thrombus formation in the fistula. A high dialyzer blood flow may have a negative impact on the central veins as well. In order to obtain a higher blood flow, the employment of large-caliber, dual-lumen venous catheters and/or the application of a strong suction force (via the catheter tip) against the vessel wall may cause damage to the vein wall, thus, promoting the development of thrombosis and stenosis.[25] The longer survival of central venous catheters in patients treated with nocturnal dialysis (using slow dialyzer blood flows in the region of 100 to 300 mL/min) than in patients maintained on rapid dialysis is consistent with this assertion.[26]

Effect of Rapid Dialysis on Cardiac Function

Subclinical myocardial ischemia occurs during hemodialysis. Zuber and colleagues first demonstrated this and noted silent ST segment depression.[27] These changes are quite common (15 to 40% of cases) and have been demonstrated in patients without known coronary artery disease. Other methods have confirmed this high prevalence of silent myocardial ischemia; these include echocardiography for the detection of regional wall motion abnormalities and positron emission tomography for the assessment of tissue perfusion.[28] One small study demonstrated that even in patients without angiographically significant coronary artery disease, standard hemodialysis (4-hour sessions thrice weekly, blood flow rate of 250 to 450 mL/min, dialysate flow rate of 500 mL/min) was associated with an acute reduction in global and segmental myocardial blood flow leading to ischemia and new areas of wall-motion abnormalities.[29] In this study, about 30% of the regions affected by wall-motion abnormality persisted in showing that abnormality at 30 minutes after the end of dialysis, displaying myocardial stunning. Repeated ischemic insults to the myocardium in ESRD patients likely contribute to the development of congestive heart failure and uremic cardiomyopathy.[28] More rapid dialysis, characterized by abrupt shifts of fluid among the body's fluid compartments and fast changes in the levels of electrolytes and other solutes may promote cardiac abnormalities.

Rapid dialysis utilizing high blood flow rates and high-flux dialyzers increases backfiltration of dialysate into the blood compartment. This, in turn, may lead to the entry of bacterial products from the dialysate into the blood, enhancing the chronic inflammatory state and accelerating atherosclerosis commonly seen in ESRD patients.[25]

Rapid Dialysis and Intradialytic Hypotension

Intradialytic hypotension (IDH) occurs in 25 to 50% of conventional hemodialysis treatments in the United States. Rapid dialysis demands that a given interdialytic weight (fluid) gain is removed from the body in a short amount of time. Higher ultrafiltration rate (UFR) achieves this goal.

Patients with large interdialytic weight gains may experience frequent episodes of hypotension for one or both of the following reasons: (1) the removal rate of the excess fluid through the dialyzer exceeds the refilling rate of the body's capillaries resulting in a reduced intravascular volume, and/or (2) the body's compensatory mechanisms, such as raised cardiac output and increased vasoconstriction, are defective (as a result of myocardial dysfunction, autonomic nervous system dysfunction, impaired secretion of vasoactive hormones or dialysis per se) or outstripped by the excessive fluid removal.[30-33] Whereas a healthy individual can tolerate a decline in circulating blood volume of as much as 20% without the ready development of hypotension, dialysis patients may become hypotensive with a much smaller decline.

Ronco et al. demonstrated that a higher UFR (from 18 mL/hr/kg to 36 mL/hr/kg) was associated with higher rates of IDH (from 8 to 60%, respectively).[34] IDH can lead to (1) arrhythmias, myocardial ischemia and infarction; (2) compromised cerebrovascular circulation with altered sensorium, blindness and stroke; (3) reduced splanchnic circulation with intestinal angina and infarction; and (4) worsening of residual renal function. Apart from bringing about IDH, rapid ultrafiltration contributes to the poor tolerance of dialysis with symptoms such as cramps, nausea, vomiting, and fatigue, both during and after dialysis. Patients often leave the dialysis unit without achieving dry weight because of (1) insufficient treatment time to remove the amount of excess fluid that had accumulated prior to dialysis (2) premature discontinuation of dialysis on account of the occurrence of the above untoward intradialytic symptoms, or (3) necessary administration of saline in an attempt to combat IDH. These patients continue to suffer from overhydration and poorly controlled hypertension during the interdialytic intervals.

Frequent occurrences of hypotensive episodes during dialysis resulting from hypovolemia or other causes may also predispose the patient to access thrombosis.[35] It is noteworthy that the average UFR was significantly lower in Europe than in the United States in the DOPPS I and DOPPS II studies. UFR greater than 10 mL/hr/kg was associated with 30% higher odds of intradialytic hypotension and an elevated risk of mortality.[36] In a similar vein, results of the USRDS Waves 3 and 4 studies also demonstrated that weight gain between dialysis treatments of more than 4.8% of body weight (eg, 3.4 kg in a 70-kg person), was associated with higher mortality.[37]

Intradialytic hypotension can be minimized by counseling the patient to limit weight gain between dialysis sessions, using bicarbonate-based dialysis solutions, lowering dialysate temperature to 35° to 36°C, and avoiding food intake immediately before and during dialysis.[30] Ideally, the fluid weight gain should not exceed 0.5 kg/day. The importance of limiting salt intake[38] to minimize the need for rapid fluid removal by ultrafiltration during dialysis was fully recognized by the pioneers of dialysis at the dawn of the dialysis era. The KDOQI[14] and the European Best Practice Guidelines (EBPG)[39] recommend a daily sodium restriction of 85 mmol (5 g NaCl) and 103 mmol (6 g NaCl), respectively, to reduce salt-induced water intake and overhydration (with resultant hypertension). If sodium restriction is observed, the necessity for quick ultrafiltration during rapid dialysis is abolished and the occurrence of IDH should be substantially curtailed.

More frequent (eg, the short daily variety, 5 to 7 times per week) and longer (eg, the nocturnal variety with 8 hours per session, 3 to 7 times per week) modalities of hemodialysis are better tolerated with a reduced incidence of intradialytic hypotensive episodes. In the case of more frequent dialysis sessions, the amount of excess fluid required for removal per session is reduced; hence, vascular volume depletion is less marked and the demand for refilling is correspondingly reduced. With the longer sessions, there is more time for a given quantity of excess fluid to be removed and for capillary refilling to take place. For these reasons, these new modalities of dialysis are capable of removing excess fluid in a manner that does not often significantly deplete the volume.[40] Consequently, these novel approaches are superior to rapid dialysis with respect to the avoidance of IDH.

Dialysis-Related Arrhythmias and Sudden Death

Sudden death is temporally related to hemodialysis, with the rates being the highest in the 12-hour period at the end of a dialysis-free weekend interval and in the 12-hour period starting with a dialysis session.[41] The majority of patients who succumbed to sudden death had suffered from congestive heart failure, cardiomyopathy, and coronary artery disease. Rapid lowering of serum potassium levels likely promotes arrhythmias in this setting of underlying heart disease In particular, the group suffering from sudden death during the 12-hour period following dialysis initiation tended to have lower serum potassium concentrations in the previous month, with about a quarter of the values being less than 4 mmol/L. This underscores the need for frequent adjustments of dialysate potassium concentrations. Patients with left ventricular hypertrophy (as evidenced by a posterior wall motion thickness of 12 mm on M mode echocardiography) were noted to have higher rates of arrhythmias during dialysis.[42] Although the development of ventricular arrhythmias did not correlate with postdialysis serum potassium values and many of the patients in this study were receiving digitalis preparations, raising dialysate potassium level from 2 to 3.5 mmol/L did reduce the frequency of intradialytic ventricular premature depolarization. Karnik et al. found cardiac arrests to be more frequent during a Monday dialysis session than during a session carried out on any other day of the week. Moreover, affected patients were about twice as likely to have been dialyzed against a dialysate containing 0 or 1 mmol/L potassium on the day of the cardiac arrest.[43]

Because cardiac arrhythmias, cardiac arrest, and sudden death are related to thrice-weekly, rapid dialysis-related changes in serum potassium levels, it has been suggested that every-other-day dialysis sessions could be beneficial in preventing sudden deaths.[41] In addition, increasing the frequency of dialysis sessions should reduce the incidence of high peaks and deep valleys of serum potassium values that can plague patients treated with rapid thrice-weekly dialysis. Careful attention to the maintenance of normal serum potassium concentrations is warranted in dialysis patients at risk for sudden death.[41]

Heightened sympathetic activity is another risk factor for sudden death and is increased in dialysis patients on rapid dialysis. A fall in blood volume, as occurs during dialysis (particularly with high ultrafiltration rates), increases sympathetic activity. Everyday dialysis regimens decrease blood pressure and sympathetic activity, as measured by serum norepinephrine levels or muscle sympathetic nerve activity.[44-45] Beta-blockers attenuate the risk for sudden death[41] but remain underutilized in dialysis patients. In recognition of the increased risk of arrhythmias and sudden death during dialysis, KDOQI recommends that automatic external defibrillators be available in all dialysis units.[46]

Benefits of Slow and Frequent Hemodialysis on Left Ventricular Hypertrophy

Both short daily and long nightly (5 or 6 times weekly) dialysis regimens have led to better blood pressure control and reversal of left ventricular hypertrophy. Left ventricular mass index (LVMI), in a crossover prospective study of short daily dialysis, was significantly reduced when evaluated by echocardiography after 6 months of treatment.[47] Frequent nocturnal dialysis resulted in an excellent blood pressure control and a regression of LVMI and also in a restoration of impaired left ventricular ejection fraction.[44] In a randomized controlled trial of 52 patients comparing nocturnal (6 times weekly) to rapid (thrice-weekly) dialysis, left ventricular mass, assessed by cardiac magnetic resonance, decreased by about 14 grams in the nocturnal group but increased by about 1.5 grams in the rapid dialysis group.[48] Possible factors contributing to the regression of left ventricular hypertrophy include improvement of hypertension through a better extracellular fluid volume control and a reduced afterload with lower levels of catecholamines, as well as decreased episodes of nocturnal hypoxemia and an improved endothelial function.[48]

Hemodialysis Access Stenosis and Venous Hypertension

Hemodialysis AV accesses often fail because of venous stenosis either at the anastomotic site (in the case of radiocephalic fistulas and grafts) or in the downstream vein (in the case of brachiocephalic fistulas and grafts). Such stenosis results from venous myointimal hyperplasia induced by turbulent flow and wall sheer stress.[49] The high blood flow demand of rapid dialysis likely increases turbulence and wall sheer stress. Stenosis is suggested by an increase in the intensity of the thrill or the pitch of the bruit on physical examination. In venous stenosis, prolonged bleeding from the access puncture site after removal of the needle may be observed. It should be noted that venous pressure data obtained at a dialyzer blood flow of 400 mL/min have limited use as a predictor of venous stenosis, in contrast to its value observed at lower flow rates.[15]

Effect of Rapid Dialysis on the Clearance of Larger Molecules and Multipool Molecules

Rapid dialysis, even while using high-flux dialyzers, does not remove sufficient amounts of the larger "middle molecules" and substances that have a multicompartement volume of distribution or are protein-bound. One example of a "middle molecule" uremic toxin is β_2-microglobulin, whose removal is time-dependent even when high-flux dialyzers are used. There is simply insufficient time in rapid dialysis for this "middle molecule" to be removed adequately.[50] Even removal of β_2-microglobulin from the body by hemodiafiltration is hampered by this molecule's slow rate of intercompartmental movement.[51] ESRD patients maintained on rapid dialysis typically have serum levels of β_2-microglobulin that are many times higher than the level of a person with normal kidney function. Chronic accumulation of β_2-microglobulin in osteoarticular tissues, blood vessels, the heart, and other tissues over many years leads to a condition known as dialysis-related amyloidosis.[52-54] The osteoarticular involvement of this form of amyloidosis with its devastating complications has received more attention than the histological finding of β_2-microglobulin deposits in the blood vessels and the heart.[53]

Inorganic phosphate is another example of a substance that is distributed in multiple compartments.[55] As it takes time for phosphate to leave various intracellular compartments (including bone) to enter the serum, there is insufficient time for rapid dialysis to optimally remove phosphate from the body. Hyperphosphatemia should be treated with phosphate binders and/or extension of dialysis duration. If hyperphosphatemia is not controlled, calcification of blood vessels,[56] the heart valves,[57] the myocardium,[58] and the coronary arteries,[59] and other body tissues can occur, particularly when the serum calcium X inorganic phosphorus product is elevated. Calcification of the cardiovascular system can cause arterial stiffness, increased pulse wave velocity, hypertension, arrhythmias, left ventricular hypertrophy, cardiac muscle dysfunction, heart failure, and death.[60-61]

Rapid Dialysis and the Dialysis Disequilibrium Syndrome

When the blood waste product concentrations are inordinately high in a severely uremic patient, a rapid and aggressive dialysis treatment can usher in dialysis disequilibrium syndrome (DDS).[32,62] Symptoms usually appear within 24 hours after completion of a dialysis session and may last for hours to days. DDS is characterized by neurological manifestations in the form of agitation, fatigue, headache, blurred vision, dizziness, disorientation, tremor, seizures, and coma. Nausea and vomiting are also common. Cardiovascular symptoms include hypertension and cardiac arrhythmias on rare occasions.[32,62] Some affected patients develop elevated intracranial pressure and cerebral edema.[32] The most likely mechanism of DDS centers on the *reverse urea effect*. The latter relates to the fact that, during dialysis, urea level falls faster in the plasma than in the brain cells, an event that leads to an osmotic gradient favoring influx of water into brain cells and development of cerebral edema.[32]

DDS is most commonly encountered with the initiation of dialysis therapy or during rapid dialysis of small children[63] or small-sized adults.

REFERENCES

1. Van Stone JC, Daugirdas JT. Physiologic principles. In Daugirdas JT, Ing TS (eds). *Handbook of Dialysis*, 2nd ed. Boston, MA: Little, Brown and Company, 1994:13-29.
2. Acchiardo SR. High-flux hemodialysis. In Bosch JP, Stein JH (eds). *Hemodialysis: High-Efficiency Treatments*. New York, NY: Churchill Livingstone Inc, 1993:105-117.
3. Collins AJ. High-efficiency treatments using conventional equipment. In Bosch JP, Stein JH (eds). *Hemodialysis: High-Efficiency Treatments*. New York, NY: Churchill Livingstone Inc, 1993:91-104.
4. Eknoyan G, Beck GJ, Cheung AK, et al. Effect of dialysis dose and membrane flux in maintenance hemodialysis. *NEJM.* 2002;347: 2010-2019.
5. Daugirdas JT, Van Stone JC, Boag JT. Hemodialysis apparatus. In Daugirdas JT, Blake PG, Ing TS (eds). *Handbook of Dialysis*, 3rd ed. Boston MA: Lippincott Williams and Wilkins, 2001:46-66.
6. Sherman RA. Recirculation revisited. *Semin Dial.* 1991;4:221-223.
7. Sherman RA. Recirculation in the hemodialysis access. In Henrich WL (ed). *Principles and Practice of Dialysis*. Philadelphia, PA: Williams & Wilkins, 1994:38-46.
8. Sherman RA, Matera JJ, Novik L, Cody RP. Recirculation reassessed: The impact of blood flow rate and the low-flow method reevaluated. *Am J Kidney Dis.* 1994;23:846-848.
9. Krivitski NM. Theory and validation of access flow measurement by dilution technique during hemodialysis. *Kidney Int.* 1995;48:244-250.
10. Lindsay RM, Burbank J, Brugger J, et al. A device and a method for rapid and accurate measurement of access recirculation during hemodialysis. *Kidney Int.* 1996;41:1152-1160.
11. Ahmad S, Misra M, Hoenich N, Daugirdas JT. Hemodialysis apparatus. In Daugirdas JT, Blake PG, Ing TS (eds). *Handbook of Dialysis*, 4th ed. Philadelphia, PA: Lippincott Williams & Wilkins, 2007:59-78.
12. Brancaccio D, Tessitore N, Carpani P, et al. Potassium-based dilution method to measure hemodialysis access recirculation. *Int J Artif Organs.* 2001;24:606-613.
13. Magnasco A, Alloatti S, Bonfant G, Copello F, Solari P. Glucose infusion test: a new screening for vascular access recirculation. *Kidney Int.* 2000;57:2123-2128.
14. National Kidney Foundation KDOQI clinical practice guidelines for vascular access: Update 2006. *Am J Kidney Dis.* 2006;48(Suppl 1): S1-322.
15. Collins DM, Lambert MB, Middleton JP, et al. Fistula dysfunction: effect on rapid hemodialysis. *Kidney Int.* 1992;41:1292-1296.
16. Besarab A, Sherman R. The relationship of recirculation to access blood flow. *Am J Kidney Dis.* 1997;29:223-229.
17. Tonelli M, James M, Wiebe N, et al. Ultrasound monitoring to detect access stenosis in hemodialysis patients: a systematic review. *Am J Kidney Dis.* 2008;51:630-640.
18. Johnson G Jr, Blythe WB. Hemodynamic effects of arteriovenous shunts used for haemodialysis. *Ann Surg.* 1970;171:715-723.
19. Ahearn DJ, Maher JF. Heart failure as a complication of hemodialysis arteriovenous fistula. *Ann Intern Med.* 1972;77:201-204.
20. von Bibra H, Castro L, Autenrieth G, McLeod A, Gurland HJ. The effects of arteriovenous shunts on cardiac function in renal dialysis patients—an echocardiographic evaluation. *Clin Nephrol.* 1978;9: 205-209.
21. Rodriguez Moran M, Rodriguez Rodriguez JM, Ramos Boyero M, et al. Noninvasive study performed with standard Doppler equipment. *Nephron.* 1985;40:63-66.
22. Ronco C, Brendolan A, Bragantini L. Technical and clinical evaluation of different short, highly efficient dialysis techniques. *Contrib Nephrol.* 1988;61:46.
23. Fan P-Y, Schwab SJ. Hemodialysis vascular access. In Henrich WL (ed). *Principles and practice of dialysis*. Philadelphia, PA: Williams & Wilkins, 1994:22-37.
24. Goodkin DA et al. an update on the dialysis outcomes and practice patterns study (DOPPS). *Contemp Dial Nephrol.* 2001;22:36-40.
25. Twardowski ZJ. Treatment time and ultrafiltration rate are more important in dialysis prescription than small molecule clearance. *Blood Purif.* 2007;25:90-98.

26. Perl J, Lok CE, Chan CT. Central venous catheter outcomes in nocturnal hemodialysis. *Kidney Int.* 2006;70:1348-1354.

27. Zuber M, Steinmann E, Huser B, et al. Incidence of arrhythmias and myocardial ischaemia during haemodialysis and haemofiltration. *Nephrol Dial Transplant.* 1989;4:632-634.

28. Selby NM, McIntyre CW. The acute cardiac effects of dialysis. *Semin Dial.* 2007;20:220-228.

29. McIntyre CW, Burton JO, Selby NM, et al. Hemodialysis-induced cardiac dysfunction is associated with an acute reduction in global and segmental myocardial blood flow. *Clin J Am Soc Nephrol.* 2008;3:19-26.

30. Bregman H, Daugridas JT, Ing, TS. Complications during hemodialysis. In Daugirdas JT, Ing TS (eds). *Handbook of Dialysis,* 2nd ed. Boston, MA: Little, Brown and Company, 1994:149-68.

31. Elias AN, Vaziri ND, Maksy M. Plasma norepinephrine, epinephrine and dopamine levels in endstage renal disease: effect of hemodialysis. *Arch Intern Med.* 1985;145:1013-1015.

32. Mujais SK, Ing T, Kjellstrand C. Acute complications of hemodialysis and their prevention and treatment. In Jacobs C, Kjellstrand CM, Koch KM, Winchester JF (eds). *Replacement of Renal Function by Dialysis,* 4th ed, revised. Dordrecht, The Netherlands: Kluwer Academic Publishers, 1996:688-725.

33. Sulowicz W, Radziszewski A. Pathogenesis and treatment of dialysis hypotension. *Kidney Int.* 2006;(Suppl 104):S36-S39.

34. Ronco C, Feriani M, Chiaramonte S, et al. Impact of high blood flows on vascular stability in haemodialysis. *Nephrol Dial Transplant.* 1990;5(Suppl 1):109-114.

35. Albers FJ. Causes of hemodialysis access failure. *Adv Renal Replacement Ther.* 1994;1:107-118.

36. Saran R, Bragg-Gresham JL, Levin NW, et al. Longer treatment time and slower ultrafiltration are associations with reduced mortality in the DOPPS. *Kidney Int.* 2006;69:1222-1228.

37. Foley RN, Herzog CA, Collins AJ. Blood pressure and long-term mortality in United States hemodialysis patients: USRDS Waves 3 and 4 Study. *Kidney Int.* 2002;62:1784-1790.

38. Twardowski ZJ. Sodium, hypertension, and an explanation of the "lag phenomenon" in hemodialysis patients. *Hemodial Int.* 2008;12:412-425.

39. EBPG guideline on haemodynamic instability. *Nephrol Dial Transplant.* 2007;22[Suppl 2]: ii22–44.

40. Ing TS, Ronco C, Blagg CR. High-intensity hemodialysis: the wave of the future? *Int J Artif Organs.* 2008;31:201-212.

41. Bleyer AJ, Hartman J, Brannon PC, Reeves-Daniel A, Satko SG, Russell G. Characteristics of sudden death in hemodialysis patients. *Kidney Int.* 2006;69:2268-2273.

42. Morrison G, Michelson EL, Brown S, et al. Mechanism and prevention of cardiac arrhythmias in chronic hemodialysis patients. *Kidney Int.* 1980;17:811-819.

43. Karnik JA, Young BS, Lew NL, et al. Cardiac arrest and sudden death in dialysis units. *Kidney Int.* 2001;60:350-357.

44. Chan CT. Cardiovascular effects of frequent intensive hemodialysis. *Sem Dial.* 2004;17:99-103.

45. Zilch O, Vos PF, Oey PL, et al. Sympathetic hyperactivity in haemodialysis patients is reduced by short daily haemodialysis. *J Hypertension.* 2007;25:1285-1289.

46. National Kidney Foundation. K/DOQI clinical practice guidelines for cardiovascular disease in dialysis patients. *Am J Kidney Dis.* 2005; 45:16-153.

47. Fagugli RM, Reboldi G, Quintaliani G, et al. Short daily hemodialysis: blood pressure control and left ventricular mass reduction in hypertensive hemodialysis patients. *Am J Kidney Dis.* 2001;38:371-376.

48. Culleton BF, Walsh M, Klarenbach SW, et al. Effect of frequent nocturnal hemodialysis vs conventional hemodialysis on left ventricular mass and quality of life. *JAMA.* 2007;298:1291-1299.

49. Roy-Chaudhury P, Kelly BS, Melhem M, et al. Vascular access in hemodialysis: issues, management, and emerging concepts. *Cardiol Clin.* 2005;23:249-273.

50. Leypoldt JK. Kinetics of beta 2-microglobulin and phosphate during hemodialysis: effects of treatment frequency and duration. *Semin Dial.* 2005;18:401-408.

51. Ward RA, Greene T, Hartmann B, Samtleben W. Resistance to intercompartmental mass transfer limits beta2-microglobulin removal by post dilution hemodiafiltration. *Kidney Int.* 2006;69:1431-1437.

52. Acchiardo S. Dialysis amyloidosis. In Nissenson AR, Fine RN (eds). *Dialysis Therapy,* 2nd ed. Philadelphia, PA: Hanley & Belfus Inc, 1993: 313-314.

53. Dember LM Jaber BL. Dialysis-related amyloidosis: late finding or hidden epidemic? *Semin Dial.* 2006;19:105-109.

54. Gal R, Korzets A, Schwartz A, Rath-Wolfson L, Gafter U. Systemic distribution of B₂-microglobulin-derived amyloidosis in patients who undergo long-term hemodialysis. *Arch Pathol Lab Med.* 1994;188: 718-721.

55. DeSoi CA, Umans JG. Phosphate kinetics during high-flux hemodialysis. *J Am Soc Nephrol.* 1993;4: 1214-1218.

56. Chertow GM, Raggi P, Chasan-Taber S, Bommer J, Holzer H, Burke SK. Determinants of progressive vascular calcification in haemodialysis patients. *Nephrol Dial Tranplant.* 2004;19:1489-1496.

57. Raggi P et al. Valvular calcification in hemodialysis patients randomized to calcium-based phosphorus binders or sevelamer. *J Heart Valve Dis.* 2004;13:134-141.

58. Rostand SG, Sanders C, Kirk KA, Rutsky EA, Fraser RG. Myocardial calcification and cardiac dysfunction in chronic renal failure. *Am J Med.* 1988;85:651-657.

59. Schoenhagen P, Tuzcu EM. Coronary artery calcification and end-stage renal disease: vascular biology and clinical implications. *Cleve Clin J Med.* 2002;69(Suppl 3):S12-20.

60. Block GA, Hulbert-Shearon TE, Levin NW, Port FK. Association of serum phosphorus and calcium x phosphate product with mortality risk in chronic hemodialysis patient: a national study. *Am J Kidney Dis.* 1998;31:607-617.

61. Weiner DE , Nicholls AJ, Sarnak MJ. Cardiovascular disease. In Daugirdas JT, Blake PG, Ing TS (eds). *Handbook of Dialysis,* 4th ed. Philadelphia, PA: Lippincott Williams & Wilkins, 2007:626-646.

62. Arief AI. Dialysis disequilibrium syndrome: current concepts on pathogenesis and prevention. *Kidney Int.* 1994;45:629-635.

63. Mian AN, Mendley SR. Acute dialysis in children. In Henrich WL (ed). *Principles and Practice of Dialysis,* 3rd ed. Philadelphia, PA: Lippincott Williams & Wilkins, 2004:617-28.

CHAPTER 28

Peritoneal Dialysis

Richard L. Feinberg and Julie A. Freischlag

In 1923, Ganter first demonstrated that peritoneal dialysis was feasible in an animal model.[1] Fifteen years later, Rhoads[2] used intermittent peritoneal dialysis to treat two patients who had nephrotic syndrome. However, it was not until the 1940s, with Palmer's development of the first permanent peritoneal catheter made of silicone rubber, that successful treatment of larger numbers of patients with peritoneal dialysis was reported.[3] In the early 1960s, subsequent modifications of Palmer's silicone catheter[4,5] allowed peritoneal dialysis to become a practical option for more widespread use in patients with renal failure.[6] In 1968, Tenckhoff and Schecter[7] invented and demonstrated a silicone catheter with two Dacron cuffs for use in patients who needed long-term peritoneal dialysis. In a modified form, this catheter remains the most frequently used catheter.[7-10] Concomitant with this evolution in peritoneal dialysis catheter design, dialysate solutions had, by then, also become commercially available. With the development of automated methods for performing dialysis runs, thereby greatly facilitating the procedure of continuous ambulatory peritoneal dialysis (CAPD), long-term peritoneal dialysis truly became an acceptable option for large numbers of patients with end-stage renal failure.[11]

In absolute terms, the number of patients who rely upon peritoneal dialysis continues to increase. In the mid-1980s, the National Institutes of Health reported[9] that more than 35,000 patients throughout the world were receiving peritoneal dialysis. In the United States alone, approximately 16,000 patients (constituting roughly 17% of the overall cohort of US patients with end-stage renal disease (ESRD) at that time) relied on peritoneal dialysis rather than hemodialysis. In the first decade of the 21st century, peritoneal dialysis is estimated to be employed by more than 120,000 patients worldwide; nevertheless, this comprises a mere 8% of the world's chronic dialysis patients—a dwindling share of the overall ESRD population relative to hemodialysis over the past 25 years.[12] Peritoneal dialysis costs less than hemodialysis and can be accomplished at home by most patients,[13] resulting in improved tolerance and a substantial advantage in the ability to maintain a functional lifestyle.[14,15] Moreover, there is evidence suggesting a significant survival advantage among patients receiving peritoneal dialysis compared with those on hemodialysis.[16,17] The two major long-term complications of CAPD remain catheter blockage and infection.

The peritoneum is the largest serosal surface in the body, with an area ranging between 1 and 2 M^2 in adults, and acts as a biologic membrane for the exchange of solids and fluids.[18] Peritoneal transport of water and solute is related to the rate of peritoneal blood flow, which ranges between 50 and 100 ml/minute. However, the *efficiency* with which water and solute are transported is more precisely a function of the actual number and distribution of capillaries within the peritoneal membrane (ie, the *vascularity* of the peritoneal membrane, rather than its total surface area).[19] The peritoneal capillary basement membrane contains *pores* of varying sizes that govern the diffusion of water, smaller solutes and macromolecules from the peritoneal cavity to the submesothelial capillary lumen and back.[20] Smaller molecules, such as urea, equilibrate in 4 hours or less, while larger molecules, such as albumin, may take twice that time to equilibrate.[21] Protein losses occur with peritoneal dialysis, averaging 6 to 12 g/day depending on the size of the patient and the frequency of the exchanges.[22] Amino acids are also lost during peritoneal dialysis, at a rate of approximately 2.0 to 3.5 g/day.[23] Serum levels of vitamins B1, B6, C, and folic acid are decreased in patients on peritoneal dialysis.[24] Glucose absorption from the dialysate mixtures is substantial. Patients on peritoneal dialysis absorb from 100 to 200 g of glucose/day, which can lead to obesity, glucose intolerance, and hypertriglyceridemia if the patient's diet is not regulated.[25]

One of the primary advantages of peritoneal dialysis over hemodialysis is that there are a number of options for conducting peritoneal dialysis that can be tailored to the needs of the individual patient and improve the quality of life. *Intermittent peritoneal dialysis* can be used effectively in the acute setting, but it is not adequate for long-term use. Malnutrition, acidosis, anemia, and poor control of the patient's hydration are side effects that occur after the first year.[26,27] This method is best reserved for the few selected patients who have some residual level of renal function. In intermittent peritoneal dialysis, 2 to 3 L of dialysate is used and peritoneal cavity "dwell" times of 20 to 30 minutes are required between each drainage of the peritoneal cavity. Usually, 10-hour sessions every other night (or 3 times a week) are necessary. Intermittent peritoneal dialysis can be done manually by the patient or by the automated reverse osmosis delivery system.

CAPD is the most widely employed method for performing peritoneal dialysis and is a low-flow, 24-hour, continuous dialysis technique that uses 2 L of dialysate with a peritoneal dwell time of 48 hours before draining.[28,29] *Continuous cycling peritoneal dialysis* (CCPD) is similar to CAPD, except that most of the cycles are performed at night, and there is only 1 diurnal cycle with a prolonged dwell time during the day in which 1500 to 2000 ml of dialysate is used.[30] Cycles also occur primarily during the night in *nocturnal peritoneal dialysis*, with 20- to 60-minute cycles over 8- to 10-hour periods. Such exchange rates require high dialysate flows. Nocturnal peritoneal dialysis is therefore best for the patient with high peritoneal transfer rates and for those who cannot tolerate large peritoneal volumes because of pain or discomfort.[31] Clearances of urea and creatine are lower in nocturnal peritoneal dialysis, and the procedure is more expensive because of the need for higher flow rates from the exchanger. *Tidal peritoneal dialysis* is an alternative method of performing peritoneal dialysis that keeps a larger reservoir of fluid in the peritoneal cavity at all times and exchanges smaller volumes.[32] It also allows the dialysate to maintain contact with the peritoneal cavity at all times. However, tidal peritoneal dialysis requires a special automated cycler that is modified by volume, and no real benefit from this type of peritoneal dialysis has yet been shown.[33]

Regardless of the form of peritoneal dialysis chosen, patient education and motivation determine success. Training sessions are required before peritoneal dialysis is instituted at home. It is also important to note that, at any point, peritoneal dialysis patients can successfully undergo renal transplantation without suffering from an increased risk of peritonitis and graft failure.[34]

Indications

Short-Term Peritoneal Dialysis

Short-term peritoneal dialysis can almost always be readily performed, especially in children, obviating the need for central venous catheterization.[35] Indications include hyperkalemia, fluid overload, metabolic acidosis, electrolyte disorders, and congestive heart failure.[36] Short-term peritoneal dialysis is also especially well-suited for patients with contra-indications to anticoagulation because, in contrast to hemodialysis, heparinization is not essential. Moreover, patients with borderline cardiovascular status can undergo peritoneal dialysis with fewer hemodynamic consequences than occur with hemodialysis—a potentially critical factor in the acute setting.[37] Finally, peritoneal dialysis may be useful as an alternative to hemodialysis in acutely ill patients with poor venous access, when establishment of a central venous access is difficult or impossible.

Drug intoxication may also be treated with short-term peritoneal dialysis when hemodialysis is unavailable or contraindicated.[38] The pH of the peritoneal dialysate can be altered to enhance anion diffusion. The addition of albumin can bind the drug and prevent its absorption.

Other indications for short-term peritoneal dialysis include profound hypothermia,[39] hypoglycemia from long-term use of hypoglycemic agents, poisoning, congenital lactic acidosis, maple sugar urine disease, urea cycle defects, hyperuricemia associated with gouty nephropathy,[40] and hepatic coma. Intraperitoneal deferoxamine has been used to chelate aluminum.[41] Patients with acute pancreatitis have been treated with short-term peritoneal dialysis,[42] but the results have not been impressive, probably because the dialysate irrigates only the intraperitoneal space and does not bathe the retroperitoneum, where most of the damaging enzymes and debris are found in acute pancreatitis.

Long-Term Peritoneal Dialysis

Suitable candidates for long-term peritoneal dialysis include patients with ESRD who are capable and competent to manage the catheter and its machine or who have a family member who can do so for them. Children are good candidates for long-term peritoneal dialysis.[43] Children who weigh less than 10 kg have very small arteries and veins, making construction of a usable hemodialysis fistula technically difficult. Patients with diabetes and congestive heart failure also do well with peritoneal dialysis,[44] as do patients who cannot be heparinized.

Contraindications

Major contraindications for peritoneal dialysis include recent abdominal surgery; inflammatory bowel disease; presence of a colostomy, an ileostomy, or an ileal conduit; extensive peritoneal fibrosis; or immunosuppression. Patients with significant neurologic deficits, psychosis, poor intellect, or poor motivation also are less suitable candidates for long-term peritoneal dialysis. Patients who are blind or who have crippling arthritis of their hands cannot be candidates for long-term peritoneal dialysis unless there is a family member or caregiver available to help them with the procedure.

Relative contraindications to peritoneal dialysis include severe chronic obstructive pulmonary disease, complications of diverticulosis, polycystic kidney disease, hyperlipidemia, obesity, and protein malnutrition. Patients who require short-term peritoneal dialysis immediately after surgery also may not be candidates for peritoneal dialysis because of surgical drains and wounds. Diaphragmatic, abdominal, or inguinal hernias may become more symptomatic during peritoneal dialysis and therefore may require repair before peritoneal dialysis.[45] Patients with severe gastroesophageal reflux may experience an exacerbation of reflux symptoms as a result of the increased intraabdominal pressure during dialysate dwells and, thus, may not be able to tolerate peritoneal dialysis.

Types of Peritoneal Catheters

One of the first peritoneal dialysis catheters to be used was a latex rubber catheter designed by Boen and associates in 1962.[4] In the same year, Weston and Roberts[46] devised a nylon catheter. Gutch and Stevens[47] first introduced silicone as a material of choice for use in peritoneal dialysis catheters. The most commonly used peritoneal access catheter today is that designed by Tenckhoff,[7,48] which consists of a soft, nonreactive silicone elastomer (Silastic) tube with multiple side holes along its innermost (peritoneal) portion and a hole in the end of the catheter (Fig. 28-1). The Tenckhoff catheter has two polyethylene terephthalate (Dacron) cuffs that help anchor the catheter in place. These Dacron cuffs initiate a local inflammatory tissue reaction, with the formation of a fibrin clot, followed

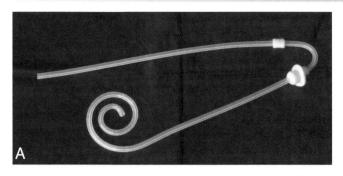

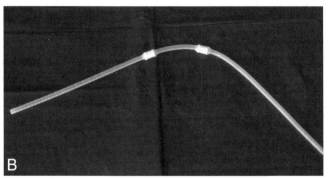

Figure 28-1.
A, Tenckhoff curl catheter: swan neck configuration. *B,* Tenckhoff straight catheter.

by the infiltration of granulocytes and fibroblasts with giant cells. Simple squamous epithelium grows around the innermost cuff over time to seal the peritoneal cavity and prevent leakage around the catheter from the peritoneal cavity. The outermost cuff is placed in the subcutaneous space, where fibrous tissue ingrowth occurs, providing a barrier to bacterial growth from the skin contaminating the catheter tunnel. Stratified squamous epithelium grows around the skin exit site as well, further sealing the catheter.[49]

Reliable data comparing various catheter configurations and design modifications are exceedingly sparse, and most reports contain small numbers of patients in retrospective comparisons. However, single-cuff catheters appear to have a lower 1-year survival rate and a higher infection rate than do the double-cuff catheters.[49] Curl-tipped catheters offer no clear advantage over straight-tipped catheters, although their advocates believe that patency time is longer. Newer types of catheters have been devised but have not been shown convincingly to have a particular advantage over the basic, double-cuff Tenckhoff catheter,[50] which has achieved catheter survival rates of 97% at 2 years and 92% at 5 years.[51] Twardowski and colleagues[52] described the swan-neck catheter, which is a variation on the classic Tenckhoff catheter in which the catheter segment between the inner and outer Dacron cuffs is formed with a sharp arch, as in the neck of a swan. The subcutaneous tunnel is formed into an acute angle, and the catheter retains that shape. It was originally thought that such a configuration could prevent tunnel infections; however, no such improvement has been documented. Nevertheless, there does appear to be a reduction in the incidence of unwanted catheter-tip migration using the swan neck configuration.[53] A polyurethane catheter (Corpak catheter) designed by

Thermedics has an inner catheter diameter 1.5 times that of the Tenckhoff catheter.[54] Good tissue ingrowth has been shown with this catheter. Polyurethane may possess more resistance to infection than Silastic. Silicone catheters become impregnated with a protein biofilm that inhibits the white blood cell function of engulfing the bacteria migrating along the catheter.[55] This process may lead to more catheter infections and is not reported as a characteristic of the polyurethane catheter.

Toronto Western Hospital has promoted the use of a catheter with two silicone disks postioned perpendicular to the catheter tube to hold the catheter in place.[56] Despite the presence of these silicone disks, obstruction from either bowel adhesions or omentum resulted in 10% outflow failure. Another new type of catheter is the Lifecath catheter, which has an intraperitoneal silicone disk that is placed just subjacent to the abdominal wall, inside the peritoneal cavity.[57] This catheter has a 6% outflow failure rate due to obstruction: the omentum can still attach itself to the disk even though it has a large port. In addition, increased leakage has been reported in some with the Lifecath catheter.[58] However, this catheter may remain patent longer than the Tenckhoff catheter because of less migration and infection.

Peritoneal Catheter Placement

Short-term peritoneal dialysis catheters can be placed percutaneously, which is efficient and less expensive than placement in the operating room. Physicians who use the percutaneous approach choose to place the catheter at McBurney's point or at a location on the left side of the abdomen just opposite to this site. A Foley catheter should be placed before the insertion of the catheter if the patient still produces urine, and an enema should be given before placement of the catheter to decompress the colon. To reduce the rate of infection, prophylactic antibiotics, targeted primarily against ordinary skin flora, should be administered before the procedure. The skin is infiltrated with lidocaine, and intravenous sedation can be used for patient comfort. A stylet or guidewire is used to advance the catheter into the peritoneal cavity The potential hazards inherent to this technique include perforation of intestine or bladder or damage to a blood vessel or solid organ.

Long-term peritoneal dialysis catheters should be placed with the patient in the operating room to ensure patient comfort and catheter sterility. Depending on the patient's preference, local, regional, or general anesthesia may be used. General anesthesia is preferred in children, because relaxation of the abdominal musculature facilitates placement of the catheter. Long-term peritoneal dialysis catheters may be inserted percutaneously using a trocar (as described above); however, we see little benefit to this method, which necessarily exposes the patient to a higher obligate incidence of inadvertent visceral and/or vascular injury. The preferred method is with an open surgical technique, which allows direct visualization of the position of the catheter and of the contents of the peritoneal cavity. The patient fasts from midnight the night before the operation, and an enema is given. Systemic antibiotic prophylaxis with a broad-spectrum antimicrobial agent is also administered; an antimicrobial effective against *Staphylococcus aureus,*

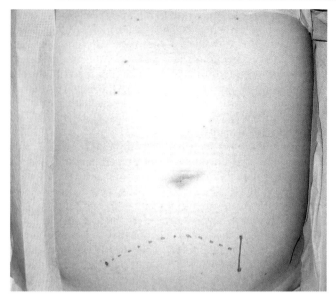

Figure 28-2.
Infraumbilical left paramedian incision overlying the left rectus muscle. Note the curvilinear path of the planned subcutaneous tunnel leading to the proposed catheter exit site in the right lower quadrant, below the belt line.

such as a first generation cephalosporin, is suitable for prophylaxis.

Specific incisions used for the insertion of peritoneal dialysis catheters have included paramedian, lower midline, and transverse in either lower quadrant. Our preferred method employs a small paramedian incision placed below the level of the umbilicus, roughly midway between the midline and the anterior superior iliac spine, directly overlying the rectus muscle (Fig. 28-2). All other considerations being equal, it is preferable to place this incision on the nondominant side (ie, left lower quadrant for right-handed individuals).The incision is carried down to the anterior rectus fascia which is incised longitudinally, and the rectus muscle is split bluntly to expose the transversalis fascia and underlying peritoneum. Blunt dissection within the rectus muscle at this level can shear the inferior epigastric artery, and care should be taken to avoid this if possible. Next, the peritoneum is grasped between clamps, lifted, and incised sharply, allowing open access to the peritoneal cavity. Particular care must be taken at this point if previous abdominal surgery has led to the formation of adhesions to the parietal peritoneum. Especially dense adhesions may preclude safe placement of the catheter, and an alternate method of dialysis may become necessary. Some authors have recommended routine omentectomy to prevent later envelopment of the catheter by the omentum which could lead to catheter occlusion[59]; however, this technique has not been widely embraced, and we do not routinely do this.

The catheter is introduced through the peritoneal opening and directed toward the pelvis, because this is the most dependent area of the peritoneal cavity in both the upright and supine positions. A guidewire passed down the lumen of the catheter may help facilitate placement of the catheter, although this is usually not necessary. A non-absorbable suture is placed on the internal aspect of the

anterior abdominal wall and tied loosely around the catheter to secure it in place in the pelvis. A purse-string suture is placed to secure the edges of the peritoneal opening to the first Dacron cuff, ensuring a watertight closure so peritoneal dialysis can be commenced early in the postoperative period. This suture is reinforced with a second purse-string suture that incorporates the transversalis fascia around the cuff to further strengthen the seal. Nonabsorbable sutures such as polypropylene (Prolene) are used.

The catheter exit site should be chosen and marked before surgery. This should be located on the side opposite that of the rectus incision (eg, right lower quadrant exit site when the catheter has been inserted through the left rectus muscle) and below the belt line for patient comfort. As the catheter exits from the peritoneum, it should be brought directly through the belly of the rectus muscle, exiting the anterior rectus sheath through a separate small puncture created in the medial leaf of the rectus fascia. The innermost Dacron cuff remains embedded within the rectus sheath, deep to the muscle. A small stab incision is next made in the skin at the previously marked exit site, and the catheter is passed from the rectus incision toward the skin exit site, care being taken not to dilate or distend the small skin opening at the exit site. The catheter is advanced through the tunnel and positioned so that the second Dacron cuff lies within the subcutaneous tunnel, at least 2 cm from the skin exit site. No sutures are placed at the exit site, as this may create an inflammatory tissue reaction that can predispose toward infection. Instead, Tegaderm is used to secure the catheter to the skin and prevent accidental dislodgment until the Dacron cuff becomes securely incorporated into the subcutaneous tissues. Irrigation of the catheter with heparinized saline at the time of the operation documents patency and flushes out any debris or blood clots. This maneuver can also help ensure that there is no leakage from around the first cuff. The fluid that is instilled should drain out of the abdominal cavity spontaneously by gravity.

The rectus fascia is closed using no. 2-0 or 0 nonabsorbable monofilament suture, and the skin is closed with an absorbable subcuticular suture. The catheter is connected to a bag of dialysate in the operating room using a titanium connector (which has been shown to reduce the incidence of catheter infection), and peritoneal dialysis is begun with a small volume. The fluid should flow freely, with no demonstrable leaks. If peritoneal dialysis does not have to be started for a period of time, daily flushes of the catheter should be performed in a sterile manner to maintain patency of the catheter. If peritoneal dialysis has to begin immediately, small volumes should be exchanged at frequent intervals with the patient in a supine and inactive position to prevent leakage from the wound. For proper healing, the patient should not lift more than 30 pounds for 2 weeks.

Laparoscopic-assisted placement of peritoneal dialysis catheters has been advocated by some authors.[60,61] Putative advantages suggested by proponents of this technique include more precise catheter placement under direct laparoscopic visualization of the abdomen and pelvis than is afforded during traditional open surgical placement. Published rates of catheter survival, as well as catheter migration and entrapment rates, have been competitive with those reported for traditional open surgical catheter insertion.[62,63] Some difficulties with catheter tunneling have been described with this technique, and it remains unclear whether the laparoscopic technique offers any tangible benefits over conventional placement, which is readily performed through a single small incision and can easily be accomplished under local anesthesia, without the need for intra-abdominal insufflation. As a result of these considerations, laparoscopic peritoneal dialysis catheter placement has still not been universally adopted.

Complications of Peritoneal Dialysis

There has been no change in the incidence of early and late complications after the placement of Tenckhoff catheters since data were first reported in the 1970s. During the first month after Tenckhoff catheter placement, the major complication is outflow failure, which occurs in 1% to 20% of cases.[64] Early catheter infections can occur but are unusual, whereas infectious complications assume a predominant role in peritoneal dialysis complications over the intermediate and long term. Outflow failure that occurs within the first few days after surgery may be caused by catheter malposition. Omentum that obstructs the catheter side holes can also cause outflow failure during the first few weeks after placement. A kink or clot in the catheter can cause both inflow and outflow malfunction. Inflow pain can also indicate malpositioning of the catheter, such as migration to the subphrenic space. If the addition of sodium bicarbonate to the dialysate composition to increase the pH does not relieve the pain experienced with infusion, the catheter may be pushing against a portion of the abdominal cavity or its contents. Most commonly, the catheter is dislodged under the diaphragm, which is confirmed by administration of a small amount of radiographic contrast via the catheter. In most cases, especially if the obstruction occurs early in the postoperative period, the catheter may have to be repositioned surgically. We have occasionally been successful in repositioning migrated catheters by means of cannulation with a stiff guidewire (Lunderquist Extra Stiff, Cook Medical; Stiff Glidewire, Terumo) under fluoroscopic guidance and manipulating the catheter back down into the pelvis, thereby avoiding the need for reoperation. However, if durable restoration of catheter function is used as the benchmark of success, this technique has been successful in only 10 to 20% of cases attempted and has not been a reliable method in our experience, although others have reported somewhat higher rates of success.[65,66]

Outflow failure continues to be the leading cause of catheter failure after 1 month, with incidence ranging from 5% to 20%. In some cases of outflow obstruction, a fibrin clot occludes the central lumen and may obstruct the catheter, or the entire length of the intraperitoneal catheter may become encased in a fibrin sheath. In such cases, either streptokinase, urokinase[67] or tPA[68] have been successfully used to lyse the fibrin clot and restore catheter patency. Most commonly, 8 mg of tPA in 10 ml of sterile water is instilled into the dialysis catheter and allowed to dwell for 60 minutes, after which the catheter is aspirated of lytic agent and 250 or 500 mL of saline are instilled and then drained from the peritoneal cavity. Needless to say, instillation of lytic agent in this manner cannot be expected to have a salutary effect on catheter malfunction due to causes other than obstruction by fibrin clot (e.g., catheter migration, compartmentalization by adhesions, omental wrapping).

However, the risks of intracatheter lytic instillation are very low, and this is often employed presumptively as the initial step in investigating sudden peritoneal dialysis catheter malfunction. If successful, heparin should be used in the dialysate for the next few days to ensure patency of the catheter.[69] If intracatheter lytic instillation proves unsuccessful in restoring a catheter to proper function, laparoscopy can be helpful in identifying the cause of the outflow failure. Such techniques, as described by Pitchford and associates,[70] may be quite helpful in removing fibrin sleeves or in repositioning a peritoneal dialysis catheter. Bowel or omentum that obstructs the catheter side holes can be easily visualized and, if present, laparoscopically guided manipulation of the abdominal contents may release the catheter and relieve the obstruction.[71] The catheter tip can even be retrieved, delivered via one of the access ports, cleaned of debris, and repositioned in the pelvis, with reports of durable success.[72] Unfortunately, in a large number of cases, open surgical re-exploration is still ultimately required to alleviate the obstruction.

Intraperitoneal bleeding can occur immediately after placement of peritoneal dialysis catheters. The most common cause of the bleeding is injury to small visceral, omental, or abdominal wall vessels. If the hematocrit of the effluent is less than 2% or if the red blood cell count is less than $60,000/cm,^3$ the bleeding is considered insignificant. Such bleeding should be monitored, and it most often resolves. To prevent clotting of the catheter while the effluent remains bloody, heparin (1000 U/2 L dialysate) should be added.[73] If a bloody dialysate is noted 1 month or longer after placement of the peritoneal dialysis catheter, one must suspect other causes, such as inflammation, which may lead to peritonitis; perforation of a viscus; or IgA glomerulonephritis, which often occurs in association with upper respiratory tract infections. Bleeding can also be seen in female patients secondary to endometriosis or during menstruation.[74,75] Diagnostic evaluation is mandatory to determine the cause of late bleeding associated with peritoneal dialysis catheters.

Leakage of dialysate from around the catheter exit site or from the midline wound may occur immediately after surgery[76] and may be manifested by edema in the abdominal wall, legs, or scrotum.[77] This represents a direct technical failure of the insertion procedure and usually results from inadequate encircling of the catheter with the purse string sutures to the peritoneum and transversalis fascia. Because large volumes of dialysate exacerbate this problem, decreasing the amount of dialysate and increasing the number of exchanges can be employed as temporary measures that allow the leak to seal without the need for reoperation.[78] Only if the inner Dacron cuff has become extruded from its original position will the pericatheter leak not seal with conservative management.

Pericatheter hernias can occur during the course of peritoneal dialysis.[79] These occur more frequently in older patients, multiparous women, and patients who had experienced leakage from the abdominal wound immediately after surgery. Most of these pericatheter hernias require surgical repair. Other preexisting hernias can be enlarged during peritoneal dialysis because of the increased intra-abdominal pressure and volume[80]; these include inguinal hernias (especially if there is a patent processus vaginalis), umbilical hernias, and incisional hernias. Acute hydrothorax on either the left or right side can occur early in the course of peritoneal dialysis if the pleuroperitoneal communication is still patent.[81] In children, an asymptomatic Bochdalek or Morgagni hernia can also be revealed once peritoneal dialysis has begun.

Other symptoms that patients might experience because of the increased intra-abdominal pressure of peritoneal dialysis include delayed gastric emptying, which may lead to gastroesophageal reflux.[82] Those with impaired pulmonary function may experience worsening of their symptoms when the peritoneal cavity is filled with dialysate fluid.[83] Cardiac output and stroke volume in patients on peritoneal dialysis are decreased secondary to decreased preload, which results from compression of the inferior vena cava. In those with marginal cardiac status, this decrease could pose a problem. However, decreasing the volume of dialysate in each dwell may help alleviate the patient's symptoms.

Metabolic complications in patients receiving peritoneal dialysis include dehydration, which can be treated with decreased osmolarity of the dialysate, and overhydration, which can be treated with decreased dwell time and increased dialysate glucose concentration. Severe hyperglycemia and the hyperosmolar state can occur in diabetic patients receiving peritoneal dialysis.[25] Protein malnutrition may result from the daily losses of protein and amino acids.[22] This can be rectified with dietary supplements, but, if treatment is unsuccessful, peritoneal dialysis may have to be terminated. The increased caloric load resulting from the absorption of glucose from the dialysate may lead to obesity, uncontrolled hyperglycemia, or hypertriglyceridemia. Changing to an osmotic agent other than glucose may help, but often peritoneal dialysis must be stopped. Depletion of important vitamins can be replenished through dietary supplements.[243]

Both osteitis and osteomalacia can develop in patients receiving peritoneal dialysis.[84] Other metabolic perturbations, such as hyponatremia, hypernatremia, hypokalemia, or hyperkalemia, can be avoided with appropriate changes in dialysate mixtures.[85] The disequilibrium syndrome, infrequently described in patients receiving peritoneal dialysis, is characterized by headaches, nausea, vomiting, hypertension, seizures, and, in rare cases, coma, secondary to cerebral edema.[86] This syndrome is thought to develop when a rapid osmotic gradient is created across the blood-brain barrier because of delay in the removal of urea. The treatment of this syndrome is supportive and can be prevented if the osmolality of the dialysate mixture is decreased.

Visceral perforation can be seen either early or late in the course of peritoneal dialysis.[87] The catheters themselves can penetrate hollow viscera, solid organs, the pelvic wall, and the retroperitoneal space.[88] Depending upon the specific organ involved, visceral perforation can be indicated by the presence of feculent effluent from the catheter, diarrhea after dialysate infusion, high volumes of urine after dialysate infusion, bloody effluent from the catheter, retention of dialysate after infusion, and polymicrobial peritonitis with a predominance of enteric organisms on culture. Visceral perforation must be addressed on an emergent basis with laparotomy, and most often the catheter must be removed for peritonitis to clear.[89]

Infectious complications of peritoneal dialysis are frequent and constitute the leading cause of hospitalization among patients on CAPD. These infections remain a leading source of morbidity for patients and lead to catheter failure in 5% to 20% of all peritoneal dialysis catheters that are placed.[9] Data collected from the National Institutes of Health National Registry documented 4.6 episodes of infection per year per patient in 1978 and 1.7 episodes per year per patient in 1982.[10] Recent data suggest a continuation of this decline in the incidence of CAPD-related peritonitis to a range of 0.3 to 0.5 episodes per patient per year.[90] The 12-month risk-rate of infection in patients receiving peritoneal dialysis is 65%.[91] The most common catheter infections include exit-site infections, deep cuff infections, and unresolving peritonitis.[92,93] It is estimated that one third of the hospitalizations of patients receiving peritoneal dialysis result from peritonitis.[16] Peritoneal dialysis is terminated in patients because of recurrent peritonitis in 25% to 60% of cases.[94,95] Some estimate that 15% of the deaths of CAPD patients result from peritonitis,[13] possibly because the catheter provides a direct route for contamination of the peritoneal cavity and secondary septicemia. The infused dialysate solutions are thought to dilute the concentrations of opsonins (IgG and C3) and peritoneal macrophages, which are needed to combat intra-abdominal infections.[96] The fluid within the abdominal cavity impairs the ability to localize infection by the omentum. Phagocytic and bactericidal white blood cell activity is also diminished by the hypertonicity and acidic nature of the dialysate.[97,98] The diagnosis of peritonitis is suggested by the presence of a cloudy effluent accompanied by abdominal discomfort.[92]

When an infection is present, the white blood cell count of the effluent increases to more than 100 white blood cells/cm^3.[99] Normally, monocytes are predominantly found in the peritoneal fluid ($\geq$70%), but, with peritonitis, the majority of white blood cells retrieved from the peritoneal cavity are neutrophils ($>$50%).[100] Some patients experience nausea and vomiting (27%), rebound tenderness (40%), fever (27%), and peripheral leukocytosis (23%).[91]

The pathogen can be cultured from the catheter fluid, which can direct the appropriate selection of antibiotic therapy. The most common pathogens found to be responsible for catheter-related peritonitis are coagulase-negative *Staphylococcus* (55% to 80%) and *S. aureus* (17% to 30%).[101] Fungal infections are also a common cause of peritonitis in these patients.[102] Contamination can originate from the patient's skin flora, nasal flora, colonized skin at the catheter exit site, and occasionally transmural contamination from the bowel. As mentioned previously, the first indication of a perforated viscus can be signs and symptoms of peritonitis. Cultures obtained from patients with a perforated viscus will reveal a polymicrobial flora with a predominance of enteric organisms and not the usual skin flora. The leading determinants of catheter loss among CAPD patients who develop peritonitis include: polymicrobial infections (these are much more likely to result in catheter loss than single-organism infections)[103]; the specific pathogen involved (among single-organism infections, those caused by gram-negative organisms and yeast species carry a significantly greater risk of catheter loss than those resulting from gram-positive organisms); and the presence of concomitant tunnel and/or exit site infections.[95]

Antimicrobial therapy instilled through the peritoneal catheter can successfully treat peritonitis in cases caused by a single organism when not associated with a perforated viscus.[104] Follow-up culture confirms eradication of the organism. Resolution of the patient's symptoms should be apparent in 3 to 5 days. Organisms that produce a biofilm or slime, an amorphous glycocalyx that can adhere to plastic surfaces, may make eradication of those bacteria more difficult.[93] The biofilm protects the bacteria from opsonization and prevents the white blood cells from engulfing the bacteria. Organisms that produce slime include coagulase-negative *Staphylococcus, S. aureus, Candida albicans,* and *Pseudomonas aeruginosa.*

The majority of patients with peritonitis can be treated initially with the instillation of intraperitoneal antibiotics, which can safely be performed as an outpatient in most cases. Hospitalization should be reserved for those patients with gram-negative infections, anaerobic infections, *Pseudomonas* infections, fungal infections, or toxic symptoms. Initially, antibiotic coverage should be broad spectrum, including coverage for *S. aureus* and gram-negative organisms. Antimicrobial therapy may be selected more precisely depending on the offending organism cultured from the peritoneal cavity. If the peritonitis does not resolve or if recurrent episodes of peritonitis occur, the catheter may be harboring the causative organisms and removal may be required in order to possibly eradicate the infection. In such cases, at least a temporary course of hemodialysis may be required until the peritonitis has resolved and a new peritoneal dialysis catheter can be placed.

Catheter tunnel infections can lead to peritonitis, or they can exist as a localized infection confined to the catheter alone. It is estimated that patients receiving peritoneal dialysis experience 1 tunnel infection episode for every 16 patient-months while on peritoneal dialysis. Increased numbers of tunnel infections are associated with poor catheter maintenance, exit-site skin irritation from tape and dressings, and undue tension placed on the catheter that causes protrusion of the outer Dacron cuff. If the exit site and the tract are erythematous without purulence, the tunnel infection can be treated with local measures, such as cleansing with hydrogen peroxide or povidone-iodine.[105] Topical antibiotic ointment, as well as systemic antibiotics, can be used. If there is frank purulence, however, it is often very difficult to eradicate the tunnel infection. Although it has rarely been successful, some advocate removal of the outer Dacron cuff to help to cure the tunnel infection.[106]

After Tenckhoff catheter placement, the peritoneum has been shown to become thickened in some patients, which leads to a loss of ultrafiltration capacity.[107,108] Peritoneal membrane dysfunction is characterized by increased peritoneal permeability, resulting in a rapid absorption of the dialysate, which alters the osmotic gradient needed for adequate dialysis. The transport of solutes remains the same, but the transfer of water does not occur. This phenomenon may be caused by the use of acetate in the dialysate solutions.[109] Treatment includes the use of shorter dwell times

with higher flow rates and the elimination of long diurnal dwell times.

Peritoneal sclerosis can also occur and lead to the abandonment of peritoneal dialysis in these patients because they can no longer achieve adequate dialysis.[110] A thickened peritoneal scar develops in these patients and envelops the intra-abdominal organs. As a result, the surface area available for dialysis is decreased. The cause is unknown but may be related to repeated bouts of peritonitis, acetate, hyperosmolar dialysate solutions, or particulate matter in the dialysate.[111] The process can be fatal if bowel obstruction and strangulation occur. No treatment is known to aid in either preventing or treating this complication.

Concluding Remarks

Peritoneal dialysis is a viable and, we believe, underutilized option for many patients with end-stage renal failure who require dialysis—especially children. Despite the frequency of the complications described herein, 60% to 90% of peritoneal dialysis catheters are still functioning at 1 year. Patient survival rates are at least equal to, and may slightly exceed, those of patients receiving hemodialysis, with 3-year survival rates of approximately 60%. Of those who survive 3 years, just over half are still maintained on peritoneal dialysis therapy. Peritoneal dialysis does not preclude the possibility of later renal allotransplantation. Ultimately, infectious complications, such as recurrent bouts of peritonitis, may result in abandoning peritoneal dialysis in a majority of patients; however, for such patients, hemodialysis may be initiated without any loss of options.

REFERENCES

1. Ganter G. Ueber die beseitigung giftiger Stoffe aus dem Blute durch Dialyse. *Munch Med Wochschr.* 1923;70:1478.
2. Rhoads JE. Peritoneal lavage in the treatment of renal insufficiency. *Am J Med Sci* 1938;192:642.
3. Palmer RA, Quinton WE, Gray JE. Prolonged peritoneal dialysis for chronic renal failure. *Lancet.* 1964;1(7335):700-702.
4. Boen ST, et al. Periodic peritoneal dialysis in the treatment of chronic uremia. *Trans Am Soc Artif Intern Organs.* 1962;8:256.
5. Tenckhoff H, Shilipetar G, Boen ST. One year's experience with home peritoneal dialysis. *ASAIO Trans* 1965;11:11.
6. Oreopoulos DG, et al. CAPD: A new era in the treatment of chronic renal failure. *Clin Nephrol* 1979;11:125.
7. Tenckhoff H, Schecter H. A bacteriologically safe peritoneal access device. *Trans Am Soc Artif Intern Organs* 1968;14:181.
8. Bullmaster JR, et al. Surgical aspects of the Tenckhoff peritoneal dialysis catheter: A seven-year experience. *Am J Surg.* 1985;149:339.
9. Steigbigel RT, Cross AS. Infections associated with hemodialysis and chronic peritoneal dialysis. In Remington JS, Swarts MN (eds). *Current Clinical Topics in Infectious Diseases.* New York, McGraw-Hill, 1987.
10. Steinberg SM, et al. *Report of the National C APD registry of the National Institutes of Health.* Washington, DC: National Institutes of Health, 1986.
11. Gutman RA. Automatic peritoneal dialysis for home use. *Q J Med.* 1978;47:261.
12. Moeller S, Gioberge S, Brown G. ESRD patients in 2001: Global overview of patients, treatment modalities and development trends. *Nephrol Dial Transplant.* 2002;17:2071-2076.
13. Rottembourg J, et al. Severe abdominal complications in patients undergoing continuous ambulatory peritoneal dialysis. *Proc Eur Dial Transplant Assoc* 1983;20:236.
14. Finkelstein AF, Wuerth D, Finkelstein SH. Quality of life assessments in hemodialysis and peritoneal dialysis patients: an important

dimension of patient choice why is the evidence favoring hemodialysis over peritoneal dialysis misleading? *Semin Dial.* 2007;20(3): 211-213.

15. Heaf J. Underutilization of Peritoneal Dialysis. *JAMA.* 2004;291(6): 740-742.

16. Collins AJ, Hao W, Xia H, Ebben JP, Everson SE, Constantini EG, Ma JZ. Mortality risks of peritoneal dialysis and hemodialysis. *Am J. Kidney Dis.* 1999;34(6):1065-1074

17. Heaf JG, Løkkegaard H, Madsen M. Initial survival advantage of peritoneal dialysis over hemodialysis. *Nephrol Dial Transplant.* 2002;17:112-117.

18. Clark AJ. Absorption from the peritoneal cavity. *J Pharmacol.* 1921;16:415.

19. Ronco C. The nearest capillary hypothesis: a novel approach to peritoneal transport physiology. *Perit Dial Int.* 1996;16:121-125

20. Rippe B. A three pore model of peritoneal transport. *Perit Dial Int.* 1999;13(suppl 2):S35-S38.

21. Nolph KD, et al. Equilibration of peritoneal dialysis solutions during long dwell exchanges. *J Lab Clin Med* 1979;93:246.

22. Rubin J, et al. Protein losses in continuous ambulatory peritoneal dialysis. *Nephron* 1981;28:218.

23. Dombros N, et al. Plasma amino acid profiles and amino acid losses in patients undergoing CAPD. *Perit Dial Bull.* 1982;2:27.

24. Blumberg A, Hanck A, Sander G. Vitamin nutrition in patients on continuous ambulatory peritoneal dialysis. *Clin Nephrol.* 1983;20:244.

25. Robson M, Rosenfeld JB. Fructose for dialysis. *Ann Intern Med* 1971; 75:975.

26. Ahmad S, Gallagher N, Shen F. Intermittent peritoneal dialysis: status reassessed. *Trans Am Soc Artif Intern Organs.* 1979;25:86.

27. Diaz-Buxo JA, et al. Experience with intermittent peritoneal dialysis and continuous cyclic peritoneal dialysis. *Am J Kidney Dis.* 1984; 4:242.

28. Oreopoulos DG, et al. A simple and safe technique for continuous ambulatory peritoneal dialysis. *Trans Am Soc Artif Intern Organs* 1978; 24:484.

29. Popovich RP, et al. Continuous ambulatory peritoneal dialysis. *Ann Intern Med* 1978;88:449.

30. Diaz-Buxo JA, et al. Continuous cyclic peritoneal dialysis: A preliminary report. *Artif Organs.* 1981;5:157.

31. Twardowski ZJ, et al. Choice of peritoneal dialysis regimen based on peritoneal transfer rates. *Perit Dial Bull* 1987;7:S79.

32. Frock J, et al. Tidal peritoneal dialysis. *Kidney Int.* 1987;31:250. Abstract.

33. Fernando SK, Finkelstein FO. Tidal PD: its role in the current practice of peritoneal dialysis. *Kidney Int Suppl.* 2006;103:S91-S95.

34. Cardella CJ, Izatt SJ. What should one do with the peritoneal dialysis catheter in a patient receiving a transplant? *Perit Dial Bull.* 1982;2:90.

35. Posen GA, Luiscello J. Continuous equilibration peritoneal dialysis in the treatment of acute renal failure. *Perit Dial Bull* 1980;1:6.

36. Raja RM, et al. Repeated peritoneal dialysis in treatment of heart failure. *JAMA* 1970;213:2268.

37. Rubin J, Bell R. Continuous ambulatory peritoneal dialysis as treatment of severe congestive heart failure in the face of chronic renal failure. *Arch Intern Med* 1986;146:1533.

38. Winchester JF, et al. Dialysis and hemoperfusion of poisons and drugs: Update. *Trans Am Soc Artif Intern Organs* 1977;23:762.

39. Reuler JB, Parker RA. Peritoneal dialysis in the management of hypothermia. *JAMA* 1978;240:2289.

40. Knochel JP, Mason AD. Effect of alkalinization on peritoneal diffusion of uric acid. *Am J Physiol.* 1966;210:1160.

41. Sorkin MI, et al. Aluminum mass transfer during continuous ambulatory peritoneal dialysis. *Perit Dial Bull* 1981;1:91.

42. Glenn LD, Nolph KD. Treatment of pancreatitis with peritoneal dialysis. *Perit Dial Bull.* 1982;2:63.

43. Stefanidis C, et al. Renal transplantation in children treated with continuous ambulatory peritoneal dialysis. *Perit Dial Bull* 1983;1:5.

44. White N, et al. The management of terminal renal failure in diabetic patients by regular dialysis therapy. *Nephron* 1973;11:261.

45. Digenis GE, et al. Abdominal hernias in patients undergoing CAPD. *Perit Dial Bull.* 1982;2:115.

46. Weston RE, Roberts M. Clinical use of stylet-catheter for peritoneal dialysis. *Arch Intern Med* 1965;115:659.

47. Gutch CF, Stevens SC. Silastic catheter for peritoneal dialysis. *ASAIO Trans.* 1966;12:106.

48. Tenckhoff H. Catheter implantation. *Dial Transplant* 1972;1:18.

49. Diaz-Buxo JA, Geissinger WT. Single cuff versus double cuff Tenckhoff catheter. *Perit Dial Bull.* 1984;4:S100.

50. Dell'Aquila R, Chiaramonte S, Rodighiero MP, Spano E, DiLoreto P, Kohn CO, Cruz D, Polanco N, Kuang D, Corradi V, De Cal M, Ronco C. Rational choice of peritoneal dialysis catheter. *Perit Dial Int.* 2007;27(Suppl 2):S119-S125.

51. Ortiz AM, Fernandez MA, Troncoso PA, Guzman S, Del Campo F, Morales RA. *Outcome of peritoneal dialysis: Tenckhoff catheter survival in a prospective study.* Adv Perit Dial. 2004;20:145-9.

52. Twardowski ZJ, et al. The need for a "swan neck" permanently bent, arcuate peritoneal dialysis catheter. *Perit Dial Bull* 1985;5:219.

53. Gadallah MF, Mignone J, Torres C, Ramdeen G, Pervez A. The role of peritoneal dialysis catheter configuration in preventing catheter tip migration. *Adv Perit Dial.* 2000;16:47–50.

54. Oreopoulos DG, et al. Catheters and connectors for chronic peritoneal dialysis: Present and future. In Atkins RC, Thomson NM, Farrel PC (eds): *Peritoneal dialysis.* New York, Churchill Livingstone, 1981.

55. Keane WF, Peterson PK. Host defense mechanisms of the peritoneal cavity and continuous ambulatory peritoneal dialysis. *Perit Dial Bull.* 1984;4:122.

56. Khanna R, et al. Experience with the Toronto Western Hospital permanent peritoneal catheter. *Perit Dial Bull.* 1984;4:95.

57. Thornhill JA, et al. Drainage characteristics of the column disc catheter: A new chronic peritoneal access catheter. *Proc Clin Dial Transplant Forum* 1980;1:119.

58. Ash SR, Slingeneyer A, Schaedin KE. Further clinical experience with the Lifecath peritoneal implant. *Perspect Perit Dial.* 1983;1:9.

59. Ogunc G, Tuncer M, Ogunc D, Yardimsever M, Ersoy F. Laparoscopic omental fixation technique versus open surgical placement of peritoneal dialysis catheters. *Surg Endosc.* 2003;17(11):1749-1755.

60. Ash SR, Wolf GC, Bloch R. Placement of the Tenckhoff peritoneal dialysis catheter under peritoneoscopic visualization. *Dial Transplant.* 1981;10:383.

61. Keshvari A, Najafi I, Jafari-Javid M, Yunesian M, Chaman R, Taromlou MN. Laparoscopic peritoneal dialysis catheter implantation using a Tenckhoff trocar under local anesthesia with nitrous oxide gas insufflation. *Am J Surg.* 2009;197(1):8-13.

62. Gajjar AH, Rhoden DH, Kathuria P, Kaul R, Udupa AD, Jennings WC. Peritoneal dialysis catheters: laparoscopic versus traditional placement techniques and outcomes. *Am J Surg.* 2007;194(6):872-875; discussion 875-876.

63. Schmidt SC, Pohle C, Langrehr JM, Schumacher G, Jacob D, Neuhaus P. Laparoscopic-assisted placement of peritoneal dialysis catheters: implantation technique and results. *J Laparoendosc Adv Surg Tech A.* 2007;17(5):596-599.

64. Khanna R, et al. Mortality and morbidity on continuous ambulatory peritoneal dialysis. *ASAIO J.* 1983;6:197.

65. Kim HJ, Lee TW, Ihm CG, Kim MJ. Use of fluoroscopy-guided wire manipulation and/or laparoscopic surgery in the repair of malfunctioning peritoneal dialysis catheters. *Am J Nephrol.* 2002;22(5-6): 532-538.

66. Savader SJ, Lund G, Scheel PJ, Prescott C, Feeley N, Singh H, Osterman FA. Guide wire directed manipulation of malfunctioning peritoneal dialysis catheters: a critical analysis. *J Vasc Interv Radiol.* 1997;8(6):957-963.

67. Palacios M, Schley W, Dougherty J. Use of streptokinase to clear peritoneal catheters. *Dial Transplant* 1982;11:172.

68. Zorzanello MM, Fleming WJ, Prowant BF. Use of tissue plasminogen activator in peritoneal dialysis catheters: a literature review and one center's experience. *Nephrol Nurs J.* 2004;31(6):695.

69. Thayssen P, Pindborg T. Peritoneal dialysis and heparin. *Scand J Urol Nephrol* 1978;12:73.

70. Pitchford, TJ, Molle JS, Price PD. Laparoscopic salvage of dysfunctional continuous ambulatory peritoneal dialysis catheters. *Surg Rounds* Oct1999;534-538.

71. Yilmazlar T, Kirdak T, Bilgin S, Yavuz M, Yurtkuran M. Laparoscopic findings of peritoneal dialysis catheter malfunction and management outcomes. *Perit Dial Int.* 2006;26(3):374-379.

72. Numanoglu A, McCulloch MI, Pool AV, Millar AJ, Rode H. *Laparoscopic salvage of malfunctioning Tenckhoff catheters.* J Laparoendosc Adv Surg Tech A. 2007 Feb; 17 (1): 128-30.

73. Furman KL, Gomperts ED, Hoclde J. Activity of intraperitoneal heparin during peritoneal dialysis. *Clin Nephrol.* 1978;9:15.

74. Blumenkrantz MJ, et al. Retrograde menstruation in women undergoing chronic peritoneal dialysis. *Obstet Gynecol.* 1981;57:667.

75. Coronel F, et al. The risk of retrograde menstruation in CAPD patients. *Perit Dial Bull.* 1984;4:190.

76. Nolph KD, et al. Factors associated with morbidity and mortality among patients on CAPD. *Trans Am Soc Artif Intern Organs* 1987;33:57.

77. Orfei R, Seybold K, Blumberg A. Genital edema in patients undergoing continuous ambulatory peritoneal dialysis. *Perit Dial Bull* 1984;4:251.

78. Twardowski ZJ, et al. Computerized tomography CT in the diagnosis of subcutaneous leak sites during continuous ambulatory peritoneal dialysis. *Perit Dial Bull* 1984;4:163.

79. Chan MK, Baillod RA, Tanner A, et al. Abdominal hernias in patients receiving continuous ambulatory peritoneal dialysis. *Br Med J.* 1981; 283:826.

80. Wetherington GM, et al. Abdominal wall and inguinal hernias in continuous ambulatory peritoneal dialysis patients. *Am J Surg* 1985; 150:357.

81. Singh S, et al. Massive hydrothorax complicating continuous ambulatory peritoneal dialysis. *Nephron* 1983;34:168.

82. Brown-Cartwright D, Smith HJ, Feldman M. Delayed gastric emptying: A common problem in patients on continuous ambulatory peritoneal dialysis. *Perit Dial Bull.* 1987;7:S10.

83. Berlyne GM, et al. Pulmonary complications of peritoneal dialysis. *Lancet.* 1966;2:75.

84. Buccianti G, Bianchi ML, Valenti G. Progress of renal osteodystrophy during continuous ambulatory peritoneal dialysis. *Clin Nephrol.* 1984; 22:279.

85. Gault MH, et al. Fluid and electrolyte complications of peritoneal dialysis: Choice of dialysis solutions. *Ann Intern Med.* 1971;75:253.

86. Port F, Johnson WJ, Klass DW. Prevention of dialysis disequilibrium syndrome by use of high sodium concentration in the dialysate. *Kidney Int* 1973;3:327.

87. Watson LC, Thompson JC. Erosion of the colon by a long-dwelling peritoneal dialysis catheter. *JAMA* 1980;243:2156.

88. Coward RA, et al. Peritonitis associated with vaginal leakage of dialysis fluid in continuous ambulatory peritoneal dialysis. *Br Med J.* 1982;284:1529.

89. Vas SI. Indications for removal of the peritoneal catheter. *Perit Dial Bull* 1981;1:149.

90. Hotchkiss JR, Hermsen ED, Hovde LB, Simonson DA, Rotschafer JC, Crooke PS. Dynamic analysis of peritoneal dialysis associated peritonitis. *ASAIO J.* 2004;50(6):568-576.

91. Gokal R, et al. Peritonitis in continuous ambulatory peritoneal dialysis. *Lancet.* 1982;2:1388.

92. Prowant BF, Nolph KD. Clinical criteria for diagnosis of peritonitis. In Atkins RC, Thomson NM, Farrel PC (eds). *Peritoneal Dialysis.* Edinburgh: Churchill Livingstone, 1981.

93. Reed WP, Light PD, Newman KA. Biofilm on Tenckhoff catheters: A possible source for peritonitis. *Proc Third Int Sym Pent Dial* 1984;176.

94. Wu G. A review of peritonitis episodes that caused interruption of continuous ambulatory peritoneal dialysis. *Perit Dial Bull* 1983;3 (suppl):S11.

95. Yang CY, Chen TW, Lin YP, Lin CC, Ng YY, Yang WC, Chen JY. Determinants of catheter loss following continuous ambulatory peritoneal dialysis peritonitis; *Perit Dial Int.* 2008;28(4):361-370.

96. Keane WF, et al. Opsonic deficiency of peritoneal dialysis effluent in continuous ambulatory peritoneal dialysis. *Kidney Int.* 1984;25:539.

97. Peresecenschi G, et al. Impaired neutrophil response to acute bacterial infection in dialyzed patients. *Arch Intern Med* 1982;141:1301.

98. Verbnigh HA, et al. Peritoneal macrophage and opsonins: Antibacterial defense in patients on chronic peritoneal dialysis. *J Infect Dis* 1983;147:1018.

99. Males BM, Walshe JJ. Amsterdam D. Laboratory indices of clinical peritonitis, total leukocyte count, microscopy and microbiological culture of peritoneal dialysis effluent. *J Clin Microbiol.* 1987;25:2367.

100. Williams P, et al. The value of dialysate cell count in the diagnosis of peritonitis in patients on continuous ambulatory peritoneal dialysis. *Perit Dial Bull* 1981;1:59.

101. Eisenberg ES, et al. Colonization of skin and development of peritonitis due to coagulase-negative staphylococci in patients undergoing peritoneal dialysis. *J Infect Dis* 1987;156:478.

102. Rault R. Candida peritonitis complicating peritoneal dialysis: A report of five cases and review of the literature. *Am J Kidney Dis* 1983;2:544.

103. Kim GC, Korbet SM. Polymicrobial peritonitis in continuous ambulatory peritoneal dialysis patients. *Am J Kidney Dis.* 2000;36(5): 1000-1008.

104. Digenis GE, et al. Morbidity and mortality after treatment of peritonitis with prolonged exchanges and intraperitoneal antibiotics. *Perit Dial Bull.* 1982;2:45.

105. Nichols WK, Nolph KD. A technique for managing exit site and cuff infection in Tenckhoff catheters. *Perit Dial Bull* 1983;.3 (suppl):S4,.

106. Poirier VL, et al. Elimination of tunnel infection. In Maher JF, Winchester JF (eds): *Frontiers in Peritoneal Dialysis.* New York, Field, Rich and Assoc, 1986.

107. Faller B, Marichal JF. Loss of ultrafiltration in continuous ambulatory peritoneal dialysis: A role for acetate. *Perit Dial Bull.* 1984;4:10.

108. Gandhi VC, et al. Thickened peritoneal membrane in maintenance peritoneal dialysis patients. *Kidney Int.* 1978;14:675.

109. Katirtzoglou A, et al. Is peritoneal ultrafiltration influenced by acetate or lactate buffers? In Maher JF, Winchester JF (eds). *Frontiers in Peritoneal Dialysis.* New York: Field, Rich & Assoc, 1986.

110. Junor BJR, et al. Sclerosing peritonitis: Role of chlorhexidine alcohol. *Perit Dial Bull.* 1985;5:101.

111. Nielsen LH, et al. Sclerosing peritonitis on CAPD: The acetate-lactate controversy. *Am J Nephrol* 1984;17:82A.

CHAPTER 29

Socioeconomic Implications of Vascular Access Surgery

Juan Carlos Jimenez and Robert S. Bennion

Rapid changes in health care delivery have accelerated in the 21st century and treatment of patients with end-stage renal disease (ESRD) continues to assume great importance. More expenditures of time, money, and resources are necessary to support the increasing number of patients with chronic kidney disease (CKD). In 2006, 110,851 new cases of ESRD were reported, signaling a 3.4% increase from 2005.[1] Prevalence rates continue to increase from a decade ago, both in the United States and internationally.[2] (Fig. 29-1) As the number of patients who require treatment continues to expand, additional strain is placed on a health care system that is already under significant stress. This chapter explores these controversial economic and social issues.

End-Stage Renal Disease Statistics

Beginning with the introduction of clinically and commercially feasible hemodialysis machines in the 1950s and spurred by invention of reliable external[3] and then internal[4] methods of gaining long-term vascular access for hemodialysis in the 1960s, treatment of ESRD has been the center of both great interest and controversy. The interest, of course, surrounded the treatment of a previously uniformly lethal

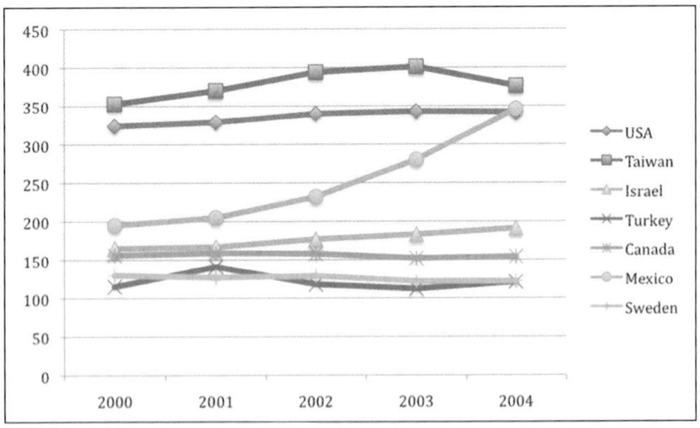

Figure 29-1.

Incidence of ESRD, by country. *ESRD,* End-stage renal disease. (Modified from National Institute of Diabetes and Digestive and Kidney Diseases. USRDS 2006 Annual Data Report. Bethesda, MD: National Institutes of Health, 2007.)

disease, whereas the controversy initially involved the process of selection of patients for this treatment because of the scarcity of both medical and financial resources.

By 1969, slightly more than 1000 patients in the United States received hemodialysis, at an annual cost of approximately $25,000 per patient.[5] Because of the prohibitive cost, selection committees were set up to decide which patients were to be offered this new form of therapy. Selection criteria for treatment included age, medical suitability, mental acuity, family environment, criminal record, economic status (income, net worth, etc.), employment record, availability of transportation, willingness to cooperate with the treatment regimen, likelihood of vocational rehabilitation, psychiatric evaluation, marital status, educational background, occupation, and future potential. Social class considerations and social worth often appeared to be more important than more equitable and less controversial criteria.[6]

With the passage of Public Law 92-603 (the Social Security Amendment Act) by the Congress of the United States in September of 1972, Medicare benefits were extended to essentially all patients with ESRD who were not already insured, such as employees of the federal government or veterans entitled to health care benefits. This extension of benefits shifted the financial burden for care of these patients from the private to the public sector and resulted in dramatic increases in access to therapy in this country. Interestingly, the actual legislation was never formally considered in the relevant House and Senate committees but was attached after only 30 minutes of discussion in the Senate as a floor amendment to a broader piece of legislation. Within three years, there were 23,000 patients receiving hemodialysis, and 3,500 renal transplantations were being performed annually.[7] In 1980, this number increased to over 50,000 patients on hemodialysis and nearly 4,700 renal transplantations.[8] By 1990, there were nearly 200,000 patients with ESRD in the United States.[9] By 2006, the number more than doubled, with 500,000 individuals living with ESRD. Of these patients, 70% were being treated with dialysis and 18,000 received renal transplants.[1]

The number of patients undergoing treatment for ESRD in 1997 was just over 350,000 patients[10] and increased to over 470,000 patients in 2004.[11] Although the largest escalation has been in the number of patients who receive hemodialysis, all treatment modalities have shown steady growth. Death, by itself, does not cause sufficient attrition

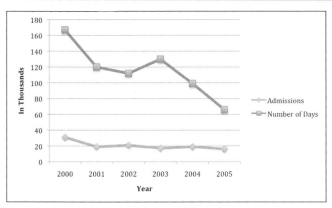

Figure 29-2.
Number of hospital admissions and number of hospital days for patients with ESRD, 2000-2005. *ESRD,* End-stage renal disease. (Modified from National Hospital Discharge Survey and National Survey of Ambulatory Surgery Reports, 2001-2005. Centers for Disease Control and Prevention. Available at http://www.cdc. gov/nchs/about/major/hdasd/listpubs.htm.)

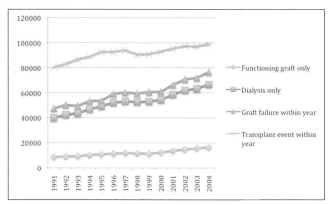

Figure 29-3.
Treatment methods (number of patients) used for ESRD between 1991 and 2004. *ESRD,* End-stage renal disease. (Modified from National Institute of Diabetes and Digestive and Kidney Diseases. USRDS 2006 Annual Data Report. Bethesda, MD: National Institutes of Health, 2007.)

to slow the growth rate. In 1997, new ESRD patients exceeded the number of patient deaths in all age groups, except in patients older than 75 years.[8] Factors that may help account for this continued increase include improvements in dialysis techniques that result in increased survival, increasing incidence of renal failure among older patients, and increased acceptance of patients into the Medicare program.[12,13] These factors have resulted in a steady expansion in the number of US patients being treated for renal failure regardless of ethnicity or socioeconomic background.

The number of hospital admissions required to treat ESRD dialysis was steady between 2000 and 2005. However, actual days of hospitalization decreased, perhaps because of the shift to outpatient procedures (Fig. 29-2).[14] Operations performed to revise existing vascular access sites between 2001 and 2005 have remained at a relatively stable rate, after a period of steady increase throughout the 1990s. The underlying cause of this may be related to the decreased number of AV grafts placed as initial access procedures in recent years, as recommended by the National Kidney Foundation through the KDOQI guidelines.[15-17]

Since the early 1980s, the number of renal transplantations performed to treat ESRD has increased steadily and has basically paralleled the growth seen in patients on hemodialysis. For the first time, in 2004, the number of deceased donor renal transplants in the United States exceeded 10,000 (Fig. 29-3).[18] Overall, there has been a noticeable trend toward better patient survival since 1985,[19] when the use of cyclosporine became widespread.[20] One-year graft survival (living patients with a functioning graft) for living donor transplants rose from 91.7% in 1995 to 95.3% in 2003. For deceased donor transplants, 1-year graft survival was 85.3% in 1995 and rose to 89.5% in 2005.[21] Unfortunately, the supply of kidneys for transplantation (especially cadaveric) remains a major concern. In 1997, cadaveric kidney transplantations were performed at the rate of 36 White male cadaveric donor grafts per 1 million population and 36.8 Black male cadaveric donor grafts per 1 million population, whereas those for White and Black females were 23.9

and 15.5 per 1 million, respectively.[19] The most recent US Renal Data System report reveals that Blacks had consistently lower transplant rates over time than did Whites and that, after controlling for age and sex, older adult patients (ages >35 years) had a markedly lower rate of transplantation than did younger patients (20 to 34 years). White and nonwhite males generally had higher transplantation rates than White and nonwhite females.[22] (Fig. 29-4)

Pediatric patients (ages 0 to 17 years) continue to have the highest renal transplantation rates.[23] In 2006, the percentage of children who received a kidney transplant within 3 years of starting ESRD treatment was 67.8%. This number is two times higher than transplant recipients in patients 20 to 39 years of age and eight times higher than patients between 60 to 69.[23] Nearly 50% of pediatric patients are

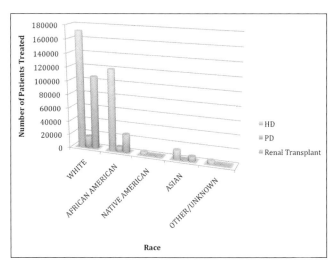

Figure 29-4.
Prevalence of treated patients with ESRD in the United States by Race, 2005. *ESRD,* End-stage renal disease. (Modified from National Institute of Diabetes and Digestive and Kidney Diseases. USRDS 2007 Annual Data Report. Bethesda, MD: National Institutes of Health, 2008.)

placed on the waiting list or undergo kidney transplant within 1 year of initiation of therapy for ESRD. This compares to a rate of 15% in all other age groups. Males are more likely to receive a transplant than females.[22] In 2001, 24.4% of White individuals with ESRD received a transplant within 3 years of ESRD registration.[22] Conversely, rates for Latino, African American, and Native American patients were 14.9%, 9.2% and 8.6%, respectively.[22]

Before extension of Medicare benefits to patients with ESRD in 1973, more than 36% of the dialysis population in the United States were being treated at home.[5] By 1980, the home dialysis population in the United States had dropped to 14% of the total, which is attributable to patients seeking treatment that was less costly and more convenient for them in dialysis facilities. With the exception of a slight increase in patients on home dialysis from 1982 to 1984, this downward trend continued so that by 1997, just over 1% of all hemodialysis in the United States was performed in the home.[24]

Cost of Treatment of End-Stage Renal Disease

Because of the prohibitive costs of treating ESRD in the 1960s and early 1970s, selection committees were created to decide which patients were to be offered therapy and which were not.[25] The intent of Congress in legislating the funding of 80% of the cost of hemodialysis in 1972 through Medicare was to remove expense as a deciding factor in the survival of patients with chronic renal failure. Senator Vance Hartke (D-Ind), whose amendment created the federal funding of renal failure, justified the expense of the program by asking, "How do we explain that the difference between life and death is a matter of dollars? How do we explain that those who are wealthy have a greater chance to enjoy a longer life than those who are not?"[25]

Although there were initial reports of cost savings after the passage of Public Law 92-603 because of more efficient use of hospital resources, the overall effect of the legislation has been an ever-escalating increase in health care expenditures. Within 5 years after implementation of the law, the annual Medicare expenditure for the treatment of patients with ESRD exceeded $1 billion, which doubled to over $2 billion 5 years later, in 1983.[7,26] In 1990, the federal funding of this disease alone had nearly tripled to $5.2 billion.[8] Between 1991 and 2004, Medicare expenditures continue to grow at an annual rate mirroring the annual growth in patients with ESRD. (Table 29-1) By 2004, the yearly per-patient Medicare payment (including hospitalization) was more than $58,000. In 2003, total expenditure (Medicare and private insurance) was approximately $27 billion.[27]

Because of the continuing increase in the cost of ESRD, efforts are focused on containing these rapidly increasing expenditures. Efforts have ranged from the application of a ceiling for reimbursed dialysis center costs,[28] a reduction in the length of dialysis treatment sessions by a factor of 3 through the use of faster, more efficient dialyzers (which reduced per session costs by 25%),[29] and reductions in the frequency and length of hospitalizations. In addition, Medicare capitation has been proposed as a method to provide cost-effective care to these patients, with payments

Table 29-1				
Medicare Expenditures in US Dollars for ESRD per Patient Year, by Treatment Modality (1991-2004)				
	Functioning Graft Only	Dialysis Only	Graft Failure Within Year	Transplant Event Within Year
1991	8,548	39,821	47,421	80,334
1992	8,998	42,254	50,127	82,868
1993	9,222	43,595	49,363	86,557
1994	10,220	46,755	53,301	88,725
1995	10,731	49,114	53,569	92,553
1996	11,332	52,009	59,059	92,623
1997	11,782	53,077	60,219	93,846
1998	11,541	52,589	59,341	90,538
1999	11,285	52,944	60,592	90,878
2000	12,189	54,295	60,745	92,941
2001	13,631	58,500	66,296	95,275
2002	14,579	61,919	70,709	97,283
2003	15,639	63,308	71,922	96,918
2004	16,376	66,650	76,500	98,968

varying with the age of the patient and with whether they are diabetic.[30] Unfortunately, the continuing addition of 10% to 15% more patients to the program each year more than offsets any cost-saving techniques, and the fiscal expenditures for the ESRD program continue to increase without much restraint.

Social Issues

As Medicare cost containment continues to occupy the minds of both lawmakers and care providers, a controversy in the treatment of patients with ESRD is the issue of the aggressive treatment of elderly patients with renal failure. In England, health care budget expenditures are more actively controlled to contain costs.[31,32] Specifically, England is particularly unlikely to aggressively treat patients older than 65 with renal failure and those who are chronically ill, although no formal laws or edicts regarding patient selection exist in the British National Health Service.[26] This rationing occurs despite evidence that 1-year survival rates in the elderly are comparable to younger patients receiving similar treatment. Because of this, England has one of the lowest hemodialysis treatment rates in Western Europe, far lower than that of the United States.

Traditionally, most other countries in the world also seem to select patients for treatment more strictly than does the United States. The exception is Japan, where the more aggressive use of therapies for renal failure has resulted in both the second highest number of patients undergoing treatment and the second highest rate of new patients undergoing treatment. In recent years, Japan actually exceeded the United States in the rate of all patients, both established and new, who are in treatment for ESRD. This observation suggests a better survival rate among Japanese

ESRD patients. Historically, high quality care for ESRD patients in Japan emerged as a result of low cost to patients and relatively high reimbursements for physicians compared with other treatments.[32] Although the incidence of newly diagnosed patients with ESRD who enter chronic treatment in the United States and Japan between 1988 and 1997 continues to increase yearly, rates in other selected countries have been essentially flat. Conversely, rates of renal transplantation in Japan are significantly lower compared with international standards.[32]

There has always been resistance to extending the use of dialysis to the older segment of the ESRD population, even in the United States.[34] However, during the 1980s, reports began to emerge indicating that well-selected patients older than 65 years tolerated dialysis as well as did younger patients and that their overall mortality rates were not significantly higher than those of individuals without renal failure.[35,36] The result was a doubling of the rate at which patients older than 55 were added to the ESRD program in the 5 years from 1983 to 1988.[9] By 1990, more than 52% of patients who received chronic dialysis treatments in this country were at least 55 years old, and by 1997 this figure had increased to nearly 60%.[9] In fact, the median age among new patients increased from 55 years in 1980 to 65 years in 1997, and the proportion of patients older than 65 in the ESRD program increased from 5% in 1973 to 34.4% in 1997.[9]

In 2004, incident ESRD rates have increased by 24% for patients aged 65 to 74 and 67% for patients greater than 75 years of age.[37] It is now recognized that, despite improvements in survival among all patients with ESRD, the overall mortality rate is high compared with the general population regardless of age. This mortality rate is comparable to that of other severe diseases (7.1 years of expected remaining life at age 49 for patients with ESRD versus 8.6 years for patients with colon cancer, 12.8 years for patients with prostate cancer, and 2.7 years patients with for lung cancer at the same age).[38] Elderly patients in particular fare poorly. Byrne and associates[39] found that the benefits of long-term hemodialysis (as defined as years of extended life) diminish sharply with advancing age, a finding quite different from earlier reports. They noted that the life expectancy of 95,394 Medicare patients who began dialysis at age 55 and older was far below that of age-matched peers, with less than 40% of patients aged 55 to 64 surviving 5 years and only 5% of patients aged 80 to 84 surviving 5 years. Fewer than 10% of all patients older than 65 were still alive 5 years after starting long-term hemodialysis. Renal failure caused by diabetes mellitus (nearly 25% of the cases) resulted in significantly ($P < .001$) poorer survival did than other causes of renal failure, such as hypertension, glomerulonephritis, and polycystic kidney disease. After 5 years, less than 18% of diabetic patients who were 55 to 64 years of age and less than 3% of those older than 80 at the start of dialysis were still living.[39]

The issue of quality of life is another important consideration in patients with ESRD. Younger patients are much more likely either to be offered transplantation or to be started on long-term ambulatory peritoneal dialysis than are older patients; both of these options certainly allow a more normal life. In 2004, 96% of all patients older than 75 with incident ESRD were treated with hemodialysis

compared with 3% who were treated with peritoneal dialysis and 1% who were treated with transplantation, whereas in the 20- to 44-year-old group, 5% of patients underwent transplant, with 85% on hemodialysis and 10% on peritoneal dialysis.[23] The time demands of dialysis, postdialysis fatigue, and enforced inactivity caused by hospitalizations, vascular access surgery, and other problems make the achievement of some level of normal activity very difficult. Hemodialysis patients aged 65 or older averaged two hospital admissions and nearly 17 days in the hospital annually.[23] Reports have shown that maintenance hemodialysis in elderly patients resulted in a significant decrease in their independent activity as measured with the Karnofsky activity scale and that few conducted any substantive portion of their lives outside their homes.[40] Interestingly, there was no difference between White and Black patients in their level of inactivity.

Although not specifically age related, the vocational status of patients with ESRD on dialysis (either hemodialysis or peritoneal dialysis) is a matter of concern. Globally, only about 25% to 30% of patients on long-term dialysis are employed,[41,42] although another study that looked specifically at patients younger than 55 found that nearly 45% of the patients were employed.[43] The two factors that were found to be significantly associated with continuing employment were the level of education of the patients (those with >12 years of school were more likely to be working, $P < .005$) and length of time on dialysis (working patients had been on dialysis an average of 44 months versus 77 months for nonworking patients, $P < .03$). These influences may be accounted for by the facts that the type and suitability of work available to less-educated, chronically ill individuals are probably rather limited and that the better-educated dialysis patient may be afforded more opportunity to seek or continue gainful employment. Interestingly, other factors such as sex, race, diabetes mellitus, mode of dialysis, and previous transplantation were not associated with employment status. Eighty percent of patients receiving hemodialysis in Japan remained employed. Possible explanations include the increasing prevalence of disability legislation discouraging reliance on public aid, and the high quality of dialysis care in Japan.[32]

The combination of high relative mortality, questionable quality of life and employment status, and high cost of treating patients with ESRD raises the specter of rationing of this expensive technology in the current era of fiscal restraint. Despite the laudable intentions of Congress when Public Law 92-603 was passed, in both the United States and other countries it is becoming apparent to some that not all patients with renal failure should be offered treatment.[44] Lowance has made the suggestion that chronologically or physiologically old patients with an estimated life expectancy of less than 2 years should be advised against dialysis.[45] In Canada, where 25% of patients with chronic renal failure are not accepted into dialysis programs, the following guidelines suggest that patients and families should be advised against chronic dialysis when there is the presence of any of the following[46]:

• Nonuremic dementia
• Metastatic or nonresectable solid malignancy or refractory hematologic malignancy

- End-stage irreversible liver, heart, or lung disease (patient confined to bed or chair and requires assistance for activities of daily living)
- Irreversible neurologic disease that significantly restricts mobility and activities of daily living
- Multisystem organ failure
- Need to sedate or restrain patient at each dialysis session to maintain functioning access

One final area of controversy and concern is the discontinuation of dialysis for any reason before biologic death or transplantation. In a study of nearly 1800 patients, 22% of all deaths resulted from the discontinuation of treatment[47]; 1 in every 11 patients had dialysis stopped, and, in patients older than 60, the frequency increased to 1 in 6. This study identified a major change in the role of the decision-maker for treatment withdrawal. The frequency with which physicians initiated the decision to withdraw treatment decreased from over 70% to less than 30% as time progressed, with the patients and their families increasingly assuming the role of decision-maker. In fact, among elderly patients, elective withdrawal from dialytic treatment is the third most common identifiable cause of death, only slightly less frequent than myocardial infarction.[38] Although there is a slightly increased tendency for women to withdraw than for men, Whites of both sexes and all age groups were two to three times more likely to withdraw from dialysis than were Blacks. This is likely a sociocultural difference.[48]

There probably is universal agreement among physicians that competent patients have the right to reject life-supporting treatment, especially if such treatment is a burden to them. Such withdrawal is not usually considered suicidal, although this right has come into question and some patients and their families have had to resort to court orders to discontinue treatment.[34] Such difficulties in terminating care, coupled with potentially increasing reluctance to initiate expensive long-term treatment in a managed-care environment, may well "force patients and their families to fight both for access to, and relief from, the medical system."[47]

REFERENCES

1. Mitka M. Report notes increase in kidney disease. *JAMA*. 2008;300: 2473-2474.
2. Coresh J, Selvin E, Stevens LA, et al. Prevalence of chronic kidney disease in the United States. *JAMA*. 2007;298:2038-2047.
3. Quinton WE, Dillard D, Scribner BH. Cannulation of blood vessels for prolonged hemodialysis. *Trans Am Soc Artif Intern Organs*. 1960; 6:104.
4. Brescia MJ, et al. Chronic hemodialysis using venipuncture and a surgically created arteriovenous fistula. *N Engl J Med*. 1966;275:1089.
5. Evans RW, Blagg CR, Bryan FA. Implications for health care policy: a social and demographic profile of hemodialysis patients in the United States. *JAMA*. 1981;245:487.
6. Abram HS: Dilemmas of medical progress. *Psychiatr Med*. 1972;3:51.
7. Roberts SD, Maxwell DR, Gross TL: Cost-effective care of end-stage renal disease: A billion dollar question. *Ann Intern Med*. 1980;92:243.
8. Data Committee of the National Forum of End-Stage Renal Disease Networks: Using end-stage renal disease facility surveys to monitor end-stage renal disease program trends. *JAMA*. 1985;254:1776.
9. National Institute of Diabetes and Digestive and Kidney Diseases. Incidence and prevalence of ESRD. In USRDS 1999 Annual Data Report. Bethesda, MD, National Institute of Health, 1999.
10. National Institute of Diabetes and Digestive and Kidney Diseases. Economic cost of ESRD and Medicare spending for alternative modalities of treatment. In USRDS 1999 Annual Data Report. Bethesda, MD, National Institutes of Health, 1999.
11. National Institute of Diabetes and Digestive and Kidney Diseases. Trends in ESRD counts and spending. In USRDS 2006 Annual Data Report. Bethesda, MD, National Institutes of Health, 2007.
12. Iglehart JK. The American health care system: the end stage renal disease program. *N Engl J Med*. 1993;328:366.
13. Parker TF, et al. Survival of hemodialysis patients in the United States is improved with a greater quantity of dialysis. *Am J Kidney Dis*. 1994; 23:670.
14. National Hospital Discharge Survey and National Survey of Ambulatory Surgery Reports, 2001-2005. Centers for Disease Control and Prevention. Available at http://www.cdc.gov/nchs/about/major/hdasd/listpubs.htm.
15. Rizzuti RP, Hale JC, Burkart TE. Extended patency of expanded polytetrafluoroethylene grafts for vascular access using optimal configuration and revisions. *Surg Gynecol Obstet*. 1988;166:23.
16. Valji K, et al. Pharmacomechanical thrombolysis and angioplasty in the management of clotted hemodialysis grafts: early and late clinical results. *Radiology*. 1991;178:243.
17. National Institute of Diabetes and Digestive and Kidney Diseases. Clinical indicators and preventive health: vascular access. In USRDS 2006 Annual Data Report. Bethesda, MD, National Institutes of Health, 2007.
18. National Institute of Diabetes and Digestive and Kidney Diseases. Transplantation. USRDS 2006 Annual Data Report. Bethesda, MD, National Institutes of Health, 2007.
19. National Institute of Diabetes and Digestive and Kidney Diseases. Renal transplantation: access and outcomes. In USRDS 1999 Annual Data Report. Bethesda, MD, National Institutes of Health, 1999.
20. Kahan BD. Transplantation timeline. *Transplantation*. 1991;50:1.
21. National Institute of Diabetes and Digestive and Kidney Diseases. Transplantation: graft survival. In: USRDS 2006 Annual Data Report. Bethesda, MD, National Institutes of Health, 2007.
22. National Institute of Diabetes and Digestive and Kidney Diseases. Transplantation: wait list, transplant and donation rates. In: USRDS 2006 Annual Data Report. Bethesda, MD, National Institutes of Health, 2007.
23. National Institute of Diabetes and Digestive and Kidney Diseases. Healthy People 2010: transplantation. In: USRDS 2006 Annual Data Report. Bethesda, MD, National Institutes of Health, 2007.
24. National Institute of Diabetes and Digestive and Kidney Diseases. Treatment modalities of ESRD treatment. In: USRDS 2006 Annual Data Report. Bethesda, MD, National Institutes of Health, 2007.
25. End-stage renal disease. In: Second Annual Report to Congress, 1980. Washington, DC: US Department of Health and Human Services, 1980.
26. Wing AJ. Treatment of renal failure in the light of increasingly limited resources. *Contrib Nephrol*. 1985;44:260.
27. Hirth RA. The organization and financing of kidney dialysis and transplant care in the United States of America. *Int J Health Care Finance Econ*. 2007;7301-7318.
28. McIlrath S. Ten percent cut in Medicare dialysis payment eyed. *Am Med News*. 1986;29:1.
29. von Albertini BV, Bosch JP. Short hemodialysis. *Am J Nephrol*. 1991; 11:169.
30. McMurry SD, Miller J. Impact of capitation of free-standing dialysis facilities: can you survive? *Am J Kidney Dis*. 1997;30:542.
31. Simmons RG, Marine SK. The regulation of high-cost technology medicine: the case of dialysis and transplantation in the United Kingdom. *J Health Soc Behav*. 1984;25:320.
32. Lamping DL, Constantinovici N, Roderick P, et al. Clinical outcomes, quality of life, and costs in the North Thames Dialysis Study of elderly people on dialysis: a prospective cohort study. *Lancet*. 2000;356: 1543-1550.
33. Fukuhara S, Yamazaki C, Hayashino Y, et al. The organization and financing of end-stage renal disease treatment in Japan. *Int J Health Care Finance Econ*. 2007;7217-7231.
34. Angell M. Respecting the autonomy of competent patients. *N Engl J Med*. 1984;310:1115.
35. Rostellar E, et al. Must patients over 65 be hemodialyzed? *Nephron*. 1985;41:152.

36. Taube DH, et al Successful treatment of middle-aged and elderly patients with end-stage renal disease. *Br Med J*. 1983;286:2018.
37. National Institute of Diabetes and Digestive and Kidney Diseases. Incidence and prevalence: geriatric nephrology. In: USRDS 2006 Annual Data Report. Bethesda, MD, National Institutes of Health, 2007.
38. National Institute of Diabetes and Digestive and Kidney Diseases. Patient mortality and survival. In: USRDS 1999 Annual Data Report. Bethesda, MD, National Institute of Health, 1999.
39. Byrne C, Vernon P, Cohen JJ. Effect of age and diagnosis on survival of older patients beginning chronic dialysis. *JAMA*. 1994;271:34.
40. Ifudu O, et al. Dismal rehabilitation in geriatric inner-city hemodialysis patients. *JAMA*. 1994;271:29.
41. Bremer BA, et al. Quality of life in end-stage renal disease: A reexamination. *Am J Kidney Dis*. 1989;13:200.
42. Evans RW, et al. The quality of life of patients with end-stage renal disease. *N Engl J Med*. 1985;312:553.
43. Holley JL, Nespor S. An analysis of factors affecting employment of chronic dialysis patients. *Am J Kidney Dis*. 1994;23:681.
44. Kjellstrand CM, Dossetor JB. Ethical problems in dialysis and transplantation. Dordrecht, the Netherlands: Kluwer Academic, 1992.
45. Lowance DC: Factors and guidelines to be considered in offering treatment to patients with end-stage renal disease: a personal opinion. *Am J Kidney Dis*. 1993;21:679.
46. Hirsch DJ, et al: Experience with not offering dialysis to patients with a poor prognosis. *Am J Kidney Dis*. 1994;23:463.
47. Neu S, Kjellstrand CM. Stopping long-term dialysis: an empirical study of withdrawal of life-supporting treatment. *N Engl J Med*. 1986;314:14.
48. Leggat JE, Swartz RD, Post FK. Withdrawal from dialysis: a review with emphasis on the black experience. *Adv Ren Replac Ther*. 1997;4:22.

CHAPTER 30

Ultrasound in Vascular Access

Jason Wellen and Surendra Shenoy

Hemodialysis is the most prevalent renal replacement therapy for patients developing end-stage renal disease (ESRD). Survival on dialysis is directly related to the adequacy of dialysis, which, in turn, substantially relies on the nature of dialysis access. Arteriovenous fistula (AVF), with superior long-term outcomes, is considered the preferred access for long-term hemodialysis (HD).[1] Compared with other industrialized countries, the prevalence rate of AVF is lowest amongst ESRD patients who are dialysis dependent in the United States.[2,3] In an attempt to increase AVF prevalence, Centers for Medicare and Medicaid Services (CMS) launched the Fistula First initiative in 2004. As a result, the incidence of AVF in the United States has risen from 27% in 2003 to over 50% and continues to increase.[4] Preoperative vessel mapping ranks high among the "change concepts" advocated by Fistula First that have contributed to this increase in AVF constructions.[5] Currently the use of ultrasound has evolved as a preferred technique for vascular mapping in planning for AVF. Besides vessel mapping, real-time ultrasound also can play an important role in other aspects of vascular access management. This chapter will discuss the use of ultrasound in planning and management of vascular access in ESRD patients.

Ultrasound

Ultrasound is the term used to describe sound waves with a frequency greater than that of audible sound. Audible sound has a frequency range of 8 to 20 kilohertz (KHz). The range of frequency of sound waves used in medical applications is from 2 to 20 megahertz (MHz). The present generation of ultrasound transducer probes, used in vascular access, has multiple piezoelectric crystals capable of emitting ultrasound waves when stimulated by electrical energy and are called linear array transducers.[6] Assuming that the sound waves travel through soft tissue at a constant speed, variable amounts of sound waves are reflected back (echo) at the interface between different soft tissues (eg, subcutaneous tissue and muscle interface) that have different acoustic impedance (tissue density that affects sound wave propagation). Assuming that sound waves travel in a straight line, the crystals that emit these waves in the transducer also sense the reflected waves and convert the sound energy back to electrical energy. Cleverly engineered handheld probes utilize computer capabilities to process the information transduced, based on the distance traveled by the wave that was emitted before it was reflected, and presents this information in a two-dimensional spatial manner on a television screen, thereby producing an image in grey scale (B mode). The speed at which the sound pulses can be generated depends on the frequency of the ultrasound. Present transducer probes have the capacity to generate and gather return-wave information at rapid rates (e.g., 5,000 times per second). This rapid change in picture frames enables the machines to scan in real time. Real-time scanners can generate images at rapid sequence and show the motion of the transducer or the tissue as it is being scanned (real-time ultrasound).[6,7]

Doppler Ultrasound

The frequency of ultrasound waves stays constant when reflected by a stationary object. On the other hand, the frequency of the waves increases or decreases if the waves are reflected by a moving object (just as the sound of a police alarm gets louder as the vehicle approaches a listener). The relationship between this alteration of frequency was first summarized and mathematically explained by Christian Doppler in 1842.[8] Early clinical application of the Doppler effect was in the evaluation of blood flow. Early-generation Doppler probes used two crystals, one continually producing the ultrasound and the other continually receiving the reflected waves (continuous wave Doppler) that are converted to audio signals. More advanced probes have crystals that can generate sound waves in short pulses and compute the reflected shifts (pulse wave Doppler). These probes can provide good depth resolution.[7,9]

Duplex Doppler is the term used for a combination of the B mode for imaging and Doppler for flow evaluation. The B mode provides imaging for accurate focusing of the Doppler to assess flows in specific locations. This is the most useful imaging modality for the functional evaluation of a vascular access. Most Duplex Doppler machines are capable of color flow that adds color to a two-dimensional image based on direction or volume of the blood flow.

Ultrasound with duplex Doppler capability can be used in various facets of arteriovenous access planning and management. The utility of this modality in preoperative vascular access planning is well established.[4,5] Intraoperatively, it can be used to image the vessels to select ideal sites for vascular anastomosis and plan precise incisions to expose vessels for access surgery.[10] Postoperatively, the duplex Doppler is an excellent tool for vascular access maturation evaluation. It helps to plan for elective interventions to facilitate early access maturation. It is also useful in evaluating access procedures with long-term problems such as stenosis, aneurismal dilations, and low fistula blood flow states.[11]

Ultrasound for Vascular Access Planning

A careful history and physical examination capturing data relevant to the success of an AVF, such as history of central and peripheral vein abuse, coagulation disorders, anatomy, and quality of available arteries and veins, continues to be the mainstay of vascular access evaluation.[12,13] However, clinical examination is of limited value in patients who are overweight and obese. Clinical examination is also not very reliable in identifying the quality of the vessel wall—and especially the amount of calcification and consequently the luminal diameter of the arteries. Ultrasound vessel mapping should always complement thorough clinical evaluation.[14] Such an approach has shown to increase the incidence of AVF placement and maturation.

Vessel Mapping

Vessel mapping is the term used for a combination of vein and arterial mapping.[15,16] This should be ideally performed or viewed in real time by the operating surgeon and should complement a thorough clinical examination. B mode ultrasonographic imaging using probes with variable frequencies from 5 to 13 MHz generally provide excellent delineation of vascular anatomy. Lowering the frequency provides better penetration. Hence, lower frequency probes are often used to visualize deeper structures. However, as depth increases, the clarity of the images is compromised. The majority of primary fistulas utilize superficial veins (cephalic in the forearm or in the upper arm) for their outflow. They also rely on brachial or radial artery for the inflow. Both the artery and the vein are superficial structures and are easy to visualize with a linear array transducer at higher frequencies with remarkable clarity.

The technique of vein mapping has been eloquently outlined in many publications, including the guidelines from the Fistula First initiative.[4,17] Results of vein mapping rely significantly on vein distention techniques. Without proper distension, a vein that is well suited for AVF creation is easily missed during the vein mapping. Applying double tourniquets (one below the elbow to occlude the superficial veins and one below the axilla to occlude the deeper vein) provides a better opportunity to maximize venous distention (Fig. 30-1). Use of gravity by leaving the extremity in dependent position (we prefer the subject sitting on a chair with arms rested on the examination couch at a lower elevation to use gravity for vein distention) and gentle tapping on the vein helps break venous spasm and dilate the veins. Similarly, the use of exercise with a tourniquet and warming the extremity can help in vein distension.[4,18] During mapping, it is important to note the size and continuity of the outflow vein. It is also important to note the relation of the vein to the artery. In the lower third of the forearm, it is not unusual for the cephalic vein to distance itself from the artery near the wrist and take a more dorsal course

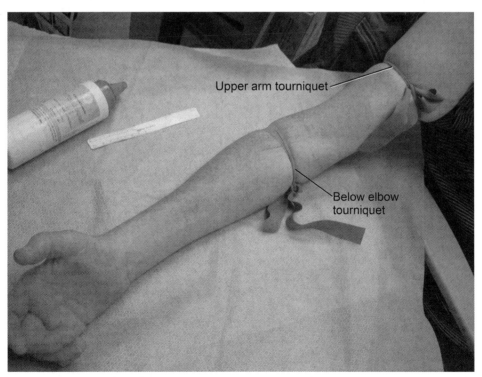

Figure 30-1.
Use of double tourniquets for vein distension.

(Fig. 30-2A). Such anatomic variations play a key role in planning incisions to identify, dissect, and mobilize veins to create a successful arteriovenous anastomosis. Ultrasound vein mapping to assess the diameter and quality of veins has shown to increase the success of fistula maturation.[5]

Arterial evaluation should include measurement of the size of the lumen and also the quality of the vessel wall.

Studies have suggested that the preexisting arterial wall disease as measured by intima-media thickness could play an important role in access patency and maturation.[19] This is also evident from successful AVF established in children with soft, healthy, thin-walled arteries that are often <2 mm in diameter.[20] It is the quality of the arterial wall that determines the capacity of the artery to dilate and accommodate

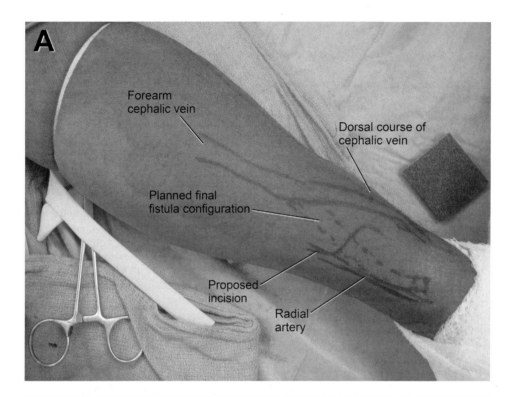

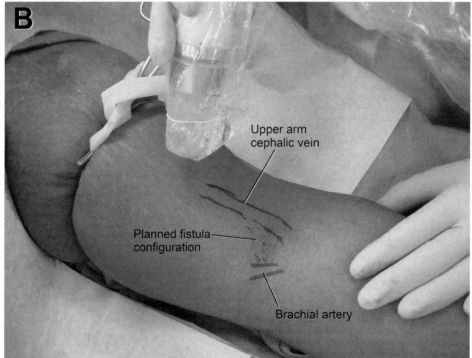

Figure 30-2.
Intraoperative vessel mapping and procedure planning using ultrasound.

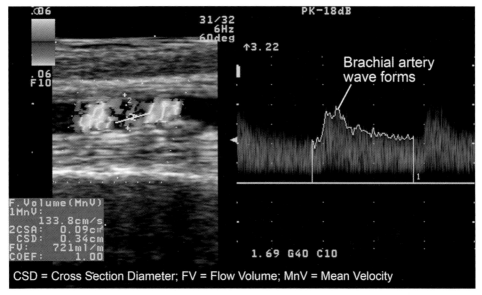

CSD = Cross Section Diameter; FV = Flow Volume; MnV = Mean Velocity

Figure 30-3.
A thick-walled narrow-caliber (3.4 mm) brachial artery with flow of 721 mL/min in a basilic transposition fistula with a 6-mm anastomosis.

the increased flow that is necessary to overcome the acute loss of resistance produced by the creation of an AVF. The wall of an artery with arteriosclerotic or atherosclerotic changes often has a limited capacity to dilate depending on the extent of the disease. In these situations, the increase in flow volumes tends to depend more on the diameter of the vessel (Fig. 30-3). Hence, larger caliber vessels with significant wall disease that are not capable of significant dilation can still provide sufficient flows necessary for dialysis. B mode ultrasound permits the surgeon to visualize the artery, evaluate the extent of calcification and the luminal diameter to make an informed critical decision on the suitability of the site in the artery that could be used for inflow to the AVF (Fig. 30-4A, B). Besides determining the luminal diameter, ultrasound imaging is very useful in assessing arterial wall calcification and stenosis. Many studies have reported increased success of AVF maturation using inflow arteries with the diameter greater than 2 mm.[21,22] Duplex Doppler evaluation of resistive indices in the artery has also been used for provocative testing (*reactive hyperemia test*) to assess the distensibility of the artery to use it as a predictor of AVF maturation.[11]

The single most important component of vessel mapping includes the appreciation of vascular anatomy in a given individual and comprehension of the spatial relationships of the artery to the vein. This becomes critical as there is often considerable variation in the normal anatomy in any given patient population forcing the surgeon to tailor an incision to achieve necessary dissection and mobilization for AVF creation. This becomes even more important during the evaluation of patients with variations in anatomy or those with multiple previous surgeries. While viewing by real time ultrasound scanning, a vascular access surgeon with the operative and clinical background is often in a position to notice subtle nuances in the surgical anatomy in a given patient. The surgeon is provided with a view of the vascular anatomy that lies beneath the skin, thereby adding

an entire new dimension to clinical evaluation while planning a vascular access procedure. In our clinical practice, using real time ultrasound as a complement to the clinical examination in the office has increased the AVF placement rate from 60% to 87% (Table 30-1).

Intraoperative Use of Ultrasound

In addition to those factors discussed above, the success of AVF also relies on surgical technique and experience of the surgeon.[23] This is evidenced by the vast range of AVF maturation failures reported in the literature.[24,25,26] Whereas vessel mapping in the clinic provides the necessary information to plan surgical intervention, the use of real time ultrasound in the operating room provides the surgeon the luxury of confirming findings of the previous assessments and marking the precise location of the artery and vein (see Fig. 30-2B). This allows precise incisions and adequate mobilization of the vein to perform the anastomosis at a planned location on the artery (see Fig. 30-2A). Using intraoperative ultrasound can thus significantly reduce negative explorations. It is particularly useful in patients who do not have clinically identifiable superficial venous anatomy. Precisely placed small incisions reduce the need for extensive tissue dissection to identify veins and thereby reduce operative time and wound morbidity.

Most operative rooms are equipped with simple ultrasound machines providing a real time image that is often used for intravenous or intra-arterial catheter placements. These transducers can be easily used for vessel mapping, to mark the vessels to be used for AVF creation, and to plan the incision (see Fig. 30-2A, B). Having an ultrasound machine with duplex adds a whole new dimension to intraoperative capabilities. Besides providing better resolution during imaging, these machines help the surgeons in assessing intraoperative arterial flows. The relationship of

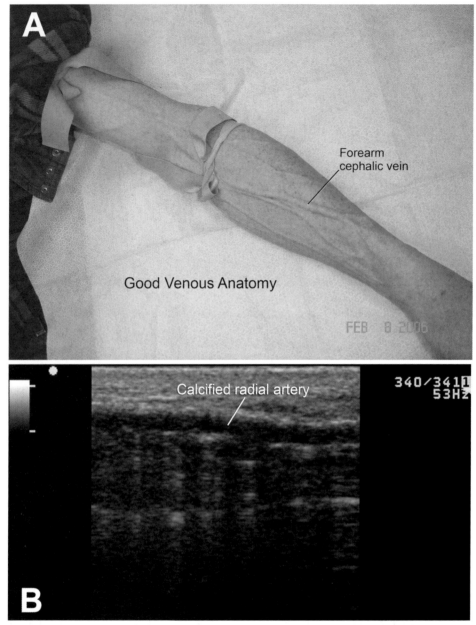

Figure 30-4.
An unexpected extensive radial artery calcification *(B)* in a patient with good superficial venous anatomy for AVF *(A)* detected by ultrasound vessel mapping.

intraoperative blood flow to fistula maturation is currently not well evaluated.[27] However, brachial artery flow volume and waveforms are very useful in detecting early access thrombosis.[11] Anecdotally, we had a patient in whom we were able to salvage a fistula that started to thrombose soon after fistula creation. This patient had decreasing flow in the brachial artery that led to re-exploration as the wound was being closed. Platelet aggregates occluding the anastomosis were cleared and the patient was treated with anticoagulants to salvage the fistula. It was later realized that the patient had an underlying hypercoagulable state. Since then, we have used the ultrasound technique to identify and salvage two more fistulas after early operative thrombosis.

Postoperative Use of Ultrasound

Ultrasound is a useful tool for identifying some postoperative problems associated with vascular access.[11] Arm edema and wound swelling are commonly encountered. Ultrasound helps differentiate tissue edema from postoperative hematoma or lymphocele. It is also useful for guiding needle aspirations of lymphoceles that occasionally compress outflow. Ultrasound can identify a tunnel hematoma from graft needle stick infiltration especially, in "early stick" situations where patients present with graft swelling. In the presence of significant edema from venous hypertension, ultrasound often shows increased pulsatility of the outflow vein extending towards central circulation, helping to make

Table 30–1

Effect of Ultrasound Evaluation on AV Access Planning

	Year	New Access	AV Grafts	AV Fistula	AVF %
Pre-DOQI era	1993	65	51	14	22
	1996	71	50	21	30
Clinical evaluation	1998	158	82	76	48
	1999	154	77	77	50
Clinical evaluation	2000	125	50	75	60
ultrasound mapping	2001	104	44	60	58
	2003	83	36	48	57
Clinical evaluation	2004	106	25	81	77
and ultrasound	2005	179	26	153	86
mapping in clinic	2006	129	17	112	87

Note. AV = arteriovenous.

the diagnosis. A surgeon well versed with viewing real-time ultrasound has innumerable opportunities for early use in postoperative evaluation of vascular access to improve patient care.

Fistula Maturation Evaluation

A mature fistula is defined as a fistula that is capable of delivering flows necessary for adequate dialyses (see Chapter 25). Establishing objective maturation criteria provides the surgeons with an opportunity to objectively evaluate maturation and electively plan interventions that could help fistulas mature. Duplex Doppler ultrasound is an ideal tool to assess fistula maturation. B mode imaging provides details pertaining to the size, diameter, length, and depth

of the outflow vein. Duplex Doppler also provides functional details by evaluating the flow patterns and flow volume. Real-time ultrasound often allows the surgeon to visualize sites of obstruction to the flow, nature of obstruction (eg, valve hypertrophy, valve dysfunction), and available collateral vessels to plan vein patch venoplasty and vein enhancement (Fig. 30-5). It also provides the surgeon an opportunity to decide if a fistulogram or a venoplasty is necessary for further evaluation and help maturation of the AVF.

Doppler Ultrasound Flow Evaluation

Duplex Doppler ultrasound is routinely used in the functional evaluation of circulation in several vascular beds.

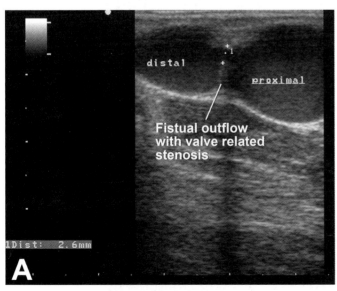
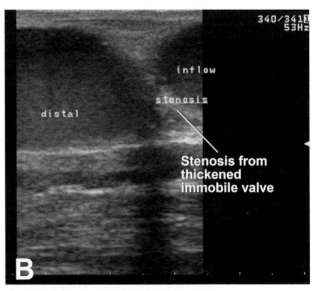

Figure 30-5.
Two longitudinal views of dilated proximal and distal vein with stenosis of lumen caused by valve thickening.

Assessing carotid arterial disease, hepatic artery, portal vein, and hepatic vein flow velocities and volumes are a few examples.[6] Doppler has the capability of assessing the flow velocity. Ultrasound imaging can reliably measure the vascular diameter. Volume flows are derived from these measurements.[10] Most modern ultrasound equipment has volume flow measurements as part of the standard parameters measured during vascular evaluation.[28]

Historically, volume flow has not been a popular parameter used for functional evaluation of the vascular system. The main reason for this is the low reliability and low accuracy of testing. Volume flow measurements are significantly dependent on equipment and technique. When compared to segmental pressure measurements, volume flows were not considered useful as an indicator of vascular disease.[29] The source of errors that could lead to inaccuracy in measurement of volume flows have been evaluated and discussed in extensive details in several previous publications.[30] Most new instruments have incorporated several steps to minimize errors in measurement and calculation of flow volumes.[28]

Measuring volume flow in AVF is a unique clinical situation. With the creation of an AVF, flow to the upper extremity bearing a vascular access conduit increases 10 to 20-fold (1000% to 2000%).[31] The observer in this situation is interested in a flow estimate rather than an accurate flow measurement. With volume flow changes of such magnitude, an error of 5 to 10% in flow estimation would be within an acceptable range (e.g., 800 mL/min vs. 720 mL/min or 860 ml/min). Moreover, measuring flow volumes 3 to 5 times and using the average of the measurements is a technique that can be used to further minimize this error. Measuring volume flow with duplex ultrasound has shown good correlation with other accepted methods of access flow measurement.[32]

Volume flow calculations using duplex Doppler rely on vascular diameter. Measuring the flow in an outflow vein of a fistula poses several problems that could account for inaccuracy with this technique. Outflow veins do not have a standard diameter. They are also easily compressible and often pose difficulty for accurate measurement of the diameter. Valves within the veins and the tributaries often produce complex flow patterns. Lastly, fistula outflow veins have markedly turbulent flow. On the other hand, major arteries in the upper limb (axillary/brachial) are most often straight and have uniform diameter. They are more deeply situated and not easily compressible. Measuring blood flow in these arteries is a reliable and reproducible technique (Fig. 30-6). Brachial artery flows in the upper extremity of a renal failure patient is usually less than 100 ml/min.[10,33] Hence the flow measurement in the feeding artery to the limb (brachial or axillary artery) can be used as a reliable indicator of fistula using the following formula:

$$AVF\ flow = Brachial\ artery\ flow - 75\ to\ 100\ mL/min$$

This is an extremely useful technique to get a reliable functional assessment of AVF to assess maturation. Volume flow measurement in the feeding artery to the limb correlates well with access flow rates and has been recommended as an accurate method to evaluate AVF.[11,33]

Use of Ultrasound for Atriovenous Graft Evaluation

Imaging an atriovenous graft (AVG) may be difficult in the early postoperative period until the expanded polytetrafluroethelene (ePTFE) graft is completely soaked. Following this, real-time ultrasound with duplex Doppler can be a useful tool in evaluating AVG to confirm tissue incorporation. It is very useful for detecting seroma, hematoma, or lymphocele accumulation, which can be subtle and pose problems with needle stick. Duplex Doppler ultrasound can also be used to estimate AVG flows by measuring inflow

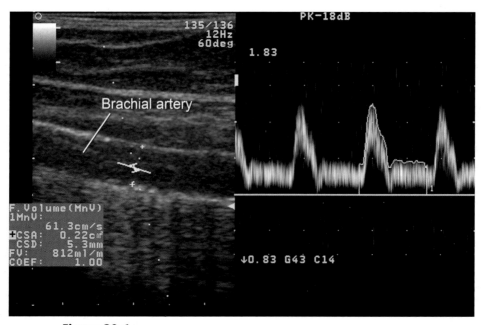

Figure 30-6.
Brachial artery flow measurement in a patient with radiocephalic fistula.

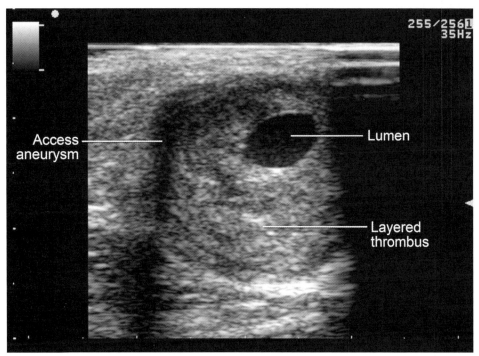

Figure 30-7.
Layered chronic mural thrombus in an aneurysm presenting as needle stick difficulty.

artery flows. Also, ultrasound is very helpful in evaluating large pseudoaneurysms filled with chronic layered thrombi, which often produce problems with needle sticks (Fig. 30-7). These are often not visualized with a contrast study, because the contrast flows only within the lumen. It is also used to look for perigraft collection and needle guided aspiration when graft infections are suspected.

Use of Ultrasound for Detection of Stenosis and Thrombosis

Duplex ultrasound is routinely used to image both the superficial and deep venous systems for evidence of thrombosis. B mode imaging can visualize a thrombus within the lumen of the veins. An acute thrombus tends to produce distention of the vein with an increased luminal diameter resulting from increased venous pressure. Compression techniques can also be used to determine if a venous thrombus is present. As opposed to a normal vein, thrombosed veins fail to collapse with Doppler probe compression.[34,35]

Ultrasound is also reliable in diagnosing stenosis in blood vessels and AV access dysfunction. The feeding artery, the anastomosis, and the entire length of the outflow vein can be scanned with relative ease with B mode scanner. Using duplex and color flow provides the examiner an opportunity for functional evaluation. Increased flow velocities caused by the stenosis are often diagnostic of a functionally significant lesion. Robin et al. showed that an increase in peak systolic velocity (PSV) ratio of 3 correlated with a 25% stenosis, as demonstrated on arteriography.[36] Though clinical examination is reliable in detecting an outflow stenosis in AVF, the ultrasound provides the operator an opportunity to evaluate the nature of stenosis and its extent to make an informed decision on appropriate management. Because of stenosis the intra-access pressure in the segment towards the inflow usually is high and makes the segment more pulsatile. The outflow vein beyond the stenosis tends to be soft and easily compressible and, hence, often difficult to evaluate. In a low-flow state subtle valve related problems can be missed. Similarly, though ultrasound based techniques to evaluate and detect central stenosis have been described, they are not always easy and reproducible. Because central stenosis requires an interventional study for evaluation and management, ultrasound can serve as a preliminary diagnostic tool to raise a suspicion of central problems.

Ultrasound can evaluate the vessel in both longitudinal and transverse axis and also delineate the vessel wall from the subcutaneous tissue and from the vessel lumen. This provides a unique opportunity for the examiner to evaluate the cause for vessel stenosis. The severity (percentage) of stenosis can easily be calculated based on the luminal diameter. Ultrasound can also clearly differentiate between extrinsic compression (such as hematoma or lymphocele) and intramural problems (such as wall thickening or venous intimal hyperplasia) and intraluminal causes (such as thrombus or valve hypertrophy). Using duplex Doppler to measure the inflow arterial flow volume and measuring the flow velocities can provide information on functional significance of the stenosis. Ultrasound also allows the observer to evaluate the state of collateral vessels available to plan for remedial surgeries such as flow diversion or vein patch venoplasty. Thus, the duplex Doppler ultrasound is an ideal tool to complement clinical evaluation of dysfunctional arteriovenous access.

Summary

The field of vascular access is going through a major change in the United States. Arteriovenous fistula is the access of choice. Vessel mapping using ultrasound has become the standard of care for preoperative planning of AV access. Ultrasound is increasingly being utilized in intraoperative planning and evaluation of AV access. Duplex Doppler ultrasound has the capability to provide functional evaluation of vascular access. It has been successfully used for fistula maturation evaluation and to identify maturation failure in AVF thus facilitating early intervention. When used in conjunction with clinical examination, real-time ultrasound scanning adds a new dimension to successful vascular access management.

REFERENCES

1. National Kidney Foundation. K/DOQI Clinical Practice Guidelines for Vascular Access: Update 2000. *Am J Kidney Dis.* 2001;37(1 suppl 1): S137-S181.

2. Sands JJ. Increasing AV fistulas: revisiting a time tested solution. *Semin Dial.* 2000;13(6):351-353.

3. Pisoni RL, Young EW, Dykstra DM, et al. Vascular access use in Europe and the United States: results from the DOPPS. *Kidney Int.* 2002; 61:305-316.

4. AV Fistula First Web site. Available at http://www.fistulafirst.org.

5. Silva MB, Hobson RW, Pappas PJ, et al. A strategy for increasing use of autogenous hemodialysis access procedures: impact of preoperative noninvasive evaluation. *J Vasc Surg.* 1998;27:302–308.

6. Fry WR. Principles of ultrasound: how waves become pictures. In Harness JK, Wisher DB (eds). *Ultrasound in Surgical Practice.* New York: Wiley-Liss Inc, 2001:1-20.

7. Wells PNT. Physics and bioeffects. In McGahan JP, Goldberg BB (eds). *Diagnostic Ultrasound.* Vol 1. 2nd ed. New York: Information Healthcare USA Inc, 2008:1-18.

8. Schuster PM. *Moving the Stars—Christian Doppler: His Life, His Works and Principle, and the World After.* Pöllauberg, Austria: Living Edition, 2005.

9. McDicken WN, Hoskins PR. Physics: principles, practice, and artefacts. In Allan P, Dubbins P, Pozniac MA, McDicken WN (eds). *Clinical Doppler Ultrasound.* London: Harcourt Publishers Ltd, 2000:1-25.

10. Shenoy S. Innovative surgical approaches to maximize arteriovenous fistula creation. *Semin Vasc Surg.* 2007;20(3):141-147.

11. Wiese P, Nonnast-Daniel B. Colour Doppler ultrasound in dialysis access. *Nephrol Dial Transplant.* 2004; 19:1956-1963.

12. Nursal TZ, Oguzkurt L, Tercan F, et al. Is Routine Preoperative Ultrasonographic Mapping for arteriovenous fistula creation necessary in patients with favorable physical examination findings? Results of a randomized controlled trial. *World J of Surgery.* 2006;30:1100-1107.

13. Davidson I, Galliene M, Saxena R, Dolmatch B. A patient centered decision making dialysis access algorithm. *J Vasc Access.* 2007;8:59-68.

14. Brimble KS, Rabbat CG, Schiff D, et al. The clinical utility of Doppler ultrasound prior to arteriovenous fistula creation. *Semin Dial.* 2001; 14:314-317.

15. Allon M, Lockhart ME, Lilly RZ, et al. Effect of preoperative sonographic mapping on vascular access outcomes in hemodialysis patients. *Kidney Int.* 2001;60:2013–2020.

16. Shemesh D, Zigelman C, Olsha O, et al. Primary forearm arteriovenous fistula for hemodialysis access—an integrated approach to improve outcomes. *Cardiovasc Surg.* 2003; 11:35–41.

17. Robbin ML, Gallichio MH, Deierhoi MH, Young CJ, Weber Tm, Allon M. US vascular mapping before hemodialysis access placement. *Radiology.* 2000;217:83-88.

18. Bethard GS. Strategy for maximizing the use of arteriovenous fistulae. *Semin Dial.* 2000; 13:291-296.

19. Ku YM, Kim YO, Kim JI, et al. Ultrasonographic measurement of intima–media thickness of radial artery in predialysis uraemic patients: comparison with histological examination. *Nephrol Dial Transplant.* 2006;21:715–720

20. Tannuri U, Tannuri AC. Experience with arteriovenous fistula for chronic hemodialysis in children: technical details and refinements. *Clinics (Brazil).* 2005;60:37-40.

21. Sedlacek M, Teodorescu V, Falk A, Vassalotti JA, Uribarri J. Hemodialysis access placement with preoperative noninvasive vascular mapping: comparison between patients with and without diabetes. *Am J Kidney Dis.* 2001;38:560-564.

22. Malovrh M. Native arteriovenous fistula: preoperative evaluation. *Am J Kidney Dis.* 2002; 39:1218-1225.

23. Fassiadis N, Morsy M, Siva M, Marsh JE, Makanjuola D, Chemla ES. Does the surgeon's experience impact radiocephalic fistula patency rates? Semin Dial. 2007;20:455-457.

24. Allon M, Robbin ML. Increasing arteriovenous fistulas in hemodialysis patients: problems and solution. *Kidney Int.* 2002;62: 1109-1124.

25. Golledge J, Smith CJ, Emery J, Farrington K, Thompson HH. Outcome of primary radiocephalic fistula for hemodialysis. *Br J Surg.* 1999;86: 211-216.

26. Biuckians A, Scott EC, Meier GH, Panneton JM, Glickman MH. The natural history of autologous fistulas as first-time dialysis access in the KDOQI era. *J Vasc Surg.* 2008;47:415-421.

27. Johnson CP, Zhu Y, Matt C, et al. Prognostic value of intraoperative blood flow measurements in vascular access surgery. *Surgery.* 1998; 124:729–738.

28. Hoskins PR, McDicken WN, Allan PL. Hemodynamics and blood flow. In Allan P, Dubbins P, Pozniac MA, McDicken WN (eds). *Clinical Doppler Ultrasound.* London: Harcourt Publishers Ltd, 27-38.

29. Carter SA. Investigation and treatment of arterial occlusive disease of the extremities. *Clin Med.* 1972;79:13-24;15-22.

30. Basseau F, Grenier N, Trillaud H, et al. Volume flow measurement in hemodialysis shunts using time domain correlation. *J Ultrasound Med.* 1999;29:177-183.

31. Shenoy S, Middleton WD, Windus D, et al: Brachial artery flow measurement as an indicator of forearm native fistula maturation. In Henry ML (ed). *Vascular Access for Hemodialysis VII.* Chicago: Precept Press, 2001:233-239.

32. Sands J, Glidden D, Miranda C. Hemodialysis access flow measurement. Comparison of ultrasound dilution and duplex ultrasonography. *ASAIO J.* 1996;42:M899–M901.

33. Lomonte C, Casuci F, Antonelli M, et al. Is there a place for duplex screening of brachial artery in the maturation of arteriovenous fistulas? *Semin Dial.* 2005;18:243-246.

34. Parsons RE, Sigel B, Feleppa EJ, et al. Age determination of experimental venous thrombi by ultrasonic tissue characterization. *J Vasc Surg.* 1993;17:470-478.

35. Esses GE, Bandyk DF. Noninvasive studies of vascular disease. In Dean RD, Yao JS, Brewster DC (eds). *Current Diagnosis and Treatment in Vascular Disease.* Norwalk, CT: Appleton and Lange, 1995: 5-21.

36. Robbin ML, Oser RF, Allon M, et al. Hemodialysis access graft stenosis: U/S detection. *Radiology.* 1998;208:655-661.

RESULTS OF VASCULAR ACCESS FOR HEMODIALYSIS

CHAPTER 31

Reflections on Four Decades of Experience in Vascular Access Surgery

A. Frederick Schild, Patrick S. Collier, and Joseph C. Fuller

The physical phenomenon of dialysis was first described and used in 1854 to separate substances in aqueous solutions based on different rates of diffusion through a semipermeable membrane. In vivo hemodialysis was performed in animals early in the 20th century. Hemodialysis was first carried out on humans in Holland by Dr. Willem Kolff during World War II. Soon afterward, Dr. Kolff came to the United States to share his discoveries from his experiments(see Chapter 1).[1]

The external arteriovenous shunt described by Quinton, Dillard, and Scribner in 1960 established the feasibility of chronic hemodialysis.[2] Just after returning from the US Army in Korea and beginning a private practice, I received a telephone call from a nephrologist. He asked if I knew how to do a "shunt." I replied, "Of course. Splenorenal or portocaval?" He said, "No, a Scribner shunt." I told him that I had never heard of that procedure. But I went to the medical school library, researched Scribner's work, and placed the first Scribner shunt of my career in 1966 (Fig. 31-1).

Later in 1966, Brescia, Cimino, and Appel proposed surgical construction of an internal arteriovenous fistula (AVF) in the forearm by side-to-side anastomosis of the radial artery and the cephalic vein. With this procedure, the arterial flow into the vein made it easily accessible for percutaneous puncture and provided the high flows necessary to support hemodialysis. Within a decade of its creation, the AVF replaced the external shunt as the preferred mode of vascular access (Fig. 31-2).[3]

The first two autologous fistulas I made remained patent and useable for 21 and 22 years, no doubt because these two patients had end-stage renal disease (ESRD) at a young age caused by hypertension, compared with today's epidemiology of ESRD in which diabetes mellitus is the major etiology and patients are more than 65 years of age. At that time, in Miami, diabetics were not placed on dialysis because of the many complications.

Before Medicare insured dialysis patients, selection committees decided who would and who would not be placed on this life-saving treatment. The patients were required to have potential for rehabilitation and to be between the ages of 18 and 50 years. In my opinion, because of the stringent selection of patients, they were healthier and more compliant with treatment, contributing to better patency and quality of life. The Social Security Amendment Act of 1973, enacted after considerable pressure from ESRD patients and their physicians, authorized Medicare to pay for chronic hemodialysis, but only after the patient had been on dialysis for 90 days. Now almost all ESRD patients were eligible for dialysis funded by Medicare without consideration of comorbidity, ultimately leading to the extensive program in place in the United States today.

Transposed saphenous veins were also used as AV conduits in the 1970s and 1980s, but are no longer in common

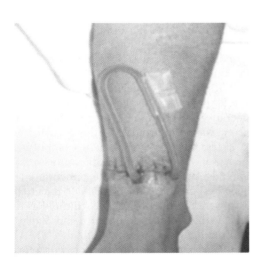

Figure 31-1.
Scribner shunt.

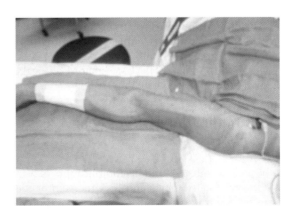

Figure 31-2.
Immediate postoperative arteriovenous fistula.

use, because after two years, only 20 to 60% of these fistulas remain functioning.[3] Thinking ahead, many physicians prefer to preserve the saphenous vein for later coronary artery or peripheral bypass surgery.

In 1973, polytetrafluoroethylene (PTFE) grafts were introduced and soon became the most commonly used artificial material for vascular grafts in hemodialysis.[3] Over the years, I have had experience with a variety of conduits for vascular access, including the Scribner shunt, bovine heterografts, autologous fistulas, umbilical vein grafts, PTFE, and polyetherurethaneurea grafts. Incremental improvements rather than major advances have been the rule in vascular prosthetic graft technology.

In 1980, a double-lumen catheter was designed and has slowly evolved to side-by-side, coaxial, and other variations.[3] These catheters are placed via the internal jugular vein and into the superior vena cava under image guidance. Although the central catheters have a safer design, the great risks of complications during introduction and late central vein stenosis and infection restrict their use. Cuffed catheters resist tunnel site infection and are accessed painlessly by staff, but their convenience may lead to longer use and central vein occlusion.

Vascular Access Requires a Multidisciplinary Approach

American Medical News reported on April 21, 2003: "Patients with chronic illnesses must navigate a complex regimen of multiple physicians and medications. *Coordination of the medical team* supports patients by improving care and avoiding hospitalizations."[4] A structured and well-organized multidisciplinary team approach appears to be the most practical and efficient way to achieve quality care for ESRD patients. Patients receiving this standard of care have earlier consultations with surgeons, enabling a higher incidence of AVF construction, because veins have not been damaged by repeated venipuncture and intravenous infusions. Since the patient will have a functioning high-flow AVF, ready for initiation of hemodialysis, dependence on temporary catheters is decreased. Further, with a team approach, complications are identified and corrected in a timely fashion, leading to increased long-term patency, fewer hospitalizations, and fewer reoperations. Early access construction continues to be a challenge, because some patients procrastinate until they have a catheter before they see a surgeon. Participating specialties include: primary care physicians, nephrologists, interventional nephrologists, interventional radiologists, anesthesiologists, surgeons, and, most important, a coordinator, who may be a nurse. This coordinator is critical to the success of a multispecialty team.

Complications of Vascular Access

Thrombosis

Thrombosis, the most common complication of vascular access, is usually caused by stenosis of the vein or the outflow vein for the graft. In AVF thrombosis, one should evaluate the proximal vein to determine type of revision. Often it can be repaired by endovascular techniques such as angioplasty or stent. Surgical revision may consist of a local

patch graft of the outflow anastomosis, a new, more proximal anastomosis, or interposition of a graft to connect to a larger vein. Regardless of treatment type, all thrombi must be removed with emphasis on the arterial plug. In some instances, the proximal vein above the graft anastomosis has enlarged so that one can create an autologous fistula.

Infection

Long-term cannulation of any vessel carries significant risks, and vascular access is no exception. The establishment of the radiocephalic AVF by Brescia, Cimino, and Appel reduced the risk relative to older methods. During the past 30 years, however, the accelerating incidence of diabetes and hypertension has led to increased need for vascular access procedures and to a corresponding increase in infection rates. Now the second most common complication in vascular access, onset of sepsis can lead to further complications such as subacute bacterial endocarditis, spine and epidural abscesses, and, in some instances, brain abscesses. Death caused by infection is estimated to occur in approximately one third of dialysis patients.

The diagnosis of infection at a vascular access site can vary depending on the physician's assessment. Recognizing that it is important to have a consistent approach to diagnosis and treatment, I diagnose infection when there are local signs of inflammation or purulence requiring intravenous antibiotics and removal of the access.

When infection in an AV fistula or graft is identified, an understanding of the cause and the typical time-course of its development can help devise treatment strategy. Infections attributable to access implantation have a low incidence. Rather, the largest number of infections occur in patients undergoing routine dialysis. When postoperative complication is defined as occurring within 30 days after surgery, retrospective review has shown that the overall postoperative infection rate was 0.51% (n = 1574). On further analysis, AVFs have 0% (n = 521). For an AV graft, the infection rate was slightly higher, with a rate of 0.86% (n = 921).[5] My conclusion is that infections most often are the result of chronic cannulation and are not a consequence of postoperative complications.

We reviewed the medical records of 1574 consecutive vascular access procedures performed on 850 patients, over a 60-month period. This included 443 new grafts, 478 graft revisions, and 521 new fistulas. Of the 963 new procedures, 54% were autologous fistulas and 46% were prosthetic grafts. In addition, 132 procedures were performed for infection in 87 patients. This data may be interpreted as an 8% postoperative infection rate. Of those, 86 were infected grafts and one was an infected AVF (this occurred two years following access surgery which was complicated by a pseudoaneurysm).[5] See Table 31-1 for sources of infection.

In this study, procedures (needle puncture sites) were found to be responsible for 50% of all infections identified. There were multiple organisms cultured as the cause of infection, with the most common being *Staphylococcus aureus* and methicillin resistant *S. aureus* (MRSA) (Table 31-2). Possible reasons may include poor antiseptic practice in preparation of the cannulation site, or not wearing sterile gloves, gowns, and masks during cannulation of the fistula. These data suggest that incidence of infection can be

Table 31–1
Sources of Infection

Source of Infection	Grafts Operated on for Infection (%)
Operative (within 30 days)	6%
Interventional Radiology (post-thrombectomy)	5%
Dialysis Center (more than 30 days post surgery)	50%
Spontaneous in Non-Functional Graft	23%
Remaining Stump of Previously Excised Graft	17%

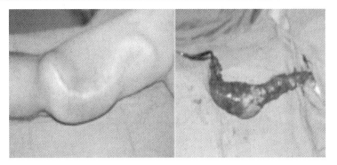

Figure 31-3.
Twenty-year-old infected arteriovenous fistula.

potentially reduced based on simple, inexpensive changes in antiseptic practices.

Thrombosed grafts may be a source of bacteremia even in the absence of local signs of inflammation. If infection is identified in nonfunctional grafts, removal is recommended. Undue delay because of prolonged antibiotic therapy is not warranted, because the presence of a foreign body will not allow complete eradication of infection with antibiotics alone. It had previously been our policy, when removing an infected graft, to leave a graft stump at the arterial anastomosis when the artery was very small and no vein was available for a patch. As many as 17% of these residual graft stumps became infected, so we now recommend that when grafts are infected they should be totally removed if technically feasible (Fig. 31-3).[5]

Despite data showing that infections are more common in grafts, the reasons may not be simple. The decision as to whether to choose a graft or a fistula is complex for additional reasons which are discussed in the following sections.

Maturation and Failure Rates in Arteriovenous Fistulas

At the present time, there are over 400,000 patients on hemodialysis in the United States. The ESRD patient group is enlarging by approximately 15% each year and doubling every 4-6 years. Total annual costs for maintenance hemodialyses are projected to exceed US$28 billion by 2010. With the number of vascular access procedures at

Other Complications

Other complications of vascular access procedures include seromas (Fig. 31-4), aneurysms (Fig. 31-5), pseudoaneurysms, proximal vein occlusion secondary to central vein stenosis (Fig. 31-6), and bleeding.

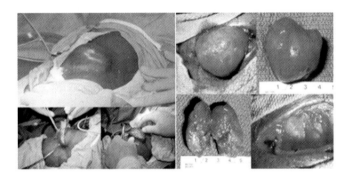

Figure 31-4.
Surgical removal of seroma.

Table 31–2
Organisms Causing Infection

Organism	Percentage of Total Infections Cultured
Staphylococcus aureus	26.32%
Negative Cultures	22.81%
Methicillin-Resistant Staphylococcus aureus (MRSA)	21.05%
Pseudomonas aeruginosa	5.26%
Staphylococcus epidermidis	3.51%
Streptococcus viridans	3.51%
Enterobacter cloacae	3.51%
Acinetobacter baumanni	1.75%
Alcanigenes xylosoxidans	1.75%
Corynebacterium	1.75%
Enterococcus	1.75%
Enterobacter faecalis	1.75%
Mycobacteria chelonae	1.75%
Serratia marcescens	1.75%

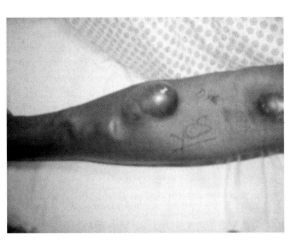

Figure 31-5.
Aneurysm in 9-year-old fistula.

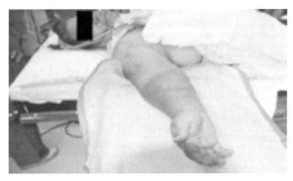

Figure 31-6.
Markedly edematous upper extremity secondary to central venous obstruction.

approximately 500,000 per year, KDOQI (National Kidney Foundation Dialysis Outcome Quality Initiative) guidelines recommend an aggressive approach to the construction of AV fistulas, in contrast to prosthetic accesses. However, it is clear that not all patients are suitable candidates for this type of vascular access procedure. In certain patients, fistulas may never mature or function, requiring additional surgeries to establish a means for dialysis.

Previously, surgeons in the United States constructed more grafts than fistulas. KDOQI now recommends that 66% of all new vascular access procedures be arteriovenous fistulas. A "Fistula First" movement has been advocated nationally, largely by nonsurgeons, perhaps unrealistically raising patients' expectations. Some surgeons have found that although AV fistulas can be constructed and remain patent, as few as half will support hemodialysis. Now the question becomes: Have we gone too far in attempting to construct AVF's in ESRD patients? Are unnecessary operations, with little chance of success, occurring because of an "ex-cathedra" directive?

We reviewed 374 consecutive AVF's in the *Journal of Vascular and Endovascular Surgery* in 2004. Of these fistulas, 31.3% either never matured or were not able to be cannulated, requiring that these patients have at least 1 additional operation. The failure rate for females was higher than that in males (41.2% and 27.2%, respectively), but increasing comorbidity did not result in major changes in failure rate. Furthermore, the brachiocephalic position matures at a higher frequency than the radiocephalic.[6,7]

Other studies show even higher failure rates for AV fistulas. Miller et al reported: "Of the 101 fistulas for which adequacy could be determined, [i.e., functional patency] 54 (or 53.5%) did not develop adequately, as defined by our prospective criteria."[8] Biuckians et al stated: "Even in the best of circumstances in which a patient is undergoing first-time access procedure, many [57%] AVF failed and of those functioning only two-thirds are working at the end of 1 year…[and KDOQI guidelines do] not necessarily translate into high AVF utilization."[9]

Findings like these raise several concerns. Should the KDOQI Guidelines be revised in terms of developing more focused criteria for AVF, or should we be more meticulous in preoperative work-up? In light of published AVF failure rates ranging from 20% to 50%, are we subjecting patients to unnecessary second operations (AVF, then prosthetic access)? Some patients do not have the vasculature necessary to sup-

port a successful fistula. These patients can often be identified by physical examination and imaging and may be better served by a nonautologous graft. AV fistulas require 4 to 12 weeks or longer to mature, but, on average, AV grafts may be used within several days. Furthermore, newer grafts that can be cannulated within 24 to 72 hours have been developed.

While waiting for the fistula to mature, patients must be dialyzed through double-lumen cuffed catheters. Double-lumen cuffed catheters are a hazard for long-term dialysis because of central venous stenosis and, especially, infection. It is estimated that infection with central venous catheters will cost over $30,000 per patient per admission as a consequence of prolonged hospitalization and expensive parenteral antibiotics for resistant microflora.[10] Lee, et al found a 50% catheter bacteremia at 6 months.[11] Summing up the risks, Allon et al reported that relative risk of death was 3.43 times greater over 1 year with a central venous dialysis catheter compared to an autologous fistula.[12]

Recently, at the University of Miami Miller School of Medicine, we compared outcomes of AV fistulas and grafts retrospectively. We reviewed 1700 consecutive cases performed by 1 surgeon at a single institution between 1997 and 2005. Patients were classified according to demographics and comorbidities. Fistula and graft survival were independently calculated from time of surgery to last contact date or loss of access (Fig. 31-7). Primary, primary assisted, and secondary patencies of grafts and fistulas were calculated.[13]

Grafts are often placed in patients with the largest number of comorbidities, previously failed fistulas, and absent distal veins. Infection, thrombosis, aneurysms, and female gender are independent prognostic factors of a poorer outcome, as shown by multivariate analysis. The type of access, however, is not a prognostic indicator of worsened outcome.[13]

Our data suggest that AV fistulas and grafts are equivalent in providing vascular access for chronic hemodialysis, as shown by univariate and multivariate analysis. Although grafts have a higher rate of thrombosis, outflow revisions are more successful compared to revisions of thrombosed fistulas.[13] Attempting AV fistulas in all chronic hemodialysis patients is unreasonable; rather, nonautologous grafts have a role in chronic renal failure. Lastly, when AV fistulas fail, a bridge graft is always a superior option to a double-lumen cuffed catheter.

Future Developments

Interrupted anastomosis (eg, clips) may be superior to a running suture anastomosis by allowing enlargement of the anastomeric lumen, and attempts are underway to develop a "glue" to hold arteries and veins together securely.[14,15] Other approaches aim to change the genetic structure of the endothelium at the venous anastomosis to prevent neointimal hyperplasia. In one method, after the anastomosis, a collagen collar is placed around the anastomosis. Then, the active biologic factors are injected between the collar and the anastomosis. Both collar and medication are biodegradable and will remain for several weeks but should not escape into general circulation. So far, this experiment has shown favorable results in animal studies. In another method designed to inhibit intimal hyperplasia, a mélange of growth factors derived from bovine endothelial cells is wrapped around the anastomosis in order to reregulate endothelial proliferation.

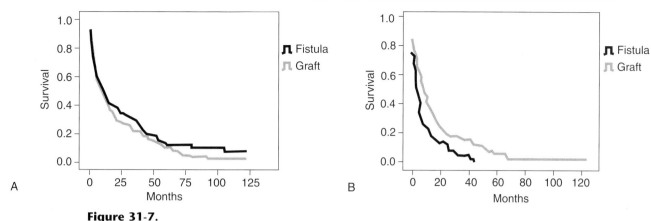

Figure 31-7.
A, Timeline showing no statistical difference between survival of primary AV fistula and primary AV graft; *B,* Comparison of revised AV fistula and revised AV graft at 120 months.[13]

New technical developments in the manufacture of grafts show considerable promise in lowering the incidence of infection, pseudoaneurysms, seromas, and thrombosis. Often the technique involves impregnation of the PTFE with a biologically active substance. Early cannulation is now possible with specialized grafts within the first 24 to72 hours with excellent results. We predict there will be fewer seromas and pseudoaneurysms as well as these grafts have a membrane that enhances clotting after needle removal.

Dos And Don'ts Of Vascular Access

Here is some practical advice for vascular access surgeons: 10 *Dos* and 10 *Don'ts* that have proved useful to me from time to time.

Top 10 "Do's" of Vascular Access:

(1) Always obtain a complete history and physical on the patient.
  • It is essential that every new patient has a complete work-up to avoid missing other pathology.
(2) Obtain Doppler duplex vein mapping when indicated.
  • Doing vascular access surgery without excellent knowledge of the patient's veins is analogous to flying an airplane when blindfolded.
  • When one has a patient with excellent veins and no history of previous catheter dialysis, vein mapping may not be essential.
(3) Remain open to use of a PTFE early cannulation graft in place of a double-lumen cuffed catheter.
  • This should be done when there are no adequate veins on physical examination or vein mapping that will allow construction of an AVF.
(4) Request early referral for access evaluation.
  • For the surgeon, it is optimal to have early referral before the patient's veins have been sclerosed during multiple hospitalizations, intravenous (IV) medications, and previous IVs.
  • Patients referred earlier are more likely to receive a functional AVF.
(5) Explain the operation to the patient in detail.
  • I feel that it puts the patient at ease if you make them aware of exactly what you are going to do.

  • I find that establishing good rapport with the patients may hold you in good stead in the future if the access fails.
(6) Use the most distal site available for access in the upper extremity.
  • Since we only have two arms, it is paramount to place the access as distal as possible in each arm.
  • This may ultimately maintain the patient on chronic hemodialysis for a longer period of time.
(7) Place the access in the upper extremity when possible.
  • Our experience with thigh grafts has not been as good as with the upper extremity. There is a higher incidence of infection.
  • If a thigh graft blows out, proximal and distal control is more challenging.
(8) Follow up with patients after surgery.
  • It is extremely important to see the patient postoperatively.
  • Patients may be seen early at 1 week to determine whether wounds are healing and the access is maturing.
  • A second visit helps determine whether the access is ready for dialysis.
(9) Communicate with the referring physician before and after surgery.
  • There is no question that communication is very important to preserve patient confidence and referrals!
  • You should write a letter and/or call the referring physician after you have seen and evaluated the patient.
  • After surgery, you should make the patient aware of what procedure you performed and the expected time to initiation of dialysis.
(10) Provide in-service education to dialysis nurses and technicians regarding sterile technique.
  • In some dialysis centers, sterile technique is not as strict as the operating room.
  • In a recently published retrospective study of 1574 consecutive patients, the most common infections (50%) were from the dialysis center.[5]

Top 10 "Don'ts" of Vascular Access:

(1) Operate on patients with HIV or hepatitis C under local anesthesia.

- We always operate upon our HIV and hepatitis C patients under general anesthesia.
  - We feel this is safer because some patients under local anesthetic and sedation become restless and move their arms or legs and can cause a cut or puncture with a needle or scalpel.
(2) Prolong the use of double-lumen cuffed catheters.
  - Prolonged use of double-lumen cuffed catheters have a high infection rate and often lead to central vein stenosis.
(3) Always rely on the vein mapping report; see the scans yourself if you have any questions.
  - We have seen reports of vein mapping that at the time of surgery were found to be different from the report.
  - Films read by residents, fellows, or "night hawks" may miss key issues.
(4) Operate on a patient that you have not seen and examined yourself.
  - It is simply unwise to perform access surgery on the basis of information provided by the referring physician.
  - You may find problems that you did not know existed, such as poor veins or calcified arteries.
  - This practice would be hard to defend in court.
(5) When obtaining consent for surgery, forget to inform every patient as well as document all of the complications that can occur with vascular access procedures.
  - If you don't, you may be very sorry when the subpoena arrives.
(6) Place an AV fistula in a patient when you know it probably will not work—but you try it anyway.
  - My old professor once said, "Don't ever do anything that you think *might* work, because 99% of the time it won't."
  - If you are really careful with your pre-op workup, you can select a successful access surgery and not cause the patient to have a second operation.
(7) Be surprised if a fistula fails to mature.
  - Because of Fistula First, many surgeons are attempting fistulas that will never mature.
  - Sometimes, even though the vein and artery look good, the fistula will fail for causes unknown. We depend on clotting deficiencies in the ESRD patient to keep the AVF open.
  - Fistula failure rates are now being reported at 30 to 50%.
(8) Operate on patients taking aspirin, clopidogrel, or warfarin.
  - Some surgeons will operate on patients taking these drugs.
  - In my experience, the platelet abnormalities of ESRD and the combination of these drugs cause oozing that is difficult to control during surgery.
  - I advise my patients not to take aspirin and/or clopidogrel for at least 10 days before surgery and to discontinue warfarin at least 5 days before surgery.
(9) Let the dialysis center cannulate the access until you decide it is ready.
  - We occasionally have seen patients in whom cannulation was carried out before the surgeon's evaluation, leading to a large hematoma and loss of the access site.
  - Then, you may have to do a second or even a third operation, prolonging the double-lumen cuffed catheter time.
(10) Schedule your access patients at the end of your surgery schedule.
  - You may be prone to making errors that could otherwise be easily avoided. At the end of the operative schedule, your brain may not be as sharp as your scalpel.

Conclusions

Vascular access procedures are among the most common operations performed in the United States. A multidisciplinary effort, vascular access surgery encompasses many difficult problems and should be only done by those dedicated to its success. Though a greater effort should be made to construct more arteriovenous fistulas than prosthetic grafts, as recommended by the KDOQI guidelines, grafts still have a place in chronic renal failure and should always be the first alternative over a double-lumen cuffed catheter. We have found that 50% of infections were attributable to the dialysis center and strongly believe antiseptic methods education should be provided by dialysis nurses and technicians regarding sterile technique.[5]

REFERENCES

1. Uribarri J. Past, present, and future of ESRD therapy in the United States. *Mt Sinai J Med.* 1999;66(1):14-19.
2. Bennion RS, Wilson SE. *Vascular Surgery: A Comprehensive Review.* 6th ed. Philadelphia: W.B. Saunders Company, 2002:652.
3. Shaldon S. Preface: Hemodialysis, vascular access, and peritoneal dialysis access. Ronco C, Levin NW (eds). *Contrib Nephrol.* 2004;142:X-XII.
4. Landa A. Collaborating for care: when joining forces helps patients. *Am Med News.* 2003;45:15.
5. Schild AF, Simon S, Prieto J, Raines J. Single center review of infections associated with 1,574 consecutive vascular access procedures. *J Vasc Endovasc Surg.* 2003;37(1):27-31.
6. Schild AF, Prieto J, Glenn M, Livingstone J, Alfieri K, Raines J. Maturation and failure rates in a large series of arteriovenous dialysis access fistulas. *J Vasc Endovasc Surg.* 2004;38(5)449-453.
7. Nguyen TH, Bui TD, Gordon IL, Wilson SE. Functional patency of autogenous AV fistulas for hemodialysis. *J Vasc Access.* 2007;8(4)275-280.
8. Miller PE, Tolwani A, Luscy CP, et al. Predictors of adequacy of arteriovenous fistulas in hemodialysis patients. *Kidney Int.* 1999;56(1) 275-280.
9. Biuckians A, Scott EC, Meier GH, Panneton JM, Glickman MH. The natural history of autologous fistulas as first-time dialysis access in the KDOQI era. *J Vasc Surg.* 2008;47(2)415-421.
10. Work J. Fistula First: has the pendulum swung too far? The unintended consequences. *Vascular Access Practicum.* Durham, NC: Duke University. 2007.
11. Lee T, Barker J, Allon M. Tunneled catheters in hemodialysis patients: reasons and subsequent outcomes. *Am J Kidney Dis.* 2005;46(3)501-508.
12. Allon M, Daugirdas J, Depner TA, Greene T, Ornt D, Schwab SJ. Effect of change in vascular access of patient mortality in hemodialysis patients. *Am J Kidney Dis.* 2006;47(3)469-477.
13. Schild AF, Perez E, Gillaspie E, Seaver C, Livingstone J, Thibonnier A. Arteriovenous fistulae vs. arteriovenous grafts: a retrospective review of 1,700 consecutive vascular access cases. *J Vasc Access Surg.* 2008;9(4):231-235.
14. Schild AF, Pruett CS, Newman MI, et al. The utility of the VCS clip for creation of vascular access for hemodialysis: long-term results and intraoperative benefits. *J Cardiovasc Surg.* 2001;9(6)526-530.
15. Shenoy S, Miller A, Petersen F, et al. A multicenter study of permanent hemodialysis access patency: beneficial effect of clipped vascular anastomotic technique. *J Vasc Surg.* 2003;38(2)229-235.

Organizing Hemodialysis Access: The Kaiser Permanente Southern California Experience

Sidney Glazer, Jean Diesto, Peter Crooks, Stephen Derose, and Michael Farooq

With the reports of the Scribner shunt[1] and Brescia–Cimino[2] arteriovenous fistula (AVF) in the 1960s, long-term hemodialysis became feasible for the first time. Initially, treatment was very selective and ideally viewed as a bridge to transplant. Committees selected the suitable patients for the limited number of machines available. By 1972, about 5000 patients were receiving hemodialysis in the United States.[3] In that year, Congress passed an amendment to Medicare extending coverage to end-stage renal disease (ESRD) patients aged less than 65 years age. With expanded indications for treatment and financial restraints removed, the population expanded rapidly to more than 325,000 Americans on chronic hemodialysis in 2008. This number is increasing at about 5% a year.[4,5] Demographics of the patient population have also changed substantially. Although there were no diabetics and an average age of 43 years in the original AVF series,[2] by 2005, diabetics were 44.9% of new patients and the mean age was 62.8 years.[6]

When the number of patients was small and their comorbidities few, organized care of vascular access was a low priority. In 1998, it was estimated that creation and maintenance of vascular access accounted for 10% of the more than $10.1 billion spent on dialysis patients.[7] Twenty-five percent of hospital admissions of ESRD patients were related to vascular access, and it was the leading cause of hospitalization in the first year on dialysis.[8] Management of access complications is much more costly than access placement. According to a United States Renal Data System (USRDS) report, total ESRD expenditures in 2005 were $32 billion, or 1.6% of health care costs. Medicare spending for ESRD in 2005 was $21.3 billion, which represented a 9.1% increase from 2004.[9] Twenty-nine percent of prevalent patients were dialyzed with a catheter at the year's end in 2006,[10] which carries a 50 to 90% higher mortality than patients using an AVF.[11] The publication of the Dialysis Outcomes Quality Initiative (DOQI) clinical practice guidelines for vascular access by the National Kidney Foundation in 1997[12] and results from the Dialysis Outcomes Practice Patterns Study (DOPPS) in 2002 put a spotlight on poor vascular access outcomes, especially in the United States.

Only 24% of patients were using a fistula in the United States, compared to 80% in Europe. Sixty percent of patients started dialysis with a catheter in the United States, compared to 31% in Europe.[13] A more organized approach to quality management of the vascular access was felt to be urgently needed by health care professionals dealing with hemodialysis patients.

The Institute for Healthcare Improvement was asked by the Centers for Medicare and Medicaid Services (CMS) to assist in developing the National Vascular Access Improvement Initiative, better known as Fistula First, in 2003. CMS considered this a high priority quality improvement project, identifying it as its first "Breakthrough Initiative." Although DOQI, later known as Kidney Disease Outcomes Quality Initiative (KDOQI), assisted in increasing the AVF prevalence rate by about 2% a year, CMS wanted a more aggressive approach to get a higher growth rate, striving for a stretch goal of 66% fistula prevalence rate by 2009.[14,15] Pay for performance is being added as an element of the program.[16] In 1978, Congress authorized the formation of ESRD Network Organizations, which encompass different areas of the country and now number 18, to serve as liaisons between the federal government and providers of patient services. They collect epidemiologic and outcomes data, such as the four Clinical Performance Measures established by CMS to deal with vascular access. This information is given back to providers as well as to CMS.[17] Fistula First developed 11 change concepts to assist clinicians and has given numerous educational presentations across the country. Their goal is to have each patient get the most suitable vascular access, which is usually a mature fistula, while minimizing the use of catheters.[14]

Medicine looked to business methods for help. After World War II, business theorists such as W. Edwards Deming helped Japan develop a continuous quality improvement (CQI) approach to production. Although each patient is unique, many of the same business principles were applicable to medical care and dialysis access in particular.[18] Using this approach, once problems are identified, a multidisciplinary team of all the important stakeholders is formed. Corrective action plans are developed and implemented to fix the problems. A database is developed to collect and analyze outcomes, which are compared to preselected benchmarks. Additional improvements are planned through continued monitoring with regular meetings of the team. Therefore, quality assurance leads to continuous quality improvement (Plan, Do, Check, and Act).[19]

Kaiser Permanente Southern California Develops a Plan

In 1996, Kaiser Permanente Southern California (KPSC) was preparing to participate in the CMS ESRD Demonstration Project, mandated by Congress to compare quality and cost outcomes between managed care and standard Medicare. The Tax Equity and Fiscal Responsibility Act of 1982 did not allow Medicare beneficiaries with ESRD to enroll in health maintenance organizations unless they were members before the onset of ESRD. We at KPSC were aware of the draft DOQI guidelines and believed that KPSC needed to improve quality and decrease the costs associated with vascular access, although we had a very limited database on access outcomes at that time.[20,21]

Kaiser Permanente is a national, nonprofit, integrated health care maintenance organization with 8.7 million members. Kaiser Health Plan and Hospitals is the insurance company and owner of the material assets. The different Permanente Medical Groups are the physician organizations that contract with Kaiser to provide physician services. There are eight regions across the country, with the two in California being by far the largest. The Southern California region has 3.2 million members. As of September 2008, 5929 patients had ESRD. Of these, 3768 patients received in-center hemodialysis, 42 were on home hemodialysis, 529 were on peritoneal dialysis, and 1590 had functioning kidney transplants. Thirty-six vascular surgeons, 32 interventional radiologists, and 71 nephrologists provided for their care.

About 1 year before the start of enrollment in the Medicare demonstration project, KPSC formed a multidisciplinary committee specifically to address hemodialysis access issues. Representatives from vascular surgery, nephrology, interventional radiology, renal nurse care managers, and administrators participated in regional meetings to define the problems, devise solutions, and evaluate data on outcomes. The issues addressed by the committee included late referral of patients with chronic kidney disease to nephrology, delays in surgery consultation and operative scheduling, excess catheter usage, predominance of graft over fistula placement, inadequate monitoring/surveillance, delays in treatment of access dysfunction, excess hospitalization for access related problems, and poor data collection.

The draft clinical practice guidelines from DOQI were adopted in large measure. The goals were to increase AVF incidence to 50% to achieve a prevalence of 40%, reduce chronic catheter use to <10%, and perform monitoring and surveillance of the access with intervention before thrombosis. Creation of uncommon autogenous fistulas not mentioned in DOQI, such as forearm transpositions and antecubital fistulas, were encouraged. The regional team developed care pathways for placement of a new access,

treatment of access dysfunction and surveillance. These included acceptable time frames to accomplish various steps in the process. However, since resources and expertise varied at each of the 13 Kaiser Permanente patient care areas in Southern California, local multidisciplinary vascular access committees were given flexibility on how to best accomplish the goals.

Nurse vascular access coordinators (VACs) are the organizational hub of the entire program at the level where interactions occur. These are usually nephrology nurses with hemodialysis experience. Desirable qualifications also include excellent organizational skills, familiarity and comfort with a computerized database, communication skills, and unflappability when dealing with several problems at the same time. Although the responsibilities vary somewhat at each medical center, the VAC is the liaison among physicians, dialysis facilities, patients, and schedulers. New problems are directly reported to the VAC, who evaluates and prioritizes them and then communicates with the appropriate physician. As the patient's advocate, the VAC organizes the medical appointments, follows up to see that scheduled visits occur and interventions are carried out in a timely fashion. The result is improvement in the quality of care, substantially reduced costs, and lower frustration levels for all parties involved.[22]

Education for providers and patients is a critical component of success. A full-day hemodialysis access symposium was held in March 1998, and another in September 2007, to update physicians and nurses on the new approaches to improve access outcomes. An ongoing series of lectures were given to small groups of staff at the various medical centers. The KPSC vascular surgeons meet as a group 4 times a year. Information shared at this meeting provides an opportunity for a vascular surgeon representative to update the local teams on regional vascular access outcomes, best practices, and new knowledge.[23] Similar regional meetings occur among the interventional radiologists, nephrologists, and renal care managers. Two videotapes were produced for patients about vascular access options and the perioperative period, encouraging patients to be proactive in their care. These are shown to predialysis patients at the "Choices" class where they learn about dialysis modalities. A recent initiative was the development of a wallet-sized card for late CKD and ESRD patients to promote vein preservation and avoid peripherally inserted central catheter (PICC) lines. Patients are being instructed to show the card to their phlebotomist or doctor. Since personnel turnover is to be expected at all levels and new knowledge is constantly being added, ongoing educational activities must be viewed as an essential component of any CQI program.

Reliable data are fundamental to any CQI project; hence the adage: if it cannot be measured, it cannot be improved. A vascular access tracking tool is completed following any vascular access encounter. This information forms the vascular access database along with monthly information from the dialysis facilities and the patient's medical record. There is always a trade-off between collecting all of the information you want versus the information you need to bring about desired change. The data should be simple, terminology consistent, and promptly entered. It needs to be reviewed on a regular basis to see how improvement plans are working and to identify new areas of concern. The results must also be fed back to the providers to improve quality and to gain their continued interest and participation.[22]

The information shared in this chapter was collected between January 1, 1997, and December 31, 2007. Data were collected on all patients starting hemodialysis and/or having any vascular access interventions. Information was taken from outpatient hemodialysis enrollment referral forms, which identified the type of access present as well as patient demographics. Monthly data reports from dialysis facilities provided the access type throughout the year. The vascular access tracking tool contains information on the indications for the intervention, what was done, who performed it, and where it occurred. It was completed at each facility by a physician or nurse whenever a surgical or radiological intervention was performed related to vascular access, and then forwarded to the regional office for data input. In the last year, Kaiser Permanente has rolled out a comprehensive computerized medical record. In the future, data input for vascular access encounters will be entered directly at the site of origin.

A report listing the incidence of AVF creation in new patients by each surgeon, identified only by code number, was provided to every surgeon and chief of service for comparison to peers. The chief used this as a quality assurance indicator during the yearly review of the surgeon's performance. Feedback to an individual on his own outcomes along with being able to see the outcomes of peers anonymously was a crucial step in the process of change. In almost all cases, this feedback plus education was sufficient to change physician behavior, as evidenced by increased use of AVF. In a few cases, high-level hospital physician administrators became involved after repeatedly attending regional meetings where data were presented showing that their facility lagged well behind others in patient vascular access outcomes. A yearly report compiled outcomes by hospital and was distributed widely. It became a source of pride or concern and served to stimulate continuous improvement.

Data on patient demographics, incidence and prevalence of hemodialysis access type, thrombosis rates, and type of replacement access were collected and analyzed. Outcomes that were assessed included the incidence and prevalence of AVFs, grafts, and catheters; proportion of replacement access with AVFs; and thrombosis rates. Prevalence calculations for AVFs, grafts, and catheters included only patients on dialysis longer than 90 days. A primary AVF or graft was defined as an initial (noncatheter) hemodialysis access procedure. Outcomes were defined as follows:

- Incidence of primary AVFs: the number of initial noncatheter access creations that were AVFs divided by the number of initial noncatheter AVFs and grafts placed during that year.
- Prevalence of AVFs: the number of patients using AVFs divided by the total number of hemodialysis patients during the year-end report card check at the outpatient dialysis facility.
- Incidence of primary grafts: the number of initial noncatheter access creations that were grafts divided by the number of initial noncatheter AVFs and grafts placed during that year.
- Prevalence of grafts: the number of patients using grafts divided by the total number of hemodialysis patients during the year-end report card check at the outpatient dialysis facility.
- Incidence of catheters: the number of patients starting dialysis with a catheter divided by the total number of patients starting on dialysis.
- Prevalence of catheters: the number of patients using a catheter at year-end divided by the total number of patients receiving dialysis at that time.
- Thrombosis rate per patient per year: all thrombosis episodes for fistulas and grafts in the year divided by the average number of hemodialysis patients for the year. The denominator was determined by taking the monthly average.

Statistical analysis of trends in proportions over time was performed using both the Mantel-Haenszel χ^2 test and the Cochran-Armitage trend test in SAS version 9.1 (SAS Institute, Cary, NC). The significance of the association between two different rates across sites of care was tested using Kendall tau rank correlation coefficients. Change in incidence rate variance across sites was normally distributed and tested by the paired t-test. The research was approved by the KPSC institutional review board.

Results

The number of hemodialysis patients treated in a given year increased from 1106 in 1997 to 4369 in 2007 (Table 32-1). More than 1000 new ESRD patients joined KPSC during the Medicare ESRD Demonstration Project, which was conducted from early 1998 through 2001. During the 11 years of the study, the average age increased from 57 to 63. Those patients older than 65 years old increased by 12.5%, whereas those younger than 65 decreased by 12.5%. Patients older than 80 years more than doubled to 10% (Fig. 32-1). The percentage of males increased from 53% to 57%. Diabetic patients increased from 57% to 66% (see Table 32-1). The number of Hispanic patients increased from 25% to 34%, whereas the White population decreased from 34% to 28%. The percentage of African Americans decreased from 32% to 25% (Fig. 32-2).

Trends in quality metrics (outcomes) showed improvement over time. AVF rates progressively increased while thrombosis rates fell and catheter rates were unchanged. The incidence of fistulas increased from 38% in 1998 to 88% in 2007. The prevalence rate increased during that time from 31% to 69%. The thrombosis rate for fistulas and grafts per patient per year fell from 0.62 to 0.34. These trends were all statistically significant ($P < .001$). The year-end prevalence rate of chronic catheters (>90 days) has remained at 14% (Fig. 32-3) while national rates have climbed to 22%.[24] Initial outpatient dialysis with a catheter has remained unchanged at 65% during the period, while the national rate increased from 71% in 2001 to 80% in 2006.[25,26] At 3, 6, and 9 months later, 40%, 29%, and 21% of KPSC patients, respectively, used a catheter (Fig. 32-4). In the United States, 52% of patients were using a catheter after 9 months.[27] Differences in AVF prevalence between the national Medicare Clinical Performance Measures, the Southern California Medicare region (Network 18), and KPSC are shown in Figure 32-5. AVF replacement access increased from 26% in 1998 to 55% in 2007 (Table 32-2).

	19-29	30-49	50-64	65-79	80+	N
1997	4%	24%	36%	31%	4%	1051
1998	4%	22%	38%	30%	6%	1768
1999	3%	23%	37%	31%	6%	2234
2000	3%	22%	38%	31%	6%	2659
2001	3%	21%	37%	33%	6%	2785
2002	3%	19%	37%	34%	7%	2929
2003	2%	19%	36%	34%	8%	2963
2004	2%	18%	35%	35%	9%	3157
2005	2%	17%	36%	36%	9%	3310
2006	2%	17%	35%	37%	9%	3488
2007	2%	16%	34%	38%	10%	3584

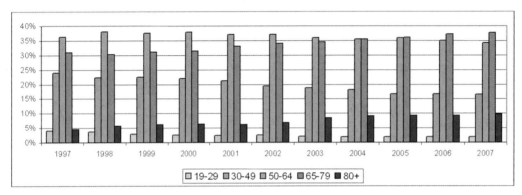

Figure 32-1.
Age distribution for hemodialysis population.

	CAUCASIAN	HISPANIC	AFRICAN AMERICAN	ASIAN	OTHER*	N
1997	34%	25%	32%	6%	3%	1075
1998	33%	26%	30%	5%	5%	1808
1999	34%	28%	27%	5%	6%	2290
2000	33%	29%	26%	5%	7%	2702
2001	32%	30%	26%	6%	7%	2833
2002	32%	32%	25%	6%	7%	2988
2003	30%	33%	25%	6%	7%	3018
2004	29%	33%	25%	6%	7%	3189
2005	29%	33%	24%	6%	7%	3337
2006	29%	34%	24%	6%	8%	3496
2007	28%	34%	25%	6%	9%	3587

*Other includes Unknown, American Indian, Indian Sub-Cont, Mid-East, Multiracial, Other, and Pacific Islander.

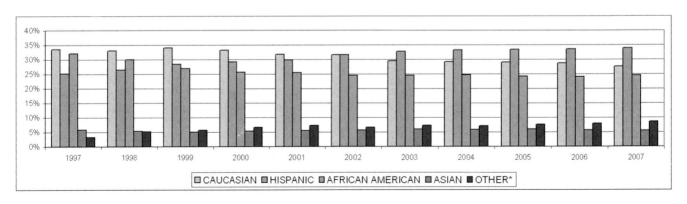

Figure 32-2.
Hemodialysis prevalence by ethnicity.

Table 32–1

Demographics

	1997	1998	1999	2000	2001	2002	2003	2004	2005	2006	2007
Hemodialysis patients	1106	2231	2773	3237	3463	3665	3785	3813	4056	4254	4369
Age (mean, years)	57.4	59.4	59.9	60.2	60.7	61.1	61.8	61.5	62.8	63.0	63.2
Male (%)	53	56	56	57	57	58	58	57	57	57	57
Diabetes (%)	57	62	58	56	57	59	61	60	60	62	66

*Hemodialysis patients includes anyone on outpatient hemodialysis during that year.

Areas with the highest AVF prevalence rates demonstrated lower thrombosis rates, a negative correlation that was statistically significant ($P = .011$; Fig. 32-6). The incidence of new fistula creation increased in the areas over time, while the variability between areas decreased from 3.6% in 1999 to 0.9% in 2007 ($P = .013$; Fig. 32-7).

Discussion

KDOQI sounded the alarm when it provided evidence-based and expert opinion-based recommendations and set goals for improvement of vascular assess outcomes. It has been Fistula First with its change concepts and ongoing educational activities, along with the 18 ESRD Networks, that have been the primary implementing force, both supported by CMS. The KDOQI and Fistula First goals of increasing fistula prevalence and access surveillance are slowly being achieved on a national basis, although catheter use has increased to an alarming 29% (22% chronic plus 7% temporary).[28]

KPSC is only one of several organizations that has already exceeded the fistula goal of 66% prevalence while keeping chronic catheter use low. The Olympia, Washington, private practice group headed by Vo Nguyen and Chris Griffith are at the 80 to 90% AVF prevalence rate, with catheters around 10%. Network 16 in the Northwest now leads the United States in vascular access outcomes by facilitating the educa-

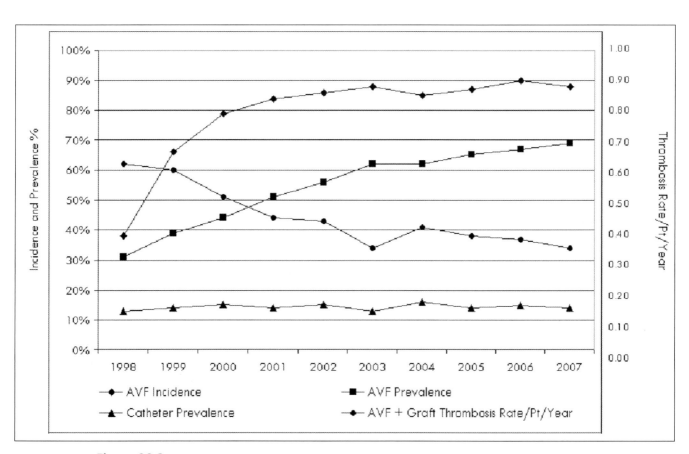

Figure 32-3.
AVF incidence, prevalence, thrombosis rate per patient per years and catheter prevalence. Differences in incidence prevalence, and thrombosis rates are significant ($P < .001$).

	% Catheter
First dialysis	65%
After 3 months of dialysis	40%
After 6 months of dialysis	29%
After 9 months of dialysis	21%

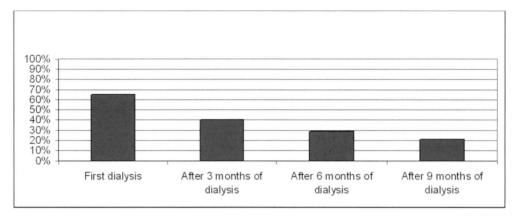

Figure 32-4.
Catheter use in new patients in 2007.

	CPM Project	Network 18	KPSC
1998	26%	20%	31%
1999	28%	24%	39%
2000	30%	28%	44%
2001	31%	31%	51%
2002	33%	36%	56%
2003	35%	38%	62%
2004	37%	42%	62%
2005	44%	44%	65%
2006	45%	49%	67%
2007	49%	52%	69%

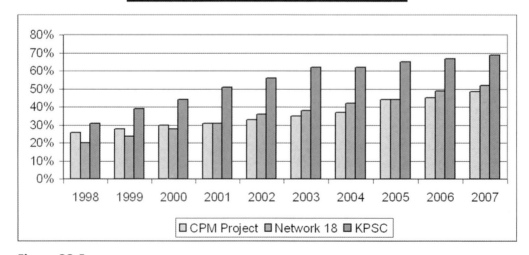

Figure 32-5.
Arteriovenous fistula prevalence. CPM, National Medicare Clinical Performance Measures; Network 18; KPSC.

Table 32–2

Hemodialysis Access Data

	1998	1999	2000	2001	2002	2003	2004	2005	2006	2007
AVF incidence (%) (first noncatheter access)	38	66	79	84	86	88	85	87	90	88
AVF prevalence (%)	31	39	44	51	56	62	62	65	67	69
Graft incidence (%) (first noncatheter access)	62	34	21	16	14	12	15	13	10	12
Graft prevalence (%)	-	47	41	35	29	25	22	21	18	18
Replacement access is new AVF (%)	26	56	58	60	54	58	58	56	57	55
Thrombosis rate per patient per year	0.62	0.60	0.51	0.44	0.43	0.34	0.41	0.38	0.37	0.34
Catheter incidence (%) (first dialysis)	-	-	53	64	69	65	67	63	65	65
Catheter prevalence (%) (>90 days at year's end)	13	14	15	14	15	13	16	14	15	14

tion of providers about the best practices of the Olympia group.[29,30] In Akron, Ohio, the use of AVFs was doubled in a year by formation of a multidisciplinary team, dialysis care pathways, education, data collection, feedback to surgeons and hospitals on vascular access outcomes, and hiring a VAC.[31] In an academic practice at the University of Alabama at Birmingham, a severe problem with multiple graft thrombosis, delayed inpatient vascular access procedures with poor outcomes, and frequent catheter use led to formation of a multidisciplinary team. Problems were identified along with plans to correct them. A computerized database of all vascular access encounters was established. A full-time

	C	H	G	M	D	K	J	F	A	B	L	I	E
2007 AVF Prevalence	85%	84%	84%	79%	73%	72%	70%	65%	63%	63%	61%	56%	42%
2007 Thrombosis Rate/Pt/Year	0.17	0.22	0.15	0.28	0.42	0.27	0.34	0.32	0.2	0.36	0.3	0.37	0.74

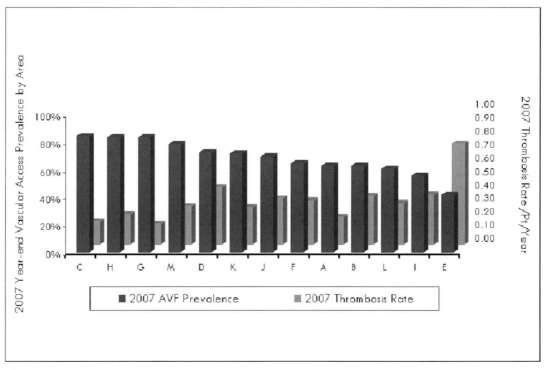

‡Thrombosis rate includes patients with fistulas or grafts.

Figure 32-6.
AVF prevalence and combined access thrombosis rates in each area for 2007. Kendall's rank tau correlation coefficient (*P* = .011).

Variability in Incidence of AVFs

Area	1999	Numerator	Denominator	2007	Numerator	Denominator
A	50%	2	4	86%	12	14
B	76%	44	58	89%	101	113
C	84%	31	37	99%	74	75
D	30%	24	79	91%	116	127
E	65%	20	31	70%	38	54
F	71%	48	68	83%	73	88
G	100%	35	35	98%	99	101
H	56%	25	45	100%	90	90
I	77%	33	43	83%	53	64
J	61%	37	61	74%	49	66
K	93%	39	42	81%	43	53
L	68%	40	59	83%	39	47

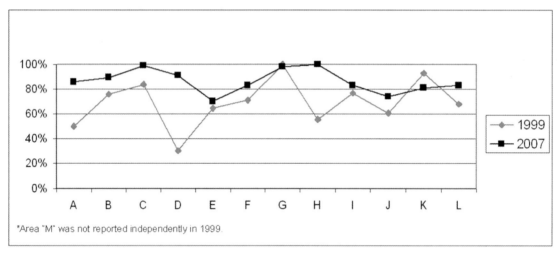

*Area "M" was not reported independently in 1999.

Figure 32-7.
Variability in incidence of AVFs between areas over time. Variability decreased from 3.6% in 1999 to 0.9% in 2007 ($P = .013$)

access coordinator tracked all procedures. Within a year, most vascular access procedures were done as outpatient procedures, more expeditiously and without the need for a catheter. Interventional radiologists declotted most grafts with a higher success rate. Surgical complication rates dropped and fistula creation in new patients increased from 33% to 69%.[32] Over a 2-year period at a West Virginia Veterans Administration Hospital, the prevalence of fistulas increased from 45% to 80%, using a team approach, vascular access tracking database, an interventional program to improve maturation, and a surveillance protocol to prevent thrombosis. Interestingly, working at another institution without these tools, the same nephrologist found vascular access a frustrating struggle with poor outcomes again.[33]

The KPSC story is similar to the others mentioned above. Success required a multidisciplinary team with representatives of all involved stakeholders. Physicians in particular were unlikely to support decisions made without their input. Advantages at KPSC included an enhanced physician education program, with 10% of the physician work week devoted to administrative and educational activities. In addition, new physicians attend orientation sessions to

become inculcated in our culture of working collaboratively to manage patients and solve problems. Vascular access team leaders not only had leadership skills but also were passionate about improving vascular access. In most programs, the opportunities to improve vascular access care were so great that everyone involved could see and celebrate their achievements. The VAC and database were central to success in dealing with these complex patients. Regular meetings of local and regional committees occurred to review outcomes data and provide ongoing education. The basic organizational structure needed in a vascular access care program is now well accepted. The challenge is to incorporate the knowledge gained in the last 10 years to further improve outcomes. The following sections discuss best practices that we propagate across the KPSC Region.

Early Referral

Advance planning for renal replacement therapy is recognized as critical to avoidance of catheter use. The DOPPS database showed that 46% of US patients did not have a permanent access in place at the time of starting dialysis with a catheter.[13] Arora showed that patients seen by a nephrologist >4 months before initiating dialysis had a 40% likelihood of having a functioning permanent vascular access for the first hemodialysis versus 4% for those seeing a nephrologist <4 months before starting hemodialysis.[34] The CHOICE study found that patients seeing a nephrologist <1 month in advance of hemodialysis used a catheter for a median of 202 days versus 19 days when patients saw the nephrologist >12 months before starting hemodialysis.[35]

KPSC has recognized the importance of chronic disease management for many years. CKD detection is embedded in the KPSC population care management program, which provides outreach and patient education for a number of chronic conditions. Whenever a serum creatinine level is determined, a calculated estimated glomerular filtration rate (eGFR) is automatically added to the result.[36] When serial creatinine levels are performed, the CKD stage is automatically determined. A patient's CKD stage is available to primary care providers, who are encouraged to send patients to "Kidney Class," a KPSC educational program in which they learn about kidney disease and treatment when the eGFR is <60. Renal providers can scan the database for patients with eGFR <30, which includes CKD stages 4 and 5. These patients are recommended to have nephrology consultation and to attend KPSC's "Choices Class," in which more detailed information is given about transplantation, peritoneal dialysis, and hemodialysis options. This class elaborates on why AVF is considered the best and catheter the worst choice for chronic vascular access. There is no consensus about which eGFR level should be used for referral to surgery for AVF creation because each patient is unique in his rate of renal function deterioration. However, there is consensus that patients should have an AVF created 6 to 12 months before the anticipated need to start hemodialysis, corresponding to an eGFR range of 20 to 30. Diabetics tend to be sent sooner while patients with hypertensive nephropathy and slower decline of eGFR are referred to surgery later. Delays may occur at any step in the process including preoperative imaging studies, surgery consultation, surgical procedure, postoperative maturation studies, and revision procedures such as angioplasty or second stage transposition. Renal case managers have the responsibility of tracking patients through the process and intervening when barriers are encountered. To this end, KPSC has developed a computerized tracking program to aid case managers in this endeavor.

Preoperative Evaluation

In the past, a graft was place if a superficial vein was not visible. Wrist and antecubital vessels were commonly explored to see if they were adequate to support a vascular access. Today, physical examination[37] is necessary but not sufficient to achieve the level of quality outcomes expected. Every patient should have vein and artery mapping with B mode or duplex ultrasound and continuous wave Doppler "Allen test" to identify the best sites for chronic vascular access location. Vein diameter >2.5 mm, artery diameter >2 mm, unsuspected peripheral venous and arterial disease and deep but usable veins are identified which change the operative plan.[38,39] Sixty-five percent of chronic catheter patients have been shown to have suitable vessels for an AVF with ultrasound,[40] and 74% of patients being treated for loop forearm graft dysfunction had suitable vessels in the same arm for an AVF.[41] Some patients with a failed arm graft will have adequate basilic or cephalic veins for AVF creation in the same extremity. If central venous occlusion is suspected because of increased collateral veins on the shoulder, upper extremity swelling, presence of a pacemaker or prolonged use of a dialysis catheter, venography is done using diluted dye and digital subtraction technique.

Several authors have shown that renal function does not deteriorate when the full strength contrast is kept at <20 mL in predialysis patients.[42] CO_2 venography is another option.[43,44] Similarly, dye angiogram is done preoperatively if questions remain after ultrasound examination. In patients presenting with a history of multiple failed previous hemodialysis access procedures, upper extremity angiogram and venogram are usually necessary in addition to ultrasound studies.[45,46] Silva and others have shown increased fistula utilization and improved vascular access patency using preoperative ultrasound mapping.[38] Many surgeons prefer to do their own mapping in the clinic. Findings are confirmed with ultrasound and vessel locations marked in the operating room with the patient under warm blankets and sedated with a rubber tourniquet on the arm just before starting the operation.

Surgical Management

Surgical judgment in AVF site selection, configuration of the access, and technical performance of the operation remain the most important factors in the construction of fistulas that mature in a timely manner.[47,48] Although at least 80% of patients can have a usable fistula, they cannot have the same one. Site selection depends on more than preprocedure imaging finding a vein with a diameter of 2.5 mm and an artery of 2 mm with minimal calcification.[38] Hakaim has shown superior maturation and patency for brachiocephalic and transposed basilic vein AVFs compared to distal radiocephalic fistulas in patients with diabetes.[49] In a meta-analysis, Lazarides found that HD patients older than 65 had better results with arm AVFs compared to distal radiocephalic AVFs.[50] An elderly diabetic on hemodialysis using a catheter may have an excellent distal radial artery and cephalic vein for an AVF. However, such a patient is more likely to have marginal quality distal vessels and should be advised to have a proximal radial or distal brachial artery based fistula, because it is more likely to be ready for use in 6-8 weeks and usually has better patency than a distal radiocephalic AVF.

If the same patient presented 6 to 12 months before the anticipated start of hemodialysis, a snuffbox or distal radiocephalic fistula might be an excellent choice even if there was a 50% chance that an intervention, whether angioplasty or surgery, will be needed before the fistula is usable. Starting distally in the upper extremity is still desirable if the patient has a life expectancy of more than 2 years. The proximal vessels enlarge while the distal fistula is working, which makes any subsequent proximal AVF more likely to succeed with minimal maturation time. Outpatient forearm fistulas created under local anesthesia have a very low morbidity and mortality rate. Although it is not conclusive, the evidence continues to mount that it is better to create an antecubital or arm fistula than to place a forearm loop or arm graft in patients without suitable forearm vessels for AVF.[51-55] There are still areas for grafts in very select patients.

The surgeon must be very knowledgeable about steal syndrome, because our population has an ever-increasing number of elderly and/or diabetic patients with peripheral arterial disease. Preoperative studies with imaging and continuous wave Doppler are critical in avoiding clinically important steal. Use of the proximal radial artery in patients whose blood flow to the hand is not dependent upon it is an increasingly popular technique to avoid both steal and unnecessarily high fistula flow,[56] which can cause left ventricular hypertrophy and accelerate intimal hyperplasia. If the brachial artery has to be used during fistula construction, the senior author (S.G.) uses a 4- × 2-mm elliptical aortic punch, in most cases, to make the opening after the artery has been hydrostatically dilated by injecting saline into it between clamps. In brachial arteries <4 mm in diameter even after dilation, the opening in the artery is only made large enough to admit a 3-mm dilator. As long as the length of the arteriotomy is kept <80% of the diameter of the artery, the anastomosis size limits flow through it. Once it is >80%, flow becomes independent of the length of the arteriotomy.[57]

When the brachial artery is <4 mm in diameter and forearm arteries are diseased, an arm access based on the proximal brachial or axillary artery is the safest way to avoid clinically important steal. This is usually done in a loop configuration. If a prosthetic graft is needed a polytetrafluoroethylene (PTFE) 4- to 7-mm stepped option is preferred for technical anastomotic reasons but has not been shown to have better outcomes than a 6-mm diameter graft.[58] Early postoperative steal is usually avoidable by proper vessel selection, technique of access construction, and intraoperative monitoring using sterile pulse oximetry and Doppler. Delayed steal or high output failure due to progressive arterial disease and/or increasing fistula flow is treated by first determining access flow. Less than 800 mL/min is considered low and greater than 1200 mL/min is considered high flow. Low flow is treated by proximalization of the inflow site, often creating a loop fistula or graft.[59] This is analogous to the direct revascularization-interval ligation (DRIL) procedure without requiring ligation of the native artery.[60] The lengthening of the dialysis access into a loop increases flow resistance, and the arterial anastomosis (flow divider) is moved proximally where the artery is larger. High flow is corrected by revision using distal inflow (RUDI) which is equivalent to banding.[61]

The surgeon must be familiar with the wide variety of AVF and graft configurations and adjuncts that have been described. KDOQI mentions the distal radiocephalic, brachiocephalic, and transposed basilic vein fistulas, but there are many other options.[15] Snuffbox,[62] ulnar-basilic,[63] forearm loop,[64] and antecubital AVFs[65] all are appropriate forearm options. The proximal radial artery bidirectional fistula may be particularly useful if the retrograde forearm portion matures. Arm loop fistulas are made when proximalization of the inflow is needed because of forearm arterial disease.

Adjunctive techniques such as patching, bifurcation advancement (V-Y advancement flap), sewing 2 veins together side-to-side or end-to-end, and transposition/superficialization are all useful at times to correct stenosis, add length, increase diameter, or to bring the vein closer to the skin surface. When attempts at correction of symptomatic central vein occlusion fail, the chronic fistula vein conduit can be excised and moved to another extremity without central vein obstruction. Transpositions are usually done in 2 stages if the vein is <4 to 5 mm in diameter.[66] These maneuvers can be time consuming, but the reward of a mature fistula in a shorter period of time makes it worthwhile.

Maturation

In comparing AVFs and grafts, there is consensus that AVFs have better patency,[67] require fewer interventions,[68,69] have a lower infection rate,[70] reduce costs,[71,72] and lower patient mortality[73] if they mature to become usable. The problem with poor maturation rate was recently highlighted in an important study by the Dialysis Access Consortium (DAC), Effect of Clopidogrel on Early Failure of Arteriovenous Fistulas for Hemodialysis.[74] This was the largest randomized, double-blind, placebo-controlled trial conducted to date on vascular access. The primary outcome found that thrombosis at 6 weeks of newly created AVFs was 12.2% with clopidogrel versus 19.5% with placebo, which was a statistically significant difference. However, the startling secondary outcome result was that 60% of fistulas in both groups did not mature enough to be usable for hemodialysis by 5 to 6 months after creation. Previous studies reported maturation failure of 8 to 53%.[75,76] At KPSC, we believe our failure to mature rate is approximately 25%, a large part of the difference between our incidence and prevalence of AVFs. A serious criticism of the DAC study was that even though interventions to improve maturation were allowed, few were done. Even when done, they did not improve the fistula suitability rate for hemodialysis. This contradicts a previous study showing that 92% of fistulas with maturation failure could be salvaged for hemodialysis use, and that 68% were still usable a year later.[77]

The DAC is planning more studies on this important topic, but we have already gathered many important findings about fistula maturation in the last few years. Blood flow in the feeding artery increases very rapidly. It is more than 600 mL/min by 2 weeks in fistulas that go on to mature, compared with <225 mL/min in those that go on to fail. At 6 weeks postoperatively, flow in successful AVFs only increased 20% more than the value at 2 weeks, while flow in unsuccessful AVFs drops 40%. Successful AVF vein size is slightly more than 4 mm in diameter at 2 weeks and increases to more than 5 mm by 6 weeks. Unsuccessful AVF vein size is 3.5 mm at 2 weeks and decreases to 3.25 mm at 6 weeks.[78] An ultrasound study by Robbin found that fistula adequacy for dialysis was 89% if vein diameter was at least 4 mm versus 44% if <4 mm. If flow volume was at least 500 mL/min, fistula adequacy was 84% versus 43% if it was <500 mL/min. If both venous diameter and flow were favorable, fistula adequacy was 95% versus 33% if both factors were unfavorable. An experienced dialysis nurse could predict eventual fistula usability 80% of the time on physical examination alone.[79] This study confirmed the finding of other studies that little change in vein diameter and blood flow occurred from 2 to 4 months after access creation. Beathard has catalogued the lesions most likely to cause maturation failure. Venous stenosis is the most common lesion, being present 78% of the time. Forty-four percent had juxta-anastomotic stenosis in the vein. Forty-six percent had an accessory vein draining flow from the main channel. Thirty-eight percent had an arterial lesion. Multiple lesions were common.[77]

It is now clear that a maturation examination should be done 4 to 6 weeks after AVF creation to see that the fistula is developing well. Physical examination is often sufficient, but if there is any doubt, a duplex scan to assess vein size, vein depth, and volume flow should be ordered. If the fistula is not developing as expected, a fistulogram is ordered and the identified problems corrected with angioplasty or surgery.[80] As noted previously, 20 mL of contrast when diluted from 1:2 to 1:4 with normal saline is adequate for the study and not associated with deterioration in renal function in predialysis patients.[42] It should be anticipated that 25% of fistulas will need an intervention before they are ready for use.[45] Waiting 3 months or more before intervening, as was commonly done in the past, only prolongs catheter use and increases complications. With an aggressive approach, maturation failure should be reduced to 10 to 15%.

Endovascular Management

The revolution in minimally invasive treatment in medical care has had an impact in vascular access care as well. These are discussed in detail in other chapters of this book. At KPSC, the vast majority of stenotic or thrombosed fistulas and grafts are sent to the interventional suite for outpatient angioplasty and/or pharmacomechanical thrombectomy.[81,82] If the access cannot be salvaged, which is uncommon, a right internal jugular tunneled catheter is usually placed at the same time and the patient referred to surgery for elective repair or new access creation within a few days. Completion contrast study from the inflow artery to the right atrium is a routine part of the fistulogram to look for unsuspected stenosis and for future access planning. In case of fistula thrombosis, is it desirable to have ultrasound and surgical evaluation before beginning the intervention. In some cases, the fistula will be diffusely sclerotic and small, requiring a new access to be created. At other times, only the first 3 cm of a distal radiocephalic AVF will be clotted and a surgical turn down of the patent cephalic vein to the radial artery 3 to 4 cm more proximally is a better long-term solution. So called "mega fistulas" with large clot burdens are safer to treat surgically because of the higher risk of major pulmonary embolus with a percutaneous approach.

For stenotic lesions, high-pressure or ultra-high-pressure balloons are often needed. Cutting balloons are used for a lesion that does not respond. If a contained rupture occurs during angioplasty without adequate expansion of the lesion, the patient is brought back for additional angioplasty 2 weeks later. On occasion, in an attempt to salvage a fistula that would otherwise be lost, balloon assisted maturation (BAM) is performed at 2 week intervals until the desired diameter is achieved. The long-term outcome of this procedure is not well known.[83] Flow studies should be done at the dialysis center to confirm correction of the clinical problem, since 20% and 40% of patients do not have sustained hemodynamic improvement when flows are measured at 1 and 4 weeks after angioplasty, respectively.[84,85] Although peripheral venous uncovered stents have not shown significant benefit, covered stents may be better.

Almost all tunneled catheters are placed and exchanged in the interventional suite. The right internal jugular vein site is the first choice with the left internal jugular vein being second for dialysis catheter location.[86] Even when the right internal jugular vein is occluded from previous catheter placement, the brachiocephalic vein is often patent and can be approached percutaneously at the base of the right neck. On rare occasions, the superior vena cava will be punctured in a similar manner for tunneled catheter placement. A catheter placed from the femoral vein into the central veins is usually used as a target.[87] Re-do catheter placement in particular may be difficult because of multiple central vein stenoses or occlusions. Excellent fluoroscopic imaging and availability of an array of wires, catheters, and balloons are necessary to safely complete the procedure.

A recent innovation in the organization of endovascular access care delivery has been the development of freestanding dedicated outpatient vascular access centers established as extensions of the physicians' offices. This simplifies credentialing and billing compared to performing the same procedures in an ambulatory surgery center or hospital. Although most staff are interventional nephrologists, some use interventional radiologists or surgeons. The centers specialize in preoperative vessel mapping and diagnostic imaging of established hemodialysis access using ultrasound and fluoroscopy. They perform a wide range of percutaneous procedures on the dysfunctional access including angiography, angioplasty, thrombectomy, stent placement, and catheter insertion. Initial reports indicate improved outcomes with fewer missed dialysis treatments, reduced hospitalization and decreased costs.[88, 89] KPSC is not using this model at present, but we are very interested to watch its evolution.

Cannulation

The ability to reliably and repeatedly cannulate the access is essential to success of the access. In the senior author's experience (S.G.), a mature fistula should be at least 8 cm in length to minimize recirculation, with a depth of 2 to 10 mm to reduce bleeding risk and achieve needle fixation. Vein size should be greater than or equal to the depth, with a 4-mm minimum size. KDOQI supports the rule of 6's—at least 6 mm diameter, less than 6 mm deep with discernible margins, and at least 600 mL/min flow.[15] The DOPPS showed that time to first cannulation varied widely between countries. In Japan and Italy, first fistula cannulation was about 30 days, in Germany 42 days, and in the United States 100 days. There was no increase in fistula failure as long as cannulation was delayed 30 days from creation.[90-92] In conjunction with efforts to speed maturation, earlier cannulation to reduce catheter dwell times is another goal. Fistula First and the ESRD Networks are working with the large dialysis providers on a CQI program to improve cannulation outcomes. Printed material, a DVD, and lectures have been provided. Three levels of certification for cannulators have been proposed, with only the most experienced sticking new fistulas. Protocols include starting with 17-gauge needles and reduced blood flows. More use of the buttonhole or same-site cannulation technique is being advocated to reduce fistula damage.[93-95] KPSC is very supportive of all these efforts. In some facilities with our patients, use of the buttonhole technique is up to 60%.

Surveillance

Although the value of surveillance of hemodialysis access using technology and intervention before failure remains controversial in regard to improving access survival, it probably leads to a 50% reduction in the thrombosis rate.[96-98] At KPSC, we noted a significant drop in our thrombosis rate as the number of AVFs increased before instituting a regular monitoring and surveillance program. Following the lead of KDOQI, we have adopted access flow surveillance as our standard.[15] Fortunately, most new dialysis machines have the ability to determine access flow built into them. Grafts with repeated flow <600 mL/min and fistulas <400 to 500 mL/min are referred for physical examination and imaging. Monitoring the access with physical examination is part of the KPSC educational program for patients, nurses, and physicians.[37] Identification of clinical problems such as difficult cannulation, prolonged bleeding after needle removal, poor flow, extremity swelling, alteration in the characteristics of the soft pulse or thrill, or reduced efficiency of dialysis are other indications for referral.

Catheter Usage

Problems with poor patency, high infection rate, and central vein occlusions are well documented with use of hemodialysis catheters.[99] Everyone agrees that the use of catheters is too high and that the initiative to increase AVF use contributed to this problem. Surgeons broadened the acceptability criteria of vessels used to construct fistulas leading to a rise in the AVF failure rate and longer catheter use.[100,101] DOQI vascular access guidelines were published in 1997[12] and Fistula First started in 2003. Total catheter use increased nationally from 19% (15% chronic plus 4% acute) in 1998 to 27% (20% chronic plus 7% acute) in 2002 to 29% (22% chronic plus 7% acute) in 2006. During the same periods, AVF prevalence increased from 25% to 36% to 47.5%, respectively. Even though Fistula First increased the fistula prevalence goal to 66%, the catheter rate, since it started in 2003, has been stable for the last 3 years, while fistula prevalence increased by one third.[28] The Clinical Performance Measures collected by the ESRD Networks look at the reasons patients are using catheters during the October through December vascular access evaluation. From 2002 to 2006, the indication "Fistula or graft maturing, not ready to cannulate" only increased from 27% to 30% while "No fistula or graft surgically created at this time" increased from 18% to 34% and "All fistula or graft sites have been exhausted" went from 12% to 19%.[102] As noted above, many programs including KPSC have been able to dramatically increase fistula use without increasing

catheters by using an organized approach which emphasizes implementing best practices.

At KPSC, we believe our chronic catheter use of 14%—and particularly the rate of patients starting dialysis with a catheter of 65%—can be substantially reduced. In 2005, our nephrologists developed the "Optimal Start" metric to help refocus the renal team on reducing catheter starts and to increase the number of new ESRD patients utilizing the best renal replacement option for them. An optimal ESRD start is defined as a preemptive kidney transplant, home dialysis (peritoneal dialysis or hemodialysis), or in-center hemodialysis with an AVF (10% of hemodialysis starts with a graft is allowed). The metric is simply the number of optimal ESRD starts over the measurement period divided by the total number of patients managed by the renal teams who reached ESRD, multiplied by 100%. Since most patients are unable to obtain a preemptive kidney transplant or utilize home dialysis, successful initiation of in-center hemodialysis with an AVF is the biggest factor in determining the percentage of Optimal Starts.

Another tool to help reduce catheter starts is the computerized tracking program mentioned earlier that is utilized by the nurse case managers. In addition to tracking the progress of AVF candidates, it also solicits reasons for "failures": patients who started outpatient hemodialysis with a catheter. This information is utilized in the renal team quality improvement process to determine where system failures occur and to stimulate the development of improved processes. Analysis of early data from this program indicated that unexpected rapid decline in renal function and patient unwillingness to have a chronic vascular access placed early were the leading causes of patients starting with a catheter.

Reducing the number of hemodialysis catheter starts involves the regular use of preoperative vessel mapping with ultrasound, the use of a wide range of fistula options, surgical evaluation at 4 to 6 weeks postoperatively with intervention at that time if maturation is not occurring, safe cannulation at 1 to 2 months postoperatively by skilled personnel, and regular follow-up monitoring and volume flow measurements. Clearly, case management through these many steps improves outcomes. If patients do start with a catheter, following the above protocol should reduce the catheter use time to a minimum. Improvements in catheter design, care, antimicrobial locking solutions, and coatings may reduce the morbidity and mortality for those who have a catheter in the future.[103,104]

Conclusions

KPSC has shown that vascular access care is well suited to the continuous quality improvement methodology. The key elements are to form a multidisciplinary team, identify the problems and their origins, establish baseline metrics and outcomes, set realistic improvement goals, develop action plans to achieve them, and create an electronic database to produce reports on a regular basis to assess progress and identify new problems. In addition, it is important to have an ongoing educational process for patients, nurses/technicians, and physicians.

Because KPSC has 13 medical care areas, each of which has different expertise and resources, flexibility was necessary in the methods used in each area to achieve the regional goals. Currently at least 1 nurse VAC is located in each area to serve as liaison among the patient, physicians, dialysis facility, and health services administration. The VAC collects data on all vascular access interventions using a tracking tool, and takes the first call when problems occur to facilitate care from the appropriate physician. Regular reports of vascular access outcomes by area and for the region as a whole are distributed to stakeholders. In the initial stages, each surgeon and their chief received coded data showing the surgeon's percentage of first-time fistula creation versus graft insertion compared to his peers. This information was used as a quality assurance indicator during the surgeon's performance review. By spreading best practices and changing paradigms, not only did the incidence of new fistula creation increase in the areas over time, but the variability between areas decreased. We were able to increase our fistula prevalence from 31% to 69% over the last 11 years while the US rate went up to 50%. The thrombosis rate per patient per year dropped from 0.62 to 0.34. The prevalent catheter rate remained 14% while the US rate increased to 22%. Our incidence of patients starting dialysis with a catheter was little changed at 65% while the US incidence is 80%. Despite a remarkable improvement in AVF use and reduction in thrombosis rate, challenges persist. Maturation failure of fistulas is about 25%, and some new patients have catheters for 6 months or more before a chronic access is ready to be used. Two thirds of patients start with a catheter. We are shifting our focus to address these remaining problems, and the importance of assessing fistula maturation at 1 month is being stressed to physicians and nurses. The quality improvement program has now been redesigned to get to the root causes of why so many patients start with a catheter. The CQI process never ends, but we do celebrate the advances that have been made thus far.

REFERENCES

1. Scribner BH, Buri R, Caner JE, Hegstrom R, Burnell JM. The treatment of chronic uremia by means of intermittent hemodialysis: a preliminary report. *Trans Am Soc Artif Intern Organs.* 1960;6:114-122.
2. Brescia MJ, Cimino JE, Appel K, Hurwich BJ. Chronic hemodialysis using venipuncture and a surgically created arteriovenous fistula. *N Engl J Med.* 1966;275:1089-1092.
3. Roberts SD, Maxwell DR, Gross TL. Cost-effective care of end-stage renal disease: a billion dollar question. *Ann Intern Med.* 1980;92:243-248.
4. US Renal Data System. 2007 Annual Data Report: Atlas of End-Stage Renal Disease in the United States. Bethesda, MD: National Institute of Diabetes and Digestive and Kidney Diseases, 2007:vol 1:Precis 21. Available at http://www.usrds.org/atlas.htm.
5. Gilbertson DT, Liu J, Xue JL, et al. Projecting the number of patients with end stage renal disease in the United States to the year 2015. *J Am Soc Nephrol.* 2005;16:3736-3741.
6. US Renal Data System. 2007 Annual Data Report: Atlas of End-Stage Renal Disease in the United States. Bethesda, MD: National Institute of Diabetes and Digestive and Kidney Diseases, 2007: vol 2: Reference Tables A.6-7:18-19. Available at http://www.usrds.org/atlas.htm.
7. Eggers PW. Medicare expenditures for fistula, graft, and catheter-access procedures. In Henry ML, Campbell DA (eds). Syllabus. The Seventh Biannual Symposium on Dialysis Access, San Antonio, Texas: ACCESS Medical Group, Ltd.; 2000:46.
8. Hakim R, Himmelfarb J. Hemodialysis access failure: a call to action. *Kidney Int.* 1998;54:1029-1040.
9. US Renal Data System. 2007 Annual Data Report: Atlas of End-Stage Renal Disease in the United States. Bethesda, MD: National Institute
10. Centers for Medicare & Medicaid Services: 2007 Annual Report, End-Stage Renal Disease Clinical Performance Measures Project. Baltimore, MD: Department of Health and Human Services, 2007:25. http://www.cms.hhs.gov/CPMProject/Downloads/ESRDCPMYear2007 Report.pdf.
11. Dhingra RK, Young EW, Hulbert-Sharon TE, Leavey SF, Port FK. Type of vascular access and mortality in US hemodialysis patients. *Kidney Int.* 2001;60:1443-1451.
12. NKF-DOQI clinical practice guidelines for vascular access. National Kidney Foundation-Dialysis Outcomes Quality Initiative. *Am J Kidney Dis.* 1997;30:S150-S191.
13. Pisoni RL, Young EW, Dykstra DM, et al. Vascular access use in Europe and the United States: results from the DOPPS. *Kidney Int.* 2002;61:305-316.
14. Gold JA, Hoffman K. Fistula First: the National Vascular Access Improvement Initiative. *WMJ.* 2006;105:71-73.
15. National Kidney Foundation clinical practice guidelines for vascular access. *Am J Kidney Dis.* 2006;48 Suppl 1:S176-S247.
16. Fistula First National Vascular Access Improvement Initiative. ESRD Vascular Access Performance Incentive Payment. Position paper submitted by the Fistula First Breakthrough Initiative 2008. Available at http://www.fistulafirst.org/pdfs/P4P.pdf.
17. ESRD Network Forum. About the Forum. Available at http://www.esrdnetworks.org/about-the-forum.
18. Berwick DM. Continuous improvement as an ideal in health care. *N Engl J Med.* 1989;320:53-56.
19. Walters BAJ PP, Bosch JP. Quality assurance and continuous quality improvement programs for vascular access care. In Ronco C, Levin NW (eds). *Hemodialysis Vascular Access and Peritoneal Dialysis Access.* Vol 142. Basel: Karger, 2004:323-349.
20. Glazer S, Crooks P, Shapiro M, Diesto J. Using CQI and the DOQI guidelines to improve vascular access outcomes: the Southern California Kaiser Permanente experience. *Nephrol News Issues.* 2000;14:21-26; discussion 27.
21. Glazer S, Diesto J, Crooks P et al. Going beyond the kidney disease outcomes quality initiative: hemodialysis access experience at Kaiser Permanente Southern California. *Ann Vasc Surg.* 2006;20:75-82.
22. Allon M. Implementing a vascular access program: improved outcomes with multidisciplinary approaches. In Gray RJ SJ (ed). *Dialysis Access: A Multidisciplinary Approach.* Philadelphia: Lippincott Williams & Wilkins, 2002:6-9.
23. Sekkarie M. Increasing the placement of native veins arteriovenous fistulae—the role of access surgeons' education and profiling. *Clin Nephrol.* 2004;62:44-48.
24. Centers for Medicare & Medicaid Services: 2007 Annual Report, End-Stage Renal Disease Clinical Performance Measures Project. Baltimore, MD, Department of Health and Human Services, 2007:14. Available at http://www.cms.hhs.gov/CPMProject/Downloads/ESRDCPMYear2007 Report.pdf.
25. 2001 Annual Report: ESRD Clinical Performance Measures Project. *Am J Kidney Dis.* 2002;39:S28.
26. US Renal Data System. 2007 Annual Data Report: Atlas of End-Stage Renal Disease in the United States. Bethesda, MD: National Institute of Diabetes and Digestive and Kidney Diseases, 2007:vol 1:Chapter 3 Patient Characteristics:100-101. Available at http://www.usrds.org/atlas.htm.
27. Centers for Medicare & Medicaid Services: 2007 Annual Report, End-Stage Renal Disease Clinical Performance Measures Project. Baltimore, MD, Department of Health and Human Services, 2007:21. Available at http://www.cms.hhs.gov/CPMProject/Downloads/ESRDCPMYear2007 Report.pdf.
28. Centers for Medicare & Medicaid Services: 2007 Annual Report, End-Stage Renal Disease Clinical Performance Measures Project. Baltimore, MD, Department of Health and Human Services, 2007:16. Available at http://www.cms.hhs.gov/CPMProject/Downloads/ESRDCPMYear2007 Report.pdf.
29. Nguyen VD, Griffith C, Treat L. A multidisciplinary team approach to increasing AV fistula creation. *Nephrol News Issues.* 2003;17:54-56, 58, 60 passim.
30. Nguyen VD, Lawson L, Ledeen M, et al. Successful multidisciplinary interventions for arteriovenous fistula creation by the Pacific Northwest Renal Network 16 vascular access quality improvement program. *J Vasc Access.* 2007;8:3-11.

31. Spuhler CL, Schwarze KD, Sands JJ. Increasing AV fistula creation: the Akron experience. *Nephrol News Issues*. 2002;16:44-47, 50, 52.

32. Allon M, Bailey R, Ballard R, et al. A multidisciplinary approach to hemodialysis access: prospective evaluation. *Kidney Int*. 1998;53: 473-479.

33. Besarab A. Resolved: fistulas are preferred to grafts as initial vascular access for dialysis. *Proc J Am Soc Nephrol*. 2008;19:1629-1631.

34. Arora P, Obrador GT, Ruthazer R, et al. Prevalence, predictors, and consequences of late nephrology referral at a tertiary care center. *J Am Soc Nephrol*. 1999;10:1281-1286.

35. Astor BC, Eustace JA, Powe NR, et al. Timing of nephrologist referral and arteriovenous access use: the CHOICE Study. *Am J Kidney Dis*. 2001;38:494-501.

36. Levey AS, Bosch JP, Lewis JB, Greene T, Rogers N, Roth D. A more accurate method to estimate glomerular filtration rate from serum creatinine: a new prediction equation. Modification of Diet in Renal Disease Study Group. *Ann Intern Med*. 1999;130:461-470.

37. Beathard G. Physical examination of the dialysis vascular access. *Semin Dial*. 1998;11:231-236.

38. Silva MB Jr, Hobson RW 2nd, Pappas PJ, et al. A strategy for increasing use of autogenous hemodialysis access procedures: impact of preoperative noninvasive evaluation. *J Vasc Surg*. 1998;27:302-307; discussion 307-308.

39. Malovrh M. The role of sonography in the planning of arteriovenous fistulas for hemodialysis. *Semin Dial*. 2003;16:299-303.

40. Sands J, Espada C, Ferrell L, Lazarus J. 65% of patients with cuffed catheters have adequate vasculature for arteriovenous fistula creation; 2000.

41. Beathard GA. Interventionalist's role in identifying candidates for secondary fistulas. *Semin Dial*. 2004;17:233-236.

42. Asif A, Cherla G, Merrill D, et al. Venous mapping using venography and the risk of radiocontrast-induced nephropathy. *Semin Dial*. 2005;18:239-242.

43. Sullivan KL, Bonn J, Shapiro MJ, Gardiner GA. Venography with carbon dioxide as a contrast agent. *Cardiovasc Intervent Radiol*. 1995;18:141-145.

44. Funaki B. Carbon dioxide angiography. *Semin Intervent Radiol*. 2008;25:65-70.

45. Huber TS, Seeger JM. Approach to patients with "complex" hemodialysis access problems. *Semin Dial*. 2003;16:22-29.

46. Hyland K, Cohen RM, Kwak A, et al. Preoperative mapping venography in patients who require hemodialysis access: imaging findings and contribution to management. *J Vasc Interv Radiol*. 2008;19:1027-1033.

47. Choi KL, Salman L, Krishnamurthy G, et al. Impact of surgeon selection on access placement and survival following preoperative mapping in the "fistula first" era. *Semin Dial*. 2008;21:341-346.

48. Saran R, Elder, SJ, Goodkin, DA, et al. Enhanced training in vascular access creation predicts arteriovenous fistula placement and patency in hemodialysis patients: results from the Dialysis Outcomes and Practice Patterns Study. *Ann Surg*. 2008;247:885-891.

49. Hakaim AG, Nalbandian M, Scott T. Superior maturation and patency of primary brachiocephalic and transposed basilic vein arteriovenous fistulae in patients with diabetes. *J Vasc Surg*. 1998;27:154-157.

50. Lazarides MK, Georgiadis GS, Antoniou GA, Staramos DN. A meta-analysis of dialysis access outcome in elderly patients. *J Vasc Surg*. 2007;45:420-426.

51. Chemla ES, Morsy MA. Is basilic vein transposition a real alternative to an arteriovenous bypass graft? A prospective study. *Semin Dial*. 2008;21:352-356.

52. Keuter XH, De Smet AA, Kessels AG, van der Sande FM, Welten RJ, Tordoir JH. A randomized multicenter study of the outcome of brachial-basilic arteriovenous fistula and prosthetic brachial-antecubital forearm loop as vascular access for hemodialysis. *J Vasc Surg*. 2008;47:395-401.

53. Lee T, Barker J, Allon M. Comparison of survival of upper arm arteriovenous fistulas and grafts after failed forearm fistula. *J Am Soc Nephrol*. 2007;18:1936-1941.

54. Matsuura JH, Rosenthal D, Clark M, et al. Transposed basilic vein versus polytetrafluoroethylene for brachial-axillary arteriovenous fistulas. *Am J Surg*. 1998;176:219-221.

55. Pflederer TA, Kwok S, Ketel BL, Pilgram T. A comparison of transposed brachiobasilic fistulae with nontransposed fistulae and grafts in the fistula first era. *Semin Dial*. 2008;21:357-363.

56. Jennings WC. Creating arteriovenous fistulas in 132 consecutive patients: exploiting the proximal radial artery arteriovenous fistula:

57. Strandness D Jr, Sumner DS. *Hemodynamics for Surgeons*. New York: Grune & Stratton, 1975:621-663.

58. Dammers R, Planken RN, Pouls KP, et al. Evaluation of 4-mm to 7-mm versus 6-mm prosthetic brachial-antecubital forearm loop access for hemodialysis: results of a randomized multicenter clinical trial. *J Vasc Surg*. 2003;37:143-148.

59. Zanow J, Kruger U, Scholz H. Proximalization of the arterial inflow: a new technique to treat access-related ischemia. *J Vasc Surg*. 2006;43:1216-1221; discussion 1221.

60. Gradman WS. Regarding Proximalization of the arterial inflow: A new technique to treat access-related ischemia. 2006;44:1134; author reply 1134-5.

61. Minion D, Moore, E, Endean, E. Revision using distal inflow: a novel approach to dialysis-associated steal syndrome. *Ann Vasc Surg*. 2005;19:625-628.

62. Mehigan JT, McAlexander RA. Snuffbox arteriovenous fistula for hemodialysis. *Am J Surg*. 1982;143:252-253.

63. Kinnaert P, Vereerstraeten P, Geens M, Toussaint C. Ulnar arteriovenous fistula for maintenance haemodialysis. *Br J Surg*. 1971;58:641-643.

64. Gefen JY, Fox D, Giangola G, Ewing DR, Meisels IS. The transposed forearm loop arteriovenous fistula: a valuable option for primary hemodialysis access in diabetic patients. *Ann Vasc Surg*. 2002;16:89-94.

65. Gracz KC, Ing TS, Soung LS, Armbruster KF, Seim SK, Merkel FK. Proximal forearm fistula for maintenance hemodialysis. *Kidney Int*. 1977;11:71-75.

66. Foran RF, Levin PM, Cohen JL, Treiman RL. Delayed vein repositioning. A procedure for improving inadequate radial-cephalic arteriovenous fistulas. *Arch Surg*. 1976;111:675-677.

67. Huber TS, Carter JW, Carter RL, Seeger JM. Patency of autogenous and polytetrafluoroethylene upper extremity arteriovenous hemodialysis accesses: a systematic review. *J Vasc Surg*. 2003;38:1005-1011.

68. Gibson KD, Gillen DL, Caps MT, Kohler TR, Sherrard DJ, Stehman-Breen CO. Vascular access survival and incidence of revisions: a comparison of prosthetic grafts, simple autogenous fistulas, and venous transposition fistulas from the United States Renal Data System Dialysis Morbidity and Mortality Study. *J Vasc Surg*. 2001;34:694-700.

69. Hodges TC, Fillinger MF, Zwolak RM, Walsh DB, Bech F, Cronenwett JL. Longitudinal comparison of dialysis access methods: risk factors for failure. *J Vasc Surg*. 1997;26:1009-1019.

70. Schild AF, Simon, S., Prieto, J., Raines, J. Single-Center Review of Infections Associated with 1,574 Consecutive Vascular Access Procedures. *Vasc Endovasc Surg*. 2003;37:27-31.

71. Lee H, Manns B, Taub K, et al. Cost analysis of ongoing care of patients with end-stage renal disease: the impact of dialysis modality and dialysis access. *Am J Kidney Dis*. 2002;40:611-622.

72. Manns B, Tonelli M, Yilmaz S, et al. Establishment and maintenance of vascular access in incident hemodialysis patients: a prospective cost analysis. *J Am Soc Nephrol*. 2005;16:201-209.

73. Astor BC, Eustace JA, Powe NR, Klag MJ, Fink NE, Coresh J. Type of vascular access and survival among incident hemodialysis patients: the Choices for Healthy Outcomes in Caring for ESRD (CHOICE) study. *J Am Soc Nephrol*. 2005;16:1449-1455.

74. Dember LM, Beck GJ, Allon M, et al. Effect of clopidogrel on early failure of arteriovenous fistulas for hemodialysis: a randomized controlled trial. *JAMA*. 2008;18:2164-2171.

75. Dixon BS. Why don't fistulas mature? *Kidney Int*. 2006;70:1413-1422.

76. Silva MB Jr, Hobson RW 2nd, Pappas PJ, et al. Vein transposition in the forearm for autogenous hemodialysis access. *J Vasc Surg*. 1997;26:981-986; discussion 987-8.

77. Beathard GA, Arnold P, Jackson J, Litchfield T. Aggressive treatment of early fistula failure. *Kidney Int*. 2003;64:1487-1494.

78. Asif A, Roy-Chaudhury P, Beathard GA. Early arteriovenous fistula failure: a logical proposal for when and how to intervene. *Clin J Am Soc Nephrol*. 2006;1:332-339.

79. Robbin ML, Chamberlain NE, Lockhart ME, et al. Hemodialysis arteriovenous fistula maturity: US evaluation. *Radiology*. 2002;225:59-64.

80. Beathard GA. An algorithm for the physical examination of early fistula failure. *Semin Dial*. 2005;18:331-335.

81. Aruny JE, Lewis CA, Cardella JF, et al. Quality improvement guidelines for percutaneous management of the thrombosed or dysfunctional dialysis access. *J Vasc Interv Radiol*. 2003;14:S247-53.

reliable, safe, and simple forearm and upper arm hemodialysis access. *Arch Surg*. 2006;141:27-32; discussion 32.

82. Clark TW, Cohen RA, Kwak A, et al. Salvage of nonmaturing native fistulas by using angioplasty. *Radiology*. 2007;242:286-292.

83. Arnold W, P. Image-guided endovascular evaluation and intervention for hemodialysis vascular access. In Davidson IJA (ed). *Access for Dialysis: Surgical and Radiologic Procedures*. 2nd ed. Georgetown: Landes, 2002:152-258.

84. Moist LM, Churchill DN, House AA, et al. Regular monitoring of access flow compared with monitoring of venous pressure fails to improve graft survival. *J Am Soc Nephrol*. 2003;14:2645-2653.

85. Schwab SJ, Oliver MJ, Suhocki P, McCann R. Hemodialysis arteriovenous access: detection of stenosis and response to treatment by vascular access blood flow. *Kidney Int*. 2001;59:358-362.

86. Trerotola SO, Johnson MS, Harris VJ, et al. Outcome of tunneled hemodialysis catheters placed via the right internal jugular vein by interventional radiologists. *Radiology*. 1997;203:489-495.

87. Wellons ED, Matsuura J, Lai KM, Levitt A, Rosenthal D. Transthoracic cuffed hemodialysis catheters: a method for difficult hemodialysis access. *J Vasc Surg*. 2005;42:286-289.

88. Beathard GA, Litchfield T. Effectiveness and safety of dialysis vascular access procedures performed by interventional nephrologists. *Kidney Int*. 2004;66:1622-1632.

89. Mishler R, Sands JJ, Ofsthun NJ, Teng M, Schon D, Lazarus JM. Dedicated outpatient vascular access center decreases hospitalization and missed outpatient dialysis treatments. *Kidney Int*. 2006;69:393-398.

90. Diskin CJ, Stokes TJ. Vascular access cannulation and the end of religion: is it time or our own human variables that determine suc-cess? *Nephrol Dial Transplant*. 2005;20:2010-2011; author reply 2011.

91. Rayner HC, Pisoni RL, Gillespie BW, et al. Creation, cannulation and survival of arteriovenous fistulae: data from the Dialysis Outcomes and Practice Patterns Study. *Kidney Int*. 2003;63:323-330.

92. Saran R, Dykstra DM, Pisoni RL, et al. Timing of first cannulation and vascular access failure in haemodialysis: an analysis of practice patterns at dialysis facilities in the DOPPS. *Nephrol Dial Transplant*. 2004;19:2334-2340.

93. Kronung G. Plastic deformation of Cimino Fistula by repeated puncture. *Dialysis & Transplantation*. 1984;13:635-638.

94. Peterson P. Fistula cannulation: The buttonhole technique. *Nephrol Nursing J*. 2002;29.

95. Twardowski Z, J. The "buttonhole" method of needle insertion takes center stage in the attempt to revive daily home hemodialysis. *Contemp Dial Nephrol*. 1997;18:18-19.

96. Paulson WD. Access monitoring does not really improve outcomes. *Blood Purif*. 2005;23:50-56.

97. Sands JJ. Vascular access monitoring improves outcomes. *Blood Purif*. 2005;23:45-49.

98. Tonelli M, James M, Wiebe N, Jindal K, Hemmelgarn B. Ultrasound monitoring to detect access stenosis in hemodialysis patients: a systematic review. *Am J Kidney Dis*. 2008;51:630-640.

99. Lacson E, Jr., Lazarus JM, Himmelfarb J, Ikizler TA, Hakim RM. Balancing Fistula First with catheters last. *Am J Kidney Dis*. 2007;50:379-395.

100. Biuckians A, Scott EC, Meier GH, Panneton JM, Glickman MH. The natural history of autologous fistulas as first-time dialysis access in the KDOQI era. *J Vasc Surg*. 2008;47:415-421; discussion 420-1.

101. Patel ST, Hughes J, Mills JL Sr. Failure of arteriovenous fistula maturation: an unintended consequence of exceeding dialysis outcome quality Initiative guidelines for hemodialysis access. *J Vasc Surg*. 2003;38:439-445; discussion 445.

102. Centers for Medicare & Medicaid Services: 2007 Annual Report, End-Stage Renal Disease Clinical Performance Measures Project. Baltimore, MD, Department of Health and Human Services, 2007:27. Available at http://www.cms.hhs.gov/CPM Project/Downloads/ESRD-CPMYear2007Report.pdf.

103. Allon M. Current management of vascular access. *Clin J Am Soc Nephrol*. 2007;2:786-800.

104. Ash SR. Fluid mechanics and clinical success of central venous catheters for dialysis—answers to simple but persisting problems. *Semin Dial*. 2007;20:237-256.

CHAPTER 33

Should the KDOQI Guidelines for First Time Dialysis Access Apply to All Patients?

Albert I. Richardson and Marc H. Glickman

Because of our aging patient population and the increased survival rate of diabetic patients, an increasing number of patients diagnosed with chronic kidney disease are developing end-stage renal disease (ESRD). Significant anatomic problems with this patient population makes arteriovenous (AV) access a difficult task for the surgeon. Access surgeons are constantly battling complications of AV access such as thrombosis, infection, and poor function. These issues are time consuming for the surgeon; they also cause substantial costs in healthcare dollars and an increase in mortality and morbidity for the patient. There is little argument that the most durable and most cost-effective form of chronic access is an arteriovenous fistula (AVF); however, achieving and maintaining autologous access remains a challenge in clinical practice.[2]

Since its inception in 1997, the Kidney Disease Outcomes and Quality Initiative (KDOQI) has provided management recommendations for physicians taking care of this complex and difficult patient population.[3] The recommendation is that autologous chronic AV access be achieved before the initiation of hemodialysis to provide the patient with the best possible conduit for dialysis with the least complications. The hierarchy for attempted access is radiocephalic, brachiocephalic, and basilic vein transposition fistulas without regard to the patient's age, sex, or other demographic features.[3] Out of the KDOQI guidelines was born the Fistula First campaign. Both KDOQI and Fistula First have set goals for patients dialyzing by an autogenous fistula at 65% by 2009.[3,4]

It is well established that AVF construction may be performed in a majority of patients, but the proportion of these accesses going on to become useful has fallen short of that achieved by our European counterparts.[5-7] There are demographic reasons that include a higher incidence of diabetes in the American populations compared to European counterparts and a generalized higher body mass index (BMI) in the American population compared to the European population. High failure rates and poor maturation has plagued American dialysis patients during the past decade, while the precise cause for the discrepancy between US and European literature remains elusive. With that being said, the answer is multifactorial at best.

We analyzed the outcomes of patients undergoing AVF versus arteriovenous grafting (AVG) as their first-time permanent access surgery to determine whether any demographic factors lead to worse outcomes in AV fistula maturation. Perhaps the KDOQI guidelines need to be modified to account for demographic analysis for establishing criteria for autogenous access placement.

With approval from the Eastern Virginia Medical School institutional review board, the CPT codes 36818, 36819, 36820, 36821, and 36825 were used to query the practice's billing database and generate a list of patients who underwent AV access surgery between January 1, 2005 and December 31, 2005. Patients who had previous access surgery were excluded from the analysis, because the focus of this study was "first access" only. Presence of a temporary or tunneled dialysis catheter was recorded, but not used to exclude patients.

Patient demographics, medical histories, imaging studies, physical examination findings, and postoperative examinations were collected from office and hospital charts and stored in a secured database. Operative notes from the initial procedure as well as subsequent procedures were reviewed for pertinent finding, complications, indications, and outcomes. All preoperative evaluations, procedures, postoperative evaluations, and interventions were performed by one of the 14 board-certified vascular surgeons or the one board-certified transplant surgeon in the practice. All initial AV access procedures were performed in the operating room; however, additional procedures were performed in one of three settings: an operating room, a hospital based endovascular suite, or an office-based endovascular access center.

A functional AVF was defined as a fistula being cannulated for at least one successful hemodialysis treatment, and a patent AVF was defined as having a palpable thrill or a bruit on auscultation. An AVF was considered abandoned if it required a major revision, including construction of a new anastomosis or placement of a jump graft, required ligation, or if a new access was required. An AVF requiring a patch angioplasty revision was not considered abandoned. Postoperative interventions were categorized as open or percutaneous, and included balloon angioplasty, mechanical thrombectomy, stent deployment, vein branch ligation or embolization, and patch angioplasty with either an autologous or prosthetic patch. The primary endpoints included AVF abandonment, renal transplantation, death or the time measurement of patency. The standards recommended by Sidaway et al. were used to define patency for this patient population.[8]

All calculations were performed using Microsoft Excel and the Excel plug-in XLstat. Categorical data was compared using χ^2 analysis, nominal data was compared using Student t test, and $P < .05$ was considered statistically significant. Kaplan-Meier survival curves were used to determine patency of the access and patient survival and used log rank testing to compare differences among curves.

Demographics

From January 1 to December 31, 2005, 239 patients underwent first-time AV access procedures. There were 168 (70.3%) AVF and 71 (29.7%) AV grafts (AVG) as seen in Figure 33-1. 62% of the AVF were placed in male patients and 70.2% of the AVG were placed in female patients ($P < .0001$). Both groups were similar with respect to preoperative clinical variables. The demographics of the AVF group compared to the United States Renal Data System (USRDS) are shown in Table 33-1 and Figure 33-2. Tunneled dialysis catheters were used in 77% of the patients in the periprocedural period for the initiation of hemodialysis. Of the 168 AVFs, 48 patients (29%) were 70 years of age or greater and we defined this as *elderly*. The distribution of ages in this study is noted in Figure 33-2.

Operative Data

The choice of location and type of access to be constructed in each patient was left to the discretion of the operating surgeon. Seventy-nine percent of the patients had preoperative vein mapping to help delineate the anatomy and guide the procedure of choice. Adequate arterial inflow was assessed with physical examination and duplex ultrasounds revealing biphasic flow through the donor artery; however, arterial size was not specifically evaluated. Average vein diameter was 3.3 (1.3 to 5.9) mm in the AVF group and 2.0 (0.8 to 4.4) mm in the AVG group ($P < .0001$). In this cohort, no basilic vein transpositions (BVTs) were constructed for first-time AV access.

Outcomes

The AVF group had 33 primary failures (19.6%) and the AVG group had 3 primary failures (8%; $P = .02$). Primary and primary assisted patency were 23% and 54% for AVF versus 18% and 35% for AVG ($P = .01$ and $P < .0001$, respectively) as shown in Figures 33-3 and 33-4. The secondary patency was 56% for AVF and 60% for AVG, which

Table 33–1

Demographics of Arteriovenous Fistula Patients Versus United States Renal Data System (USRDS) Patients

	EVMS, % (No.; N = 168)	USRDS, % (N = 335,963)
Mean age, years	59.2	62.6
Sex		
Male	62 (104)	55
Female	38 (64)	44
Race/Ethnicity		
White	33 (55)	55
African American	62 (105)	36
Hispanic	2.4 (4)	14.5
Asian/Pacific Islander	2.4 (4)	4.3

EVMS, Eastern Virginia Medical School.

Results

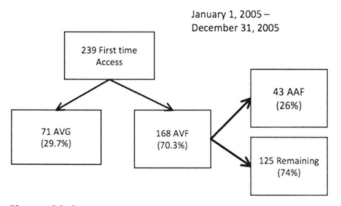

Figure 33-1.
Patients undergoing first-time arteriovenous (AV) access surgery. AVG, arteriovenous graft; AVF, arteriovenous fistula; AAF, African American female patients.

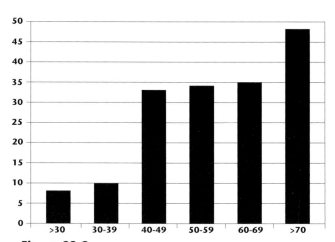

Figure 33-2.
Distribution of patients according to 10-year age categories.

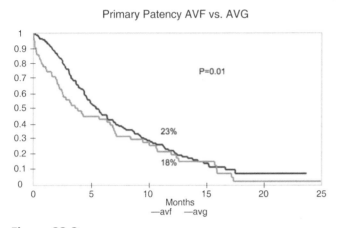

Figure 33-3.
Primary patency of arteriovenous fistula (AVF) versus arteriovenous graft (AVG).

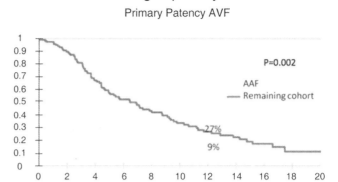

Figure 33-5.
Primary patency of arteriovenous fistula (AVF) in African American female patents versus the remaining cohort of patients.

was not significantly different. The AVF group had an average intervention rate of 0.91 interventions/year, whereas the AVG group had a yearly intervention rate of 1.53 ($P < .001$). In subgroup analysis, it was noted that primary failure in African American female patients was significantly higher (36% versus 16.7%; $P = .013$) than the remaining AVF cohort; primary patency rates were significantly worse (9% versus 27%; $P = .002$), and more interventions were required in these patients (Fig. 33-5). African American female patients with AVG had similar patency rates as non–African American female patients.

At the end of the data collection, 23 (48%) of the elderly patients were deceased compared to 24 (20%) of the non-elderly patients. When survival was viewed with Kaplan-Meier survival curves, the 18-month survival was 50% for elderly versus 75% for non-elderly patients ($P = .004$). This is represented in Figure 33-4. Of the 23 deceased elderly patients, the average time to death was 13.1 months. Only eight (35%) had their AVF accessed, and one of the eight had a radiocephalic fistula.

A substantial decrease in primary assisted and secondary patency of the elderly versus non-elderly patients became apparent when patency of the fistula was examined. The

primary assisted patency was 39% and 69% at 12 months for elderly versus non-elderly, respectively ($P = .0002$). The secondary patency was similar at 38% and 68% for elderly versus non-elderly, respectively ($P = .004$), as represented in Figures 33-6 and 33-7.

During the past decade, vascular access management as a component of the KDOQI guidelines has changed drastically. Since inception of the guidelines in 1997, the construction and utilization of AVF for chronic access has increased.[9,10] However, access surgeons have been unable to attain the goal to have two thirds of dialysis patients dialyzing via an AVF by 2009. Despite the steady progress towards these goals, there has yet to be a demonstrable decrease in the mortality and morbidity in this difficult patient population.[1] Although these guidelines have forced access surgeons to reevaluate the methods used to create hemodialysis access, the question remains: does it apply to all patient populations?

Our review focused on first-time AV access over the course of 1 year. It was found that 70% percent of patients had an autologous fistula constructed as their first-time chronic dialysis method, and the ratio of radiocephalic arteriovenous fistula (RCAVF) to brachiocephalic arteriove-

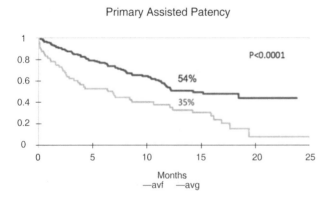

Figure 33-4.
Primary assisted patency of arteriovenous fistula (AVF) versus arteriovenous graft (AVG).

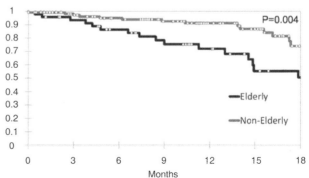

Figure 33-6.
Patient survival—elderly versus non-elderly.

Primary Assisted Patency
Elderly vs. Non-Elderly

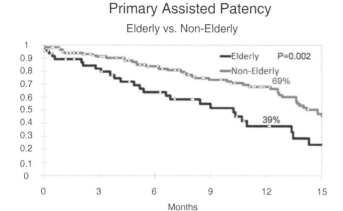

Figure 33-7.
Primary assisted patency—elderly versus non-elderly.

nous fistula (BCAVF) created is consistent with the ratio reported in the literature.[11] The reason for the lower number of RCAVF is related to vein size on preoperative vein mapping, which may be a result of the number of female patients undergoing first-time AVF access.[11-14] No patients in this cohort underwent BVT as a first attempt at chronic AV access. Although BVT remains in each surgeon's armamentarium, it is rarely performed as a first attempt at AV access in our practice, and it is usually reserved as the next step after failed RCAVF or BCAVF.

Peterson et al. reported rates of primary failure in AVF construction to be 40%.[2] Three factors were associated with increased primary failure in their study: female gender, RCAVF, and age 65 years or older.[2] There are racial differences that affect the outcomes of surgical procedures, particularly infrainguinal bypasses. The effect of race on the success of other vascular procedures, particularly infrainguinal revascularization, has been well studied, and findings suggest that those of African American race have experienced worse outcomes than other groups.[15-17] Although some of these differences may be attributed to more advanced or diffuse disease, after control for these variables, the disparity between ethnicities still holds true.[17] These factors, especially the combination of African American race and female gender, lead to poor results in autologous fistula construction. In this patient population, it appears that AVG may be the preferred primary access of choice, because autogenous fistulas have resulted in poor outcomes in these patients.

In our review of elderly patients, we found these patients to have a much reduced overall survival compared with the younger cohort of patients undergoing dialysis. Primary assisted patency and secondary patency in the elderly group was 30% less than for the non-elderly at 12 months. These poor outcomes lead us to believe that this patient population needs to be approached differently from younger patients undergoing dialysis. A patient 70 years or older undergoing dialysis for the first time has a statistically higher one-year mortality and fistula failure rate than the general patient population.

It is well established that autologous fistula construction may be performed within all patient populations. However, the question remains: should it be the first line in all sub-

groups of patients? Data suggest that African American female patients have a limited benefit secondary to their increased primary failures and may experience decreases in primary patency. The elderly patient population also has a higher failure rate, and we need to reassess our approach to this patient population. Access surgeons and nephrologists should carefully weigh all access options when dialysis is initiated and determine which method of chronic access best suits these patients. It is difficult to recommend that fistulas should be first for all patients. As more data to corroborate these findings becomes available, the KDOQI guidelines should be revisited.

REFERENCES

1. US Renal Data System. 2006 Annual Report: Atlas of End-Stage Renal Disease in the United States. Bethesda, MD: National Institutes of Health 2006.
2. Peterson WJ, Barker J, Allon M. Disparities in fistula maturation persist despite preoperative vascular mapping. *Clin J Am Soc Nephrol.* 2008;3(2)437-441.: Epub Jan 30, 2008.
3. National Kidney Foundation Kidney Disease Outcomes and Quality Initiative (KDOQI). Clinical Practice Guidelines for Hemodialysis Adequacy, Update 2006. Available at http://www.kidney.org/Professionals/kdoqi/pdf/hemodialysis_adequacy.pdf.
4. Fistula First. Tools for Professionals. Available at http://www.fistulafirst.org/professionals/tools.php.
5. Biuckians A, Scott EC, Meier GH, Panneton JM, Glickman MH. The natural history of autologous fistulas as first-time dialysis access in the KDOQI era. *J Vasc Surg.* 2008;7(2):415-421; discussion 420-421.
6. Shrestha PC, Asher J, Shrestha SM, et al. Survival of arteriovenous fistula for dialysis at different centers in the North of England. *J Vasc Access.* 2007;8(4):231-234.
7. Rayner HC, Besarab A, Brown WW, Disney A, Saito A, Pisoni RL. Vascular access results from the Dialysis Outcomes and Practice Patterns Study (DOPPS): performance against Kidney Disease Outcomes Quality Initiative (KDOQI) Clinical Practice Guidelines. *Am J Kidney Dis.* 2004;44(5 suppl 2):22-26.
8. Sidawy AN, Gray R, Besarab A, et al. Recommended standards for reports dealing with arteriovenous hemodialysis accesses. *J Vasc Surg.* 2002;35(3):603-610.
9. Robbin ML, Gallichio MH, Deierhoi MH, Young CJ, Weber TM, Allon M. US vascular mapping before hemodialysis access placement. *Radiology.* 2000;217(1):83-88.
10. Silva MB Jr, Hobson RW 2nd, Pappas PJ, et al. A strategy for increasing use of autogenous hemodialysis access procedures: impact of preoperative noninvasive evaluation. *J Vasc Surg.* 1998;27(2):302-307; discussion 307-308.
11. Berman SS, Gentile AT. Impact of secondary procedures in autogenous arteriovenous fistula maturation and maintenance. *J Vasc Surg.* 2001; 34(5):866-871.
12. Dixon BS, Novak L, Fangman J. Hemodialysis vascular access survival: upper-arm native arteriovenous fistula. *Am J Kidney Dis.* 2002;39(1): 92-101.
13. Kalman PG, Pope M, Bhola C, Richardson R, Sniderman KW. A practical approach to vascular access for hemodialysis and predictors of success. *J Vasc Surg.* 1999;30(4):727-733.
14. Miller CD, Robbin ML, Allon M. Gender differences in outcomes of arteriovenous fistulas in hemodialysis patients. *Kidney Int.* 2003; 63(1):346-352.
15. Huber TS, Wang JG, Wheeler KG, et al. Impact of race on the treatment for peripheral arterial occlusive disease. *J Vasc Surg.* 1999;30(3): 417-425.
16. Chew DK, Nguyen LL, Owens CD, et al. Comparative analysis of autogenous infrainguinal bypass grafts in African Americans and Caucasians: the association of race with graft function and limb salvage. *J Vasc Surg.* 2005;695:e1-8.
17. Rowe VL, Kumar SR, Glass H, Hood DB, Weaver FA. Race independently impacts outcome of infrapopliteal bypass for symptomatic arterial insufficiency. *Vasc Endovasc Surg.* 2007;41(5):397-401.

Ten Mistakes to Avoid in Dialysis Access Surgery

Eric D. Ladenheim

Dialysis access surgery can be intellectually challenging one moment and emotionally frustrating the next. The surgeon can maximize his or her professional satisfaction by learning from past mistakes. Here are 10 mistakes the author has observed during his 17 years of practicing dialysis access surgery, presented to help the reader avoid some of these pitfalls.

Skipping the Vascular Mapping

When suitable vessels for an autogenous arteriovenous fistula (AVF) are not clearly evident on the physical examination, vascular mapping should be done.[1] I suspect some surgeons skip it because of overconfidence in their clinical examination acumen.

Be very wary of omitting the vascular mapping. On occasion, mapping is inconvenient because of unusual circumstances which may include the unavailability of equipment during the initial evaluation or the patient being seen in a correctional facility, rehabilitation hospital, or skilled nursing facility. Although most dialysis access surgeons have developed systems for performing or obtaining vascular mapping on patients referred to their office, many acute care hospitals unfortunately do not offer useful vascular mapping services. This can pose a serious dilemma when the referring physician is pressuring the surgeon to place an arteriovenous (AV) access before hospital discharge and vascular mapping.

The ideal solution is to work with the hospitals at which you practice and assist them in offering these services. Useful protocols are mentioned in Chapter 30 of this volume and at the Fistula First website.[2] Should vascular mapping services be the "turf" of the peripheral vascular lab, the cardiovascular department or the radiology department? It may be expedient to let local hospital politics dictate this. The most important thing is to work with the department that will provide the services to ensure that relevant and essential data are reported.

A definite plan should already have been made for the surgery before the patient reaches the operating room; however, if there is still any uncertainty regarding the peripheral veins or runoff, contrast venography can be done with a peripheral intravenous (IV) catheter and mobile imaging equipment. Duplex ultrasound and venography are complementary, not competing, examinations (Table 34-1). Duplex

Table 34–1		
Comparison of Venography versus Ultrasound		
	Venography	**Duplex Ultrasound**
Measuring vessel size	Fair	Excellent
Identifying central venous stenosis	Excellent	Gives indirect dues
Measuring vessel depth	Poor	Excellent
Identifies focal stenosis	Excellent	Fair
Applicable to pre-ESRD patients	Caution required	Applicable
Assessment of arteries	No	Excellent

ultrasound is not perfect, and I have seen many significant venous strictures missed by duplex ultrasound but revealed by venography. For example, I once misidentified a prominent deep radial vein as the median antebrachial vein. In performing venography, the peripheral IV cannula is placed on the volar forearm, and the injection may fail to fill the median antebrachial vein or the entire cephalic system. Precise measurements are more difficult to make with venography than ultrasound. Also, venography can be an inefficient use of valuable operating room time. Minimize its use by performing preoperative Doppler ultrasound mapping.

Ignoring Arterial Steal and Hoping it Will Get Better

Severe arterial steal leads to gangrene and limb loss; moderate steal leads to pain and disability; and mild steal leads to reliance on gloves or mittens. Patients who are obliged to wear mittens to ameliorate their symptoms are frequently questioned about this and are often eager to discuss their negative experiences with surgery and with the surgeon.

Surgeons may ignore mild or moderate arterial steal in the hope that it will go away. Often, this reflects uncertainty as to what to do. There is still a widespread lack of familiarity with instrumentation for quantifying access flow. Further indications for a flow restrictive procedure versus a distal revascularization and interval ligation are unclear. My personal approach is to first measure access flow using duplex methodology. If the patient is symptomatic and access flow is high (greater than 1000 mL/min), I do a restrictive procedure and reduce access flow to about 600 mL/min. If the access flow is lower, I obtain a fistulogram and arteriogram in preparation for a distal revascularization and interval ligation. I generally ligate the access if there is profound or progressive weakness. Chapter 22 details the principles of recognition and correction of arterial steal. Obtaining access to flow measurement instrumentation is invaluable in formulating a plan.

When moderate or severe steal presents in the early postoperative period (less than 30 days), symptoms tend to worsen, because flow increases as the access matures. Symptoms persist in the late postoperative period, and there is little to be gained by waiting to see if they abate.

Never Using the Dominant Arm

AVFs should be placed in the arm with the best vessels regardless of which arm is dominant. It makes little sense to place a compromised fistula or, worse, an arteriovenous graft (AVG) in an extremity without doing vascular mapping on the contralateral side. Patients appreciate a thorough, systematic physical examination by their vascular access surgeon, and I have found that the process of the surgeon personally mapping the vessels brings the patient, surgeon, and family together with the common goal of finding the best solution to the dialysis access problem.

I have regretted overlooking the dominant arm several times. An extreme but good example is the limb paralyzed from cerebral infarction. If the surgeon becomes trapped in the mindset that he *must* place the access on the paralyzed side, difficulties can rapidly multiply. The weak side may be contracted and difficult to operate on, and the fistula will be difficult to expose for cannulation. The vessels tend to be smaller on the weaker side. I have erred by placing an AVG in such a patient without mapping the dominant arm, only to find, after it failed, that a radiocephalic fistula was possible in the dominant arm.

Although it might seem obvious, the ideal time to assess which arm has the best vessel for an AVF is before the first AV access is placed and when the patient's hopes and confidence are high. After one or more failed procedures in the nondominant arm, I have found it becomes harder for the patient to accept switching to the dominant side. In addition, subconsciously or consciously the surgeon may feel that switching arms after a failed procedure is the same as admitting he made a mistake in placing the access in the nondominant arm. These technical and emotional difficulties can be avoided by adopting the rule that AV fistulas should be placed in the arm with the best vessels regardless of dominance.

Using Rapidly Absorbable Suture to Ligate Errant Fistulas

When large AVFs need to be ligated, they should be divided and ligated with nonabsorbable suture material. Here is an illustrative example:

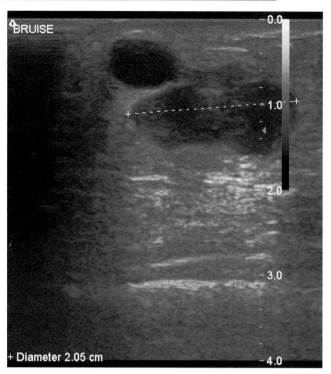

Figure 34-1.
Posterior hematoma compresses fistula but does not cause downward displacement.

An 82-year-old man with stage 4 chronic kidney disease was referred for creation of an AVF. After evaluation, including vascular mapping, he underwent creation of a left-arm brachiocephalic fistula. On the first postoperative day, he presented to our office with finger pain, a cool hand, poor capillary refill, and hand weakness. Access flow by duplex methodology was 1150 mL/min. The diagnosis was severe arterial steal. The full range of treatments for steal were discussed, but we agreed that ligation of the fistula would be in his best interest. Ligation of the fistula in continuity was done under local anesthesia with 2-0 plain gut. He had immediate improvement in his symptoms, but after 5 days he presented again with recurring symptoms. The physical examination showed a strong thrill in the fistula and signs of recurrent arterial steal. On exploration of the wound, the knot was intact but the suture had parted. The fistula was divided and re-ligated with nonabsorbable (silk) suture.

Although solid evidence supports the use of absorbable suture in vascular surgery,[3-5] the AVF seems to be a unique application. Fistulas tend to be large, thick-walled, and bulky vessels. Once ligated, they continue to be exposed to pulsatile arterial pressure. When ligated in continuity, sometimes blood will continue to flow through the ligated vessel. Take no chances. When they need to be closed, divide and ligate with nonabsorbable suture.

Trying to Cannulate an Arteriovenous Fistula That Is Too Small or Too Deep

The *rule of 6s* describes criteria for cannulation of the AVF: more than 6 mm in diameter, less than 6 mm deep, and at least 6 weeks of maturation have passed since creation.

Unfortunately, even if this rule is followed, infiltrations of varying severity are common. My patients often find that the first cannulation of a new AVF often goes much more smoothly than the second or third. The reason for this is unclear, but may have to do with the increased care and attention surrounding the first cannulation. Infiltrations can occur when the needle leaving the fistula or blood leaks around the needle. When imaged by duplex ultrasound, hematomas will be seen either anterior or posterior (Fig. 34-1) to the fistula. Of these, anterior hematomas are the most common and are more troublesome, because they displace the fistula deeper beneath the skin.

A fistula that initially clearly meets criteria for cannulation can become entrapped in a vicious cycle of infiltration, resulting in deep displacement of the fistula, (Fig. 34-2), more difficult cannulation, more infiltration, and deeper displacement. Common sense calls for breaking the cycle by resting the fistula until it meets criteria for cannulation again. Two to four weeks may be needed for healing.

In the typical patient, the anxiety associated with the cannulation procedure diminishes over time; but, in patients subjected to repeated attempts at difficult cannulation of a small or deep fistula, anxiety may magnify to the point that a strong attachment develops to the bridging catheter and the patient may refuse to have it removed. In such cases, we offer the patient emotional reassurance and objective feedback about the health of the fistula as the patient is guided towards the goal of trouble-free cannulation of the AV access and removal of the bridging catheter.

Once a Graft, Always a Graft

To assume that a patient with a graft must have poor peripheral veins is missing an opportunity to potentially construct an AV fistula. Not only may there be an excellent runoff vein from the existing graft that can be converted into a fistula, but there may be excellent veins that were overlooked on physical examination. Mapping may never have been done. There are opportunities at every graft failure for evaluation for an autogenous AVF.[6] Certainly, before a revision of an AV graft is contemplated, an autogenous AVF should be considered. However, even if the intervention on the failing graft is successful, this is an excellent opportunity to map the patient for a new fistula.

Take the example of a forearm loop graft based on the brachial artery with antecubital runoff to the upper arm cephalic vein. Graft salvage can be achieved in a variety of ways:

- Percutaneously: balloon angioplasty, stenting, or stent graft
- Surgical revision: patch graft angioplasty; jump graft to cephalic, brachial, or basilic vein
- New autogenous AVF based on cephalic runoff or other vein.

The ideal time for discussion of the advantages of conversion of the graft to a fistula is before the graft fails. The discussion should include the patient, family, nephrologist, and surgeon. Once the graft fails, the path of least resistance is usually to attempt graft salvage procedures. Repeated attempts can lead to patient expectations of graft salvage

with any thrombotic event and resistance to conversion to a fistula. Should the patient develop such an attachment to a failing graft, we use a similar counseling strategy used to wean patients from the bridging catheter.

Concluding an Arteriovenous Access Procedure With Only a Weak Doppler Signal

Vascular access surgeons have long been intuitively aware that newly constructed fistulas and grafts with slow flow experience early failure. Studies using ultrasound transit time or duplex measurement of access flow have borne this out.[7-9] Won et al. reported that the radiocephalic fistula had a wide range of intraoperative flow rates ranging 50 to 500 mL/min and found that fistulas with a flow of less than 160 mL/min had a significantly higher early failure rate than those with flow rates greater than 160 mL/minute. In his study, all fistulas with a flow rate of less than 70 mL/min failed within a month. A similar result was found by Berman,[10] who found that a threshold value of 179 mL/min for radiocephalic and 308 mL/min for brachiocephalic AVFs predicted maturation to a functional access.

Every dialysis access surgeon has a choice of methods to use for assessing the adequacy of the procedure. Qualitative measures include palpation of the access and auscultation of a bruit or listening with continuous wave Doppler. Quantitative assessment of the flow may be measured directly by ultrasound transit time, duplex ultrasound, or electromagnetic flow meter. It is my practice to perform intraoperative fistulography when uncertainty remains after noninvasive assessment.

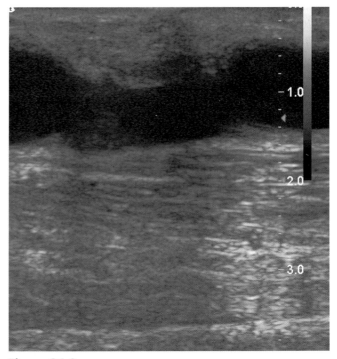

Figure 34-2.
Hematoma compressing fistula and forcing it down to 10-mm depth.

Palpation of the access is the simplest noninvasive assessment measure. When there is a swing point narrowing, the pulse will increase proximally and decrease distally. Unfortunately, most anastomotic errors cannot be distinguished from spasm or clot by palpation. At higher flow rates, physical examination of the access can accurately rate the flow on the basis of the character and distribution of the thrill.[11] However the low-flow detection threshold for the thrill is poorly characterized in the literature. Similarly, uncertainty exists regarding the low threshold for detection of a bruit. My experience, gained with intraoperative flow measurement by duplex of the last 50 autogenous AVFs, suggests the lower threshold for detection of a bruit is about 125 to 150 mL/min. For palpation of a thrill, it is slightly higher: 150 to 175 mL/min. However, qualitative evidence of some flow can be detected by continuous wave ultrasound at levels below 25 mL/min.

The implications are that palpation of a thrill at the initial procedure is associated with flows that predict probable maturation of the fistula. A bruit but no palpable thrill represents flow in the gray zone between fistulas that mature and those that do not. The fistula (or graft) with a flow detectable by continuous wave Doppler but no audible bruit or palpable thrill is likely to fail.

Never Performing the Transposed Brachiobasilic Arteriovenous Fistula

Reasons sometimes cited for not doing vein transpositions are:

"The veins are too thin-walled—there are bleeding problems with cannulation."
"The incisions are too big—they have too much morbidity."
"A forearm prosthetic graft could be placed now and the fistula created later."

The reader should refer to Chapter 13 for an excellent discussion of the technique and utility of transposed brachiobasilic AVF. The goal of the procedure should be to move the vein superficially into a safe spot for cannulation (laterally) and away from the incision. Simple elevation of the vein is technically easier, but it does not move the vein laterally and away from the incision. The lateral position moves it away from the brachial artery and the medial cutaneous nerve, allowing the arm to be in a more convenient position for cannulation and allows for easier compression after the needles are removed.

Some of these deep veins are indeed thin-walled, and it can be difficult to ascertain this by physical examination or even Doppler ultrasound. Thin-walled veins are fragile and hard to work with. Dialysis access surgeons should become familiar with doing the procedure either as a one- or a two-stage procedure. The two-stage procedure allows borderline small veins or thin-walled veins to be prepared for transposition. Some surgeons deal with the uncertainty of vein wall thickness by routinely doing the procedure as a two-stage procedure. I also utilize the two-stage procedure if the vein to be transposed is 3 mm in diameter or less. In the case of larger veins, I begin as distally as possible, preferably in the forearm, and expose the vein to assess its quality and decide whether to do a one- or two-stage procedure.

The incisions are indeed large, but they are less troublesome than leg incisions. Adequate incisions will allow for dissection of the vein from accompanying nerves and allow for secure ligation of all branches without placing sutures in the vein itself. Intraoperative (or preoperative) Doppler ultrasound marking speeds up the procedure and allows for precise positioning of the incisions, avoiding problematic skin flaps. I do not have enough experience with endoscopic basilic vein harvesting to advocate its use.

For the surgeon lacking confidence in the transposed brachiobasilic AVF, the AVG might appear to be an attractive alternative. Tactics than can help improve use of transposition AVFs include:

- Regular use of preoperative vascular mapping
- Using Doppler ultrasound to mark the vein intraoperatively (or immediately preoperatively)
- Making adequately large incisions
- Harvesting vein from the forearm/upper arm to obtain enough length for a lateral tunnel
- Having a skilled assistant
- Using general anesthesia
- Scheduling enough time for the procedure to avoid the stress of affecting other cases

Doing Thrombectomy Without Any Imaging Studies to Learn Why the Access Failed

Surgical thrombectomy of the clotted arteriovenous graft was a common procedure until the mid-and late 1990s, when percutaneous methods of declotting arteriovenous accesses outside of the operating room became common.[12-17] This was our traditional method of non–image guided surgical thrombectomy that is rarely performed today:

1. An incision is made near the venous anastomosis.
2. The venous end is declotted first with a balloon embolectomy catheter.
3. The caliber of the venous outflow is assessed by feeling the drag of the balloon embolectomy catheter and observing the venous back bleeding.
4. If anastomotic stenosis seems likely, the first line of treatment is treated by coaxial dilatation with steel vessel dilators.
5. Once venous back bleeding is established, the arterial inflow is declotted with the balloon embolectomy catheter. The endpoint for arterial inflow thrombectomy is recovery of the platelet/fibrin "plug" and the occurrence of brisk arterial bleeding.
6. The graft or fistula is repaired with vascular suture often using a patch angioplasty and the success assessed by palpation of the thrill or auscultation of the bruit.

Most of the time, this non–image guided procedure did allow dialysis access to continue for several months.[18] Early failures were managed by patch angioplasty or a jump graft to a more proximal vein. Recurrent failures were investigated with radiologic fistulography.

The successes of non–image guided surgical thrombectomy notwithstanding, percutaneous methods have become dominant in recent years. Medical advantages include less blood loss and complete imaging of the dialysis access system. Practical advantages are that they can be accomplished quickly and as an outpatient procedure. Their profitability is evidenced by the rapid increase in numbers of free-standing access centers.[19] Most referrals seen in our practice for thrombosed arteriovenous accesses now come after the patient has had one (or several) failed percutaneous procedures. This is where the surgeon can serve the patient best by utilizing the full range of reconstructive and imaging methods. After a failed percutaneous thrombectomy and angioplasty, the likelihood of simple surgical thrombectomy without imaging being successful is very low.

Fortunately, a roadmap to the surgical reconstruction is available by review of the imaging from the previous percutaneous procedures. Although my preference is for intraoperative fistulogram after reconstruction to check the technical adequacy of the revision, careful physical assessment can be combined as needed with continuous wave ultrasound, duplex scanning, or flow measurement with success.

Lysing Too Many Valves With the Proximal Radial Artery Arteriovenous Fistula

The proximal radial artery (PRA) can provide a reliable source of inflow for autogenous AVFs of the upper extremity. Outflow can be to the upper arm, forearm, or a combination of both. It has also been successful in patients whose only superficial vein is the median antebrachial vein of the forearm after disruption of its most central valve in the proximal forearm. However, careful consideration should be given to what the subsequent outflow will be (Fig. 34-3). A paucity of superficial runoff from the fistula along with overzealous disruption of the median antebrachial vein valves can lead to peripheral venous hypertension of the hand (Fig. 34-4).[20]

Large studies of the PRA AVF have shown venous hypertension to be a rare event. Bachleda reported a total of 574 proximal forearm fistulas were constructed with only 18 patients showing symptoms of venous hypertension.[21] In

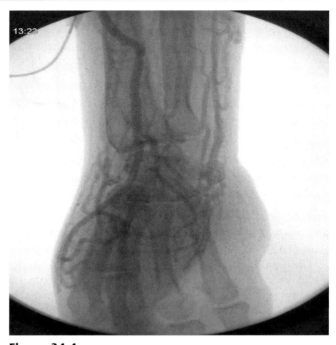

Figure 34-4.
Venous hypertension after lysis of all median antebrachial valves with LeMaitre valvulotome.

recent years, the PRA AVF has been constructed more frequently, however, it is not the PRA that promotes venous hypertension; rather, the outcome is dependent on the quality of the venous outflow.

The temptation to perform complete valve lysis of the median antebrachial vein in the forearm should be resisted. I no longer attempt to lyse all median antebrachial veins but, rather, limit valve lysis to one or two sets to allow for more limited forearm runoff.

REFERENCES

1. Vascular Access Work Group. Clinical practice guidelines for vascular access. *Am J Kidney Dis.* 2006;48(suppl 1):S248-S273.
2. Griffith C, Robinson K, Krug R, et al. Duplex of Upper Extremity Vessels Prior to AVF Surgery. Fistula First, 2005. Available at http://www.fistulafirst.org/pdfs/AVFMapprotocol.doc.
3. Merrell SW, Lawrence PF. Initial evaluation of absorbable polydioxanone suture for peripheral vascular surgery. *J Vasc Surg.* 1991;14(4):452-457; discussion 457-459.
4. Myers JL, Campbell DB, Waldhausen JA. The use of absorbable monofilament polydioxanone suture in pediatric cardiovascular operations. *J Thorac Cardiovasc Surg.* 1986;92(4):771-775.
5. Occhionorelli S, De Tullio D, Pellegrini D, et al. Arteriovenous fistulas for hemodialysis created using a long-term absorbable suture: a safe solution and a measure to minimize myointimal hyperplasia. *J Vasc Access.* 2005;6(4):171-176.
6. Beathard GA. Strategy for maximizing the use of arteriovenous fistulae. *Semin Dial.* 2000;13(5):291-296.
7. Won T, Jang JW, Lee S, Han JJ, Park YS, Ahn JH. Effects of intraoperative blood flow on the early patency of radiocephalic fistulas. *Ann Vasc Surg.* 2000;14(5):468-472.
8. Lin CH, Chua CH, Chiang SS, Liou JY, Hung HF, Chang CH. Correlation of intraoperative blood flow measurement with autogenous arteriovenous fistula outcome. *J Vasc Surg.* 2008;48(1):167-172.
9. Wong V, Ward R, Taylor J, Selvakumar S, How TV, Bakran A. Factors associated with early failure of arteriovenous fistulae for haemodialysis access. *Eur J Vasc Endovasc Surg.* 1996;12(2):207-213.

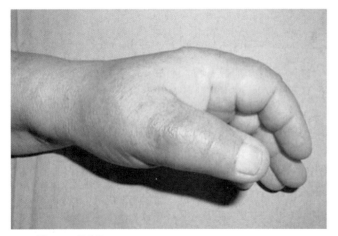

Figure 34-3.
Hand swollen from peripheral venous hypertension.

10. Berman SS, Mendoza B, Westerband A, Quick RC. Predicting arteriovenous fistula maturation with intraoperative blood flow measurements. *J Vasc Access*. 2008;9(4):241-247.

11. Agarwal R, McDougal G. Buzz in the axilla: a new physical sign in hemodialysis forearm graft evaluation. *Am J Kidney Dis*. 2001; 38(4):853-857.

12. Dougherty MJ, Calligaro KD, Schindler N, Raviola CA, Ntoso A. Endovascular versus surgical treatment for thrombosed hemodialysis grafts: a prospective, randomized study. *J Vasc Surg*. 1999;30(6):1016-1023.

13. Bakken AM, Galaria II, Agerstrand C, et al. Percutaneous therapy to maintain dialysis access successfully prolongs functional duration after primary failure. *Ann Vasc Surg*. 2007;21(4):474-480.

14. Beathard GA, Welch BR, Maidment HJ. Mechanical thrombolysis for the treatment of thrombosed hemodialysis access grafts. *Radiology*. 1996;200(3):711-716.

15. Beathard GA. Thrombolysis versus surgery for the treatment of thrombosed dialysis access grafts. *J Am Soc Nephrol*. 1995;6(6):1619-1624.

16. Bittl JA. Percutaneous therapy of dialysis access failure. *Catheter Cardiovasc Interv*. 2002;56(2):157-161.

17. Bush RL, Lin PH, Lumsden BA. Management of thrombosed dialysis access: thrombectomy versus thrombolysis. *Semin Vasc Surg*. 2004; 17(1):32-39.

18. Marston WA, Criado E, Jaques PF, Mauro MA, Burnham SJ, Keagy BA. Prospective randomized comparison of surgical versus endovascular management of thrombosed dialysis access grafts. *J Vasc Surg*. 1997; 26(3):373-380; discussion 380-381.

19. Mishler R, Sands JJ, Ofsthun NJ, Teng M, Schon D, Lazarus JM. Dedicated outpatient vascular access center decreases hospitalization and missed outpatient dialysis treatments. *Kidney Int*. 2006;69(2):393-398.

20. Ladenheim E. Excessive use of the Lemaitre valvulotome for median antebrachial valve lysis resulting in venous hypertension of the hand. Presented at 11th Symposium, Vascular Access for Hemodialysis; Orlando, FL; May 8-9, 2008.

21. Bachleda P, Kojecký Z, Utikal P, Drác P, Herman J, Zadrazil J. Peripheral venous hypertension after the creation of arteriovenous fistula for haemodialysis. *Biomed Pap Med Fac Univ Palacky Olomouc Czech Repub*. 2004;148(1):85-87.

VASCULAR ACCESS FOR CRITICAL CARE, CHEMOTHERAPY, AND NUTRITION

CHAPTER 35

Placement of Indwelling Venous Access Systems

James E. Wiseman, Gail T. Tominaga, and James G. Jakowatz

The need to control the rising cost of health care has driven a general trend from costly inpatient care to less costly outpatient care management. In conjunction with this trend, long-term venous access is assuming increased importance in surgical and medical practice for hemodialysis and the infusion of total parenteral nutrition (TPN), multiagent chemotherapy, antibiotics, and blood products.

Peripheral access with needles or polyethylene catheters is the most commonly used method for short-term administration of iso-osmolar solutions or noncaustic medications. Peripheral venous access in the chronically ill and debilitated patient has several limitations, including venous sclerosis, thrombosis, infection, infiltration, and extravasation. The incidence of these problems increases with the administration of hyperosmolar or vesicant solutions. To avoid these problems, alternative means of vascular access have been used.

Central venous access is the preferred method of circulatory access for long-term use. A large central vein allows high flow and liberal administration of hyperosmolar solutions not tolerated by smaller peripheral veins. Indications for chronic central access include:

- TPN in patients unable to tolerate enteral nutrition
- Patients receiving vesicant chemotherapy (eg, doxorubicin hydrochloride)
- Patients receiving continuous infusion therapy
- Patients receiving intensive chemotherapy, for which blood products, nutritional support, and antibiotics are anticipated
- Pediatric patients
- Patients with difficult to access or maintain or exhausted (ie, "used up") peripheral veins
- Patients receiving long-term antimicrobial therapy (eg, those with endocarditis and fungal infections)

Arteriovenous (AV) fistulas have been used as a more reliable means of access in nonuremic patients.[1] Reported infection rates were favorably low at 0% to 3%. They have not gained widespread use as a result of the high rate of failure related to thrombosis in the nonuremic patient with normal platelet function.[2,3] Bridge fistulas have been described with conduits between superficial veins and arteries when direct AV fistulas are not feasible.[4] The preferred conduit material is autogenous saphenous vein, although polytetrafluoroethylene (PTFE), fluoropolymer (Teflon), umbilical vein, and bovine carotid artery have also been used.[5,6,7] The benefit of access convenience is countered by the increased thrombogenicity compared with direct fistulas. The poor durability of direct and bridge fistulas led to the development of artificial indwelling access systems. Various types of long-term central venous catheters have been developed, including the Broviac, Hickman, and Groshong catheters and totally implantable subcutaneous ports.

Development of Long-Term Venous Access

The first intravenous infusion was performed using a cannula made from a quill by Sir Christopher Wren in 1657. After experimental work with dogs, Robert Boyle transfused animal blood into humans in 1663. Richard Lower performed the first successful human transfusion in 1667 and introduced sheep blood into the circulation of Arthur Coga.[8] At that time, interest in circulation was modest and progress toward improved methods of venous access was slow.

In 1929, Forssmann, a German urologist, introduced a catheter from a peripheral vein into his right atrium and confirmed catheter position by radiography.[9] The importance of this technique was not recognized until after World War II.

Percutaneous subclavian venipuncture was first described in 1951 by Aubaniac, a French military surgeon, for the resuscitation of patients.[10] The first percutaneous placement of a subclavian vein catheter was reported in 1956.[11] As the use of this procedure increased, complications such as thrombosis, phlebitis, and sepsis became more frequent. With progress in industrial technology, materials that coupled greater pliancy with reduced thrombogenicity became available, and complication rates decreased.

Seldinger described a new technique for catheter insertion in 1953. Direct venipuncture involved introduction of a guidewire through the needle. After removal of the needle, the catheter was introduced over the guidewire.[12] This technique gained widespread acceptance in vascular access surgery. With the use of softer catheters, however, the peel-away introducer sheath has modified this technique.

In 1968, Dudrick reported the use of percutaneous infraclavicular subclavian catheterization for the administration of hypertonic parenteral nutrition solutions.[13] This led to the development of a long-term, indwelling, right atrial silicone elastomer ((Silastic; Dow Corning Corp., Midland, MI) catheter by Broviac, Cole, and Scribner in 1973 for home TPN.[14] These catheters were inserted directly via cutdown technique into the cephalic or internal jugular vein. The catheter was then tunneled subcutaneously, with the external end of the catheter exiting the skin on the lower anterior chest wall. Advantages included decreased thrombogenicity and a reduced infection rate thought to be secondary to the bacterial barrier provided by the subcutaneous tunnel and fibrous adhesions to the polyethylene terephthalate (Dacron; INVISTA, Wichita, KS) cuff.

In 1979, Hickman modified the Broviac catheter by increasing the catheter size to facilitate care of patients undergoing bone marrow transplantation.[15] The larger-bore catheter had greater internal diameter (ID) and a thicker wall, which increased durability. To avoid the external component of the Broviac and Hickman catheters, a totally implantable device consisting of a small-volume, subcutaneous injection port and Silastic catheter was developed in 1982.[16]

Peripherally inserted central venous silicone elastomer catheters (PICCs) were first reported in 1975 by Horshal.[17] He reported on the placement of 36 catheters with a 22% phlebitis rate. Bottino and associates[18] reported a 23% incidence of phlebitis and a 1% incidence of catheter-related sepsis in 87 catheters placed in 81 hospitalized oncology patients. This rate compares favorably with that of peripherally inserted central polyvinyl catheters, which have a 40% phlebitis rate at 6 days when used for hyperalimentation.[19] These PICCs declined in popularity with the advent of Broviac and Hickman catheters, as well as totally implantable devices.

Types of Catheter

Temporary central venous polyethylene catheters were popularized in the hospital setting in the 1970s. Long-term success with central venous catheters of Teflon, polyethylene, and polyvinyl chloride has been limited by unacceptable rates of sepsis and thrombosis. Advances in catheter technology have made silicone rubber catheters available. Advantages of the silicone catheter include greater flexibility, decreased thrombogenicity,[20-22] and decreased incidence of sepsis compared with polyethylene catheters. Silicone catheters are more expensive but have a longer life expectancy than polyethylene catheters.

In 1973, Broviac, Cole, and Scribner introduced a silicone rubber right atrial catheter (1.0 mm ID, 2.2 mm external diameter [ED]) for prolonged parenteral alimentation.[14] Hickman and colleagues[23] modified the Broviac catheter, making it larger (1.6 mm ID, 3.2 mm ED) to draw blood samples and infuse drugs, intravenous solutions, and blood products. Broviac and Hickman catheters are 90 cm long, are radiopaque, and have a Dacron cuff 30 cm from the Luer lock at the external end (Figs. 35-1 and 35-2). Available Broviac catheters range in size from 2.7F (0.5 mm ID) with a single lumen to 7F (0.8 and 1.0 mm ID) with a double lumen. Hickman catheters come with one, two, or three lumens and one or two Dacron cuffs placed on the extravascular segment. These are available in sizes from 8F (1.5 mm ID) to 9.6F (1.6 mm ID) with a single lumen, from 9F (0.7 mm ID, 1.3 mm ID) to 12F (1.6 and 1.6 mm) with a dou-

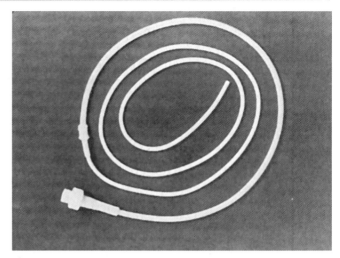

Figure 35-1.
Standard Broviac catheter. Note the external Luer fitting, the Dacron cuff, and the open-ended intravascular portion of the catheter.

ble lumen, and in 12.5F with a triple lumen (1.0, 1.0, and 1.5 mm ID). These catheters are also available with a VitaCuff (VitaPhore Corp., Menlo Park, CA) antimicrobial cuff located either 4 cm from or immediately adjacent to the Dacron cuff. The catheter is placed into a central vein and then tunneled subcutaneously with the Dacron cuff distant from the venipuncture site. This Dacron cuff was designed to prevent infection by promoting tissue fibroblastic ingrowth and forming an anatomic barrier to organisms ascending along the outer aspect of the catheter.[24] Subsequent studies,[25,26] however, have shown that tunneling catheters do not decrease catheter sepsis and that the origin of most catheter sepsis is bacteria migrating intraluminally from the infected hub.[26,27] The Broviac and Hickman catheters are available in cutdown or percutaneous kits from various manufacturers.

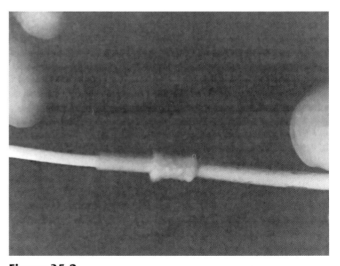

Figure 35-2.
Dacron cuff of the Dacron Broviac catheter. It provides for tissue ingrowth to prevent infection and to secure the catheter to the skin.

The Broviac and Hickman catheters require weekly heparin flushes to avoid thrombosis. The Groshong catheter requires weekly saline flushes when not in use. It is a thin-walled Silastic catheter (1.5 mm ID, 2.5 mm ED) with a pressure-sensitive, three-way valve.[28] The proposed advantage is the Groshong valve, which reduces the risk of air embolism, reduces the opportunity for blood reflux, and eliminates the need for catheter clamping and heparin flushes. It is available with one or two lumens and in percutaneous or cutdown kits.

Implantable central venous access devices (ICVADs) were developed in an attempt to further reduce complications associated with central venous access.[16] These devices consist of a Silastic catheter attached to a port with a self-sealing silicone septum. ICVADs are available with one or two ports, in titanium or plastic. The port is implanted subcutaneously and is accessed with the use of a specially designed noncoring needle known as a *Huber needle*. This needle has a deflected point and an opening on the sidewall to avoid taking a core of silicone from the diaphragm during each puncture. The integrity of the septum is maintained for 1500 to 2000 cannulations. A 90° Huber needle is used for continuous infusion. Because they are totally implanted, ICVADs eliminate the need for daily catheter care. When not in use, the system requires flushing every 4 to 8 weeks. Catheter obstruction by thrombosis is rare when an adequate protocol for catheter care is maintained.

There has been a resurgence in use of of the PICC. The standard PICCs are available in 4F or 5F, single or double lumen, and with or without a Groshong valve. A modification of this is the peripheral implantable port (Port-a-Cath PAS Port; Deltec Inc., St Paul, MN). The PAS (peripheral access system) Port is smaller than other systems (5.6 g in weight, 26.7 mm in length, 16.5 mm in width, 7.4 mm in height, and 6.6 mm in diameter for the self-sealing silicone septum). The device consists of a miniature titanium port and a 5.8F polyurethane catheter specifically designed for forearm implantation. These devices have been used for the infusion of chemotherapeutics, antibiotics, antivirals, antifungals, and blood products. A Cath-Finder (Smith's Medical MD Inc., St Paul, MN) tracking system has been developed to aid catheter placement.[29] Winters and associates[30] reported the use of the P.A.S. Port in 14 patients. There were 19 complications in 14 patients (3.88 per 1000 catheter days), with an infection rate of 3% (0.2 per catheter days), port-pocket cellulitis in 3% (0.2 per catheter days), phlebitis in 12.5% (0.8 per 1000 catheter days), and thrombosis in 6.2% (0.4 per 1000 catheter days). Johnson and Didlake[31] reported on 61 P.A.S. Port devices placed in 56 patients. The patients had a 13.1% complication rate, a 6.6% infection rate, and a median event-free patency of 278 days. Although the authors report the PICC ports to be less expensive and comparable to standard subcutaneous ports, the experiences reported in the literature involve small patient populations.

Choice of Device

Broviac and Hickman catheters are similar, with the main difference being size. The Hickman catheter, with its larger ID, is more durable. Complication rates are similar.

Pasquale and associates[32] compared Groshong with Hickman catheters and found no significant difference in septic complications and thrombus formation but found catheter malfunction rates higher with Groshong catheters.

The decision of whether to place a transcutaneous catheter or an ICVAD depends on several factors. Both systems allow for simultaneous venous access. For example, if the patient requires chemotherapy and hyperalimentation, a multilumen catheter or a double-port ICVAD can be placed. There are certain situations when one method of venous access is preferred over the other. If the vascular access device is to be used for a short period of time (ie, <3 months), a catheter should be used; they are easier to insert and remove. Catheters are easy to access through a Luer fitting at the end of the external portion of the catheter. It is simple to instruct patients in how to access them, and for frequent home use, the transcutaneous catheter is probably the device of choice. They also do not require a needle for access, which is an advantage for health care personnel, who may be required to access ICVADs in patients who have, for example, tested positive for human immunodeficiency virus.

Catheters are often preferred in children because cannulation of the port may be problematic. The avoidance of a needle is more acceptable both to the patient and to medical personnel, who may otherwise have to struggle with an uncooperative child while attempting to access a port with a needle. In a prospective comparison of totally implanted devices with external catheters in pediatric patients, the ports were easier to care for and more readily accepted by patients but only in children older than 11 years.[33] Another advantage is the almost complete absence of drug extravasation. In every report of experience with implantable ports, there is a small (approximately 5%) incidence of drug extravasation caused by the difficulty of accessing ports, particularly in obese patients or because the needle backs out of the rubber septum after having been accessed correctly. The need to anchor the port against bony structures to resist the pressure required for needle access makes the transcutaneous catheter more desirable in obese patients.

The major drawback of the transcutaneous catheter is the external component, which requires constant care, alters the patient's self-image, and can be caught and dislodged or torn. A damaged catheter may be repaired using a kit that is appropriate for the size of the catheter. A dislodged catheter should be removed and, if necessary, replaced.

Subcutaneous ports have the advantage of requiring less maintenance. The *port-catheter* system is totally implantable. It requires no care by the patient when it is not in use. There is no external portion that can be damaged or dislodged. It interferes minimally with self-image, allows almost unlimited normal activity, and is ideal for intermittent long-term therapy. ICVADs appear to have increased longevity,[34] lower complication rates,[33-35] and improved cosmetic appearance. The disadvantages are that they are more difficult to insert and remove, require trained personnel and a special needle to access the device, and require repeated punctures through the skin. Health care personnel are intended to intermittently access these devices. Continuous infusion via the port-catheter system requires the prolonged placement of a Huber needle. Unless the needle site is changed at least weekly, infection and necrosis around the needle site occur, exposing the port and necessitating explanation.

Withdrawal of blood for sampling can be accomplished through ICVADs. Often, the ability to withdraw blood is lost a short time after implantation. This loss may result from the catheter tip lodging against the vessel wall or the development of a fibrin sheath that acts as a one-way valve. Ease of blood sampling is also compromised by the narrow lumen of the 19-gauge Huber needle used to access implantable ports. The port must be carefully flushed with heparinized saline after blood sampling.

Infection rates are often cited as reasons to recommend one device over the other. Traditionally, the risk of infection associated with the use of a particular catheter has been expressed as the number of catheter related blood-stream infections (CRBSIs) per 100 devices used. More recently, however, the Centers for Disease Control and Prevention has recommended that this should be reported as CRBSIs per 1000 intravascular device (IVD)-days. The advantage of this classification is apparent when comparing to short-term central venous catheters, with the risk of CRBSIs per 100 devices used being dramatically higher. When described in terms of CRBSIs per 1000 IVD-days, however, this risk proves to actually be considerably lower. Infection rates for transcutaneous catheters are difficult to compare directly with rates for implantable port-catheter systems. Infections of the pocket and the port are seen only with the port-catheter systems, while exit-site infection and tunnel infection are seen only with transcutaneous catheters. However, the risk of either bacteremia or fungemia occurring with the use of tunneled catheters has been reported at 34% with CRBSI per 1000 IVD-days of 2.14, with the corresponding risk associated with the use of implanted ports reported as 4% with CRBSI per 1000 IVD-days of 0.096. Overall risk of infection has been reported as high as 43% versus 8% with respective CRBSIs per 1000 IVD-days of 2.767 and 0.211, respectively.[36] These differences are less pronounced in certain patient groups, including those with cancer and other causes of neutropenia.[30] It is reasonable, then, that the risk of infection should influence the choice of catheter utilized.

There is some controversy regarding whether ports or catheters are better for the infusion of hyperalimentation. Many argue that the hyperalimentation fluid in the infusion port may increase the risk of infection. One series found that an infection rate of 23% in patients receiving home parenteral nutrition through a subcutaneously implanted catheter versus 10% in patients receiving this therapy through a tunneled catheter.[37] This is contradicted by the work of Pomp et al.,[4] who found a 13% infection rate with ports compared with the 11% to 42% infection rate with Hickman catheters previously reported in the literature. Because most patients on TPN require daily catheter use for prolonged periods of time, multiple punctures of the skin and port would be required if an ICVAD is used for this purpose. This practice could result in skin breakdown, which may possibly explain the increased infection rates. In addition, the risk of extravasation of hyperosmolar TPN fluid is higher with ports than with catheters.

It is difficult to determine the superiority of subcutaneous ports over catheters, or vice versa. The device chosen should be tailored to the needs of the patient, with the advantages and disadvantages of each weighed.

Catheter Placement

Two techniques have been described for catheter insertion: (1) the *cutdown* method using the cephalic, internal, or external jugular vein as described by Heimbach and Ivey[23] and (2) the *percutaneous* method using a guidewire and peel-away introducer described by Cohen and Wood.[38] The latter technique may substantially reduce operating time at the expense of the potential complications of pneumothorax, hemothorax, vascular trauma, thoracic duct injuries, and bleeding.

The choice of cutdown versus percutaneous catheter placement should be individualized based on the patient's body habitus, venous anatomy, and coagulation status. The cutdown method may be preferred in the obese patient and in patients with thrombocytopenia or coagulopathy.

Often venous access in the upper torso is precluded because of anatomic constraints, such as burns to the upper body, cervicothoracic trauma, planned radiation therapy to the mediastinum, bilateral radical neck dissection, infected median sternotomy incisions, and venous thrombosis. In addition, the long-term presence of central venous catheters may lead to the formation of fibrin sheaths with subsequent stenosis of the vessel. Venous occlusion may also occur when these lines become infected, rendering the vessel unusable.[9] In these circumstances, cannulation of the inferior vena cava can be successfully performed.[39,40] The access is obtained by saphenous vein cutdown with a subcutaneous tunnel to the abdominal wall. The catheter tip is placed below the renal veins. Infection rates have been comparable with those of catheters placed in the superior vena cava; however, there appears to be an increased risk of iliofemoral thrombosis. Williard and colleagues[40] reported on 31 catheters placed infraumbilically in 26 patients and found a statistically significant difference in central vein thrombosis compared with catheters placed in the superior vena cava (13% versus 1.5%). It is not clear whether these patients would benefit from low-level anticoagulation.

Successful translumbar insertion of an inferior vena cava Hickman catheter has been reported in two patients with thrombosis of the upper great vessels.[41] The translumbar approach has also been used for placement of central venous catheters into the azygous vein either directly[29] or through ascending lumbar veins.[42] Other strategies include cannulation of a hepatic vein[43] or the gonadal vessels[44] via a retroperitoneal approach in patients with thrombosis of both the superior vena cava and bilateral iliofemoral veins.

Patients who have had previously placed central lines often have clinically silent venous thrombosis. To avoid this problem, these patients can be evaluated preoperatively with Doppler ultrasonic imaging of vascular structures.[31]

Traditionally, surgeons have placed long-term central venous access catheters in the operating room; however, there have been reports of catheter placement by interventional radiologists in the radiology suite. Morris and associates[45] reported on the successful placement of 102 infusion ports in the interventional radiology suite. They report major complications in 13.6% (0.88 per 1000 access days), catheter-related infection in 5% (0.31 per 1000 access days), and refractory thrombosis rates of 4% (0.25 per 1000 access days). These results are comparable to those of surgically placed ports.

Although central venous catheters are placed in the emergency department, the operating room, interventional radiology suite, and other inpatient and outpatient locations, it is essential to follow strict aseptic precautions in all. The practitioners should wear caps, masks, sterile gowns and gloves. The patient should be prepared and draped as for a major operation. These precautions significantly lower catheter infections.

Placement Techniques

The most common sites for open insertion of long-term venous catheters are the external jugular vein, the internal jugular vein, the cephalic vein at the deltopectoral groove, and the saphenous vein near its junction with the femoral vein. The most common sites for percutaneous insertion of long-term venous access devices are the internal jugular, external jugular, subclavian, and femoral veins. All of these procedures can be performed with the patient under local anesthetic with or without intravenous sedation. General anesthesia is not necessary but may be warranted in selected cases. We prefer to perform these procedures in a formal operating room where aseptic techniques are optimized.

Preoperative neck examination of the patient is very important. Patients with mass lesions near the thoracic inlet or with evidence of previous venipuncture in the neck may have a partial thrombosis or stenosis of the ipsilateral neck veins. It is also important to know whether the patient has had previous surgery on the neck, because the external jugular vein may have been ligated. Cannulation of ipsilateral neck veins should be avoided in patients with upper extremity AV fistulas for hemodialysis.

Cutdown Techniques

External Jugular Vein

Preoperative neck examination of the patient is performed to assess the size and location of the external jugular veins. A simple Valsalva maneuver distends the neck veins and provides a good idea of the size and branching of the vein. The patient is placed in the Trendelenburg position. After the appropriate injection of a local anesthetic agent, a 1- to 2-cm incision is made transversely over the visible external jugular vein, approximately 1 to 3 cm above the clavicle. The platysma is divided, and the vein is skeletonized by blunt and sharp dissection. At this time, it is wise to ligate any collateral veins to prevent unwanted bleeding or catheter placement into a tributary that will not lead centrally. A 2-cm segment of vein is isolated between two untied silk sutures. Attention is then turned to the catheter exit site for the catheter or implantable disk. The customary location is on the anterior chest wall, inferior to the cutdown site. This is generally 2 cm above the point that is midway between the lateral border of the sternum

and the areola. In females, a higher and more lateral position is occasionally required to avoid breast tissue. For a Broviac or Hickman type of catheter, a stab incision is made after the injection of a local anesthetic agent. For the implantable disk, a 3- to 4-cm transverse incision is made. The pocket for the disk is usually made cephalad to its incision and should be large enough for the entire disk to fit above (or below) the incision. The disk, now attached to its catheter or the external catheter, is flushed with heparinized saline.

The local anesthetic agent is then injected subcutaneously from the exit-site incision to the external jugular vein cutdown site. Using the tunneling device included with most catheter kits, the catheter is brought subcutaneously to the external jugular vein site in the neck. The Dacron cuff of the external catheter is placed approximately 1 cm proximal to the stab incision. Catheter length is determined by laying the catheter along the sternum and cutting it at Louis' angle (the junction of the manubrium to the sternum), which marks the usual junction of the superior vena cava and the right atrium.

The cephalad side of the external jugular vein can now be tied with the previously placed silk suture, and then a small venotomy is made. The catheter can be placed through the venotomy and advanced. The catheter should pass easily. Occasionally, it is necessary for the patient to turn his or her head to the left or right to facilitate insertion. The catheter is checked for adequate backflow of blood, flushed with heparinized saline, and tied in place with the previously placed silk suture. A portable chest radiograph (if fluoroscopy is not used) is obtained at this time to document central placement of the catheter in the superior vena cava.

The external catheter is sutured to the chest wall at its junction with the skin. The implantable disk is sutured to the fascia of the pectoralis major muscle (not merely to the subcutaneous fat) with at least three nonabsorbable sutures, which ensure that the disk does not migrate or invert to an upside-down position that makes access impossible. The pocket incision is then closed in two layers with absorbable sutures. The neck wound is closed with absorbable sutures, also in two layers, and ensures that the platysma is closed. An upright chest radiograph is taken to confirm catheter position and absence of pneumothorax. The catheter may then be used immediately.

Internal Jugular Vein

The internal jugular vein is isolated in the anterior neck between the sternal and clavicular heads of the sternocleidomastoid muscle. A 3- to 4-cm incision is made here, approximately 2 cm above the clavicle. The platysma is divided, and using blunt dissection, the internal jugular vein is exposed. It is important to divide all of the fibers around the adventitia of the vein and to clearly isolate the vein wall, preventing a posterior vein injury. The internal jugular vein may be quite large; therefore, meticulous dissection to completely isolate the vein is mandatory. Posterior internal jugular vein injuries result in hemorrhage that is difficult to control. Again, the vein is isolated between two heavy silk sutures. At this point, the operator must decide if a purse-string suture around the impending venotomy will be used or if the cephalic portion of the vein will simply be ligated. If the vein will be ligated, the opposite internal jugular vein must be intact. If the opposite vein is patent, the internal jugular vein may be safely ligated. If ligation is not possible, a 4-0 or 5-0 monofilament, nonabsorbable purse-string suture is placed around the potential venotomy site. The remaining procedure is performed in the same manner as for external jugular vein catheter placement.

Cephalic Vein

The usual location for the cephalic vein cutdown is in the deltopectoral groove. The antecubital fossa location of the cephalic vein is best reserved for placement of the PICCs. The cephalic vein lies in the groove formed at the junction of the deltoid and pectoralis major muscle where the humerus meets the clavicle. After injecting a local anesthetic agent, a 3-cm incision is made in the deltopectoral groove. The vein is usually found at the base of this groove, on top of the muscle fascia and below the subcutaneous fat. Again, a 2-cm segment of vein is isolated between two silk ties in preparation for cannulation. The catheter exit or port site is determined and completed in the exact manner as previously described. The catheter is measured, tunneled, and placed into the cephalic vein and advanced centrally. This technique is probably best performed with the aid of C-arm fluoroscopy, because the cephalic vein cutdown is a more peripheral site and catheter placement up the neck veins or other collaterals is possible. The closure is performed as previously described.

Saphenous Vein

For placement of a central, long-term venous access catheter or port via the lower extremity, a saphenous vein cutdown near the groin is performed. The saphenous position allows easy access to the femoral vein without exposing the femoral vein itself. Radiographic control with C-arm fluoroscopy and a small amount of radiopaque contrast material is helpful for correct positioning of the catheter below the renal veins. The groin, ipsilateral abdomen, and chest are prepped. A 2- to 3-cm longitudinal incision is made approximately two finger-breadths medial and two finger-breadths inferior to the femoral pulse in the upper medial thigh. The saphenous vein is dissected free of surrounding tissues, and a 2-cm segment is isolated between two silk sutures. This portion of the saphenous vein should be well below its junction with the femoral vein.

After isolation of the vein, the exit site for the catheter or port must be prepared. In general, the exit site should be above the groin. The ipsilateral chest wall provides a clean and stable site that also allows for easy use and care by the patient. The position on the chest wall lies several centimeters above the costal margin in the anterior axillary line. A simple stab incision for a catheter and a 3- to 4-cm incision for a port pocket are made. The catheter is tunneled from the chest wall to the groin cutdown site, and an appropriate length is measured. The tip of the catheter is usually placed

below the renal veins. A rough measure of this position is cutting the tunneled catheter on the anterior abdominal wall at a point 2 to 3 cm above the umbilicus. The catheter is placed into a saphenous venotomy and threaded in completely. Here, the C-arm fluoroscopy is valuable for correct placement. Exit site closure, vein site closure, and catheter or port securement are completed in the manners already described.

Percutaneous Technique

Percutaneous kits are available for Broviac, Hickman, and port catheters. These kits include a peel-away sheath introducer with vessel dilator, 12-ml disposable syringe, 18- or 19-gauge 2-inch extra-thin-walled needle, 50-cm (0.38- or 0.32-inch) Flexible stainless steel J-shaped guidewire with tip straightener, 33-cm tunneler, clamp or clamps, and injection cap or caps.

Subclavian Vein

The curve of the left subclavian vein is much less acute than that of the right subclavian vein and should be selected unless the patient has had previous left clavicular fracture or a previous left subclavian venous device. For subclavian vessel cannulation, the patient is positioned with a towel roll placed vertically between the shoulder blades to drop the shoulders back. The patient is placed in the supine position. The neck and periclavicular area are cleaned and sterilely draped. The point along the clavicle approximately two thirds the distance from the sternal notch is located. This point is usually at the deltopectoral groove. The area 2 cm inferior to this point along the clavicle is infiltrated with local anesthetic agent. The patient is then placed in the Trendelenburg position to avoid air embolus. An 18-gauge (or a 19-gauge), thin-walled needle is percutaneously introduced into the subclavian vein infraclavicularly with the needle perpendicular to the sagittal plane and parallel to the coronal plane, directed slightly above the sternal notch. The subclavian vein is located between the clavicle and the first rib. Care is taken to avoid the subclavian artery, which is located posterosuperior to the vein. When venous blood is aspirated, the flexible stainless steel J-shaped guidewire is threaded through the needle. The guidewire is stabilized, and the needle is removed. The position of the guidewire is verified with fluoroscopy. A small incision is made in the skin adjacent to the wire.

For placement of a long-term venous catheter, the next step is to locate and create the exit site of the catheter. As previously described, this site is usually 3 to 4 cm inferior to the initial venipuncture site. In females, care is taken to avoid placing the exit site in the breast tissue. After the appropriate administration of a local anesthetic agent, the tunneling device is then used to create a subcutaneous tunnel between the exit and venipuncture sites. The catheter is connected to the tunneling device and introduced from the exit site to the initial venipuncture site. The catheter is positioned so that the Dacron cuff is located in the tunnel. Placement of the Dacron cuff only 2 cm within the subcutaneous tunnel facilitates eventual catheter removal. The catheter is cut to length so that the tip is located at the junction of the superior vena cava and right atrium. The dilator is placed over the guidewire only about 3 to 4 cm through the skin. The purpose of the dilator is to dilate the subcutaneous tissues. It should not be placed to the hilt. The guidewire should move easily through the dilator at all times. After initial dilation, the peel-away sheath introducer with dilator is threaded over the guidewire. Again, the dilator and overlying sheath are inserted only 4 to 5 cm together over the guidewire. The sheath is then inserted to the hilt while maintaining the dilator and guidewire stationary. The guidewire and the dilator are removed. Free venous backflow should be noticed at this point. The catheter is then placed into the introducer sheath. Once the catheter is fully introduced, the peel-away introducer sheath is divided and removed.

Fluoroscopy or plain radiographs are used to confirm the location of the catheter tip. The initial venipuncture site is closed with absorbable suture followed by Steri-Strips (3M Corp., St Paul, MN). The catheter exit site is secured with nonabsorbable suture. All catheter lumens are then flushed with heparinized saline, and sterile dressings are dressed.

For implantable port placement, the port site is determined after the guidewire is introduced into the vein. The port is usually placed between the midclavicular line and the lateral border of the sternum, approximately 2 to 4 cm inferior to the clavicle. In females, the port is often placed higher and more lateral to avoid the breast tissue. For cosmetic purposes, it is preferred to avoid placing the port too high or next to the sternal notch. The catheter is tunneled to the venipuncture site and trimmed to the proper length. The peel-away sheath introducer with dilator is threaded over the guidewire. The guidewire and dilator are then removed, and the surgeon's thumb or other digit is placed over the end of the peel-away sheath catheter. Good venous backflow should be noticed at this point. The catheter is placed through the introducer sheath, and the peel-away introducer sheath is divided and removed. The venipuncture site is sutured with absorbable sutures and dressed with Steri-Strips. The port site is then checked for hemostasis. The port is secured to the pectoralis fascia at three sites using nonabsorbable suture. The subcutaneous tissues are closed with absorbable suture, and the skin is reapproximated. The port is punctured through the skin using the Huber needle. Good venous blood should be aspirated and then the port flushed with heparinized saline. Sterile dressings are then placed. Fluoroscopy or plain radiographs are used to confirm the location of the tip of the catheter in the superior vena cava.

Internal Jugular Vein

For percutaneous placement into the internal jugular vein, a towel roll should be placed transversely across the shoulders to extend the neck. Carotid pulsations should be palpated. The vein is located in a coronal plane posterior to the sternocleidomastoid muscle above the first rib insertion of the scalenus anticus and parallel to the axis of the sternocleidomastoid. The internal jugular vein is most easily accessed at the apex of the triangle formed by the sternal and clavicular heads of the sternocleidomastoid muscle. The vein is located with a 22-gauge needle initially before cannulation with the larger 18-gauge needle, which accommodates the guidewire. The initial direction of the needle is lateral to the carotid artery, 30° to the sagittal plane, and parallel to the coronal plane, aiming toward the ipsilateral nipple. Once the vein is cannulated, the guidewire is introduced and the needle is removed. The remainder of the procedure is similar to that described earlier.

Femoral Vein

For percutaneous placement into the femoral vein, the groin and ipsilateral abdomen and lower chest are cleaned and draped. The femoral artery is palpated. The femoral vein is located medial to the femoral artery. Once the femoral vein is entered, the guidewire is introduced and the needle is removed. For long-term catheter devices, the catheter exit site may be located in the lower abdomen. A technique similar to that described previously is followed. For implantable ports, the port site should be located on a firm surface, such as the lower chest wall.

Peripherally Inserted Central Venous Silicone Elastomer Catheter Lines

The placement of PICC lines is performed using sterile technique. The nondominant arm is preferred unless otherwise contraindicated. A 4-cm transverse incision is made in the antecubital fossa 2 to 3 cm distal to the elbow crease. The antecubital venous complex is visualized, and a branch communicating with the basilic vein is selected for cannulation. The cephalic vein is used if the basilic vein cannot be cannulated. Catheter position is confirmed using an electromagnetic tracking system (Cath-Finder) that is preassembled with the PAS Port catheter. The locator wand of the unit indicates the initial course of the catheter and confirms ultimate tip position. When the catheter is in the desired location, the sensing wire is removed, the catheter is cut to length, and the system is completed by attaching the catheter to the connector ring mechanism of the port. The port and catheter are flushed with heparinized saline using a Huber needle. The port is positioned in a subcutaneous pocket in the volar surface of the forearm. All incisions are closed with absorbable suture.

Placement Under Radiographic Guidance

Ultrasound

In 1990, Lameris et al[46] reported a decrease of complications associated with subclavian vein cannulization from 10% to 0% when ultrasound was used to visualize the vessel. That same year, Mallory et al. reported a decrease in the failure rate of internal jugular catheter placement from 35% to 0% when ultrasound was used.[28] Since that time the use of sonographic guidance for visualization of the subclavian vein before or during line placement has not been widely adopted. By contrast, in many institutions it has become standard in the catheterization of the internal jugular vein. The reader is referred to guidelines from Institute of Medicine of the National Academies.[47] The primary advantages of the use of ultrasound for the placement of central venous catheters include the safety associated with direct visualization of the vessel without making an incision, shorter operating time, and decreased complications with lower failure rates. These advantages, however, are dependent upon the experience and competence of the individual performing the procedure. In addition, use of ultrasound frequently requires the participation of a second, similarly skilled surgeon.

Fluoroscopy

The placement of central venous catheters under fluoroscopic guidance saw its advent in 1989 when Robertson et al. reported their experience with 60 catheters placed utilizing this strategy.[48] The advantages of employing this modality are significant: cannulation of the vein may be immediately confirmed by venography instead of relying on the visual characteristics of the withdrawn blood. Likewise, the appropriate length of catheter needed can be directly measured as opposed to using the surgeon's estimate. Using fluoroscopy, complications of line placement such as pneumothorax, bleeding and malpositioning, although equivalent to traditional methods in occurrence, may be promptly identified and expeditiously addressed. However, the procedure requires the availability of costly equipment and is again highly dependent upon the experience of the operator. Nevertheless, the use of fluoroscopy in the placement of long-term central venous catheters has become widespread and is the method of choice in many major institutions.

▨ Concluding Remarks

Long-term venous access devices provide safe and effective means of central venous access. Placement technology continues to advance to allow for safe implantation of these devices.

REFERENCES

1. Ries CA, et al. Arteriovenous fistulas for vascular access in patients with hematologic disorders. *N Engl J Med.* 1976;295:342.
2. Engels LGJ, et al. Home parenteral nutrition via arteriovenous fistulae. *JPEN.* 1983;7:412.
3. Wobbes T, et al. Five years' experience in access surgery for polychemotherapy. *Cancer.* 1983;52:978.
4. Pomp A, Caldwell MD, Albina JE. Subcutaneous infusion ports for administration of parenteral nutrition at home. *Surg Gynecol Obstet.* 1989;169:329.
5. Chinitz JL, Yokoyama T, Bower R. Self sealing prosthesis for arteriovenous fistula in man. *Trans Am Soc Artif Intern Organs.* 1972;18:452.
6. Dardik H, Ibrahim M, Baier R. Human umbilical cord-a source for vascular prosthesis. *JAMA.* 1976;236:2859.
7. Raaf JH. Vascular access grafts for chemotherapy: Use in forty patients at M.D. Anderson Hospital. *Ann Surg.* 1979;190:614.
8. Gordon HE. Historical development of vascular access procedures. In Wilson SE (ed). *Vascular Access Surgery.* 2nd ed. St. Louis, MO: Mosby, 1988.
9. Falk A, et al. Placement of tunneled hemodialysis catheters across stenotic and occluded central veins. *J Vasc Access.* 2003;4:3.
10. Aubaniac R. L'injection intraveineuse sous-claviculaire: Avantages et technique. *Presse Med.* 1952;60:1456.
11. Kerri-Szantu M. The subclavian vein, a constant and convenient intravenous injection site. *Arch Surg.* 1956;72:179.
12. Seldinger SI. Catheter replacement of the needle in percutaneous arteriography. *Acta Radiol (Stockh).* 1953;39:368.
13. Dudrick SJ, Wilmore DW, Vars HM, Rhoads JE. Long-term total parenteral nutrition with growth development and positive nitrogen balance. *Surgery.* 1968;64:134.
14. Broviac JW, Cole JJ, Scribner BH. A silicone rubber atrial catheter for prolonged parenteral alimentation. *Surg Gynecol Obstet.* 1973;136:602.
15. Hickman RO, et al. A modified right atrial catheter for access to the venous system in marrow transplant recipients. *Surg Gynecol Obstet.* 1979;148:871.
16. Niederhuber JE, et al. Totally implanted venous and arterial access system to replace external catheters in cancer treatment. *Surgery.* 1982;92:706.
17. Horshal VL. Total intravenous nutrition with peripherally inserted silicone elastomer central venous catheters. *Arch Surg.* 1975;110:644.
18. Bottino J, et al. Long-term intravenous therapy with peripherally inserted silicone elastomer central venous catheters in patients with malignant diseases. *Cancer.* 1979;43:1937.
19. MacDonald AS, Master SKP, Moffitt EA. A comparative study of peripherally inserted silicone catheters for parenteral nutrition. *Can Anaesth Soc J.* 1977;24:263.
20. Jaques PF, Mauro MA, Keefe B: Ultrasound guidance for vascular access: Technical note. *J Vasc Intern Radiol.* 1992;3:427.
21. Stenquist O, et al. Stiffness of central venous catheters. *Acta Anaesthesiol Scand.* 1983;27:153.
22. Welch GW, et al. The role of catheter composition in the development of thrombophlebitis. *Surg Gynecol Obstet.* 1974;138:421.
23. Heimbach DM, Ivey TD. Technique for placement of a permanent home hyperalimentation catheter. *Surg Gynecol Obstet.* 1976; 143:634.
24. Wagman LD, Kirkemo A, Johnston MR. Venous access: A prospective, randomized study of the Hickman catheter. *Surgery.* 1983;95:303.
25. Forssmann W. Die Sondierung des rechten Herzens. *Klin Wochenschr.* 1929;8:2085.
26. Sitges-Serra A, Linares J. Tunnels do not protect against venous catheter related sepsis. *Lancet.* 1984;1:459.
27. Sitges-Serra A, Linares J, Garan J. Catheter sepsis: The clue is the hub. *Surgery.* 1985;97:355.
28. Mallory DL, et al. Ultrasound improves the success rate of internal jugular vein cannulation: A prospective, randomized trial. *Chest.* 1990;98:157.
29. Pearl JM, Goldstein L, Ciresi KF. Improved methods in long term venous access using the P.A.S. port. *Surg Gynecol Obstet.* 1991; 173:313.
30. Winters V, et al. A trial with a new peripheral implanted vascular access device. *Oncol Nurs Forum.* 1990;17:891.
31. Johnson JA, Didlake RH. Peripherally-placed central venous access ports: Clinical and laboratory observations. *Am Surg.* 1994; 60:915.
32. Pasquale MD, Campbell JM, Magnant CM. Groshong versus Hickman catheters. *Surg Gynecol Obstet.* 1992;174:408.
33. Ross MN, et al. Comparison of totally implanted reservoirs with external catheters as venous access devices in pediatric oncologic patients. *Surg Gynecol Obstet.* 1988;167:141.
34. Stanislav GV, et al. Reliability of implantable central venous access device in patients with cancer. *Arch Surg.* 1987;122:1280.
35. Shaw JHF, Douglas R, Wilson T. Clinical performance of Hickman and Portacath atrial catheters. *Aust NZ J Surg.* 1988;58:657.
36. Groeger, JS, et al. Infectious morbidity associated with long-term use of venous access devices in patients with cancer. *Ann Intern Med.* 1993; 119:1168.
37. Mueller BU, et al. A prospective randomized trial comparing the infectious and noninfectious complications of an externalized catheter versus a subcutaneously implanted device in cancer patients. *J Clin Oncol.* 1993;10:1943.
38. Cohen AM, Wood WC: Simplified technique for placement of long term central venous silicone catheters. *Surg Gynecol Obstet.* 1982; 154:721.
39. Curtas S, Bonaventura M, Meguid MM: Cannulation of inferior vena cava for long term central venous access. *Surg Gynecol Obstet.* 1989; 68:121.
40. Williard W, et al. Long-term vascular access via the inferior vena cava. *J Surg Oncol.* 1991;46:162.
41. Denny DF, et al. Translumbar inferior vena cava Hickman catheter replacement for total parenteral nutrition. *AJR.* 1987;148:621.

42. Jaber MR, et al. Azygous vein dialysis catheter placement using the translumbar approach in a patient with inferior vena cava occlusion. *Cardiovasc Intervent Radiol.* 2008;31:S206.

43. Crummy A, et al. Percutaneous transhepatic placement of a Hickman catheter. *Am J Roentgenol.* 1998;153:1317.

44. Coit DG, Turnbull ADM: Long-term central vascular access through the gonadal vein. *Surg Gynecol Obstet.* 1992;175:362.

45. Morris SL, Jacques PF, Mauro MA. Radiology assisted placement of implantable subcutaneous infusion ports for long-term venous access. *Radiology.* 1992;184:149.

46. Lameris JS, et al. Percutaneous placement of Hickman catheters: comparison of sonographically-guided and blind techniques. *Am J Roentgenol.* 1990;155:1097.

47. Kohn LT, Corrigan JM, Donaldson MS (eds). *To Err Is Human: Building a Safer Health System.* Committee on Quality in America, Institute of Medicine. Washington, DC: National Academy Press, 2000.

48. Robertson LJ, et al. Radiologic placement of Hickman catheters. *Radiology.* 1989;170:1007.

CHAPTER 36

Vascular Access for Trauma, Emergency Surgery, and Critical Care

Richard Brad Cook and Jonathan R. Hiatt

Appropriate vascular access is essential for treatment of trauma victims, patients undergoing emergency surgery, and critically ill patients who require intensive care. Both venous and arterial access are often needed for acute resuscitation, administration of medications, physiologic monitoring, sampling of arterial and venous blood, dialysis and hemofiltration, and parenteral nutrition.

The clinician must determine the need for vascular access procedures in various settings and weigh the attendant risks and benefits. In the emergency department, the physician must select appropriate infusion catheters for resuscitation based on the location and severity of injury. In the intensive care unit (ICU) and before beginning in the operating room, catheters must be selected to monitor and optimize resuscitation.

This chapter considers the clinical indications, techniques for placement, and potential complications of invasive lines and monitors. A proper understanding of the risks and benefits of vascular access is vital for decision making in the emergency department and ICU. Informed consent should be obtained whenever possible before undertaking these invasive procedures.

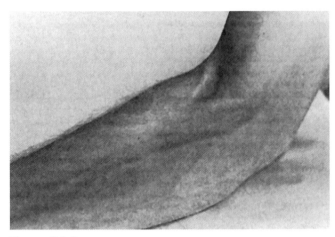

Figure 36-1.
Veins in the antecubital fossa represent access sites of first choice for trauma resuscitation.

Trauma

Optimal management of the trauma victim requires rapid resuscitation followed by diagnosis and treatment of injuries. The mechanism and extent of injuries determine the relative importance of each of these efforts. Although two intravenous lines and a blood sample for cross-match may be all that are required for the emergency department's evaluation of a patient with penetrating trauma to the lower abdomen, this workup would be inadequate for a patient who has sustained high-energy blunt trauma with a large spectrum of potential injuries. For head trauma, monitoring of central venous and arterial blood pressures are necessary for goal-directed resuscitation. Major vascular injuries, such as an aortic transection, may require arterial pressure monitoring above and below the diaphragm.

After securing the airway and assuring adequate oxygenation and ventilation, the foremost priority in the care of the trauma victim is to restore circulation. Outcome from trauma depends on the timely restoration of normal intravascular volume.[1] Isotonic crystalloid fluid resuscitation is the current standard approach in the United States,

although research with hypertonic saline solution is ongoing.[2] Therefore, vascular access that allows rapid volume administration must be obtained quickly and safely. The first initial approach is to obtain two large-bore (16-gauge or larger) intravenous catheters in a peripheral upper extremity vein. The preferred location is within the antecubital fossa (Fig. 36-1). Other accessible veins are located at the wrist, the dorsum of the hand, and the saphenous vein in the leg.

Simultaneous access should be attempted by at least two qualified providers. A standard 16- or 14-gauge angiocatheter can allow respective flow rates of up to 370 to 410 mL/min and 490 to 580 mL/min when infused using a commercial rapid infusion system.[3] Although peripheral venous access may be obtained rapidly and avoids the potential complications of central access, venous infiltration and extravasation into soft tissues can occur more easily than with central venous cannulation with potential risk of compartment syndrome. Peripheral catheters should be avoided in any crushed, burned, or fractured extremity.

When the patient exhibits signs of hemorrhagic shock or when two reliable large-bore intravenous catheters cannot be obtained, alternative forms of access are needed. We favor percutaneous cannulation of the femoral vein with a trauma infusion catheter as a first choice (Fig. 36-2). Rapid infusion catheters specifically designed for trauma resusci-

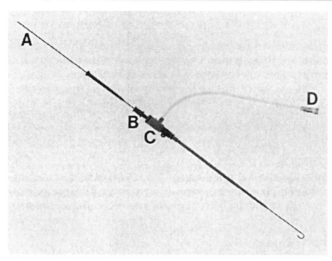

Figure 36-2.
Components of trauma infusion catheter. *A,* Guidewire. *B,* Dilator. *C,* Introducer sheath. *D,* Intravenous aspiration and infusion port.

tation are available in 7.5 to 8.5 French sizes and provide flow rates of approximately 450 to 500 mL/min when used with a pressure bag or rapid infusion device.

Femoral venous cannulation can be performed safely and rapidly in experienced hands using the Seldinger technique (Fig. 36-3).[4] If possible, the leg is abducted and externally rotated to optimize access to the femoral vessels. The right leg provides easiest access for a right-handed operator. The

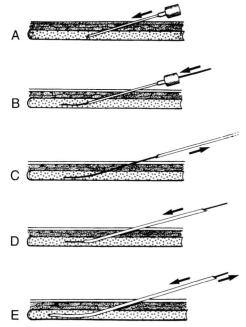

Figure 36-3.
The Seldinger technique for the placement of intravascular catheters. *A,* A needle is used to locate the vessel to be cauterized. *B,* A guidewire is threaded through the needle and into the vessel. *C,* The needle is withdrawn while stabilizing the guidewire. *D,* The catheter is advanced over the guidewire using a twisting motion. *E,* The guidewire is removed, leaving the catheter in place.

infrainguinal area is prepared with chlorhexidine and draped in a sterile fashion. While the femoral artery is palpated with one hand, the introducer needle is inserted medial to the artery at a 45° angle from the skin and is directed parallel to the course of the artery below the inguinal ligament. Negative pressure is applied to the syringe until dark, nonpulsatile blood is aspirated. While the needle is anchored with one hand, the syringe is removed and a J-tipped guidewire is inserted. A small incision is made over the guidewire with a no. 11 blade scalpel and the catheter and dilator are inserted. Periodic small to-and-fro movements of the wire prevent kinking and assure safe passage as the dilator is advanced. The dilator is removed and the catheter is advanced to the hub, secured to the skin with suture, and dressed.

If arterial puncture inadvertently occurs, as evidenced by return of bright, pulsatile blood, the clinician should consider whether or not the patient will require invasive arterial monitoring or frequent arterial blood gas measurement. If so, and if time permits, he or she should open a femoral arterial catheter kit, insert the smaller femoral arterial guidewire, and proceed with arterial catheter insertion. In most instances the needle is removed from the artery and pressure is held to minimize formation of a hematoma. It is important to identify arterial puncture before dilation and cannulation with a large device.

Percutaneous cannulation of the subclavian or internal jugular vein represents an alternative method for vascular access in the trauma patient. Subclavian access carries additional risk of inadvertent entry into the pleural space and injury to the lung when compared with femoral cannulation. This risk may be increased in the trauma setting, where patient positioning and clinical conditions are often suboptimal. Consequently catheters should be placed on the side of a chest injury to avoid damaging the pleural cavity. Suspected injuries to the clavicle or subclavian vessels represent contraindications to this approach. The internal jugular vein is used rarely since most trauma patients are treated with a rigid cervical collar at the outset of management. Furthermore, placement of such a catheter in a combative patient can be hazardous.

Intraosseus infusion has been studied as a safe, easy, and effective method for vascular access in children, and newer devices are available for use in adults.[5] The intraosseus infusion system includes a 15.5 gauge specialized intraosseus needle 25 mm in length with a knob and a stylet (Fig. 36-4).[6] Preferred sites for use are 1 to 2 cm below the tibial tuberosity on the flat anteromedial surface of the tibia and 1 to 2 cm proximal to the medial malleolus on the medial aspect of the tibia. After the area is prepared in a sterile fashion and local anesthesia is instilled, the intraosseus needle is driven into the cortex of the bone using constant pressure and rotational force. Successful intraosseus puncture is indicated by a sudden loss of resistance as the cortex is penetrated. The inner stylet is then removed and replaced by a syringe that withdraws blood and confirms positioning. Saline solution should then be freely injected without any local signs of swelling, which would suggest active extravasation. All fluids and medications may be given via the intraosseus route. This technique can be learned quickly by clinicians and accomplished in less than 40 seconds, making it also suitable for prehospital access.[7]

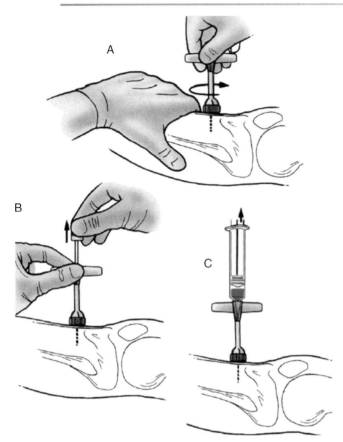

Figure 36-4.
Technique for intraosseus access. *A,* An intraosseus needle is driven into to bone using a downward twisting motion. *B,* The inner stylet is removed. *C,* Blood is withdrawn with a syringe to confirm positioning. An infusion may then be attached. (Used with permission from Reichman EF, Simon RR. *Emergency Medicine Procedures.* New York: McGraw-Hill, 2004.[6])

A venous cutdown is an alternative route for vascular access (Fig. 36-5). Although cutdown allows the placement of large-bore catheters by direct visualization, it takes rela-

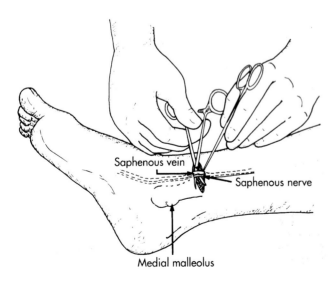

Figure 36-5.
Distal saphenous vein cutdown.

tively longer to perform when compared to percutaneous central venous access.[8] Contraindications to saphenous vein cutdown include previous saphenous vein harvest for coronary artery bypass or vascular surgery and injury proximal to or at the anticipated cutdown site.

The classic technique for venous cutdown, first described by Kirkham in 1945,[9] uses the greater saphenous vein at the ankle as the preferred site. After skin preparation and infiltration with a local anesthetic agent, a transverse incision is made 2 cm anterior to the medial malleolus of the tibia. The vein is dissected from the subcutaneous tissue and cleaned for a length of approximately 2 cm. The vein is ligated distally and controlled proximally with 2-0 silk suture. Polyethylene tubing is then cut in a gentle bevel, and a venotomy is made near the distal tie. The tubing is threaded into the vein, guided by a plastic catheter introducer if needed, and is secured using the proximal tie. It may not be possible to aspirate blood from the vein; proper positioning is confirmed on the basis of easy passage of the catheter, free and unobstructed flow of solution, and the absence of subcutaneous swelling more proximally in the leg. The skin is closed, the catheter is secured with 3-0 nylon suture, and dressings are applied.

A modified technique for venous cutdown can be performed more quickly and is technically easier than the classic approach.[10] This technique utilizes a Seldinger wire-guided dilator to access the vein for passage of an infusion catheter. After the skin is prepared and anesthetized, a transverse incision is made along the tibial surface approximately two fingerbreadths proximal to the medial malleolus. The incision should be made through the skin only as the vein is located in a superficial position. A curved hemostat may be passed along the tibia with the tip pointed against the cortex to pick up the subcutaneous tissue and greater saphenous vein. The hemostat is then turned with the tip pointing upward and opened widely so that the vein can be identified. With the vein tethered by the hemostat, a small (1 to 2 mm) venotomy is made using a no. 11 scalpel blade. A guidewire containing a mounted infusion catheter and dilator is then inserted into the vein under direct vision. The dilator and guidewire are removed followed by the hemostat, and a secure tape dressing is applied. If time permits, the skin may be closed with sutures.

With infusion catheters in place, active resuscitation can proceed. When the patient is transported to the operating room or ICU, additional vascular access may be obtained in a more controlled setting.

Emergency Surgery

When preparing a patient for an emergency operation, the physician strives to optimize hemodynamic and other physiologic parameters within the confines of the surgical disease and the associated medical problems. Hypovolemia from dehydration and sepsis are common with acute surgical disease. Proper management is directed at venous access and volume repletion with careful attention to correction of electrolyte and coagulation abnormalities. Patients with significant gastrointestinal or other bleeding require evaluation and management similar to the trauma victims, including selection and placement of catheters for resuscitation.

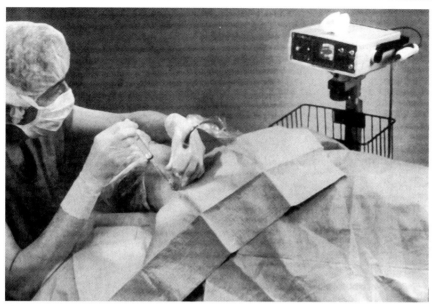

Figure 36-6.
Ultrasound-guided right internal jugular venous catheter insertion using a portable ultrasound device (Site-Rite II). (Courtesy of Dymax Corp, Pittsburgh, PA.)

Early preoperative hemodynamic optimization has demonstrated improved outcome in trauma, high-risk surgery, and sepsis.[11-13] Central venous pressure monitoring via the subclavian or internal jugular vein is the preferred method to guide preoperative resuscitation prior to emergency surgery. In addition, invasive arterial monitoring is useful for frequent assessment of arterial oxygen and carbon dioxide concentration, arterial pH, and to guide the effectiveness of vasoactive medications in real time.

Critical Care

Vascular access in the critical care setting allows for venous and arterial monitoring and provides a route for hemodialysis, administration of parenteral nutrition, and acute cardiopulmonary resuscitation. With the high acuity of illness in the modern ICU, the placement and maintenance of lines and recognition and treatment of the complications of invasive monitoring demand continuous monitoring of the patient and invasive catheters. Vascular access for hemodialysis is further described in Chapter 16.

Central Venous Access

For trauma victims and patients undergoing emergency surgery, venous access with a central catheter is the mainstay of therapy for the critically ill patient. The internal jugular vein can be cannulated using ultrasonography guidance, and this technique has resulted in reduction in the rates of unsuccessful catheterization, carotid artery puncture, and hematoma formation.[14]

For internal jugular vein catheterization, the patient is placed in the Trendelenberg position with the head turned 45° away from the site of cannulation. The skin should be prepared with chlorhexidine and barrier drapes should en-

compass the entire patient (Fig. 36-6). The physician should wear a sterile gown, gloves, hat, and mask with a face shield.[15] Important landmarks include the apex of the triangle formed by the two heads of the sternocleidomastoid muscle and the clavicle (Fig. 36-7). The internal jugular vein runs deep to the sternocleidomastoid muscle and through this triangle before joining the subclavian vein to become the brachiocephalic vein.

An ultrasound probe is used to locate the internal jugular vein and the more medial carotid artery. The carotid artery is usually smaller, deeper, pulsatile, and noncompressible when pressure is placed on the probe (Fig. 36-8).

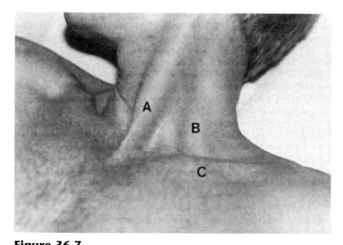

Figure 36-7.
Surface anatomy of the neck for percutaneous central venous catheterization. Sternal (A) and clavicular (B) heads of the sternocleidomastoid muscle and the clavicle form a triangle within which the internal jugular vein lies. Approach to subclavian vein is infraclavicular (C).

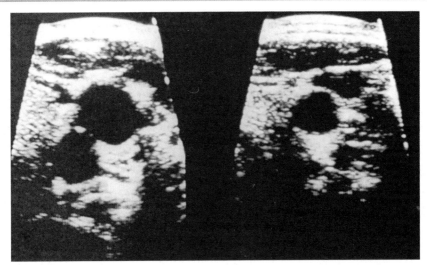

Figure 36-8.
Left, Ultrasound image of the right internal jugular vein, lying superior to the internal carotid artery. *Right,* Compression of the right internal jugular vein by the ultrasound probe. The internal carotid artery inferior to the vein remains patent.
(Courtesy of Dymax Corp, Pittsburgh, PA.)

After the skin and subcutaneous tissues are infiltrated with local anesthetic, an 18-gauge needle is inserted into the vein under direct vision. To reduce resistance, a small stab incision may be placed in the skin by a no. 11 scalpel blade before needle insertion. The vein is usually superficial and often within a depth of 1.5 cm. The needle should be inserted at 20 degrees above the plane of the skin and aimed toward the ipsilateral nipple. If an ultrasound probe is unavailable, a 22-gauge finder needle may be used to cannulate the vein while the index and middle fingers of the nondominant hand palpate the carotid artery.

For the subclavian approach, the patient is positioned and prepared in a manner similar to the internal jugular approach. A rolled towel may be placed longitudinally between the shoulder blades to open the angle between the clavicle and rib cage. The landmark for needle insertion is the infraclavicular groove, which is located between the middle and lateral one third of the clavicle. The skin is punctured and the needle is advanced in the direction of the sternal notch until the tip of the needle abuts the clavicle at the junction of its medial and middle thirds. The needle is then passed beneath and parallel to the clavicle and advanced under gentle negative pressure until venous blood is aspirated.

At this point, both for internal jugular and subclavian cannulation, the syringe is removed, and a J-tip guidewire is inserted through the needle and into the vein. To prevent air embolism, care must be taken to occlude the lumen whenever possible. The guidewire should pass easily into the superior vena cava and should never be forced if resistance is encountered. Should ventricular ectopy appear on the cardiac monitor as the guidewire irritates the myocardium, the guidewire should be withdrawn to the superior vena cava to avoid dysrhythmia. Once the wire is inserted, the needle is removed and a nick is made in the skin over the guidewire using a no. 11 scalpel blade to allow passage of the dilator. The dilator should be held close to the skin, and a twisting

motion should be used to facilitate passage. The guidewire should be held at the tip at all times to prevent migration into or out of the vessel, and gentle to-and-fro movement of the wire helps confirm and maintain safe intravenous position. The dilator is withdrawn, and the catheter is threaded over the guidewire into the vein. All ports of the catheter should be flushed with normal saline solution before insertion to decrease the resistance of the guidewire within the catheter lumen and to decrease the risk of air embolism. After the guidewire is removed, venous blood should be aspirated from all ports of the catheter to remove any remaining air, and each port should be flushed with saline solution to prevent thrombosis and occlusion. The waveform on a transduced pressure tracing also confirms venous versus arterial placement. Once flushed, the catheter should be sutured into position with the tip at the junction of the superior vena cava and right atrium, which usually lies 16 to 18 cm from the point of insertion. Either gauze and tape or transparent polyurethane dressings are equivalent for prevention of catheter-related infection.[16] A chest radiograph must be obtained to confirm proper placement and the absence of complications.

The pulmonary artery catheter (PAC) was introduced in 1970 and allows direct measurements of cardiac output, oxygen consumption, pulmonary artery systolic, diastolic, and wedge pressures with a flow-directed, balloon-tipped device (Fig. 36-9). Newer models allow continuous assessment of right ventricular volumes and venous oxygenation. Despite more than 20 years of randomized controlled trials and other studies, pulmonary artery catheters have not been proven to improve outcomes in critically ill patients and their use has decreased substantially in the United States over the past decade.[17-19] Additionally, newer methods of noninvasive monitoring, such as transcutaneous oxygen and carbon dioxide tensions, may supplant the PAC as safer alternatives to obtaining more sophisticated physiologic measures.[20] Research is still ongoing to determine

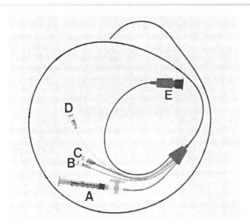

Figure 36-9.
A pulmonary artery (Swan-Ganz) catheter.

whether PACs may be beneficial to a subset of patients when placed early in the course of resuscitation.[21]

If a PAC is to be used, a larger introducer mechanism is needed that is similar to a trauma infusion catheter but has an additional venous side port to allow infusion while the pulmonary artery catheter is in place. Subclavian or internal jugular venous access is obtained as described previously. The introducer mechanism is then advanced over the guidewire and into the vein. The dilator and guidewire are removed simultaneously, which leaves the introducer sheath in place. Again, proper positioning is confirmed by aspiration of blood through the infusion port. The port is connected to an intravenous infusion, and the sheath is secured to the skin with suture. The PAC may then be introduced through the sheath. With the balloon inflated, passage of the catheter through the right atrium, right ventricle, and pulmonary artery is guided by the characteristic waveforms on the pressure monitor.

Arterial Access

A radial artery catheter at the wrist is used when continuous arterial access is indicated for blood pressure monitoring and for repeated arterial blood gas analyses. The radial artery may be cannulated by direct percutaneous puncture or by cutdown. Integrity of the ulnar artery contribution to palmar flow should be confirmed by palpation, Doppler signal, or Allen test before puncture of the radial artery. Relative contraindications to arterial catheterization include bleeding disorders and severe peripheral vascular disease. Arterial puncture should be avoided at sites with audible bruits or local signs of infection. Femoral or dorsalis pedis arteries are second-line options for arterial catheter placement.

In the direct method of arterial cannulation, the wrist is secured in an extended position using a rolled towel and tape. The area is prepared and draped in a sterile fashion, and a 20-gauge, 2-inch, over-the-needle-catheter is inserted through the skin and directed at a 45° angle towards the artery with a single forward movement. After the anterior wall of the artery is punctured, as indicated by a brisk return of blood, the needle is advanced 1 mm farther into the lumen, and the catheter is threaded into the artery. Successful placement of the catheter is verified by pulsatile

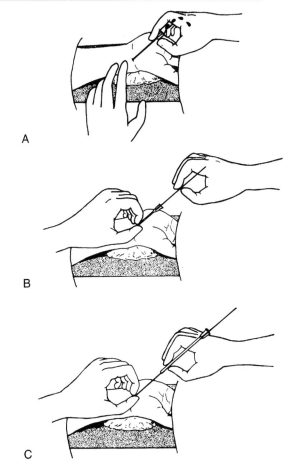

Figure 36-10.
Radial artery catheterization using the guidewire technique. *A,* A 20-gauge angiocatheter is inserted at a 45-degree angle to the wrist. The angiocatheter is advanced until arterial blood returns into the hub. *B,* The inner angiocatheter needle is removed while the angiocatheter is stabilized with the nondominant hand. The 0.018-inch guidewire is advanced with the dominant hand well beyond the end of the angiocatheter. *C,* The catheter is advanced over the guidewire into the vessel, after which the guidewire is removed.

blood return and a transduced arterial waveform through the catheter.

In addition to the Seldinger technique for radial artery cannulation (Fig. 36-10), an increasingly popular modified Seldinger technique has been described, in which a guidewire of diameter 0.018-inch is threaded through the needle following arterial puncture.[22] A catheter that is aligned over a needle is then advanced over the guidewire, and afterwards the guidewire and needle are removed from the catheter. The wire-guided method is equivalent to the direct method with respect to success rate and insertion times.[23] However, the use of ultrasound guidance increases the rate of success at first attempt and may decrease the overall insertion time for both techniques.[24]

A radial artery cutdown allows the cannulation of the artery under direct vision. Following skin preparation and local anesthesia, a transverse incision is deepened through the subcutaneous tissue, and the artery is found superficial to the bone. The artery is controlled with silk suture but if possible should not be ligated. A 2-inch angiocatheter is brought through a skin puncture site at a point distal to the main incision and advanced into the wound. The artery is then cannulated via direct puncture; the angiocatheter is connected to a pressure transducer and secured to the skin with suture. The wound is closed with nylon suture and dressed in a sterile fashion before securing the catheter.

Access for Intravenous Nutrition

Critically ill patients often exhibit altered physiology, characterized initially by an early shock state followed by a prolonged period of hypermetabolism with increased metabolic rate and negative nitrogen balance. Although the inciting event may vary, the physiologic response is typical. As malnutrition is known to be associated with increased morbidity and mortality in the critically ill patient, adequate nutritional support must be provided.[25] Although enteral nutrition is preferred, it is contraindicated in the severe shock state, severe peritonitis, and when the gut is nonfunctional due to obstruction or ischemia. Parenteral nutrition may improve outcomes as a supplement to enteral nutrition when the patient is underfed, which is common during the first week in the ICU, but is not used with severe sepsis or septic shock.[26,27] Once patients have reached a point of hemodynamic stability, total parenteral nutrition (TPN) is administered as a continuous infusion into the superior vena cava or femoral vein via a central venous catheter. Because of its hypertonicity, TPN causes thrombophlebitis and venous sclerosis if infused in a peripheral vein. Moreover, given its high glucose concentration, duration of TPN administration is a risk factor for catheter-related infection, and a dedicated catheter or port is recommended if possible.[28] If patients require long-term parenteral nutrition, a more permanent central catheter should be placed.

Access for Cardiopulmonary Resuscitation

Cardiopulmonary resuscitation, which may also be conducted in the emergency department, the operating room, or the ward as well as the ICU, represents a special and particularly acute phase of intensive care. Adequate and reliable venous access is essential, yet may be extremely challenging because of ongoing chest compressions, intubation efforts, and peripheral venoconstriction. As with the trauma patient, percutaneous access of the femoral vein is the preferred and safest technique.

▰ Complications

The overall incidence of complications for central venous catheters is 15% and can be subdivided into infectious complications, mechanical complications related to placement or removal, and thrombotic events.[29] Many complications may be preventable if proper technique is used and evidence-based guidelines for insertion and use are followed.[30] With more than 5 million central venous catheters placed annually in the United States, recognition and prevention of catheter-related complications could have an important effect on improving medical care.[31]

Infectious Complications

Catheter-related blood stream infections (CRBSI) represent one of the most common nosocomial infections and are caused by central venous catheters in 90% of cases.[32] The use of central venous catheters results in approximately 250,000 CRBSIs annually, with an increase in duration of hospital stay and a three-fold increase in mortality.[33]

Multiple factors contribute to the development of catheter-related infections, including migration of skin flora into the catheter site, contamination of the port site during manipulation or use, contamination of infused products, and colonization of intraluminal thromboses.[34] Risk factors for the development of CRBSIs have been studied extensively and include operator inexperience, failure to use a full sterile barrier during insertion, replacement of the catheter using a guidewire, catheters placement for more than 7 days, and heavy colonization of the insertion site.[35] The rate of infection is not affected by the number of ports within an individual catheter.[36]

In 2002, the Centers for Disease Control and Prevention (CDC), in coordination with the Society of Critical Care Medicine and other medical societies, published evidence-based guidelines for the prevention of catheter-related bloodstream infections.[15] Recommendations included routine hand washing before insertion, the use of full barrier precautions and aseptic technique during insertion, skin disinfection with a chlorhexidine-based solution, and the use of antibiotic-coated catheters if the rate of catheter-related infection exceeds 3.3 per 100 catheter days at a particular institution. Clinicians should evaluate the need for a central venous catheter daily and promptly remove the device when deemed unnecessary. Additionally, the risk of catheter-related infection is lower with subclavian insertion than with internal jugular or femoral insertion. In keeping with recommendations, it is our practice to replace any catheter placed in the emergency department within 24 hours, although routine scheduled catheter changes should be avoided.[37]

Mechanical Complications

Mechanical complications during placement and removal of central venous catheters are less common but potentially morbid. Arterial puncture, hematoma, and pneumothorax are the most common mechanical complications during central venous catheter insertion and are more common in patients with skeletal deformity or who have had previous catheters or procedures at the site of insertion.[38,39] Less frequent complications include guidewire migration into the venous or pulmonary circulation, cardiac dysrhythmia, nerve injury, pseudoaneurysm or arteriovenous fistula formation, and air embolism.

As noted previously, mechanical complication can be reduced significantly by using ultrasound guidance during internal jugular vein cannulation. Clinicians must recognize difficult anatomy or unfavorable body habitus and should seek assistance from a more experienced operator, especially after two failed attempts at venipuncture or catheter passage.

Thrombotic Complications

Intravascular catheters contribute to turbulent flow and represent a foreign body nidus for thrombus formation. The reported rate of catheter-related thrombosis varies widely from 2 to 26% and is increased in patients with hypercoagulable states, infusion of hypertonic solutions, when the diameter of the catheter approaches that of the vessel, and when catheterization of the vessel is prolonged.[29,40] Catheter-related thrombosis can be reduced by subclavian vein cannulation, as thrombosis rates are higher with femoral and internal jugular sites.[41]

Summary

Safe and prompt vascular access is a crucial aspect of modern care of hospitalized patients. Mastery of the indications and techniques for placement of a variety of intravascular catheters are essential for best practices. Strict adherence to evidence-based recommendations, meticulous attention to sterile technique, and early recognition and proper management of complications will yield optimal results in trauma surgery and critical illness.

REFERENCES

1. Tisherman SA, Barie P, Bokhari F, et al. Clinical practice guideline: endpoints of resuscitation. *J Trauma.* 2004;57:898-912.
2. Cooper DJ, Myles PS, McDermott FT, et al. Prehospital hypertonic saline resuscitation of patients with hypotension and severe traumatic brain injury: a randomized controlled trial. *JAMA.* 2004;291:1350-1357.
3. Barcelona SL, Vilich F, Cote CJ. A comparison of flow rates and warming capabilities of the Level 1 and Rapid Infusion System with various-size intravenous catheters. *Anesth Analg.* 2003;97:358-363.
4. Tsui, JY, Collins AB, White DW, et al. Videos in clinical medicine. Placement of a femoral venous catheter. *N Engl J Med.* 2008;358:e30.
5. LaRocco BG, Wang HE. Intraosseus infusion. *Prehosp Emerg Care.* 2003;7:280-285.
6. Reichman EF, Simon RR. *Emergency Medicine Procedures.* New York: McGraw-Hill, 2004.
7. Brenner T, Bernhard M, Helm M, et al. Comparison of two intraosseous infusion systems for adult emergency medical use. *Resuscitation.* 2008;78:314-319.
8. Westfall MD, Price KR, Lambert M, et al. Intravenous access in the critically ill trauma patient: a multicentered, prospective, randomized trial of saphenous cutdown and percutaneous femoral access. *Ann Emerg Med.* 1994;23:541-545.
9. Kirkham JH. Infusion into the internal saphenous vein at the ankle. *Lancet.* 1945;2:815-817.
10. Klofas, E. A quicker saphenous vein cutdown and a better way to teach it. *J Trauma.* 1997; 46:985-987.
11. Bishop MH, Shoemaker WC, Dram HB, et al. Prospective randomized trial of survivor values of cardiac index, oxygen delivery, and oxygen consumption as resuscitation endpoints in severe trauma. *J Trauma.* 1995;38:780-787.
12. Boyd O, Grounds M, Bennett ED. Preoperative increase of oxygen delivery reduces mortality in high risk surgical patients. *JAMA.* 1993; 270:2699.
13. Rivers E, Nhuyen B, Havstad S, et al. Early goal-directed therapy in the treatment of severe sepsis and septic shock. *New Engl J Med.* 2002; 345:1368-1377.
14. Randolph AG, Cook DJ, Gonzales, CA, et al. Ultrasound guidance for placement of central venous catheters: a meta-analysis of the literature. *Crit Care Med.* 1996;24:2053-2058.
15. O-Grady NP, Alexander M, Dellinger EP, et al. Guidelines for the prevention of intravascular catheter-related infections. CDC. *MMWR Recomm Rep.* 2002;51:1-29.
16. Gilles D, Carr D, Frost J, et al. Gauze and tape and transparent polyurethane dressings for central venous catheters. *Cochrane Database Syst Rev.* 2003;3:CD003827.
17. Shah MR, Hasselblad V, Stevenson LW, et al. Impact of the pulmonary artery catheter in critically ill patients. *JAMA.* 2005;294:1664-1670.
18. Harvey S, Young D, Brampton W, et al. Pulmonary artery catheters for adult patients in intensive care. *Cochrane Database Syst Rev.* 2006;3:CD003408.
19. Wiener RS, Welch HG. Trends in the use of the pulmonary artery catheter in the United States, 1993-2004. *JAMA.* 2007;298:423-429.
20. Shoemaker WC, Wo CCJ, Chien LC, et al. Evaluation of invasive and noninvasive hemodynamic monitoring in trauma patients. *J Trauma.* 2006;61:844-854.
21. Kern JW, Shoemaker WC. Meta-analysis of hemodynamic optimization in high-risk patients. *Crit Care Med.* 2002;30:1686-1692.
22. Mangar D, Thrush DN, Connell GR, et al. Direct or modified Seldinger guide wire-directed technique for arterial catheter insertion. *Anesth Analg.* 1993;76:714-717.
23. Ohara Y, Nakayama S, Furukawa H, et al. Use of a wire-guided cannula for radial arterial cannulation. *J Anesth.* 2007;21:83-85.
24. Levin PD, Sheinin O, Gozal Y. Use of ultrasound guidance in the insertion of radial artery catheters. *Crit Care Med.* 2003;31:481-484.
25. O'Brien JM, Phillips GS, Ali NA, et al. Body mass index is independently associated with hospital mortality in mechanically ventilated adults with acute lung injury. *Crit Care Med.* 2006; 34:738-744.
26. Heidegger CP, Darmon P, Pichard C. Enteral vs. parenteral nutrition for the critically ill patient: a combined support should be preferred. *Curr Opin Crit Care.* 2008;14:408-414.
27. Elke G, Schadler D, Engel C, et al. Current practice in nutritional support and its association with mortality with septic patients—Results from a national, prospective, multicenter study. *Crit Care Med.* 2008; 36:1762-1767.
28. Chen HS, Wang FD, Lin M, et al. Risk factors for central venous catheter-related infections in general surgery. *J Microbiol Immunol Infect.* 2006;39:231-236.
29. Merrer J, De Jonghe B, Golliot F, et al. Complications of femoral and subclavian venous catheterization in critically ill patients: a randomized controlled trial. *JAMA.* 2001;286:700-707.
30. Barbarth S, Sax H, Bastmeier P. The preventable proportion of nosocomial infections: an overview of published reports. *J Hosp Infect.* 2003; 54:258-266.
31. Raad I. Intravascular-catheter-related infections. *Lancet.* 1998;351: 893-898.
32. Maki DG, Kluger DM, Crnich CJ. The risk of bloodstream infection in adults with different intravascular devices: a systematic review of 200 published prospective studies. *Mayo Clin Proc.* 2006;81:1159-1171.
33. Garrouste-Orgeas M, Timsit JF, Tafflet M, et al. Excess risk of death from intensive care unit-acquired nosocomial bloodstream infections: a reappraisal. *Clin Infect Dis.* 2006;42:1118-1126.
34. Rodriguez-Paz JM, Pronovost P. Prevention of catheter-related bloodstream infections. *Adv Surg.* 2008;42:229-248.
35. Safdar N, Kluger DM, Maki DG. A review of risk factors for catheter-related bloodstream infection caused by percutaneously inserted, noncuffed central venous catheters: implications for preventive strategies. *Medicine (Baltimore).* 2002;81:466-479.
36. Ma TY, Yoshinaka R, Banaag A, Johnson B, et al. Total parenteral nutrition via multilumen catheters does not increase the risk of catheter-related sepsis: a randomized, prospective study. *Clin Infect Dis.* 1998;27:500-503.
37. Cook D, Randolph A, Kernerman P, et al. Central venous catheter replacement strategies: a systematic review of the literature. *Crit Care Med.* 1997;25:1417-1424.
38. McGee DC, Gould MK. Current Concepts: Prevention complications of central venous catheterization. *N Engl J Med.* 2003;348:1123-1133.
39. Mansfield PF, Hohn DC, Fornage BD, et al. Complications and failures of subclavian-vein catheterization. *N Engl J Med.* 1994;331:1735-1738.
40. Henriques HF, Karmy-Jones R, Knoll SM, et al. Avoiding complications of long-term venous access. *Am Surg.* 1993;59:555-558.
41. Timsit JF, Farkas JC, Boyer JM, et al. Central vein catheter-related thrombosis in intensive care patients: Incidence, risk factors, and relationship with catheter-related sepsis. *Chest.* 1998;114:207-213.

Complications of Percutaneous Vascular Access Procedures and Their Management

Karen Woo, Thomas B. Kinney, and Robert J. Hye

Although the development of the ability to access the central venous system for administration of medications, parenteral nutrition, and hemodialysis has been invaluable, a number of significant complications are encountered as a consequence. Some of the most important and serious complications occur at the time of catheter insertion and are related to technical considerations, anatomic abnormalities, or disorders of coagulation. Acute complications most often occur when a needle, dilator, sheath, or catheter tip is advanced on a trajectory that causes injury to the vein and adjacent structures. Although some of these complications can be minimized by the use of a cutdown technique, most patients and practitioners prefer percutaneous insertion.[1] Late complications are more often a consequence of the presence of the intravenous device with associated risks of infection and thrombosis.

Death is rarely reported as a complication of venous access procedures, but it has been described as a result of air embolization, tension pneumothorax, massive hemothorax, cardiac perforation and tamponade, and catheter sepsis.[2] The advantages of access to the venous system clearly exceed the disadvantages related to complications, but it is imperative that the indication be definite and that every effort be made to correct complications through prompt recognition and appropriate management. Even so, a penetrating injury to the heart or vessels of the thoracic outlet is often lethal.

Acute Complications

The relationship between technical errors and complications of catheter insertion is underscored by studies that show physician inexperience is an important correlate of the complication rate for subclavian venous cannulation.[3,4] In a report by Bernard and Stahl,[3] subclavian catheters inserted by inexperienced physicians (<50 procedures each) resulted in a complication rate of 8%, and insertion by a more experienced group (>50 procedures each) resulted in a complication rate of 0%. These complications involve needle or catheter injuries to the pleura, lung, vascular or nerve structures in the neck, thoracic inlet, mediastinum, and heart (Table 37-1).

Table 37–1
Acute Complications of Central Venous Catheters
Thoracic
Pneumothorax Tension pneumothorax Subcutaneous emphysema Hemothorax Hydrothorax Hemomediastinum Hydromediastinum Tracheal perforation
Arterial
Subcutaneous hematoma Arterial laceration Arteriovenous fistula Pseudoaneurysm
Venous
Venous laceration Air embolism Catheter embolism
Lymphatic
Thoracic duct laceration
Cardiac
Right ventricular infarction Arrhythmia Perforation and tamponade
Neurologic
Brachial plexus Stellate ganglion Phrenic nerve Vagus nerve Recurrent laryngeal nerve
Catheter misplacement

Table 37-2

Complications of 1794 Reported Percutaneous Central Venous Cannulations

Complication	No. (%)
Failure to place	51 (2.8)
Arterial puncture	52 (2.9)
Pneumothorax	9 (0.5)
Venous perforation	5 (0.3)
Lost wire	4 (0.2)
Thoracic duct injury	2 (0.1)
Hemothorax	1 (0.1)
Brachial plexus injury	1 (0.1)
Pneumomediastinum	1 (0.1)
Stroke	1 (0.1)
Total	127 (7.1%)

Signs and symptoms of these complications may take minutes or hours to develop and may be nonapparent or extremely subtle on initial postcatheterization chest radiographs. The onset of vascular injury may be insidious and life threatening, particularly in elderly and/or frail individuals, with a later and sudden collapse in vital signs. The keys to successful management of these complications are awareness, prompt recognition even with a delayed presentation, and expeditious therapy. Table 37-2 provides a summary of the relative frequency of these complications in a group of 1794 catheterizations from a prospective study.[5] In this compilation of data, there were a total of 127 complications, including failure to place the central line, for an overall rate of 7.1%. The most common mechanical complications, followed by pneumothorax, were failure to place the central line and arterial puncture.

The key to management of these complications is prevention. Use of imaging during the procedure has significantly reduced the incidence of acute complications due to technical error. Ultrasound guidance of the venous puncture is now standard.[6-8] Liberal use of fluoroscopy and contrast medium is also essential in preventing technical complications as well as recognizing complications when they occur.

Pneumothorax

Pneumothorax occurs as a consequence of the angle or depth of needle advancement such that there is disruption of the parietal, visceral, or mediastinal pleura. This allows air to collect in the pleural space, with subsequent partial or total collapse of the lung. Tension pneumothorax occurs when there is an accumulation of air under pressure in the pleural space. This develops when the injured tissue forms a one-way valve that allows air to enter the pleural space, but prevents it from exiting. The result is collapse of the ipsilateral lung, shift of the mediastinum, compression of the contralateral lung, and impairment of venous return to the heart. In the setting of a tension pneumothorax, symptoms can progress rapidly to acute severe respiratory distress, with or without cardiovascular collapse, and ultimately to death if unrecognized and untreated.

Pneumothorax should be suspected when there is aspiration of air into the syringe while the needle is being advanced. Physical examination of the chest should be performed after all percutaneous attempts at central venous catheter placement are made. The primary physical finding of a pneumothorax is normal or increased tympany to percussion with decreased breath sounds. In some cases, subcutaneous emphysema may be present.

If acute, severe symptoms and signs of pneumothorax develop, the patient should have tube thoracostomy performed immediately and be placed on oxygen by mask. In the setting of tension pneumothorax, decompression of the pleural space by a catheter covered needle can be lifesaving. The needle should be placed in the second intercostal space in the midclavicular line. More frequently, the air leak is relatively small, and the pneumothorax develops over a period of several hours. In such cases, there is time to confirm the diagnosis and to determine its size with a chest radiograph (Fig. 37-1). The best examination to detect a pneumothorax is an end-expiratory upright chest radiograph.[9]

When a small pneumothorax is encountered (<15%) and there are no symptoms or signs of respiratory compromise, watchful waiting with repeated chest x-rays is appropriate. If symptoms develop or there is an apparent size increase on subsequent chest radiographs, tube thoracostomy should be performed immediately. If the pneumothorax is initially noted to be large (>15%), tube thoracostomy is the safest course regardless of whether symptoms are present. An alternative to tube thoracostomy is a mobile thoracic vent device that is more comfortable for the patient and allows the patient to remain ambulatory. Aspiration of the pneumothorax through a small catheter is appropriate for some individuals but it increases the risk of recurrence and necessitates close patient observation. If the central

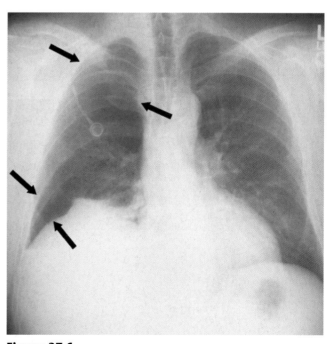

Figure 37-1.

Chest radiograph demonstrating a right pneumothorax (arrows) secondary to percutaneous right subclavian catheterization for placement of port.

venous catheter is well positioned and functioning appropriately, there is no reason to remove it because of the presence of a pneumothorax. Finally, the patient should not undergo bilateral attempts at venous catheterization until pneumothorax has been ruled out on the initial side by either physical examination or chest radiography before attempts are made at catheterization on the second side. Ignoring this dictum invites the potential disaster of bilateral pneumothoraces.

Hemothorax

Percutaneous insertion of central venous catheters may be complicated by the development of a hemothorax when the back wall of a vein or artery and the parietal pleura are perforated by an advancing needle tip, dilator, or sheath.[2] The subclavian vein or artery, innominate vein or even the superior vena cava may be involved. The lack of effective tamponade combined with negative respiratory pressure may result in a large blood loss through a small puncture. Clinically, patients may develop some respiratory compromise accompanied by dullness to percussion and decreased

breath sounds on the affected side. A declining hematocrit measurement and evidence of fluid in the pleural cavity on chest radiograph strongly support the diagnosis (Fig. 37-2A). Diagnosis can be confirmed with needle aspiration of blood from the pleural space, although when the diagnosis is obvious, the placement of a large-bore chest tube is both confirmatory and therapeutic. Significant hemothoraces should be drained to prevent entrapment of the lung. Drainage of the pleural space with a tube thoracostomy is generally adequate therapy. Rarely, bleeding must be controlled surgically or, if possible, percutaneously with the use of covered stents (see Fig. 37-2B, C).

Hydrothorax

During the placement of central venous catheters, it is possible for the catheter tip to penetrate the back wall of the vein and the parietal pleura such that the tip resides in the pleural space. This penetration can occur either ipsilateral or contralateral to the site of catheter placement. If fluids are infused, a hydrothorax results, which may be indicated by symptoms such as respiratory distress caused

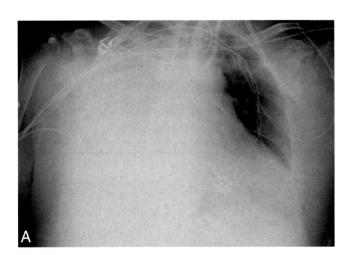

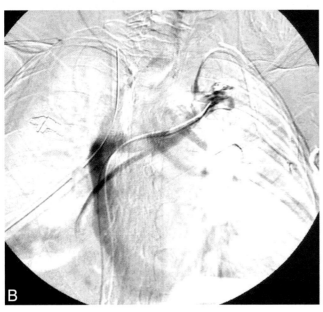

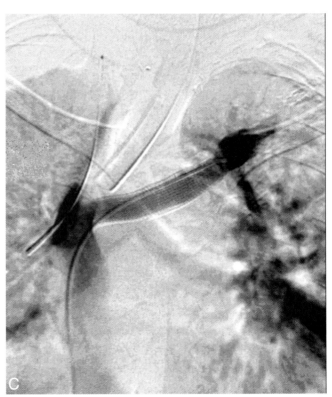

Figure 37-2.
A, Chest radiograph of massive right hemothorax secondary to left internal jugular tunneled dialysis catheter placement. B, Angiogram demonstrating catheter in A pulled back into the distal left internal jugular vein with extravasation of contrast from the innominate vein. C, Completion angiogram showing repair of injury to innominate vein by placement of a covered stent.

by compression of the lung or may be noted as an incidental finding on a chest radiograph. A thoracentesis should be performed. Removal of sanguineous fluid chemically consistent with the infusate is diagnostic, and treatment consists of thoracentesis with removal of as much of the fluid as possible. The misplaced catheter should also be removed. This condition rarely requires tube thoracostomy. This complication is avoided by confirmation of easy aspiration of blood from the catheter or injection of contrast under fluoroscopy to confirm intraluminal catheter position before use.

Hemomediastinum and Hydromediastinum

It is also possible for a stiff catheter tip or a part of the delivery system to penetrate the wall of the innominate vein or superior vena cava, resulting in bleeding or infusion of fluid into the mediastinum. In very rare instances, arterial laceration of the subclavian or carotid arteries may occur, producing massive and potentially lethal hemomediastinum and hemothorax. The diagnosis of hemomediastinum is suggested by the presence of chest pain and radiographic evidence of mediastinal widening.[10] Removal of the catheter suffices as treatment in most cases. If there is evidence of ongoing bleeding or a major arterial injury, surgical exploration and repair through a median sternotomy may be required.

One mechanism of injury that may occur after appropriate placement of the guidewire is for the dilator to push the mid portion of the guidewire, creating a loop, perforating the side wall of the central vein or even the artery. This laceration of the vessel wall may result in major intrathoracic hemorrhage that is impossible to control in time to save the patient's life. Fluoroscopic guidance of the guidewire placement and observation during insertion of subsequent instruments reduces the risk of this complication. Dilators and sheaths should be introduced to the least depth possible to accomplish catheter insertion.

Subcutaneous Hematoma

Hemorrhage from punctured or lacerated vessels in the cervical and clavicular area is often manifest as subcutaneous hematoma, with or without bleeding from the skin puncture site. To avoid this complication, thrombocytopenic patients should be transfused platelets to maintain the platelet count >50,000 per deciliter.[11] Intravenous unfractionated heparin should be stopped 3 hours before catheter insertion. International normalized ration (INR) should also be corrected to below 1.5.[11]

In the event that a hematoma occurs, prolonged compression of 15 minutes or greater, with or without catheter removal, usually suffices to control the bleeding unless there is a major vascular injury.[11] It is also beneficial to elevate the patient's upper body to decrease venous pressure. If direct pressure with catheter removal is inadequate to control the bleeding, surgical intervention must be considered. The presence of a thrill or bruit suggests the possibility of an arteriovenous fistula being present, and the presence of a pulsatile mass indicates the possibility of a pseudoaneurysm. Stent graft prostheses that can be delivered endoluminally should be considered in the management of these complications. Balloon occlusion catheters may be

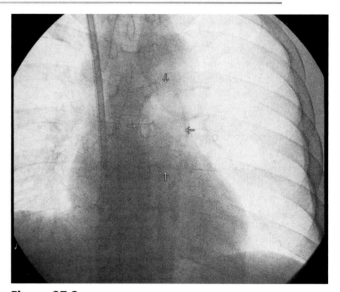

Figure 37-3.
Fluoroscopic image of large air embolus in pulmonary outflow tract.

used to temporarily tamponade bleeding from a puncture wound of the subclavian artery.

Air Embolism

Air embolism is a rare but potentially lethal complication of central venous access.[2,12] (Fig. 37-3). It generally occurs as a consequence of air entering the catheter either before attachment of the infusion tubing or when the tubing disconnects.[13-16] Air embolization has also been reported to occur through cracks in the catheter or its hub. In addition, it has been reported as occurring through the catheter tract after the removal of a central venous catheter.[17] Negative intrathoracic pressure results in air being sucked into the open catheter or catheter tract, where it enters the central venous system and ultimately obstructs the right ventricular outflow tract. Massive air embolism usually manifests with the abrupt onset of cardiovascular collapse or respiratory distress with cyanosis.

Given the near 50% mortality rate of massive air embolism, prevention is clearly more desirable than treatment. It is therefore critical that all personnel involved with placement and maintenance of central venous catheters be aware of the possibility of this complication and take measures to prevent it. In general, patients should be well hydrated and placed in the Trendelenburg position with the head 15° below the horizontal plane during catheter insertion. Patients should be instructed to hum audibly when catheters are inserted or when the intravenous tubing is disconnected for any reason, which assures the clinician that positive intrathoracic pressure is being generated. The use of peel-away sheaths with one-way valves during insertion of the catheter significantly reduces the risk of air embolism. Needles and catheters should never be allowed to be open to the air for longer than a fraction of a second by those who place or manipulate them. Patients should also be informed of the possibility of critical complications should their catheter and tubing become disconnected. They should be instructed to cap the open catheter with a thumb or finger and to call for help immediately. Finally, it is good policy to place an occlusive dressing over the skin puncture site when the catheter is removed to allow adequate sealing of the tract and prevention of air entrance.

If sudden cardiorespiratory collapse develops during catheter insertion or in a patient with a central venous catheter, air embolism must be strongly considered as the diagnosis. The classic physical finding is that of a mill wheel–churning type murmur over the anterior precordium, caused by the frothing of air and blood at the pulmonic valve. Rapid action must be taken to prevent progression to fatal shock or development of a neurologic deficit as a consequence of low cardiac output. Further embolization must be prevented by capping or clamping the catheter while the patient is simultaneously placed in the Trendelenburg and left lateral decubitus position (*Durant maneuver*).[16] This position displaces air away from the pulmonic valve, thereby relieving the right ventricular outflow obstruction. Attempted aspiration of air through the central venous catheter after it has been advanced into the heart has been advocated and shown to be of some benefit experimentally.[18] If the patient has had a cardiorespiratory arrest and does not respond to initial closed chest resuscitation, immediate left anterolateral thoracotomy with needle aspiration of the right ventricle followed by cardiac massage may be lifesaving.

Catheter or Wire Embolism

Catheter embolism is a rare complication that occurred more frequently when the catheterthrough-needle introduction systems were commonly used. Withdrawal of the catheter through the needle introducer could result in shearing of the catheter and subsequent embolization. Catheter embolization now mostly occurs when fractures develop in chronically indwelling catheters, usually at sites of stress such as the thoracic inlet.[19,20] Catheter embolism is diagnosed whenever an incomplete catheter is removed from a patient. A chest radiograph generally confirms the diagnosis. The catheter tip may remain lodged in the vena cava; however, it may also migrate into the right side of the heart or the pulmonary artery. (Fig. 37-4A) Wire embolism occurs when control of the wire is lost during the procedure. (Fig. 37-5A,B) Guidewires can also be transected during withdrawal through access needles. Resistance to wire removal mandates fluoroscopic imaging and may require removal of the wire and needle as a unit. Fortunately, many embolized catheters and wires can be expeditiously removed in the angiography suite with use of a wire snare retrieval system[21,22] (see Fig. 37-4B). Occasionally, a patient is discovered to have a catheter embolus that has been present for many years. These are generally asymptomatic and have been incorporated into body structures at the site of their lodgment. In this setting, it is not necessary to attempt removal of the catheter.

Cardiac Arrhythmia, Perforation, Tamponade, and Infarction

Cardiac complications related to central venous catheterization are relatively rare. Soft, flexible catheters are unlikely to perforate the heart or major vessels, although this is possible with the more-rigid, larger-diameter catheters used for hemodialysis access. When perforation does occur, it is most often due to guidewires, dilators, and rigid introducers with the catheter following through.

Arrhythmia is associated with overinsertion of the guide wire or catheter. Patients who have a history of a cardiac arrhythmia or those with altered plasma electrolytes are at a higher risk. The problem can be minimized by using guide wires that have distance markings as well as using fluoroscopy to determine the location of the tip of the catheter.[23] The development of cardiac arrhythmias during or after the placement of central venous catheters mandates that the catheter position be checked fluoroscopically and that the catheter withdrawn if the tip is near or traversing the tricuspid valve. If serious arrhythmias occur during insertion, the catheter should be immediately withdrawn. This procedure generally results in prompt resolution of the arrhythmia. Rarely, patients will develop arrhythmias that require chemical or electrical cardioversion. One study of 300 patients who underwent an implantable port reported the incidence of this to be 0.9%.[24]

As mentioned, it is possible to penetrate the myocardium with a stiff guidewire or other rigid components of catheter insertion systems. Such penetration may result in acute pericardial tamponade from bleeding or fluid infusion into the pericardial space. Signs and symptoms of pericardial tamponade can develop rapidly and include shock and cyanosis with marked cervical venous distention. Tachycardia and muffled heart sounds are generally present, and a large globular cardiac silhouette may be present on a chest radiograph. Any intraluminal catheter devices should be removed and pericardiocentesis or a pericardial window created. Mortality rates from tamponade may exceed 50%; thus, prompt recognition and treatment are essential.[25,26] If the tamponade recurs after pericardiocentesis or a window is created, median sternotomy with formal cardiac repair may be necessary. An unusual complication, right ventricular infarction, has been reported as a consequence of infusion of hypertonic solution through catheters whose tips are lodged in the trabeculae of the right ventricular wall.[27]

Thoracic Duct Laceration

Percutaneous catheterization of the superior vena cava via the left internal jugular or the subclavian approach carries a small risk of thoracic duct laceration. Cirrhotic patients are more prone to the development of this complication. If a lymphatic leak becomes apparent, the catheter should be removed and a pressure dressing should be applied. Nearly all such leaks resolve spontaneously.

Nerve Injuries

The brachial plexus is the nerve structure that is most vulnerable during percutaneous catheterization by virtue of its large size and proximity to the subclavian vein and artery.[3,28] Acute upper extremity pain referred along neural anatomic pathways is suggestive of impingement on the brachial plexus and necessitates immediate withdrawal of needles or catheters. Permanent injury is rare. The vagus, recurrent laryngeal, and phrenic nerves are also in proximity to sites of placement of central venous catheters, especially those directed to the internal jugular vein. These are small nerves, and they are infrequently injured. The development

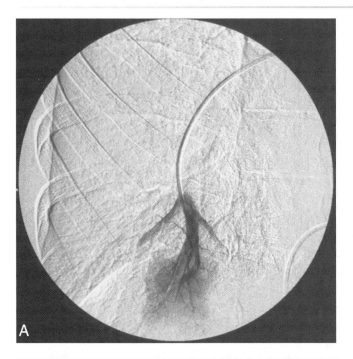

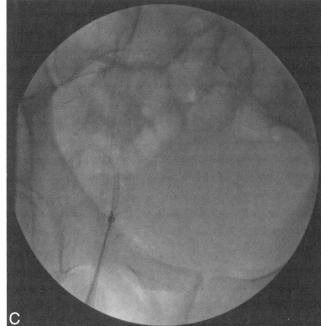

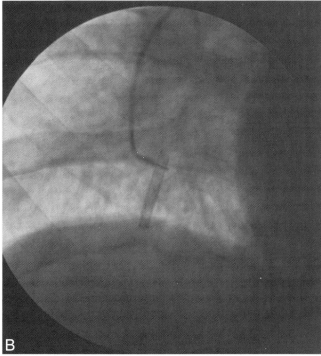

Figure 37-4.
A, Pulmonary angiogram of embolized tip of dialysis catheter lodged in a small branch of the right pulmonary artery. *B,* Angiogram showing catheter tip being snared in the pulmonary artery. *C,* Angiogram demonstrating catheter tip being removed from the right femoral vein.

of hoarseness after catheter placement suggests injury to the vagus or recurrent laryngeal nerve. Phrenic nerve injuries are generally asymptomatic and are incidentally identified during radiographic examination.[29] The development of Horner's syndrome has also been reported by inadvertent trauma to the stellate ganglion during percutaneous cannulation of the internal jugular vein.

Catheter Misplacement

In a prospective study of 1619 patients, the incidence of catheter tip malposition, defined as extrathoracic or ventric-

ular positioning, was 3.3%.[30] An unfavorable anatomic site occurs in as many as 6% to 8% of central venous catheter insertions,[31] with the incidence of catheter malposition being greater with peripherally inserted central catheters (PICC) than any other type of central venous catheter.[11] Catheter misplacement is generally discovered only on post-placement radiographic evaluation. This situation underscores the importance of early and routine verification of proper positioning of all central venous catheters and lines. Fluoroscopy can be an invaluable aid in minimizing the occurrence of misplacement. If there is a question as to the location of the tip of the catheter, contrast dye can be

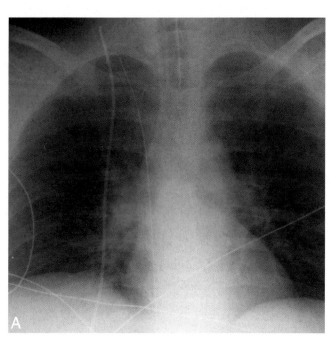
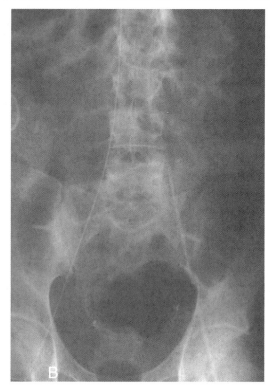

Figure 37-5.
A, Chest radiograph of embolized guide wire. *B,* Abdomen radiograph showing remainder of embolized guide wire.

injected through the catheter to help define the anatomy. Difficulty in advancing catheters or guidewires should alert the operator of the possibility of misplacement.

If the catheter tip is left to reside in the subclavian, axillary, jugular, or even hepatic veins, intimal injury by the catheter tip or the infusion solution frequently causes thrombosis of the vein.[32,33] Upper extremity venous occlusions related to semipermanent venous access devices may occur in this setting. Thrombotic complications can be minimized by confirming that the catheter tip is placed in the right atrium or superior vena cava. Stiff catheters or introducers left abutting the wall of the superior vena cava or more peripheral veins can erode through the wall and produce a hemomediastinum or hydromediastinum. Ideally, central venous catheters should have their tips placed at the junction of the superior vena cava and right atrium or in the upper right atrium to minimize complications related to misplacement.[34]

Catheters intended for a vein may be placed into the subclavian or carotid artery without the practitioner realizing the misplacement. This can occur in a hypotensive or poorly oxygenated patient from whom bright red, pressurized blood is not returned. Further, infusion of total parenteral nutrition solutions can cause major injury to the extremities and central nervous system. A simple method of determining whether the catheter is placed intra-arterially or intravenously is to transduce the pressure through the catheter to see if the waveform is an arterial or a venous waveform. Another method is to send a sample from the catheter for a blood gas test to determine whether the values are consistent with an arterial or venous blood gas test. The majority of catheters inadvertently placed intra-arterially

can simply be removed and pressure held for a prolonged period of time (15 to 20 minutes.) If this fails, operative repair of the arteriotomy is required.

Late Complications

Late complications are those that manifest after a catheter has been in place for some time, usually for at least several days (Table 37-3). Naturally, there is some overlap between acute and late complications, and some late complications are a manifestation of initial catheter misplacement. The catheter material, type of catheter (whether it is totally implantable or protrudes through the skin), site of placement, catheter care, and nature of the patient's underlying disease are important factors in the development and type of late complications. Acute complications that were discussed earlier may also present as late complications and include air embolism, cardiac perforation, hydrothorax, and hydromediastinum. Complications that occur almost exclusively as late events are related to thrombosis and infection.

Catheter Occlusion

Catheter occlusion is the most frequent and frustrating late complication of central venous catheters, accounting for discontinuation of as many as one third of venous catheters.[1,29,31,35] Line occlusion is more common with PICC lines than non-PICC lines.[36] Blockage generally occurs as a consequence of the development of a fibrin sleeve or plug at the catheter tip. Impending occlusion is often heralded by the inability to withdraw blood from the catheter while the

Table 37-3

Late Complications of Central Venous Catheters

Catheter obstruction

Thoracic

Hydrothorax
Hydromediastinum

Venous

Air embolism
Central vein thrombosis
Superior vena cava syndrome
Hepatic vein thrombosis

Cardiac

Arrhythmia
Perforation and tamponade
Coronary sinus thrombosis

Lymphatic

Lymphatic fistula
Chylothorax

Septic

Catheter sepsis
Septic thrombosis
Suppurative thrombophlebitis

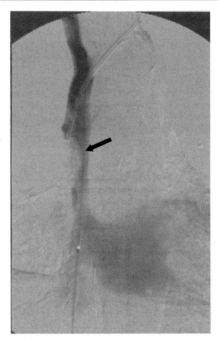

Figure 37-6.
Fluoroscopic image of thrombus at end of catheter.

ability to infuse fluids is retained. In the past, forceful irrigation of a heparinized saline solution has been advocated to relieve the obstruction. Although this may provide some temporary benefit with catheters needed only for short-term access, it is rarely definitive therapy for long-term catheters and can cause catheter rupture. Local infusion of fibrolytic agents has been advantageous to some in the salvage of occluded central venous catheters.[2,17,37] Most commonly, a dilute solution of fibrinolytic agent is injected and allowed to dwell in the catheter for 2 to 3 hours. The catheter is then irrigated and flushed, with removal of any residual clot, until patency is restored. Guidewires should never be passed through catheters in an effort to relieve an obstruction due to the risk of dislodging part or all of the occlusion and causing an embolic event.

Because of the frequency of recurrent occlusion and the difficulty in delivering highly concentrated fibrinolytic agent to the fibrin sheath around the tip of the catheter, techniques have been developed to eliminate the fibrin sheath. These techniques generally involve the insertion of a wire snare device through another venous access site, such as the femoral vein. The fibrin sheath is then stripped from the catheter and removed. An alternative technique is the use of angioplasty balloons to rupture the sheath. Should these measures fail, the only alternative is removal of the old catheter and placement of a new catheter, if still required. The extent of the attempt at catheter salvage is obviously dictated by the patient's need for central venous access and the availability of alternative sites.

Central Venous Thrombosis and Pulmonary Embolism

Catheter-related thrombosis of the internal jugular, subclavian, or innominate veins occurs more frequently than is commonly appreciated (Fig. 37-6). Unless there is an associated embolic or infectious complication, many patients are asymptomatic because of the excellent collateral venous drainage channels in the upper extremities and neck.[10] In patients who are symptomatic, there is mild to moderate edema of the affected extremity, a sensation of tightness or heaviness, and an increased subcutaneous collateral venous pattern. Catheter-associated thrombosis has also been demonstrated to have an association with infection.[38] Patients who have had multiple central venous access sites and have had multiple venous thromboses may have more severe symptoms and signs. In addition, in patients in whom complete thrombosis of the superior vena cava occurs, there are signs and symptoms of superior vena cava syndrome of varying severity.

Clinical evidence of subclavian vein thrombosis occurs in less than 5% of catheterized patients. In patients studied venographically, however, the frequency of partial or complete thrombosis may be as high as 50%.[39] Factors predisposing to the development of thrombosis include the nature of the infusate solution, duration of catheterization, the presence of infection or a hypercoagulable state, and catheter size, composition, and tip position. The use of softer catheters and heparin in the infusate solution has been reported to reduce the incidence of venous thrombosis.[20,40] The use of low dose warfarin prophylaxis is not recommended.[11] For patients at high risk of developing a thrombosis, therapeutic warfarin may be considered.[30]

Patients who have indwelling central venous catheters and show evidence of arm, neck, or facial swelling;

prominent collateral venous patterns; signs or symptoms of embolic complications; or unexplained fever should be suspected of having venous thrombosis. Duplex scanning generally is diagnostic, but occasionally venography is required for definitive diagnosis and determination of the extent of thrombosis. Conventional therapy consists of anticoagulation and elevation of the symptomatic body part. The catheter should be removed in most circumstances. In patients with long term need for central venous access and limited available sites for catheterization, anticoagulation therapy with the catheter left in place can be considered.[23] Depending on the location, extent of thrombosis, and need for catheter salvage, thrombolytic therapy may be considered.

If pulmonary embolism is suspected, the diagnosis is made by using the conventional modalities of ventilation or perfusion scanning, computed tomography angiography, or pulmonary arteriography. Again, treatment consists of immediate anticoagulation, initially with heparin, and then catheter removal and later conversion to warfarin. In general, the prognosis for catheter-related venous thrombosis is good. Most patients' symptoms improve with time; the thrombosed venous segments recanalize, and relatively few patients experience chronic severe sequelae. Those who do are primarily individuals who have had multiple catheters and have long-term need for venous access. Hemodialysis patients in particular are prone to long-term complications related to chronic venous occlusion.

Peripherally inserted central catheters have been shown to have a higher incidence of thrombosis in patients with hematologic malignancies.[41] PICC lines made of silicon rubber have been associated with a lower risk of thrombosis than those made of polyurethane.[42]

Catheter-Related Infection

There are three categories of catheter-related infections: blood stream infection, exit site infection, and tunnel infection. A catheter-related blood stream infection is defined as at least two blood cultures positive with the same organism, obtained from at least two separate sites at different times in association with evidence of colonization of the catheter with the same organism, which can only be positively determined by removing the catheter. Catheter-related blood stream infections manifest themselves by fever and tachycardia, although signs of frank sepsis, including rigors, tachypnea, mental status changes, and shock may also occur. The incidence of line sepsis in the literature ranges from 2% to 33%.[36] An exit site infection is diagnosed by the presence of erythema, tenderness, and, occasionally, discharge at the insertion site. A tunnel infection presents with pain and induration along the tract of the catheter.[11] Immunocompromised patients may show minimal signs of infection; therefore, a high index of suspicion is required in those patients. Catheter-associated infections may produce a constant low-grade fever, although fever spikes can occur during times of catheter manipulation and flushing.

The predominant organism isolated from infected lines is *Staphylococcus epidermidis*.[43,44] Other major organisms associated with line sepsis are gram-positive cocci such as *S. aureus* and enterococci, both of which are becoming increasingly resistant to antibiotics. Gram-negative bacilli, including *Pseudomonas* species, *Klebsiella pneumoniae*, *E. coli*, and *Enterobacter* species, have also been isolated from infected lines.[44] Fungal infections, predominantly *Candida* species, are associated with broad spectrum antibiotic therapy and renal impairment.[36] Consequences of bacteremia include infective endocarditis and metastatic abscesses.

Ideally, the management of line sepsis includes the removal of the infected catheter.[10,35,45] Initial empirical antibiotic therapy should include broad spectrum coverage of both potentially resistant strains of gram-positive organisms as well as gram-negative organisms. This coverage should be adjusted to a focused regimen when culture results become available. Amphotericin B or capsofungin, which has a more favorable toxicity profile, should be used if there is evidence of disseminated fungal infection or if patients demonstrate persistent fungemia after catheter removal.[11]

In general, new catheters should not be inserted until all signs of sepsis or bacteremia have been resolved. This delay may not be possible in critically ill patients. Nevertheless, many physicians prefer to wait until blood cultures return with "no growth" results before inserting a long-term venous access catheter. As patients who require central venous catheters are often immunocompromised, they are susceptible to the usual sources of sepsis in addition to their venous catheters. Therefore, a diligent search for other causes of infection in these patients is required. In patients who have limited central venous access sites and the source of sepsis is in question, it may be appropriate to change the catheter over a wire and await the culture results from the removed catheter tip while giving antibiotic therapy.

Occasionally, patients can be treated successfully with antibiotic therapy administered through the catheter. The decision to attempt salvage of a suspected infected catheter should not be made lightly. The patient should show minimal signs of infection (usually fever only), be physiologically fit to tolerate low-grade infection, and have a compelling reason (e.g., limited alternative access sites) to justify this approach. Either failure of the patient to respond to therapy within 24 to 48 hours or clinical deterioration necessitates removal of the catheter. Although such a course of management is at times appropriate and can be successful, it is important to recognize that the safest course of action is most often to remove the catheter.

The most significant factor in minimizing catheter-related infections is careful, aseptic initial placement of the catheter with maximum sterile barrier conditions that include mask, cap, sterile gloves, sterile gown, and large drape[11] followed by similarly strict antiseptic catheter maintenance by experienced health care providers using established protocols.[10,35] Cleansing of the skin before catheter insertion with 2% aqueous chlorhexidine has been shown to be superior to iodine or alcohol in reducing the infection rate.[46] Avoidance of hematomas at the time of catheter placement is a critical aspect in minimizing the risk of infection. In addition, the use of long subcutaneous tunnels and the placement of the cuff portion of cuffed catheters near, but not at, the skin exit site are thought to reduce the risk of infection. Routine replacement of catheters as a means of reducing catheter sepsis has not been shown to be effective and is not recommended.[11] Whether the type of long-term catheter that is used (external or port) affects infection risk has been debated, with most clinicians favoring the totally implantable port.[47] Antiseptic impregnated catheters may offer some initial resistance to contamination.

The development and introduction of multilumen catheters for the delivery of drugs, total parenteral nutrition, and intravenous fluids in critically ill patients have resulted in an increase in the incidence of catheter-related sepsis compared with that associated with single-lumen catheters.[48] This increase is undoubtedly because of a reduced ability to prevent catheter contamination, particularly when the catheter is being used for intravenous nutritional support. Nevertheless, the advantages of multilumen catheters justify their continued use as long as the potential for increased infection risk is recognized and every method is used to reduce environmental and skin contamination.

Septic Thrombosis and Suppurative Thrombophlebitis

Septic thrombosis and suppurative thrombophlebitis represent an additional potentially lethal complication of central venous catheterization. They most often occur in burn and other severely immunocompromised patients.[10,49,50] The introduction of long-term catheters introduced into the antecubital fossa vein increased the frequency of these complications in the veins of the upper arm.

Septic thrombosis of the great veins should be suspected when there is evidence of both infection and thrombosis or when sepsis does not resolve promptly after the removal of an infected catheter. Catheter-related thrombosis is a common complication of *S. aureus* catheter-related bacteremia—up to 71% in one report.[38] As such, patients with central venous catheter–associated *S. aureus* bacteremia

should undergo venous duplex to detect relatively asymptomatic thromboses that may be a nidus for infection.[38] Gram-negative organisms are increasingly responsible for this complication, whereas *C. albicans* is a common isolate in burn patients. Positive blood cultures and demonstration of venous thrombosis by duplex scanning or venography are diagnostic. In the periphery, expression of pus from the puncture site or through a limited exploratory incision may require removal of the involved segment of vein for cure. In the absence of purulent discharge, initial treatment with heat, elevation, and antibiotics is appropriate, with excision reserved for those patients who fail to respond to treatment within 24 to 48 hours. With involvement of the subclavian veins or larger veins of the thorax, excision is not practical, and treatment with anticoagulation and aggressive antibiotic therapy should be instituted.[51] Fogarty balloon catheter thrombectomy combined with anticoagulation and antibiotic therapy may be a useful adjunct in patients who fail to respond to more conservative therapy. As is true of most life-threatening complications, a high index of clinical suspicion, prompt diagnosis, and institution of therapy are the keys to a successful clinical outcome.

Catheter Migration

Secondary catheter migration/malposition complicates up to 6% of patients with central venous catheters.[52] (Fig. 37-7A) Factors predisposing to this complication are vigorous irrigation of the catheter, Valsalva maneuvers, coughing, hyperextension of the shoulder, and conditions that

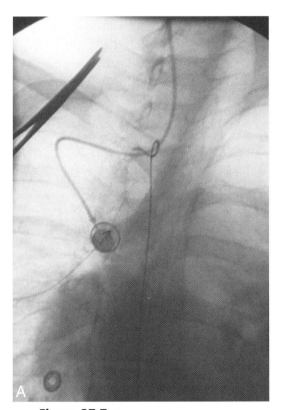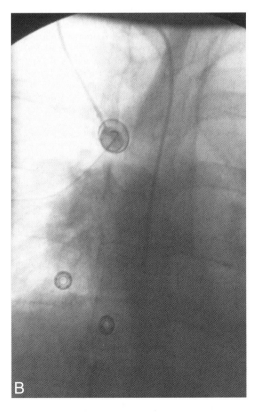

Figure 37-7.
A, Fluoroscopic image of catheter tip that has migrated into the right internal jugular vein and is being repositioned percutaneously with a snare. *B,* Fluoroscopic image of successfully repositioned catheter.

lead to dilatation of the central great veins. Presenting symptoms include shoulder, anterior chest, neck or head pain during infusion of solutions that irritate the veins. When the tip of the catheter is malpositioned in a proximal vein, the risk of venous thrombosis increases with the infusion of solutions that are potentially sclerosants. As such, secondarily migrated catheters should be removed or repositioned. A high rate of success, up to 93%, has been reported with interventional repositioning of the catheter tip (see Fig. 37-7B).[52]

Concluding Remarks

Clearly, prevention is the ideal form of management of complications of percutaneous vascular access. At the same time, there are certain complications such as catheter-related infection that can be unavoidable. The clinician must maintain a high level of suspicion, so that when complications do occur, early diagnosis and prompt treatment can ensue. In considering treatment options, minimally invasive catheter-based methods can now be used to treat a variety of complications and result in less stress to the patient than an open procedure. As such, percutaneous treatment of complications should be employed whenever feasible.

REFERENCES

1. Riella MC, Scribner BH. Five years' experience with a right atrial catheter for prolonged parenteral nutrition at home. *Surg Gynecol Obstet.* 1976;143:205-208.
2. Borja AR. Current status of infraclavicular subclavian vein catheterization: review of the English literature. *Ann Thorac Surg.* 1972;13:615-624.
3. Bernard RW, Stahl WM. Subclavian vein catheterizations: a prospective study. I. Noninfectious complications. *Ann Surg.* 1971;173:184-190.
4. Herbst CA. Indications, management, and complications of percutaneous subclavian catheters: an audit. *Arch Surg.* 1978;113:1421-1425.
5. Schummer W, Schummer C, Rose N, et al. Mechanical complications and malpositions of central venous cannulations by experienced operators. A prospective study of 1794 catheterizations in critically ill patients. *Intensive Care Med.* 2007;33:1055-1059.
6. Karakitsos D, Labrapoulos N, De Groot E, et al. Real-time ultrasound guided catheterization of the internal jugular vein: a prospective comparison to the landmark technique in critical care patients. *Crit Care.* 2006;10:R162.
7. Feller-Kopman D. Ultrasound-guided internal jugular access: a proposed standardized approach and implications for training and practice. *Chest.* 2007;132:302-309.
8. Leung J, Duffy M, Finckh A. Real-time ultrasonographically guided internal jugular vein catheterization in the emergency department increases success rates and reduces complications: a randomized, prospective study. *Ann Emerg Med.* 2006;48:540-547.
9. Giacomini M, Iapichino G, Armani S, et al. How to avoid and manage a pneumothorax. *J Vasc Access.* 2006;7:7-14.
10. Ryan JA, Abel RM, Abbot WM, et al. Catheter complications in total parenteral nutrition: a prospective study of 200 consecutive patients. *N Engl J Med.* 1974;290:757-761.
11. Bishop L, Dougherty L, Bodenham A, et al. Guidelines on the insertion and management of central venous access devices in adults. *Int Jnl Lab Hem.* 2007;29:261-278.
12. Ordway CB. Air embolus via CVP catheter without positive pressure: presentation of case and review. *Ann Surg.* 1974;179:479-481.
13. Flanagan JP, Gradisar IA, Gross RJ, et al. Air embolus: a lethal complication of subclavian venipuncture. *N Engl J Med.* 1969;281:488-489.
14. Hoshal VL Jr, Fink GH. The subclavian catheter. *N Engl J Med.* 1969; 281:1425.
15. Levinsky WJ. Fatal air embolism during insertion of CVP monitoring apparatus. *JAMA.* 1969;209:1721-1722.

16. Durant TM, Oppenheimer MJ, Lynch P, et al. Body position in relation to venous air embolism: a roentgenologic study. *Am J Med Sci.* 1954; 227:509-520.:
17. Paskin DL, Hoffman WS, Tuddenham WJ. A new complication of subclavian vein catheterization. *Ann Surg.* 1974;179:266-268.
18. Alvaran SB, Toung JK, Graff TE, et al Venous air embolism: comparative merits of external cardiac massage, intracardia aspiration, and left lateral decubitus position. *Anesth Anal.* 1978;57:166-170.
19. McMenamin EM. Catheter fracture: a complication in venous access devices. *Cancer Nurs.* 1993;16:464-467.
20. Van der Hem KG, Meijer S, Werter CJ, et al. "Spontaneous" catheter fracture and embolization of a totally implanted venous access port. *Neth J Med.* 1991;38:262-264.
21. Block PC. Transvenous retrieval of foreign bodies in the cardiac circulation. *JAMA.* 1973;224:241-248.
22. Bessoud B, de Baere T, Kuoch V, et al. Experience at a single institution with endovascular treatment of mechanical complications caused by implanted central venous access devices in pediatric and adult patients. *AJR.* 2003;180:527-532.
23. Lowell JA, Bothe A. Venous access- preoperative, operative and postoperative dilemmas. *Surg Clin N Amer.* 1991;71:1231-1246.
24. Brothers TE, Von Moll LK, Neiderhuber JE, et al: Experience with subcutaneous infusion ports in three hundred patients. *Surg Gynecol Obstet.* 1988;166:295-301.
25. Bolasny BL, Shepard GH, Scott HW Jr. The hazards of intravenous polyethylene catheters in surgical patients. *Surg Gynecol Obstet.* 1970; 130:342-346.
26. Brandt RL, et al. Mechanism of perforation of the heart with production of hydropericardium by a venous catheter and its prevention. *Am J Surg.* 1970;119:311-316.
27. King TC, Saffitz JE. Acute right ventricular infarction resulting from intracardiac infusion of hyperosmotic hyperalimentation solutions. *Am J Cardiol.* 1985;55:1659-1660.:
28. Ramdial P, Singh B, Moodley J, et al. Brachial plexopathy after subclavian vein catheterization. *J Trauma.* 2003;54:786-787.
29. Takasaki Y, Arai T. Transient right phrenic nerve palsy associated with central venous catheterization. *Br J Anaesth.* 2001;87:5101-5101.
30. Pikwer A, Baath L, Davidson B, et al. The incidence and risk of central venous catheter malpositioning: a prospective cohort study in 1619 patients. *Anaesth Intensive Care.* 2008;36:30-37.
31. Christensen KH, Nerstron B, Boden H. Complications of percutaneous catheterizations of the subclavian vein in 129 cases. *Acta Chir Scand.* 1967;133:615-620.
32. Langston CS. The aberrant central venous catheter and its complication. *Radiology.* 1971;100:55-59.
33. Raffensperger JG, Ramenofsky ML. A fatal complication of hyperalimentation: A case report. *Surgery.* 1970;68393-394.
34. Henriques HF III, Karmy-Jones R, Knoll SM, et al. Avoiding complications of long-term venous access. *Am Surg.* 1993;59:555-558.
35. Sariego J, Bootorabi B, Matsumoto T, et al. Major long-term complications in 1,422 permanent venous access devices. *Am J Surg.* 1993;165: 249-251.
36. Ghabril MS, Aranda-Michel J, Scolapio JS. Metabolic and catheter complications of parenteral nutrition. *Nutrition.* 2004;6:237-334.
37. Hurtubise MR, Bottino JC, Lawson M. Restoring patency of occluded central venous catheters. *Arch Surg.* 1980;115:212-213.
38. Crowley AL, Peterson GE, Benjamin DK, et al. Venous thrombosis in patients with short- and long-term central venous catheter associated Staph aureus bacteremia. *Crit Care Med.* 2008;36:385-390.
39. Bozzetti F, Scarpa D, Terno G, et al. Subclavian venous thrombosis due to indwelling catheters: a prospective study of 52 patients. *J Parenter Enteral Nutr.* 1983;7:560-562.
40. Padberg TI, Ruggievo J, Blackburn GL, et al. Central venous catheterization for parenteral nutrition. *Ann Surg.* 1981;193:264-270.
41. Cortelezzi AN, Moia M, Falanga A, et al. Incidence of thrombotic complications in patients with hematological malignancies with central venous catheters: a prospective multicenter study. *Br J Hem.* 2005; 129:811-817.
42. Galloway S, Bodenham AR. Long-term central venous access. *Brit J Anaes.* 2004;92:722-734.
43. Safdar N, Maki DG. Inflammation at the insertion site is not predictive of catheter-related bloodstream infection with short-term, noncuffed central venous catheters. *Crit Care Med.* 2002;30:2632-2635.
44. Bevc S, Pecovnik-Balon B, Ekart R, et al. Non-insertion-related complications of central venous catheterization- temporary vascular access for hemodialysis. *Renal Failure.* 2007;29:91-95.

45. Sanders RA, Sheldon GF. Septic complications of total parenteral nutrition: a five-year experience. *Am J Surg.* 1976;132:214-220.

46. Maki DG, Ringer M and Alvarado CJ. Prospective randomized trial of povidone iodine, alcohol and chlorhexidine for prevention of infection associated with central venous and arterial catheters. *Lancet.* 1991;338:339-343.

47. Groeger JS, Lucas AB, Thaler HT, et al. Infectious morbidity associated with long-term use of venous access devices in patients with cancer. *Ann Intern Med.* 1993;119:1168-1174.

48. Pemberton LB, Lyman B, Lander V, et al. Sepsis from triple-lumen vs. single-lumen catheters during total parenteral nutrition in surgical or critically ill patients. *Arch Surg.* 1986;121:591-594.

49. McDonough JJ, Altemeier WA. Subclavian venous thrombosis secondary to indwelling catheters. *Surg Gynecol Obstet.* 1971;133:397-400.

50. Stein JM, Pruitt BA Jr. Suppurative thrombophlebitis: a lethal iatrogenic disease. *N Engl J Med.* 1970;282:1452-1455.

51. Pruitt BA Jr, Stein JM, Foley FD, et al. Intravenous therapy in burn patients: suppurative thrombophlebitis and other life-threatening complications. *Arch Surg.* 1970;100:399-404.

52. Gebauer B, Teichgraber UK, Podrabsky P, et al. Radiological interventions for correction of central venous port catheter migrations. *Cardiovasc Intervent Radiol.* 2007;30:216-221.